OXFORD MEDICAL PUBLICATIONS

Nutrition for developing countries

From 'Song of Lawino', by Okot p'Bitek, of Uganda.

Come, brother,
Come into my mother's house!
Pause a bit by the door,
Let me show you
My mother's house.

Look,
Straight before you
Is the central pole.
That shiny stool
At the foot of the pole
Is my father's revered stool.

Further on
The rows of pots
Placed one on top of the other
Are the stores
And cupboards.
Millet flour, dried carcasses
Of various animals,
Beans, peas,
Fish, dried cucumber . . .

Look up to the roof,
You see the hangings?
The string nets
Are called cel.
The beautiful long-necked jar
On your left
Is full of honey.

That earthen dish
Contains cimsim paste;
And that grass pocket
Just above the fireplace
Contains dried white ants.

Here on your left
Are the grinding stones:
The big one
Ashen and dusty
And her daughter
Sitting in her belly
Are the destroyers of millet
Mixed with cassava
And sorghum.

       *   *   *

When the baby cries
Let him suck milk
From the breast.
There is no fixed time
For breast feeding.

When the baby cries
It may be he is ill;
The first medicine for a child
Is the breast.
Give him milk
And he will stop crying,
And if he is ill
Let him suck the breast . . .

Reprinted with permission of the East African Publishing house, P.O. Box 30571, Nairobi, Kenya.

Nutrition for Developing Countries

SECOND EDITION

Felicity Savage King

and

Ann Burgess

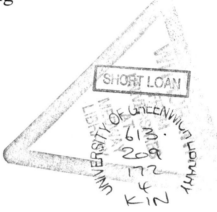

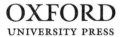

OXFORD
UNIVERSITY PRESS

OXFORD
UNIVERSITY PRESS

Great Clarendon Street, Oxford OX2 6DP

Oxford University Press is a department of the University of Oxford.
It furthers the University's objective of excellence in research, scholarship,
and education by publishing worldwide in

Oxford New York

Athens Auckland Bangkok Bogotá Buenos Aires Calcutta
Cape Town Chennai Dar es Salaam Delhi Florence Hong Kong Istanbul
Karachi Kuala Lumpur Madrid Melbourne Mexico City Mumbai
Nairobi Paris São Paulo Singapore Taipei Tokyo Toronto Warsaw

with associated companies in Berlin Ibadan

Oxford is a registered trade mark of Oxford University Press
in the UK and in certain other countries

Published in the United States
by Oxford University Press Inc., New York

First edition © Oxford University Press, 1972
Second edition © Felicity Savage King and Ann Burgess, 1993

The moral rights of the author have been asserted
Database right Oxford University Press (maker)

First published 1993
Reprinted 1995 (twice), 1998, 2000

A catalogue record for this book is available from the British Library

Library of Congress Cataloging in Publication Data
(Data available)
ISBN 0 19 262233 1

Printed in Great Britain
on acid-free paper by
Butler & Tanner, Frome, Somerset

Foreword

Maurice King, *Department of Public Health Medicine, University of Leeds*

In the late 1960s there was little that a health or nutrition worker in Africa could read to tell him how to improve the nutrition of his community. At the request of the late Ewan Thomson, then Director of the National Food and Nutrition Commission of Zambia, and with little previous experience of nutrition, my wife (Felicity Savage King) and I boldly tried to fill this gap, and were fortunate in being able to enlist the help of Leslie and Ann Burgess and David Morley. Two experimental editions were necessary before there was anything fit to print. But when the first edition did appear, it was such a success that it sold over 50 000 copies and has remained in print for nearly 20 years, besides being widely adapted and translated. Meanwhile, it has slowly become out of date; in what it said, such as the emphasis it placed on protein; in what it did not say, which was quite a lot; and in the way in which it was written.

In 1982 Ann Burgess and my wife started work on a new edition with much help from colleagues in Africa, the United Kingdom, and elsewhere. A generous grant from the Commonwealth Foundation made the work possible. Here after many delays and interruptions is the fruit of their labour. Although I have often tried to look over my wife's shoulder as she wrote, I have had to contain my curiosity until the manuscript was complete. As I read it, I am delighted with the clarity, simplicity, humanity, and completeness of what they have done. The second edition is nearly twice the size of the first, its language is much improved, and it has many new illustrations. It has retained the good ideas of the first edition, particularly the 'food paths' and the things which block them, while rejecting some of its curiosities, such as likening amino acids to the letters in a sentence. Lest I lose all contact with the child that I begat, I have been allowed to write this 'Foreword'. I wish the second edition a long and a useful life.

My own interests have now moved to other fields. I have, however, a compelling interest in the nutrition of the world as a whole and with one particularly serious food block, which is the relationship between land and people.

When we wrote the first edition of this book in 1972, there were 3.8 billion people in the world; now, 20 years later, there are 5.4 billion. This is nearly two billion more mouths to feed. Unless we starve first, the world population is probably going to double to 11 billion, and could triple to 17 billion. Meanwhile, almost all the land that can usefully be ploughed has been ploughed. By the year 2000 there will only be about a tenth of a hectare (about a quarter of an acre) for each of us, with the prospect of further decline thereafter. We can try to grow more food by farming the land more productively and using more fertilizer, but there are many difficulties, especially lack of water.

Ultimately, all the energy that we eat comes from the sun. If we mostly eat this energy as grain, we each need 200 kg a year. If we feed grain to animals and eat their meat, milk, and eggs, we can use up to 800 kg a year. The world produces an average of about 300 kg for each of us, and feeds about a third of this to the animals that we eat. If we ate this grain, instead of the animals, the world could feed about half as many people again, or about 8 billion, but it could not feed twice as many.

Population is already a serious block in the food path, and there are now many communities in which one of the most important causes of malnutrition is too many people and not enough land. One answer to this is better sharing of the food that we have; another is family planning. This is why family planning is increasingly important for improved nutrition, and why a key chapter in this book addresses the problems of nutrition, the environment, and family size. The technicalities of contraception are outside the scope of this book, but the need to discuss with families and communities the urgency of limiting the number of their children as part of nutrition education is well within it, and should make the book particularly relevant to some of the most pressing problems of our time.

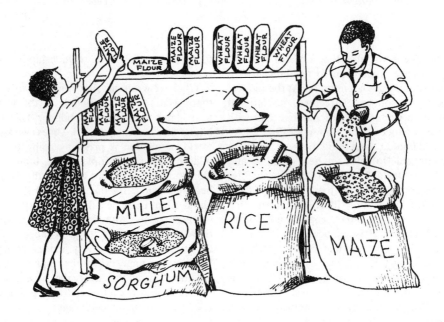

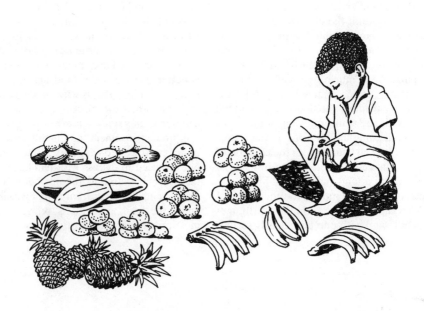

Preface

Many children do not get enough of the right foods to eat. They do not grow well, they become ill, many die or they do not grow up as clever, as healthy, or as tall as they should be.

These words introduced the first edition of *Nutrition for developing countries* when it was published in 1972. Although there are now nearly 2 billion more people, the general trend has been for the prevalence of malnutrition to decrease gradually, except in areas of political, economic, or climatic crisis. But, because there are now more people, there are now, in total, more malnourished people.

The extent, causes, and consequences of poor nutrition are now better understood, and so are the ways to prevent and manage it. Low food intake and infection are the immediate causes of malnutrition. But the underlying causes are a combination of unfair distribution of food between and within communities, poor family food security, particularly the inability to obtain enough food, poor living conditions, inadequate health care, lack of education, heavy physical work, and frequent childbearing. The function of some nutrients is better known. Lack of iodine, for example, has been recognized as causing varying degrees of poor mental development, not only goitre and cretinism. Vitamin A has been shown to protect against infection, as well as against xerophthalmia. Lack of energy and a range of nutrients, rather than protein deficiency alone, has been recognized as the nutritional cause of growth failure in children.

Methods of combating nutrition have also changed, and there is now more emphasis on community-based primary health care. Nutrition activities are being incorporated in development programmes, and planners are using nutritional outcomes, such as improved growth, to evaluate the impact of these programmes. In local and central governments a new generation of well educated and motivated planners has arisen to develop these programmes.

All this requires that the elements of nutrition be understood by a range of workers, most of whom do many other things, but all of whom are in part 'nutrition workers'. Thus, although this book is likely to be most useful to health workers and home economists, it is also for agricultural extension officers, social workers, and school teachers. All these people, in their capacity as nutrition worker, are the 'you' whom we address in the text. We hope this book will give you a core of practical nutritional knowledge as well as essential theory, to build upon as necessary, according to your particular specialty. We hope too that it will also be useful to college students and their lecturers.

The first edition was sometimes criticized for not describing the medical management of severe malnutrition, so this time we have included such a chapter. It is at a higher technical level than other parts of the book, but we felt that it was justified because the information is not easily available from other sources. Although the book is not specifically written for doctors, there is little else available for them on practical nutrition, and we hope that they too will find the book useful and that this chapter addresses one of their important needs.

The first edition was written in Zambia, for use mainly in Central and East Africa, but it was found useful in other parts of Africa, and even on other continents. We would have liked this time to write a book useful anywhere in the world. But there are too many local and cultural factors in nutrition for this to be possible. So we have once again written for East and Central Africa, which is the area that we know best. But we hope that many parts of the book, such as the basic nutrition, will be of use elsewhere, and that other parts can be adapted to different areas without too much difficulty.

The first edition used joules rather than Calories, since it seemed a pity that readers who had been introduced to SI units at school should have to switch to Calories when they studied nutrition. However, applied nutrition has still to fully adopt joules, and since the use of both units would be confusing, this edition is entirely in Calories.

English, in common with many other languages, has no singular personal pronoun which is independent of gender. To overcome this problem, we use 'she' for about half the children we talk about, and 'he' for the other half. We hope this helps to emphasize that girls are often at a greater disadvantage than their more fortunate brothers.

We have done our best to make this book correct, relevant, and easy to use. This is one reason why it has taken so long to write. But no book is perfect, and new advances are being made in nutrition all the time. So we hope that you will think carefully as you read, and ask yourselves, 'Is this true? Is it still true today? Is it relevant to the place where I work?'

Writing this book has been hard work. We have learnt much from the many people who have helped us, and from the communities we have worked with and visited. Many new ideas in nutrition developed as we wrote. We looked round and wrote down the most useful things we found. Once again, we have provided the paper and ink for the ideas of others. So this is not our book but theirs and yours.

If a book like this is to live and develop, it must throw out old material, and bring in new ideas, as one edition succeeds another. This calls for a partnership between readers and writers. So we look forward to hearing what you liked and what you did not. Your ideas can be included in a third edition. It may also be time that we handed over this task to colleagues in Africa. Would any of you like to do it?

Leeds, England   F.S.K.
Glenisla, Scotland   A.B.
August 1992

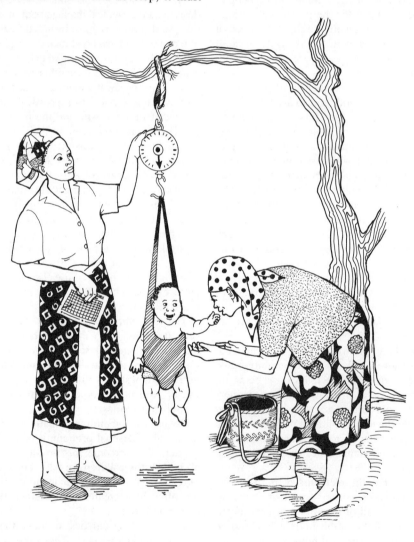

Acknowledgements

Very many people helped us to prepare this book by commenting on draft chapters, supplying information, or inspiring us through their work or writings. We are particularly grateful to Maurice King who graciously allowed us to take his book and change it so much, and the late Ewan Thomson who encouraged us to embark on the revision. We thank the other co-authors of the first edition, David Morley and Leslie Burgess, for their support during the preparation of this one as well as our consultants, Ruth Oniang'o and Charity Dirorimwe who helped to revise the first (and often subsequent) drafts of most chapters.

In addition we want to thank other colleagues who helped with various sections of the book: Hilda Kigutha and Joy Redhead for all the chapters on 'Nutrients' and 'Foods', Chapters 1–6; Clare Schofield and Bob Weisell for 'Energy needs', Sections 2.7–2.12; Elaine Monsen and Eduardo DeMaeyer for 'Iron', Section 4.10; Ali Kiduku for 'Keeping food safe and clean', Chapter 7; Ann Ashworth and Alan Jackson for 'Management of severe malnutrition in children', Chapter 17; Nazarit Mirza, Festus Kavishe, and Lauren Blum for 'Vitamin A deficiency', Chapter 18; Frits van der Haar, Festus Kavishe, and John Dunn for 'Iodine deficiency disorders', Chapter 21; Sheila Lakhani for 'Preventing obesity', Sections 22.8–22.9; Pam Goode for 'Home gardens', Sections 24.9–24.14; staff of the African Medical Research Foundation for 'Working with communities and families', Chapters 26 and 27; and also Alice Ngesa who commented on several chapters.

Many other people contributed comments and information and we would particularly like to thank David Alnwick, Helen Armstrong, Jacqui Babcock, Ken Bailey, Chris Bates, Michael Blake, Neville Belton, Anne-Jacqueline Berio, Paula Bertolin, Freda Chale, Marrietta Chapa, June Copeman, Peter Cox, Mai El Nadeef, Linda Ettangata, Grace Ettyang, Norah Gibson, Michael Golden, Jill Gordon, Ralph Hendrickse, Marilyn Hoskins, John Hubley, Ad Jansen, Urban Jonsson, Nandita Kielmann, Eric Kwered, Margaret Kyenkya, Julian Lambert, Jackie Landman, Michael Latham, Elisabeth Linusson, Zohra Lukmanji, Elizabeth Macha, Grace Maina, Firoze Manji, John Mason, John McDonald, Nelson Muroke, Penina Ochola, Andrew Prentice, Barbara Purvis, Vicky Quinn, Sonya Rabeneck, Hans Rosling, Eva Sarakikya, Alfred Sommer, Louise Sserenjogi, Paget Stanfield, Wilma van Steenberger, Andrew Tomkins, and Njoki Wainyima.

Special thanks too to our artists: Celly Bacon for the drawings which characterized the first edition, and a number that are new, including Wambui and her friends; Sara Kiunga-Kamau for more than a hundred pictures of individuals, families, and communities; Jill Last for the series of market scenes; Beth Rogers for most of the diagrams; Daphne Paley-Smith for the breastfeeding diagrams and others of infants feeding; Ivanson Kayaii for a number of African children, adults, and scenes; and Dominic King for the cells (Fig. 2–15) and the mice (Fig. 5–15). Thanks also to Gill Tremlett for the story 'Two Schools' in Chapter 20.

We are grateful to the following people and organizations for the use of their illustrations. Full references for specific publications or teaching materials are given in Appendix 6.

- African Medical Research Foundation, Kenya for Figs 7–3, 9–3, and 24–4 taken from Burgess (in press) and figures in Chapter 10 taken from Savage King (1992);
- Child-to-child Trust, Institute of Education, London for Figs 10–5 and 23–14;
- Food and Agricultural Organization of the United Nations for Figs 6–8, 7–4, 14–36, 19–7, 21–6, 25–3, 28–6, 29–1, 29–2, 29–3, 29–5; 29–6, 29–8, 30–6, 30–7, 31–1, and 31–2, which are taken from FAO (1984);
- Hesperian Foundation, Palo Alto, California for Figs 19–2 and 19–3 taken from Werner (1979);
- Hesperian Foundation, Palo Alto, California for Fig. 22–11 taken from Dickson (1983);
- International Eye Foundation for Figs 19–1 and 19–4;
- Jackie Landman for Fig. 17–8;
- Teaching Aids at Low Cost (TALC) for illustrations from the slide set 'Weaning foods and energy' (TALC 1985) (Figs 11–4, 11–5, and 16–4); the thinness chart (Fig. 14–29); the insertion tape (Fig. 14–35), and cleaning teeth (Fig. 22–10);
- Tear Fund for permission to use the drawing of the Maendeleo stove (Fig. 24–3) from *Footsteps* (1990), no. 5, p. 12;

- UNICEF, Kenya for Figs 8–6, 11–6, and 11–9 taken from illustrations from the chart set 'Good growth prevents malnutrition' (Kenya Ministry of Health/UNICEF 1987);
- United Nations University for Fig. 24–12 taken from Niñez B. (1985).

The following figures were adapted from illustrations from various sources.

- Figure 10–27 was adapted from an illustration by Rose O'kongo in Burgess (in press).
- Figure 11–1 was adapted from illustrations in Hofvander and Underwood (1987) and Greiner (1988).
- Figure 11–12 was adapted from UNICEF, New York and Kenya.
- Figure 11–20 was adapted from Kenya Ministry of Health/UNICEF (1987).
- Figure 11–3 was adapted from the slide set 'Weaning foods and energy' (TALC 1985) and from Kenya Ministry of Heath/UNICEF (1986).
- Figures 13–7 and 16–13 were adapted from King *et al.* (1979).

- Figure 16–5 was adapted from a drawing by Dr S.N. Chaudhuri in Swaziland Ministry of Health/UNICEF (1988).
- Figure 22–6 was adapted from Perisse *et al.* (1969).
- Figure 24–2 was adapted from an illustration provided by the Valley Trust and TALC.
- Figures 24–5, 24–6, 24–7, 24–9, and 24–10 were adapted from FAO (1988c).
- Figure 26–2 was adapted from McMahon *et al.* (1980).

This long list of friends and colleagues shows that the book has been a co-operative enterprise. However, the final responsibility for the contents, and hence any errors, rests with us, the principal authors.

Our most profound and grateful thanks are to the Commonwealth Foundation, who by a generous grant made it possible to commission so many illustrations and to publish the book at an affordable price. They have patiently borne with us through ten years of delays and interruptions. We can only hope that they, as well as our readers, will find the book worth waiting for.

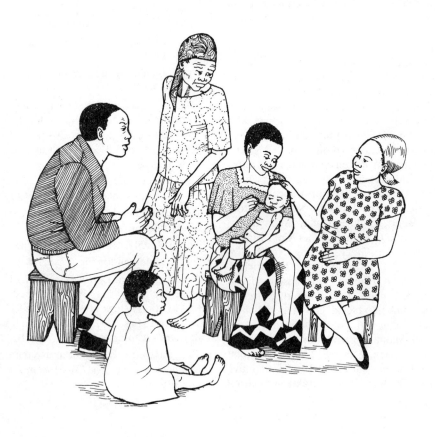

Contents

1 Nutrients and how the body uses them

1.1 INTRODUCTION

Nutrition is the study of foods and how our bodies use them. It is concerned with how food is produced, processed, handled, sold, prepared, shared, and eaten and with what happens to food in the body—how it is digested, absorbed, and used. If you are a nutrition worker, you need to know about foods, but to help people who are undernourished you also need a lot of practical knowledge about good meals and about how to help families and work with communities.

This book starts with the nutrients, which are the parts of food that our bodies use. This first chapter and Chapters 2–4 explain why we need nutrients and how much of each kind we need. Chapter 5 then describes the different types of food, especially those grown in Africa, which might be found in a typical market and the nutrients that they provide. Many more foods these days are processed so that it is necessary to know something about the methods used to process them (Chapter 6) and how to keep foods clean and safe so that eating them does not make people ill (Chapter 7).

When you know about nutrients and foods, you can see in Chapter 8 how to use the different kinds of food to prepare meals for the family that provide all the nutrients that different members of the family need. Chapter 9 describes how to buy and budget for food and how to help families to get good value for the money that they spend.

Two of the most important tasks of nutrition workers are to encourage breastfeeding (Chapter 10) and to help parents to introduce young children to solid food in the safest way (Chapter 11). You also need to know how to feed older children and adults (Chapter 12) and sick people, especially sick children (Chapter 13).

A child's growth is a good indicator of her nutrition, so you should understand growth and development (Chapter 14) and how to use growth charts to promote healthy growth (Chapter 15). Chapter 16 describes how a child who does not eat enough and is often ill is undernourished and fails to grow properly. You need to know how to help families to feed these children better so that they do not become more malnourished.

You may also need to manage children with severe protein–energy malnutrition, who may need treatment in hospital (Chapter 17). Women are at high risk of undernutrition, especially when they are childbearing, so you must be able to help them (Chapter 18). You may need to prevent or treat people with vitamin A and other vitamin deficiencies (Chapter 19), nutritional anaemia (Chapter 20), and iodine deficiency (Chapter 21). As more people come to live and work in cities, some of those who have enough to eat suffer the diseases associated with overnutrition. You need to understand how to prevent them (Chapter 22).

Chapter 23 introduces the idea of 'food paths' and follows the path of foods from the plants where they grow to our bodies which eat, digest, and use them. Chapter 24 describes some of the many factors which can block the food paths and cause undernutrition. Blocks vary from place to place but two of the most important ones are harm to the environment and increasing population. We are none of us able to remove all the blocks, but we need to know about those that we can remove, and it is useful to be able to understand those that are the responsibility of other workers. Chapter 25 describes family food security and how you can improve it.

You will need to work with communities (Chapter 26) or the most needy families in a community (Chapter 27) to help them solve their nutrition problems. There are many different ways to do this. Chapter 28 tells you about some ways to help people learn about nutrition. You may need to organize a group feeding programme (Chapter 29) or a school nutrition programme (Chapter 30).

Many of you will be training workers in nutrition, either in pre-service or in-service courses or on the job. Chapter 31 tells you how to plan this training, and at the end of each chapter there are a number of ideas for training exercises ('Things to do'). The appendices at the end of the book give some of the more detailed technical information that you may need. Because it is difficult to keep up to date with developments in nutrition, Appendix 6 lists the most useful books, newsletters, and teaching materials available. Appendix 6

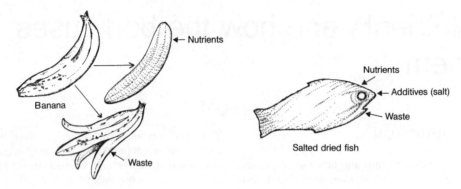

Fig. 1–1 Foods are made of *nutrients, waste*, and *other substances*.

also gives the addresses of organisations from which you can get more information about nutrition.

But—to start at the beginning. It is necessary first to consider what nutrients are and how the body uses them.

1.2 WHAT FOOD IS MADE OF

Nutrients are the part of the food which the body uses:

* to build tissues;
* to produce energy;
* to keep healthy.

Waste is the part of the food that we cut off or throw away, such as peel and stones from fruit.

Other substances:

* *Anti-nutrients* are substances in foods that are natural poisons or *toxins* (for example, the poison in bitter cassava) or that interfere with the digestion, absorption, or use of nutrients in the body (for example, anti-nutrients in beans).

* *Food additives* are chemicals which are added to some processed foods, such as canned foods, bottled drinks, sausages, etc. Additives may:
  * improve the taste or appearance of the food;
  * improve its nutritive value;
  * make the food keep longer.

* *Contaminants* are chemicals, poisons, micro-organisms, and dirt which get into food by accident and spoil it.

* *Harmless micro-organisms* may be yeasts or bacteria, such as those which ferment food.

1.3 NUTRIENTS

The types of nutrients are:

* sugars
* starches   } (carbohydrates)
* fibre

* fats

* proteins

* vitamins
* minerals   } (micronutrients)

* water

Sugars, starches, and fibre are often grouped together as they are all *carbohydrates*.

Vitamins and minerals are needed in very small amounts and they are sometimes called *micronutrients*.

Almost all foods are a *mixture of nutrients*. They contain different amounts of sugar, starch, fibre, fat, protein, minerals, vitamins, and water.

The food composition tables in Appendix 1 give the amounts of nutrients and waste in different foods.

Figure 1–2 compares the amounts of sugar, starch, fibre, fat, protein, and water, in rice, milk, and ground-nuts. It is not possible to show vitamins and minerals on this kind of diagram, because they always occur in very small amounts. For example, 100 g of boiled rice contains about:

* 0.08 g of minerals, which is the same proportion as 1 grain of rice in about 1250 grains!
* 0.004 g of vitamins, which is the same proportion as one grain of rice in 25 000 grains!

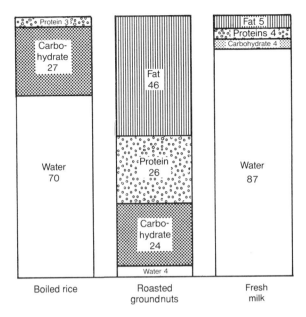

Fig. 1–2 Nutrients in 100 grams (g) of different foods.

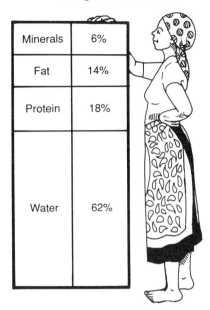

Fig. 1–3 What we are made of.

How the body uses nutrients

The body uses nutrients:

- to build the body, produce fluids, and repair tissues;
- to produce energy so that the body can keep alive and warm and so that it can move and grow;
- to help chemical processes;
- to protect the body from disease.

1.4 USING NUTRIENTS TO BUILD TISSUES

A person who weighs 50 kg, consists of about 31 kg of water, 9 kg protein, 7 kg fat, and 3 kg minerals.

Thus, besides water, the most important building nutrient is *protein*.

Fat is important too, both to build cells and to build energy stores. Some minerals are important, for example, calcium to build bone and teeth and iron to build blood.

Why we need nutrients to build the body

For growth

A child starts life as a single cell inside his mother. The cell absorbs nutrients; it grows and divides into two cells. The cell uses some nutrients as building materials

for the new cell and other nutrients as fuel for energy to do the work of building (see Fig. 1–4).

Each new cell absorbs more nutrients to grow larger and divide again. The cells continue to absorb nutrients and to grow and divide until there are millions of cells which form different *tissues* such as skin, muscle, and bone.

The child's body also makes the fluids such as blood which nourish and protect the cells.

For pregnancy

During pregnancy, a woman needs body-building nutrients to:

- provide the baby and placenta with nutrients to grow;
- increase the size of her uterus and breasts;
- make more blood and stores of fat and other nutrients.

To secrete fluids

The body has to keep making fluids, such as saliva, other digestive juices, tears, and breast milk, because they are used up.

To replace cells

Most cells live only a short time. The body must build new cells to replace those that die. The need to replace cells continues throughout life, (see Fig. 1–5).

Skin is a good example. The outside layer of skin is

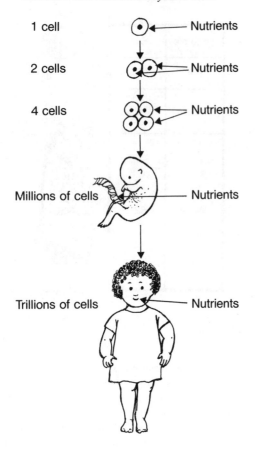

1 cell — Nutrients

2 cells — Nutrients

4 cells — Nutrients

Millions of cells — Nutrients

Trillions of cells — Nutrients

Fig. 1–4 Using nutrients to grow from a single cell into a child.

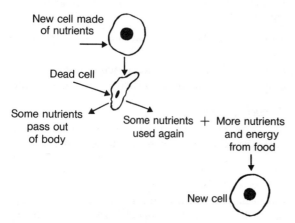

New cell made of nutrients

Dead cell

Some nutrients pass out of body

Some nutrients used again + More nutrients and energy from food

New cell

Fig. 1–5 Why the body needs nutrients to replace old cells.

already dead. All the time, new cells are growing under the dead cells to replace them. When you wash and dry yourself, you remove some of the dead cells.

If you wear shoes for a long time you get holes in the soles. But if you walk without shoes, you do not get holes in your feet, because new skin cells grow under the old cells to replace them.

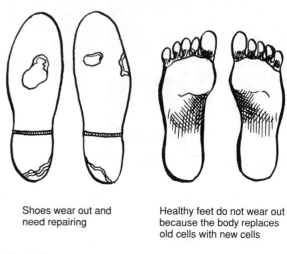

Shoes wear out and need repairing

Healthy feet do not wear out because the body replaces old cells with new cells

Fig. 1–6

To repair tissues

After injury or illness, the body makes new cells to repair the damaged tissues.

So everyone needs nutrients to replace cells and body fluids from the moment they are conceived until they die.

1.5 USING NUTRIENTS TO PRODUCE ENERGY

When you turn on the engine of a car, the petrol combines with oxygen and 'burns' to make energy. The energy makes the car move, and it also makes the engine warm.

The body 'burns' nutrients to make energy. Sometimes people are surprised to learn that nutrients are 'burning' inside their bodies. Nutrients really do burn—but in a different way from a fire so that there is no flame or smoke.

Starch, sugar, and fat are made of the elements carbon, hydrogen, and oxygen. When they 'burn' in the cells, they combine with oxygen from the air that we breathe in. They release energy, and they change into carbon dioxide and water which we breathe out.

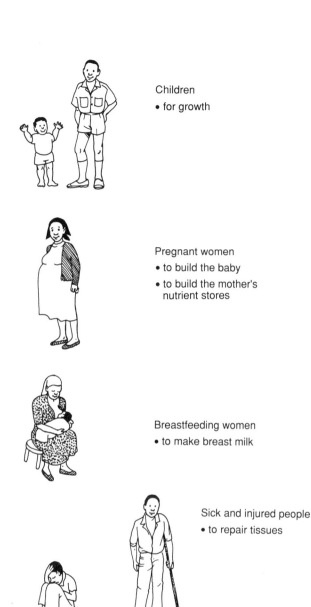

Children
- for growth

Pregnant women
- to build the baby
- to build the mother's nutrient stores

Breastfeeding women
- to make breast milk

Sick and injured people
- to repair tissues

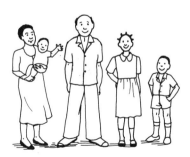

Everyone
- to replace fluids and old cells

Fig. 1–7 Who needs nutrients to build tissues?

```
      to keep        to keep
       alive          warm
          \          /
to fight ___  The body uses ___ to build new
infection       ENERGY            tissues/cells
          /          \
      to move       to secrete
      and work        fluids
```

Fig. 1–8 How the body uses energy.

How the body uses energy

To keep alive

When you stop a car, you can keep the engine running or you can turn it off altogether. If you leave the engine running, it uses a little petrol. It only stops burning petrol if you turn the engine off.

Our bodies are 'turned on' and using energy from the moment of conception until we die, just to keep alive. Even when people are asleep they use energy:

- to pump blood around the body;
- to breathe;
- to digest food;
- to excrete waste, such as urine.

To keep warm

Our bodies are warm, even if we are asleep. Keeping warm uses energy.

To build tissues

The body uses nutrients such as starch to provide the energy for building. This is in addition to using nutrients such as protein and iron as building materials for the tissues.

To secrete fluids

The body uses energy to secrete fluids such as saliva and breast milk.

To repair tissues

After injury or illness, the body uses energy to repair damaged tissues.

To move and work

We need energy to move muscles, to move our bodies, to walk, to talk, to play, to run, and to work.

When a person runs or works hard, he burns more nutrients to make the energy that he needs. Some of the energy is made into heat so that he feels hotter. If you feel cold, one way to get warmer is to move about—to do some work or to go for a run—so that you burn more nutrients.

The nutrients which provide energy

Starch, sugar, and fat all provide energy. Foods which contain a lot of carbohydrate and fat are sometimes called 'energy foods'. *Protein* can also provide energy. But if we eat enough carbohydrate and fat, our bodies keep most of the protein for building new cells.

How we measure energy

We measure energy in *calories* in the same way that we measure weight in grams. In nutrition, we use *kilo-calories* (like kilograms). We can write kilocalories as Calories* or **kcal** for short.

The amount of energy which nutrients give

Figure 1–9 shows how much energy the body gets when it burns 1 g of different nutrients.

Calories per gram

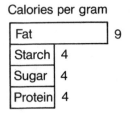

Fig. 1–9 Energy in different nutrients.

Fat gives more energy than starch, sugar, or protein. One spoonful of pure fat gives slightly more energy than two spoonfuls of pure sugar. Thus we need to eat *more* sugar, or starch, or protein, than fat to get the same number of Calories.

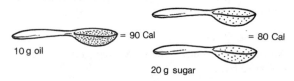

Fig. 1–10 One spoonful of oil gives more energy than two spoonfuls of sugar.

---

* Some scientists measure energy in *joules*. We used joules in the first edition of this book, but most people find them difficult, so we use Calories here.

1.6 USING NUTRIENTS TO HELP CHEMICAL PROCESSES

Chemical processes, or *reactions*, take place all the time in all the cells and body fluids. They are what make the body function. Chemical processes:

- digest food;
- 'burn' nutrients for energy;
- use energy to move muscles;
- build new cells;
- secrete fluids.

Some nutrients are used to make these processes happen—in particular, water, some proteins, some micronutrients. For example,

Oxygen +	$\longrightarrow$	**ENERGY +**
sugar	*B vitamins make*	**carbon dioxide +**
	this process	**water.**
	happen	

Enzymes are chemicals which digest food, and which make many other chemical processes happen. Enzymes are a special kind of protein, and they often work with vitamins or minerals.

Hormones are chemicals which control body processes. For example thyroid hormone, which contains the mineral *iodine*.

1.7 USING NUTRIENTS TO PROTECT THE BODY AGAINST INFECTION

The body needs nutrients to *resist* and *fight* infection, and to *recover* from infections.

The cells and fluids on body surfaces must function properly to resist infection. They need enough protein and vitamin A. Fibre helps to keep the gut healthy.

Antibodies in the blood, the lining of the intestine, and other tissues help to fight infections. Antibodies are a special kind of protein.

Different kinds of *white blood cell* are also essential to fight infections. They are made from protein and other nutrients in the same way as other cells.

People burn more nutrients for energy when they fight infections, especially if they have a fever. Some micronutrients and proteins destroy harmful chemicals ('*free radicals*') produced during infection, and prevent them from damaging tissues (see Section 17.2).

During an infection, some cells die and tissue may

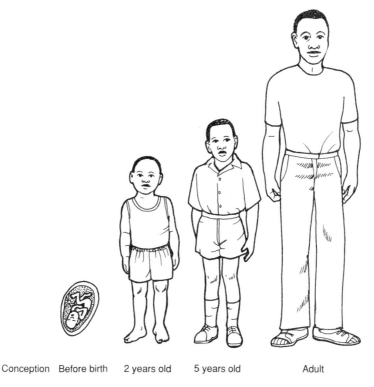

Conception   Before birth   2 years old   5 years old   Adult

Fig. 1–11 To grow from a single cell to an adult requires energy, protein, and other nutrients.

be damaged. The body has to make new cells and repair the tissues. This uses energy, protein, and other nutrients.

THINGS TO DO

To show how the nutrient content of food varies

1. Choose a few common foods, for example rice, beans, milk, cooking oil, and a vegetable or fruit.
   Ask trainees to:
   a. use the food composition tables in Appendix 1 to find out how much water, carbohydrate (starch and sugar), protein, and fat there is in 100 g of each food.
   b. Draw a diagram like Fig. 1–2 to show how much of each nutrient the different foods contain.

To show how fat is more energy-rich than starch

2. Choose 1–2 fat-rich foods (such as margarine or oil) and 1–2 starchy foods (such as rice or cassava).
   Ask trainees to:
   a. use the food composition tables in Appendix 1 to find out how many grams of each food contains 100 Calories.
   b. Measure these amounts of food and compare them. Discuss why the different amounts of food give the same number of Calories.

USEFUL PUBLICATION

Davidson, R. and Eastwood, M. A. (1986). *Human nutrition and dietetics* (8th edn). Churchill Livingstone, Edinburgh.

2 Carbohydrates, fats, and energy

2.1 SUGARS AND STARCHES

Sugars and starches are different sorts of carbohydrate.

Sugars

Sugars are the main type of carbohydrate in sugar cane, refined sugar, ripe fruit, milk, and honey. Notice that there are *nutrients* called sugars, and a *food* called sugar.

Sugar ⟨ **a group of nutrients (glucose, sucrose, etc.)**

food sugar (refined sugar).

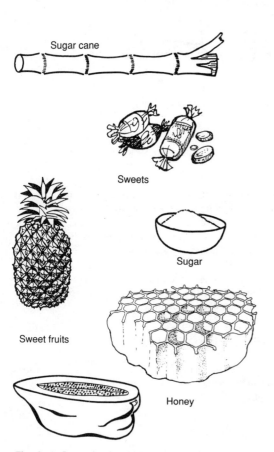

Sugar cane

Sweets

Sugar

Sweet fruits

Honey

Fig. 2–1 Some foods which contain sugar.

There are several sorts of sugars in foods. For example,

● The sugar in milk is *lactose*.
● The sugar in sugar cane and refined sugar is *sucrose*.
● The sugars in ripe fruit and honey are *glucose* and *fructose*.

Glucose and fructose are 'simple sugars'. The body's cells can only use simple sugars.

Some sugars are made of two simple sugars. Lactose and sucrose are examples.

● Lactose is made of glucose and galactose.
● Sucrose is made of glucose and fructose.

When they are digested, lactose and sucrose break down in the gut to simple sugars. For example:

● Lactose breaks down into glucose and galactose.
● Sucrose breaks down into glucose and fructose.

Starches

Starches are the main sort of carbohydrate in cereals (such as rice, maize, and wheat), starchy roots (such as cassava, yams, and potatoes), and starchy fruits (such as cooking bananas). Each starch molecule is made of many glucose molecules.

When starch is digested in the gut, it breaks down into glucose. The glucose is absorbed into the blood and goes to the cells to provide energy.

Starch is stored in *starch grains* inside plant cells. When a starchy food is boiled the starch grains absorb water. They swell up and may break. This makes the starch easier to digest. It may make the food swell up. Cooked starchy foods which contain a lot of water are called *bulky foods*.

Sugar and starch needs

There are no separate values for starch or sugar needs. They are used for energy, so they are covered by *energy needs* (see Sections 2.7–2.12).

Sucrose is made of glucose and fructose

Lactose is made of glucose and galactose

Starch is made of many glucose molecules

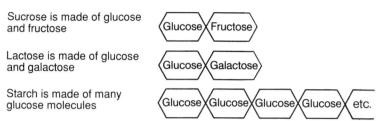

Fig. 2–2

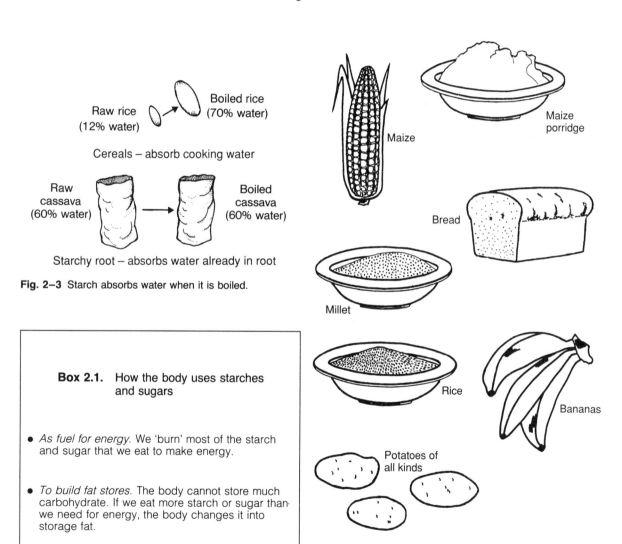

Raw rice (12% water) → Boiled rice (70% water)

Cereals – absorb cooking water

Raw cassava (60% water) → Boiled cassava (60% water)

Starchy root – absorbs water already in root

Fig. 2–3 Starch absorbs water when it is boiled.

Box 2.1. How the body uses starches and sugars

- *As fuel for energy.* We 'burn' most of the starch and sugar that we eat to make energy.

- *To build fat stores.* The body cannot store much carbohydrate. If we eat more starch or sugar than we need for energy, the body changes it into storage fat.

- *To build cells.* A little carbohydrate is used to build cells.

Maize

Maize porridge

Bread

Millet

Rice

Bananas

Potatoes of all kinds

Cassava

Fig. 2–4 Some good sources of starch.

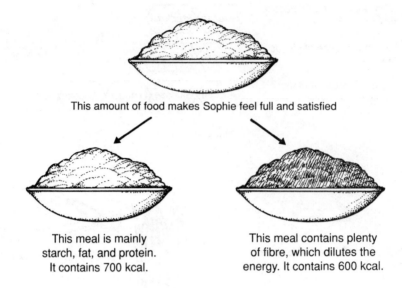

This amount of food makes Sophie feel full and satisfied

This meal is mainly
starch, fat, and protein.
It contains 700 kcal.

This meal contains plenty
of fibre, which dilutes the
energy. It contains 600 kcal.

Fig. 2–6 Fibre dilutes the energy in a meal.

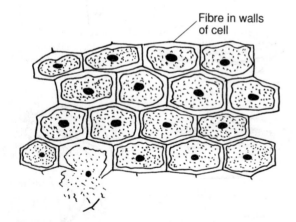

Fibre in walls
of cell

Fig. 2–5 Some plant cells. Fibre comes from the walls of plant cells.

2.2 FIBRE

Dietary fibre is a mixture of different carbohydrates which are not digested like other nutrients by humans. These carbohydrates occur only in the cell walls of plants. Nutritionists sometimes call dietary fibre *unavailable carbohydrate*, or *resistant polysaccharides*.

There is fibre in all *unprocessed* plant food—cereals, roots, legumes, oil seeds, fruits, and vegetables. However, *processing* may break down the cells and remove some or all of the fibre.

There are different sorts of fibre which we can group as:

- *soluble* fibre;
- *insoluble* fibre.

Plant foods contain different amounts of each kind. For example, legumes, fruits, and oats contain mainly soluble fibre. Most other cereals contain mainly insoluble fibre.

Some starch is still undigested when it reaches the large intestine. This is called *resistant starch* and it has many of the same effects as fibre.

How fibre helps the body

The gut does not digest and absorb fibre in the same way as other nutrients. Fibre stays in the gut, and most passes out in the faeces. Soluble fibre ferments in the large intestine and produces fatty acids and other substances. The body absorbs and uses some of these for energy.

Fibre is an important nutrient for the following reasons.

Fibre makes food **bulky** (bigger)

Fibre takes up space in a food.

- If there is no fibre, there are more of the other nutrients in each mouthful of food, so a person may eat more energy-giving nutrients before they feel full and satisfied.
- If there is fibre in a food, a person may feel full and satisfied after they have eaten less of the other nutrients.

This can help a person who is overweight to eat less. But it may make it more difficult for a young child with a small stomach to get enough nutrients (see Section 11.7).

Fibre slows digestion of a meal

When people eat *unprocessed* plant food, they have to chew it well in their mouths and mash it in their stomachs to break open the cell walls. Then the digestive juices can get at the nutrients to digest them.

When people eat a *processed or refined* food (such as refined flour, or sugar), the food is ready for digestion and absorption as soon as they eat it.

Thus an unprocessed food, with fibre in it, stays longer in a person's mouth and stomach and is digested more slowly. The person does not feel hungry again so quickly.

Fibre slows absorption of nutrients

Soluble fibre soaks up and holds water and makes the food in the gut thicker. This slows down absorption of nutrients. It is better for the body if nutrients enter the blood slowly and evenly, than if they come all at once.

Fibre makes the faeces soft and bulky

This may be the most important effect of insoluble fibre and resistant starch. With some of the water that they soak up, they pass into the large intestine, to pass out with the faeces.

The fibre, resistant starch, and water make the faeces bulkier and softer. Fermentation of soluble fibre also makes the faeces bulkier. When faeces are soft and bulky:

- They pass more easily and quickly, preventing constipation.
- They keep the wall of the gut more healthy.
- Diseases of the gut, such as cancer, and haemorrhoids (piles) are less likely to develop.

Fibre soaks up harmful substances

Fibre may soak up any harmful substances in the gut, so that they pass out in the faeces.

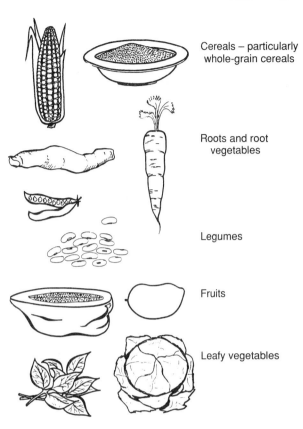

Cereals – particularly whole-grain cereals

Roots and root vegetables

Legumes

Fruits

Leafy vegetables

Fig. 2–7 Useful sources of fibre.

Fibre affects blood cholesterol

Soluble fibre seems to reduce the level of LDL (low-density lipoprotein) cholesterol in blood, but not HDL (high-density lipoprotein) cholesterol (see Section 2.5).

Fibre and food processing

Processing (see Chapter 6) may remove *all* the fibre:

- When oil is extracted from oil seeds such as groundnuts or when sugar is extracted from sugar cane, all the fibre is removed.

Processing may remove *some* of the fibre:

- When cereals (maize, rice, or wheat) are milled, much of the outside of the grain is removed. In highly milled or refined flours much of the fibre is removed. In wholegrain flours, more of the fibre remains.
- When legumes, vegetables, or fruit are skinned, some of the fibre is removed.

Processing may *alter* the fibre. Grinding and mashing squash or break cell walls so the nutrients spill out and the food is softer—for example, groundnut paste or mashed beans. When a person eats the food, she digests and absorbs the nutrients more quickly and easily. The fibre remains in the food and can have some of its effects, but not all of them.

Fibre needs

There are no recommended values at present, but a guideline is that adults should eat about 30 g fibre each day.

Fibre reduces the absorption of iron and some other minerals, so pregnant women and young children and other groups at risk of anaemia should not eat too much.

Too much fibre also makes children's meals bulky, so that they may not get enough Calories and other nutrients.

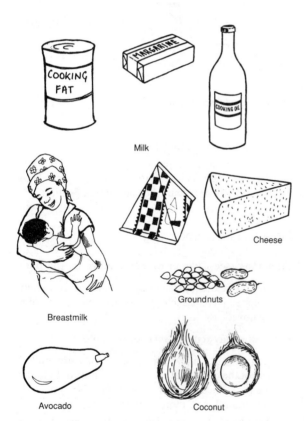

Milk

Breastmilk

Cheese

Groundnuts

Avocado

Coconut

Fig. 2–8 Some good sources of fat.

2.3 FATS

We use the word 'fat' to mean a group of nutrients (sometimes called *lipids*) and to mean a particular type of fat in food.

Fat
- A group of nutrients (fatty acids, cholesterol, etc.)
- Food fat which is hard at cool temperatures (butter, cooking fat, ghee)

Oil   Food fat which is liquid at cool temperatures (maize oil, 'salad oil', red palm oil)

Fats, or lipids, provide more Calories per gram than any other nutrient. They are the most *concentrated* form of energy.

Sources of fat

- Fats and oils including maize oil, palm oil, coconut oil, margarine, butter, ghee, cooking fat;
- Fatty animal foods including meat, chicken, fatty fish, milk, and cheese;
- Fatty vegetable foods including groundnuts and soybeans.

Sometimes it is easy to see which foods contain fat. For example, you can see and feel the fat in foods like butter, oil, fatty meat, and cream on top of milk. In other foods, such as groundnuts, the fat is mixed with other nutrients and you cannot see it.

How the body uses fat

Figure 2–9 shows the different ways in which the body uses fat from food.

- Fat is a concentrated source of energy. One gram of fat provides twice as much energy as 1 g carbohydrate.
- Fat is also an important energy store in the body.
- But fat is also needed for other things, for example, for building cells, and to help body processes, and to help absorption of vitamin A.

Box 2.2 explains the different kinds of fat in the body.

2.4 FATTY ACIDS

Most fats consist mainly of *fatty acids*. Three fatty acid molecules combine with a glycerol molecule to make a *triglyceride*. During digestion, triglycerides are broken down to fatty acids and glycerol.

Box 2.2. Fat in the body

Cell fat

- *Part* of all cells
- Mostly in brain and nerves
- Contains large amounts of essential fatty acids

Storage fat

- *Inside* special storage cells
- Mostly under skin and inside abdomen
- Contains smaller amounts of essential fatty acids
- Forms body's store of energy
- Insulates body (like a blanket) to keep it warm
- Protects delicate organs like the kidneys

There are at least 40 different fatty acids. Figure 2–10 shows that each is made of a chain of carbon and hydrogen atoms. Each fatty acid is different because:

- The chains of carbon atoms may be different lengths (long-, medium-, and short-chain fatty acids).
- There may be one or more *double bond* (or double link) between the carbon atoms. A fatty acid with a double bond contains less hydrogen.
- The chains of carbon atoms in fatty acids with double bonds are usually bent (*cis* fatty acids). If fat is processed, the chain may become straight (*trans* fatty acids).

These differences affect what the fat looks like and what it does in the body.

Saturated and unsaturated fatty acids

If a fatty acid has no double bonds and so contains the maximum amount of hydrogen, we call it a *saturated fatty acid*.

If a fatty acid contains one double bond we call it a *monounsaturated fatty acid*.

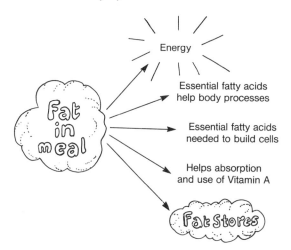

Fig. 2–9 How the body uses fat from food.

If a fatty acid contains two or more double bonds we call it a *polyunsaturated fatty acid* (see Fig. 2–10).

Essential fatty acids

The body can make most fatty acids from carbohydrates, but there are two polyunsaturaed fatty acids that it cannot make. These are *linoleic* and *linolenic* acids. The body needs them to build cells, particularly the cells of the brain and nerves, and to help body processes. They are called *essential fatty acids* because we have to eat enough of them in our food.

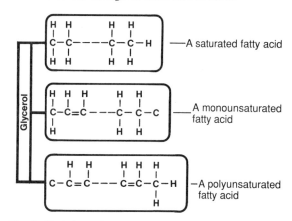

Fig. 2–10 A fat molecule made of three fatty acids joined by glycerol. This is a *triglyceride*. This triglyceride consists of one saturated fatty acid, one mono-unsaturated fatty acid, and one polyunsaturated fatty acid.

The mixture of fatty acids in fats

Fats consist of a mixture of saturated and unsaturated fatty acids. Figure 2–11 shows the proportion of saturated and unsaturated fatty acids in some fats.

Fats which contain a large proportion of saturated fatty acids are usually harder at cool temperatures than fats which contain a small proportion. For example, butter and beef fat are harder than sunflower seed oil.

Fats which contain a large proportion of saturated fatty acids are called 'saturated fats'.

Examples of saturated fats are the fats from:

● the meat and milk of animals;
● coconut.

Fats which contain a large proportion of unsaturated fatty acids are called 'unsaturated fats'. Examples are the fat from:

● fish;
● oil seeds such as sesame and sunflower;
● cereals and legumes (maize oil and groundnut oil);
● breast milk.

Cis and trans fatty acids

Unsaturated fatty acids which occur naturally are '*cis*' fatty acids. When unsaturated fats are processed the '*cis*' fatty acids may be changed to '*trans*' fatty acids. The body uses '*trans*' fatty acids as if they were saturated. The body cannot use '*trans*' linolenic or '*trans*' linoleic acids as essential fatty acids.

Processing fats

Unsaturated fats can be hardened to make margarine, vegetable ghee, or cooking fat. To do this the double bond is broken and hydrogen is added, or *cis* fatty acids are changed to *trans* fatty acids.

2.5 CHOLESTEROL AND HEART DISEASE

In the cells and blood of humans and animals there are small amounts of another type of lipid called *cholesterol*. We need cholesterol to build cells, to make some hormones and body fluids, and for some body processes.

Proteins carry cholesterol and fatty acids in the blood. These 'fat–protein' molecules are called 'lipoproteins'. Two important lipoproteins which carry cholesterol are called *high-density lipoprotein cholesterol (HDL cholesterol)* and *low-density lipoprotein cholesterol (LDL cholesterol)*.

A high level of LDL cholesterol in the blood may increase the risk of heart disease. A high level of HDL cholesterol decreases the risk (see Section 22.7).

The type and amount of fatty acids that we eat is one thing which affects the types and levels of cholesterol in the blood. It is the fatty acids in the food, more than the cholesterol, which affect blood cholesterol.

Some saturated fatty acids seem to increase the level of LDL cholesterol in the blood—but not all. Some mono- and polyunsaturated fatty acids seem to lower cholesterol—but they cannot do this if they are '*trans*' fatty acids, or if they have been hardened because then

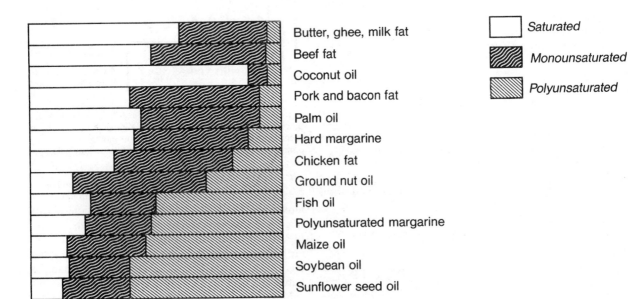

Butter, ghee, milk fat
Beef fat
Coconut oil
Pork and bacon fat
Palm oil
Hard margarine
Chicken fat
Ground nut oil
Fish oil
Polyunsaturated margarine
Maize oil
Soybean oil
Sunflower seed oil

Saturated
Monounsaturated
Polyunsaturated

Fig. 2–11 Saturated, monounsaturated, and polyunsaturated fatty acids in different fats.

they become saturated. The different unsaturated fatty acids have different effects on the levels of LDL and HDL cholesterol. A lot more research is needed on diet and heart disease, so watch out for developments.

2.6 FAT NEEDS

There are no exact values for fat needs, because the body can make most fatty acids, cholesterol, and other fats from carbohydrate.

If we eat more starch, sugar, fat, or protein than we need for energy, the body changes it into storage fat. The amount of storage fat varies, so people with a little storage fat are *thin*, and people with a lot of storage fat are *fat*.

However, everyone needs to eat some fat because everyone, especially children, needs essential fatty acids. Also, fat makes meals less bulky and helps the absorption of some vitamins. But too much fat can lead to obesity and other health problems (see Chapter 22).

A general guideline is that about 20–35 per cent of Calories should come from fat (see Appendix 2). Not more than 10 per cent of Calories should come from saturated fat. A diet should never contain less than 10 per cent of Calories from fat.

2.7 ENERGY NEEDS

The amount of energy that people need to get from their food in order to keep healthy and active varies (see Figs. 2–12 and 2–13). To measure energy needs, nutritionists in the past estimated what people *ate*. Now, they estimate the energy that people *use*.

Variation between individuals
The tables of energy needs (Table 2.4 and Appendix 2) give the *average* needs of individuals of different types. For example, they tell you the average energy requirements of active young men. But this does not tell you exactly what each young man needs, because individuals vary. Some need more, and some need less than the average. This is called *individual variation* (see Fig. 2–14).

Different energy needs
Fig. 2–15 shows that we can divide energy needs into:

Energy needs vary with:

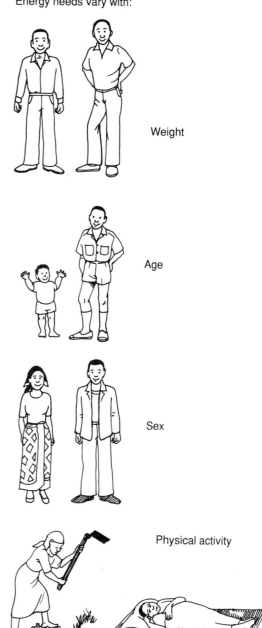

Weight

Age

Sex

Physical activity

Fig. 2–12 Energy needs vary.

- energy to keep alive at rest—this is called the *basic metabolic rate* or BMR;
- energy for activity.

BMR + Energy for activity = Total energy needs.

Energy needs increase during:

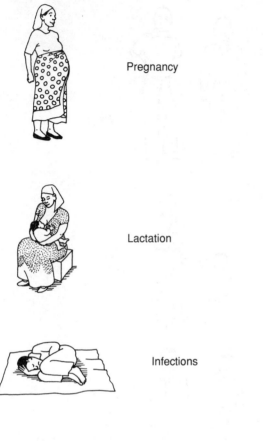

Pregnancy

Lactation

Infections

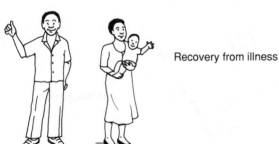

Recovery from illness

Fig. 2–13 Energy needs increase during these events.

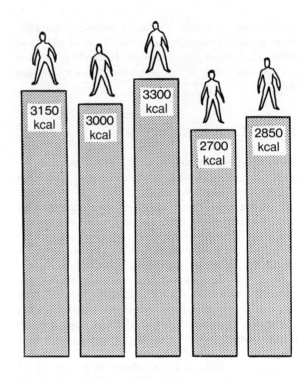

Fig. 2–14 Individual variation in energy needs.

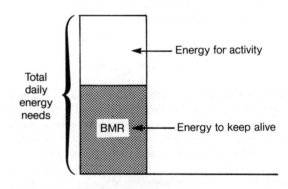

Fig. 2–15 Total daily energy needs.

2.8 ENERGY FOR THE BASAL METABOLIC RATE (BMR)

The BMR is the rate at which the body uses energy for the chemical processes that keep us alive and warm and that build tissues and secrete fluids. The BMR is the rate at which the body uses energy when we are com-

pletely at rest and not moving at all. It is a little less than the rate at which it uses energy when we sleep. The BMR is measured in *kcal/day* (24 hours) or *kcal/hour*.

How the BMR varies

The BMR varies with the person's weight, age, and sex.
It also varies with the *composition* of the person's

body, that is with the proportion of muscle and fat in the body. Muscles and organs like the heart use more energy than fat.

Part of the variation of BMR is due to differences in the energy used *per kilogram body weight*.

The BMR is:

- higher in large people than in small people of the same age, because larger people have bigger hearts and more muscle and other tissues;

- lower in old people than in young people of the same weight;

- higher in men than in women of the same weight and age. Men contain a higher proportion of muscle to fat than women;

- lower in fat people than in thin people of the same age and weight.

The BMR per kilo is higher in children than in adults.

Table 2.1 gives some examples of average BMRs for different types of people. (The table does not include children, because their energy needs are calculated in a different way.)

Table 2.1. Some average BMRs for adolescents and adults (kcal/person/day)

Weight (kg)	Adolescents (10–17 years)		Adults (18–30 years)	
	Boys	Girls	Men	Women
40	1351	1234		
45	1439	1295		
50	1526	1356	1444	1231
55	1614	1417	1521	1305
60			1597	1378
65			1674	1451
70			1750	

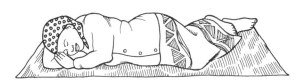

Fig. 2–16 Hannah sleeping. Her BMR is 1308 kcal/day, or 54.5 kcal/hour.

Appendix 2 explains how to calculate BMRs yourself.

Examples

Hannah is 33 years old and weighs 55 kg. Table A2.2 in Appendix 2 shows that the average BMR for women of her weight and age is 1308 kcal/day, or 54.5 kcal/hour.

Hannah has a husband called Tom. He is 40 years old and weighs 60 kg. The average BMR for men of the same age and weight as Tom is 1575 kcal/day or 65.6 kcal/hour. Tom has a higher BMR than Hannah because he weighs more and is a man.

2.9 ENERGY FOR ACTIVITY

When we are asleep, we use energy at a little more than the BMR. But when we are awake and moving, the rate at which we use energy increases. The more active we are, the faster we use energy.

The *total* amount of energy that people use when they are active depends on:

- *The type of activity.* A 'heavy' activity such as digging or chopping wood uses energy faster than a 'light' activity such as sewing or reading.

- *How hard the person does the activity.* When people do some activities, especially heavy ones, they usually stop for rests. The number and length of the rests affects the amount of energy that they use.

- *The person's BMR.* A person who has a high BMR uses more energy for the same activity than a person with a lower BMR. A large person with more muscles and other tissues needs more energy to move them. For example, if Tom and Hannah both climb a hill, Tom uses more energy than Hannah.

Activity factors

To calculate energy needs during a particular activity, you have to multiply the BMR by an *activity factor*.

The activity factor depends on the amount of extra energy that a person uses to perform the activity. Table 2.2 lists activity factors for different activities.

Examples

The activity factor for sweeping is 1.7. The average BMR for women of the same age and weight as Hannah is 54.5

kcal/hour. So the rate at which Hannah uses energy while sweeping is about

$$54.5 \times 1.7 = 92.7 \text{ kcal/hour.}$$

The activity factor for hoeing is 6.5. So the rate at which Hannah uses energy while hoeing is

$$54.5 \times 6.5 = 354.3 \text{ kcal/hour.}$$

The average BMR for men of the same age and weight as Tom is 65.6 kcal/hour. Thus the approximate rate at which Tom uses energy while hoeing is

$$65.6 \times 6.5 = 426.4 \text{ kcal/hour.}$$

Tom uses more energy than Hannah for the same activity because his BMR is higher.

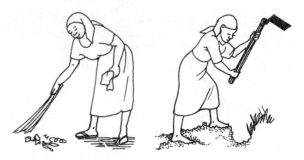

Sweeping – 93 kcal/hour   Hoeing – 354 kcal/hour

Fig. 2–18 The energy that Hannah uses for sweeping and hoeing.

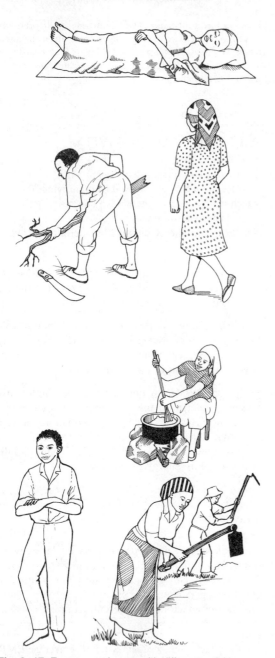

Fig. 2–17 Energy needs vary with different activities.

	Hannah		Tom
24		Sitting, talking, and social activity	
	6.5		9.5
18			
	2	Food preparation	
		Travelling	1
	3	Housework	0.5
12			
	3	Agriculture work	3.5
	1	Washing, dressing	1
6			
	8.5	Sleeping	8.5
	Hours		Hours

Fig. 2–19 Hannah's and Tom's activities during 24 hours.

Table 2.2. Activity factors for different activities

Sleeping	1.0
Sewing	1.1
Office work	1.2
Playing cards/bao	1.5
Washing dishes	1.5
Sweeping	1.7
Cooking	1.8
Walking	2.9
Planting groundnuts	3.1
Washing clothes	3.2
Scrubbing floor	3.2
Weeding	5.0
Labouring	5.4
Pounding grain	5.6
Playing football	6.0
Chopping wood	6.1
Hoeing or digging	6.5
Walking uphill with load	8.8

The activity factors do not allow for rests during the activity, when less energy is used. The factors which allow for rests are called the 'integrated energy indices'.

2.10 DAILY ENERGY NEEDS

People do not sweep or hoe all day and all night. They sleep and rest, eat and talk, and engage in many other activities which use energy at different rates.

To find out the total daily energy needs you need to know both the type of activity and the time that people spend on each. Figure 2–19 shows the average time spent on different activities over 24 hours by people like Hannah and Tom.

Physical activity levels

It would take too long to measure everyone's different activities to calculate their total daily energy needs.

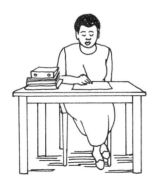

Fig. 2–20 Mary's energy needs are 2040 kcal/day.

Instead, we use factors based on people's average levels of activity, or occupation, during 24 hours. These are called *physical activity levels (PAL)*. Table 2.3 gives some examples.

Table 2.3. Physical activity levels for women and men aged 18–60 years

	Level of physical activity			
	Light	Moderate	Heavy	'Average'*
Women	1.56	1.64	1.82	1.67
Men	1.55	1.78	2.10	1.82

*The 'average' value is based on the proportion of people doing light, moderate, and heavy work in a typical low-income country.

Examples of occupations for each physical activity level

PAL	Typical occupation
Light	People working in offices, students, unemployed
Moderate	Shop assistants, domestic servants, housewives, tradesmen, drivers
Moderate-to-heavy	Farmers, fishermen, labourers, forestry workers

How to calculate average daily energy needs

Multiply the person's BMR by his or her PAL.

BMR × PAL = daily energy needs.

Examples

Hannah does housework and cultivates her fields. She has a moderate physical activity level, so her PAL is 1.64. The BMR for women like Hannah is 1308 kcal/day.

So Hannah's daily energy needs are

$$1308 \times 1.64 = 2145 \text{ kcal/day.}$$

Tom also has a moderate physical activity level, so his PAL is 1.78. The BMR for men like Tom is 1575 kcal/day.

So Tom's daily energy needs are

$$1575 \times 1.78 = 2804 \text{ kcal/day.}$$

Mary is Hannah's younger sister. Her BMR is about the same as Hannah's but she works in an office and has a light physical activity level. Her PAL is 1.56.

Thus Mary's daily energy needs are

$$1308 \times 1.56 = 2040 \text{ kcal/day.}$$

Remember that these are *average values* for people like Hannah, Tom, and Mary and that people vary.

2.11 ADDITIONAL ENERGY NEEDS FOR WOMEN

During pregnancy

A woman needs extra Calories during pregnancy to build up her own tissues, to build fat stores to make breast milk, to build the baby and the placenta, and because of the extra work that her body has to do.

It is difficult to say exactly how much extra food a woman needs during pregnancy. Her gut absorbs nutrients better and her body uses them more efficiently than when she is not pregnant. The amount of extra energy that a pregnant woman needs may not be as much as people formerly thought. Nutritionists are still not sure exactly how much to recommend but we suggest that:

- Well nourished women with light–moderate activity levels have an extra 100 kcal/day.
- Well nourished women with heavy activity levels have an extra 200 kcal/day.
- Undernourished women have an extra 200–285 kcal/day.

It is particularly important that pregnant undernourished women and adolescent girls have enough Calories to avoid having low birth weight babies, and to ensure a good supply of breast milk.

Example

When Hannah is pregnant her daily energy needs are about

$$2145 + 100 = 2245 \text{ kcal/day.}$$

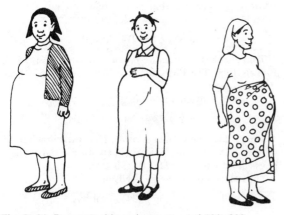

Fig. 2–21 Pregnant girls and women need 100–200 Calories extra each day.

During lactation

During the first 6 months of lactation women use about 700 kcal per day to make breast milk.

A well nourished lactating mother gets about 200 kcal/day from the fat that she stored during pregnancy. The additional energy needs of lactation for at least the first 6 months are about 500 kcal/day.

However, a woman's total needs may not increase as much as this. Women may use less energy for their own body processes during lactation, so their own daily energy needs may decrease. This is not yet fully understood.

Additional needs probably continue at the same level until the child is 1 year old or more, and then they gradually decrease as the child takes less breast milk.

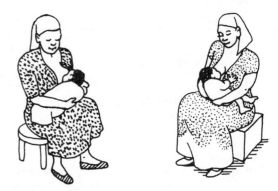

Fig. 2–22 Lactating girls and women need about 500 Calories extra each day.

When Hannah breastfeeds her 3-month-old baby, her daily energy needs will *probably* be about

$$2145 + 500 = 2645 \text{ kcal/day.}$$

2.12 ENERGY NEEDS OF CHILDREN

There is not yet enough data to work out activity factors and PALs for children under 10 years old. So to calculate the energy needs of children we use '*energy allowances*'. Appendix 2 gives energy allowances by age.

These provide enough energy for:

- growth;
- play and other physical activities;
- energy to fight infections;
- catch-up growth following infections.

Daily energy needs = weight × energy allowance per day.

Energy allowances decrease with age because the rate of growth slows down as children become older.

Example
The average weight of a group of 3–4-year-old boys is 16 kg. The energy allowance for boys of this age is 99 kcal/kg/day. So the average daily energy need of these boys is

16 kg × 99 kcal = 1584 kcal/day.

You can see that young children need a *large amount* of energy—*more than half* the needs of many adults. This is very important when we consider the kind of meals that young children should have in Chapters 8 and 11.

The body weights used in the calculation can be:

- the average weight of the actual children you are interested in;

or

- the average weight of healthy children of the same age and sex (*reference weights*, see Appendix 5). (This usually gives a higher value for daily energy needs and so allows more Calories for growth.)

Tables of energy needs

Table 2.4 and Appendix 2 give tables of energy needs using the weights and activity levels from an African country as an example.

Energy values for your own country should be prepared using national values for body weights and activity levels if possible.

Table 2.4. Approximate daily energy needs for different sex and age groups

Age (years)	Weight (kg)	Energy (kcal)
Children—both sexes		
0–1	7.3	800
1–3	11.9	1250
3–5	15.9	1510
5–7	19.6	1710
7–10	25.9	1880
Boys		
10–12	34.0	2170
12–14	43.2	2360
14–16	54.5	2620
16–18	63.6	2820
Girls		
10–12	35.4	1925
12–14	44.2	2040
14–16	51.5	2135
16–18	54.6	2150
If pregnant		+200
Men—active		
18–60	65.0	2944
> 60	65.0	2060
Women—active		
Childbearing age	55.0	2140
Pregnant	55.0	2240
Lactating	55.0	2640
> 60	55.0	1830

Taken from Appendix 2.

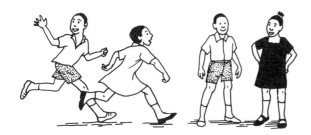

Fig. 2–23 Children need energy for growth and activity.

THINGS TO DO

Show that starch absorbs water when boiled

1. Put a small amount of raw rice in a glass. Measure the same amount of rice, boil it until cooked, and drain it. Ask trainees to compare the volume of raw and cooked rice. Discuss why the volume has increased.

Show how starch changes to simple sugars during digestion

2. Give trainees small pieces of bread to chew slowly. Ask them if it begins to taste sweeter. Explain that an enzyme called amylase in saliva digests the starch into glucose.

Decide whether the carbohydrate in food is starch or sugar

3. Display examples or pictures of milk, a variety of cereals, roots, legumes, and fruits. Ask trainees to arrange the foods so that those in which the carbohydrate is starch are in one group and those in which it is sugar are in another group.

Show the amounts of starch, sugar, and fat in local foods

4. Ask trainees to list some of the foods they ate yesterday. Together choose a few of these foods and use the food composition tables in Appendix 1 to find the amounts of starch, sugar, and fat in 100 g of each food. For example: millet flour, cowpeas, groundnuts, milk.

Discuss which foods are rich in fibre

5. Display examples of pictures of maize, bread, beans, fruit, milk, egg. Ask trainees to discuss:

   a. Which foods contain fibre;
   b. How the fibre helps to keep the body healthy.

Calculate energy needs for different types of people

6. Ask trainees to calculate which type of people have the highest energy need:

   • young men with an average BMR of 1500 kcal who do light work;
   • women with an average BMR of 1300 kcal who do heavy work.

   [Answer: women. Young men: PAL is 1.55, so they need 1500 × 1.55 = 2325 kcal. Women: their PAL is 1.82, so they need 1300 × 1.82 = 2366 kcal.]

7. A group of labourers aged 18–24 years old employed mostly in digging have an average weight of 65 kg. Ask trainees to calculate their average daily energy needs. [Answer: 1674 (BMR) × 2.10 (PAL) = 3515 kcal/day.]

8. Compare the average energy needs of young women in these groups:

   • urban women with an average weight of 55 kg doing light work in an office;
   • rural women with an average weight of 50 kg doing moderate work in the fields and house.

   [Answer: Urban women: 1305 (BMR) × 1.56 (PAL) = 2036 kcal/day. Rural women: 1231 (BMR) × 1.64 (PAL) = 2019 kcal/day.]

9. Use Appendix 2 to calculate the daily energy needs of 2–3-year-old girls with an average weight of 13 kg. Compare their needs with the needs of the adult women in question 8. [Answer: 13 (weight) × 102 (energy allowance) = 1326 kcal/day.]

USEFUL PUBLICATIONS

Davidson, R. and Eastwood, M. A. (1986). *Human nutrition and dietetics* (8th edn). Churchill Livingstone, Edinburgh.

FAO (1980). *Dietary fats and oils*, Food and Nutrition Series, no. 20. FAO, Rome.

James, W. P. T. and Schofield, E. C. (1990). *Human energy requirements: a manual for planners and nutritionists*. Published for FAO by Oxford University Press, Oxford.

WHO (1985). *Energy and protein requirements*, Technical Report Series, no. 724. WHO, Geneva.

3 Protein

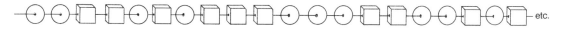

Fig. 3–1 A protein is like a necklace made of amino acids.

3.1 INTRODUCTION

Protein contains nitrogen as well as carbon, hydrogen, and oxygen. The body cannot make protein from carbohydrate or fat, because they contain no nitrogen. So we must eat enough protein.

All animals and plants contain protein, but the proteins in each of them are different. For example, the proteins in rice are different from the proteins in beans. The proteins in red blood cells are different from the proteins in muscle cells or brain cells. Different enzymes and antibodies are all different, special proteins.

To understand why each protein is different, look at how proteins are made.

3.2 AMINO ACIDS

Each protein molecule is made of chains of *amino acids* joined together. There are 20 different amino acids. Different proteins are made from different numbers of these amino acids arranged in different patterns.

When proteins are digested, they break down into amino acids which pass through the gut wall into the blood (Fig. 3–2). The blood carries the amino acids to the cells, and the cells build some of them into new proteins. The cells must get enough of each different amino acid to make the protein that the cell needs.

One way to understand amino acids is to imagine that they are like beads. You can join beads together to make a necklace. When amino acids are joined together they make a molecule of protein. If you have 20 different sorts of beads, you can make hundreds of different sorts of necklace. In the same way, 20 amino acids can make hundreds of different proteins.

If you break several necklaces, you have a lot of loose beads, and you can mix them together in a new pattern and make a different necklace.

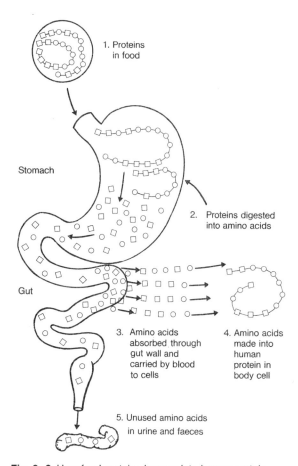

1. Proteins in food

Stomach

2. Proteins digested into amino acids

Gut

3. Amino acids absorbed through gut wall and carried by blood to cells

4. Amino acids made into human protein in body cell

5. Unused amino acids in urine and faeces

Fig. 3–2 How food protein changes into human protein.

When food is digested, the amino acids from all the different proteins become loose and mixed together in the gut, and later in the blood. The cells join the amino acids together in new patterns to make human proteins.

9 essential amino acids   11 non-essential amino acids

          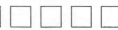 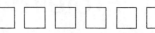

Fig. 3–3 The 20 amino acids.
Me, methionine; Is, isoleucine; Le, leucine; Ly, lysine; Pf, phenylalanine;
Th, threonine; Tf, tryptophan; Va, valine. Histidine (Hi) is essential for infants.

A human protein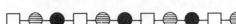

Egg protein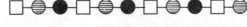

Bean protein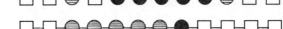

Maize protein

Fig. 3–4 Simplified diagrams of protein molecules. (Really, each protein contains hundreds of amino acids.)

 = Methionine   = Lysine

Essential and non-essential amino acids

There are 11 amino acids which the body can make from other amino acids—if there is enough protein. They are called *non-essential* amino acids.

There are eight amino acids which the body cannot make, and one amino acid (*histidine*) which babies cannot make. Newborns may also need *taurine*. These are called *essential amino acids* (Fig. 3–3). We must eat enough of each of these amino acids so that we can make human proteins.

3.3 COMPLETE AND INCOMPLETE PROTEINS

Most animal proteins contain almost the same proportion of each essential amino acid as human proteins. Because of this proteins in eggs, milk, meat, and fish are sometimes called *complete* proteins.

Proteins in plants often contain much smaller amounts of one or more essential amino acids than animal and human proteins—for example, the maize and bean proteins in Fig. 3–4. The bean protein has less methionine, and the maize protein has less lysine than egg or human protein. Proteins from plants are sometimes called *incomplete* proteins.

Mixing different incomplete proteins

However, the amounts of essential amino acids in different plants vary. For example, although maize protein contains only a little lysine, it contains a lot of methionine. Although bean protein contains only a little methionine, it contains a lot of lysine.

The diagram in Fig. 3–5 shows how the body can use most of the amino acids in egg protein to make a human protein—both proteins contain almost the same amount of essential amino acids.

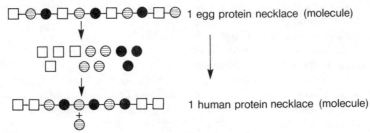

1 egg protein necklace (molecule)

1 human protein necklace (molecule)

Fig. 3–5 Rearranging amino acids in egg protein to make human protein.

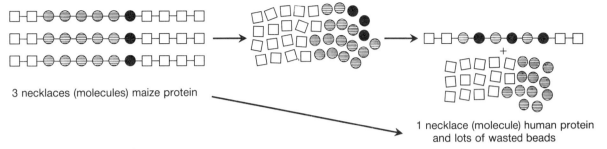

3 necklaces (molecules) maize protein

1 necklace (molecule) human protein and lots of wasted beads

Fig. 3–6 Three molecules of maize protein make only one molecule of human protein.

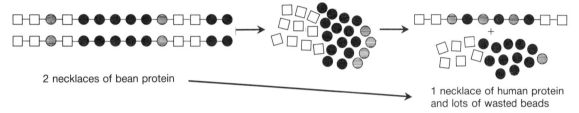

2 necklaces of bean protein

1 necklace of human protein and lots of wasted beads

Fig. 3–7 Two molecules of bean protein make only one molecule of human protein.

But if a person eats only maize, she gets plenty of methionine but little lysine. She must eat very large amounts of maize to eat enough lysine to make human protein (Fig. 3–6).

If she eats only beans, she gets enough lysine but not enough methionine. She must eat very large amounts of beans to get enough methionine to make human protein (Fig. 3–7).

But, if the person eats maize and beans *together*, she can get enough lysine and enough methionine from a normal-sized meal (see Fig. 3–8).

So maize and beans help each other to give all the essential amino acids needed to make human proteins. Encourage people to eat a mixture of foods so that the different proteins in a meal can 'help each other' to provide enough essential amino acids.

Protein from animals is usually expensive. But plant foods can give us all the protein we need if we eat:

● a mixture of plant foods;
● enough plant proteins.

Amino acid score

Meals that contain plenty of animal protein provide enough of all the essential amino acids. So almost all the protein in the meal can be used to make human protein. We say that the **amino acid score is 100**.

Meals that contain a lot of cereals or roots and some legumes, but only a little animal protein do not provide enough of some essential amino acids. So not all the protein can be used, and the amino acid score is lower. The exact score depends on the mixture of foods eaten. If 75 per cent of the protein can be used, the **amino acid score is 75**.

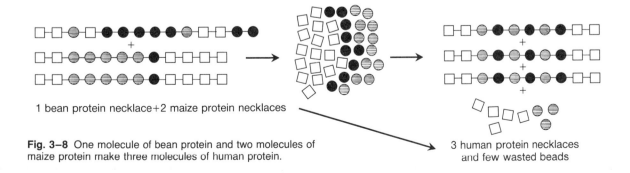

1 bean protein necklace+2 maize protein necklaces

3 human protein necklaces and few wasted beads

Fig. 3–8 One molecule of bean protein and two molecules of maize protein make three molecules of human protein.

Meals that contain mainly cereals or roots and very small amounts of legumes provide very small amounts of several essential amino acids, and the score is even lower. The **amino acid score may be about 60**.

If a child's meals have a low amino acid score, he needs to eat *more* protein than if his meals had a high amino acid score.

3.4 HOW THE BODY USES PROTEIN

The body uses protein:

- *To build new tissues and fluids*, especially for growth in children and pregnant and breastfeeding women.

- *To replace lost amino acids*. When cells in the body die, the protein in them breaks down into amino acids. The body uses some amino acids again, but some are lost in the urine. So everyone needs some protein to replace these lost amino acids. During illness amino acids may be lost faster than normal.

- *To help the cells to work*. Enzymes which make the chemical processes in the body happen are special proteins.

- *To protect the body against infections*. Antibodies which help to kill viruses and bacteria are special proteins.

- *As fuel for energy*. A person uses protein from food for energy if:

  - She eats more protein than she needs for building cells and fluids and for making her cells function. If her body does not need the protein for energy it changes it into fat.

  - She does not eat enough starch, sugar, or fat to provide all the energy she needs. This means that there is less protein available for body building. But it is more important to have energy to stay alive than to build new cells.

The body cannot store extra protein—though sometimes it uses the muscles as a store. When a person does not eat enough, she uses her muscles to provide protein for important purposes—for example, as fuel for energy or to make breast milk. This is one reason why people who do not eat enough become thin, and why children who do not eat enough stop growing.

3.5 PROTEIN NEEDS

Table 3.1 and Appendix 2 show the protein needs for different kinds of people. Figure 3–10 shows how protein needs depend on a person's size, age, and sex, and, for women, on whether they are pregnant or breastfeeding.

Protein needs also vary according to the *type of protein* and the *amount of fibre* in meals:

- People need less protein if they eat *complete* proteins (with a high amino acid score) than if they eat *incomplete* proteins (with lower amino acid score). For example, the daily protein needs of 1–3 year old children are about 14 g if they eat complete protein and about 23 g if they eat incomplete protein.

- The amount of fibre in a meal affects the amount of protein which is digested into amino acids and absorbed. If a meal contains only a little fibre, *more* protein is digested. If a meal contains a lot of fibre, *less* protein is digested.

However, fibre is important in other ways for people's health, so this is not a reason to eat less fibre.

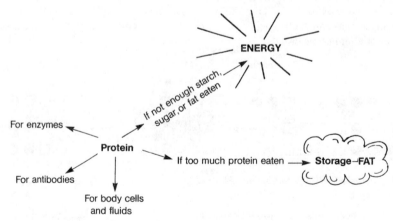

Fig. 3–9 How the body uses protein.

Protein needs depend on:

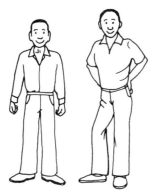

Size–Big people need more protein than smaller people because they have to replace more cells and other tissues

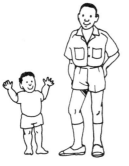

Age–children need more protein for growth. Younger children need more protein per kilogram body weight than older children because they are growing faster

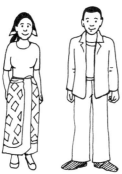

Sex–men have more muscle and less fat than women so they need more protein to replace muscle cells

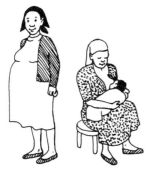

Pregnancy–a pregnant woman needs extra protein for the growth of the baby and placenta and to increase her own blood and tissues. Over the 9 months of pregnancy, she needs about 6–7 g extra protein each day

Lactation–a breastfeeding woman needs extra protein to make breast milk. She needs about 18–21 g extra each day.

Fig. 3–10 Different sorts of people have different protein needs.

Table 3.1. Daily protein needs for different sex and age groups

Age (years)	Weight (kg)	Protein (g)*
Children—both sexes		
0–1	7.3	12
1–3	11.9	23
3–5	15.9	26
5–7	19.6	30
7–10	25.9	38
Boys		
10–12	34.0	50
12–14	43.2	64
14–16	54.5	75
16–18	63.6	84
Girls		
10–12	35.4	52
12–14	44.2	62
14–16	51.5	69
16–18	54.6	66
If pregnant		+7
Men—active		
18–60	65.0	57
> 60	65.0	57
Women—active		
Childbearing age	55.0	48
Pregnant	55.0	55
Lactating	55.0	68
> 60	55.0	48

*These values assume that all groups (except 0–1-year-old breastfed children) are eating very little animal protein, and large amounts of fibre (see Appendix 2). Children who are breastfed for 2 years need less protein.

THINGS TO DO

Foods which contain protein

1. Show several samples or pictures of foods which contain protein. Ask trainees to pick out those which contain:

- complete (animal) proteins;
- incomplete (plant) proteins.

Ask them to suggest a meal using incomplete proteins only.

Explain amino acids and proteins using 'beads' and 'necklaces'

2. To do this exercise, you need at least three different sorts of 'beads' and some string. Different sorts of bottle tops make good beads, and you can arrange them in rows like a string of 'beads'. Or you can make holes in them and put them on a string.

Divide the trainees into four groups.

a. Give each group some string and an identical pile of three sorts of 'beads'—say five red, five blue, and five green beads. Ask groups to make a necklace. Compare the necklaces. Most will be different showing how different proteins can be made from the same amino acids.

b. Choose two sorts of beads to be essential amino acids, say red and blue beads. Use the other beads, say the green ones, to be non-essential amino acids. Make a 'necklace' of beads as in Fig. 3–1 to represent a *human protein*. Use three red, three blue, and four green beads.

Give Group 1 three necklaces, each of which is made of three red beads, three blue beads, and four green beads, but in a different order from the *human protein* necklace. Tell them that this is *milk protein*.

Give Group 2 three necklaces, each of which contains seven red beads, two blue beads, and five green beads. Tell them that this is *bean protein*.

Give Groups 3 and 4 three necklaces, each of which contains one red bead, five blue beads, and six green beads. Tell them that this is *maize protein*.

- Now ask each group to unthread one necklace and to try to make the human protein necklace. Only Group 1 can do this.

- Then ask each group to find out how many necklaces they use to make a human protein necklace. Group 2 will use two necklaces, and groups 3 and 4 will each use three necklaces. Ask them to count the number of wasted beads.

Explain that this shows that you need to eat about twice as much bean protein or three times as much maize protein as milk protein to make the same amount of human protein. The other amino acids are wasted.

c. Ask groups 2, 3, and 4 to rethread their necklaces to make maize and bean protein again. Ask each group to unthread one necklace and then put all the beads together and find out how many human protein necklaces they can make and how many beads are left over.

This demonstrates that you can make more human proteins from a certain quantity (say 10 g) of a mixture of maize and bean proteins than you can from the same amount of maize protein, or the same amount of bean protein alone. Fewer amino acids are wasted from the mixture of maize and bean proteins.

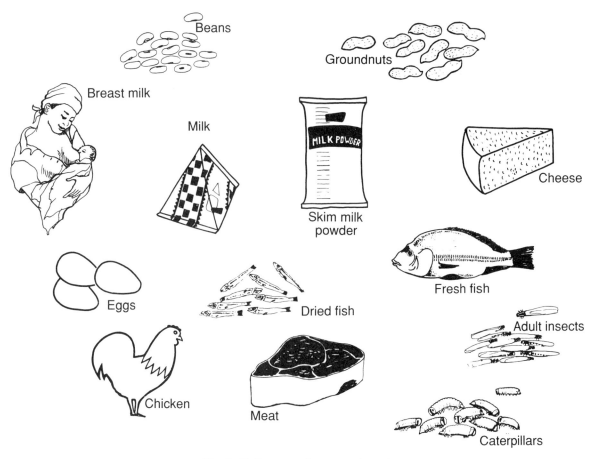

Fig. 3–11 Some good sources of protein.

'Role play' proteins and amino acids

3. This exercise may be done in different ways, depending on the age and experience of the trainees. It may be done by a whole class as a group exercise, or some trainees may demonstrate amino acids to the rest of the class.

Tell each trainee that he or she is an amino acid. If appropriate you can give them names of different amino acids. Choose a leader to explain what is happening. Ask trainees to:

a. Join hands together to show how a protein is made of amino acids. Let them do this in different orders and with different numbers of trainees to show how different proteins have different patterns of amino acids.

b. Stop holding hands and move around to show how protein is digested.

c. Go one by one into another room or part of the class-room to show how amino acids pass through the gut wall.

d. Join hands again in a different order to show how to build human protein.

Calculate protein needs

4. Ask trainees to look in Table 3.1 and find out the individual daily protein needs for the following sorts of people:

a. 3–5-year-old children with an average weight of about 16 kg;

b. Young men with an average weight of about 65 kg.

Then ask them to calculate the protein needs per kg body weight for an individual of each group. Discuss their answers.

[Children—daily need = 26 g = 1.63 g/kg body weight. Young men—daily need = 57 g = 0.88 g/kg body weight. Children need more protein per kg body weight because they are growing.]

USEFUL PUBLICATIONS

Davidson, R. and Eastwood, M. A. (1986). *Human nutrition and dietetics* (8th edn). Churchill Livingstone, Edinburgh.

WHO (1985). *Energy and protein requirements*, Technical Report Series, no. 724. WHO, Geneva.

4 Micronutrients and water

4.1 VITAMINS

Vitamins are chemical compounds that the body needs in small amounts to help it function properly. The important vitamins are:

- vitamin A (retinol and carotene);
- the B vitamins:
  - thiamine or vitamin B_1;
  - riboflavin or vitamin B_2;
  - niacin or nicotinic acid;
  - folate or folic acid;
  - pyridoxine or vitamin B_6;
  - pantothenic acid;
  - biotin;
  - vitamin B_{12} or cyanocobalamin;
- vitamin C or ascorbic acid;
- vitamin D or calciferol;
- vitamin E or tocopherols.

In this book we discuss vitamin A, folate, and vitamin C in detail, because these are the vitamins that people are most likely to lack. We mention thiamine, niacin, riboflavin, and vitamin D because deficiencies occur occasionally.

4.2 VITAMIN A

Why people need vitamin A

- *To prevent infections.* Vitamin A helps the body to resist infections. It helps to keep all the cells on the surface of the body healthy so that it is difficult for micro-organisms to enter the body. These body surfaces include:
  - the skin;
  - the surface of the eye;
  - inside the mouth;
  - the cells which line the gut;
  - the cells which line the respiratory tract.

  Vitamin A destroys *free radicals* and so helps to prevent tissue damage during infection (Section 17.2).

- *To keep the eye healthy.* Vitamin A keeps the front of the eye (the conjunctiva and cornea) strong, clear, and wet. It helps the eye to see in dim light (i.e. dusk or candlelight) (see Chapter 19).

- *To help children to grow properly.*

The two forms of vitamin A

There are two forms of vitamin A in foods:

- *Retinol* which is colourless and found only in animal foods. Retinol is the form of vitamin A which our bodies use most.

- *Carotene* which is yellow and which is found mainly in yellow or green plant foods. There is a little carotene in some animal foods such as milk. There are several sorts of carotene but the most important one is called *beta carotene*. Carotene destroys free radicals.

The body changes much of the carotene to retinol. Six molecules of carotene make one molecule of retinol.

Fat, protein, zinc, and vitamin E help the body to absorb or use vitamin A.

How we measure vitamin A

Because there are two types of vitamin A in food, we measure vitamin A (both carotene and retinol) as retinol equivalents. Because people need very small amounts of vitamin A, we measure it in *micro*grams (μg). 1 gram = 1 000 000 μg. The short way to write 'μg retinol equivalents' is RE.

1 μg retinol = 1 μg retinol equivalent = 1 RE.
6 μg beta carotene = 1 μg retinol equivalent = 1 RE.

Some vitamin A medicines and supplements are still measured in International Units (IU).

One RE = 3.33 IU retinol or 10 IU beta carotene
One IU retinol = 0.3 RE;
One IU beta carotene = 0.1 RE.

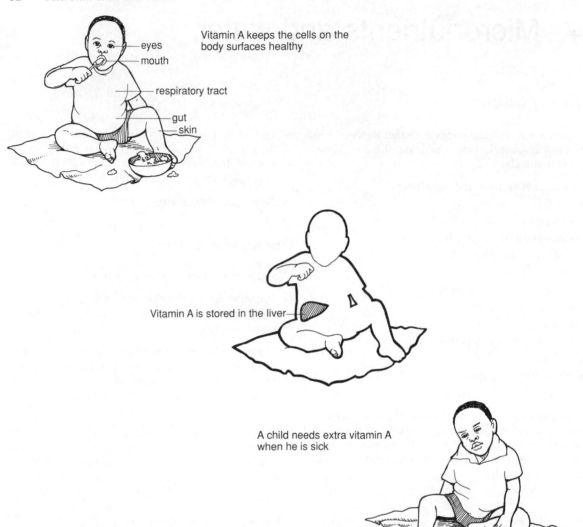

eyes
mouth
respiratory tract
gut
skin

Vitamin A keeps the cells on the body surfaces healthy

Vitamin A is stored in the liver

A child needs extra vitamin A when he is sick

Fig. 4–1 Vitamin A.

Important sources of vitamin A

- *Mainly as retinol*:
  - breast milk—colostrum in particular is very rich in vitamin A;
  - animal milk;
  - liver from animals, birds, and fish—small fish which are eaten whole with their livers are good sources of vitamin A;
  - kidney;
  - eggs;
  - butter and animal ghee.

- *As carotene*:
  - red palm oil (the carotene makes the oil red);
  - orange and yellow fruits, particularly mangoes and pawpaws;
  - orange vegetables such as carrots and pumpkins (dark orange vegetables contain more vitamin A than yellow ones);
  - dark-green and medium-green leaves, for example spinach, amaranthus, kale and leaves of cassava, cowpeas, sweet potato, and beans; in these leaves,

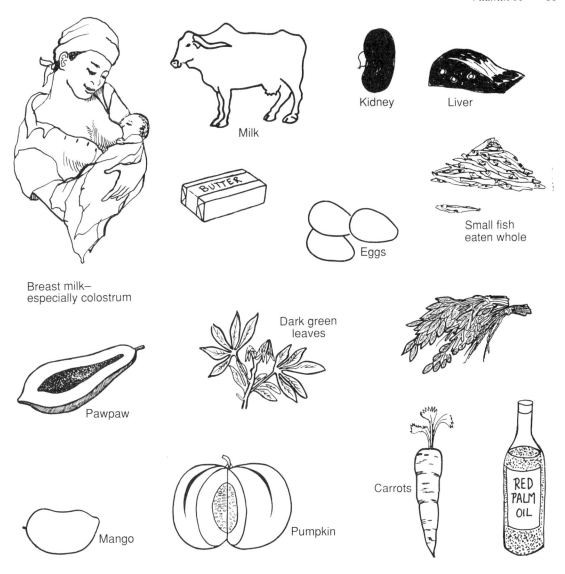

Milk

Kidney   Liver

Small fish
eaten whole

Eggs

Breast milk—
especially colostrum

Dark green
leaves

Pawpaw

Carrots

RED PALM OIL

Mango   Pumpkin

Fig. 4–2 Some good sources of vitamin A.

yellow/orange carotene mixes with green chlorophyll and makes it darker. So a dark green leaf contains more vitamin A than a light green leaf.

- yellow maize, yellow sweet potatoes, and bananas contain some vitamin A. People who eat a lot of these foods may get most of their vitamin A from them.

Some foods have vitamin A added to them such as some margarines, vegetable ghee, and dried milks.

Compared to other vitamins, vitamin A is quite stable. Some vitamin A is lost if foods are exposed to air and high temperatures (for example, sun-drying and some kinds of cooking) or when fats go 'bad' (rancid).

Vitamin A stores

Humans, animals, birds, and fish store vitamin A in their livers. This means that:

- Livers of animals, birds, and fish are very good sources of vitamin A.

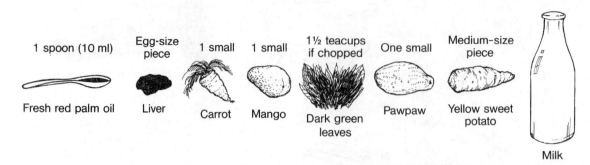

Fig. 4–3 Amounts of different foods which contain approximately 500 RE vitamin A.

Table 4.1. Daily vitamin A needs for different sex and age groups

Age (years)	Weight (kg)	Vitamin A (RE)
Children—both sexes		
0–1	7.3	350
1–3	11.9	400
3–5	15.9	400
5–7	19.6	400
7–10	25.9	400
Boys		
10–12	34.0	500
12–14	43.2	600
14–16	54.5	600
16–18	63.6	600
Girls		
10–12	35.4	500
12–14	44.2	600
14–16	51.5	550
16–18	54.6	500
If pregnant		600
Men—active		
18–60	65.0	600
> 60	65.0	600
Women—active		
Childbearing age	55.0	500
Pregnant	55.0	600
Lactating	55.0	850
> 60	55.0	500

• If a person eats a lot of vitamin A at one time (for example during the mango season) she stores it in her liver. The liver can store enough vitamin A to last up to 6 months. This means that it does not matter if we eat very little vitamin A on some days, provided that we eat plenty on other days.

Vitamin A needs

Table 4.1 and Appendix 2 show the amount of Vitamin A needed by different people on average each day. These amounts are enough to keep most people healthy and give them some to store in the liver.

4.3 THIAMINE

Thiamine helps the body 'burn' nutrients to release energy. People who lack thiamine develop beriberi (Section 19.11). Sources of thiamine include:

• meat, poultry, fish;
• liver;
• wholegrain cereals;
• legumes;
• oil seeds;
• milk;
• eggs.

4.4 RIBOFLAVIN

Why people need riboflavin
Riboflavin also helps the body to 'burn' nutrients to release energy. People who lack riboflavin may have cracked lips, sores at the corners of their mouths, and a rough skin.

Sources of riboflavin

Important sources are:

- milk;
- eggs;
- liver, meat, and fish.

Foods which are useful sources if people eat large amounts include:

- wholegrain cereals;
- green leaves;
- legumes.

Riboflavin is destroyed by daylight.

4.5 NIACIN

Why people need niacin

Niacin helps the body to 'burn' nutrients to release energy. People who lack niacin get pellagra (Section 19.12).

Sources of niacin

Most foods contain some niacin, but the best sources are:

- liver, meat, and fish;
- groundnuts;
- milk;
- wholemeal wheat, millet, and parboiled or un-polished rice.

Maize and sorghum are *not* good sources of niacin. The niacin in maize and sorghum is bound to large molecules, and the body cannot absorb it.

4.6 FOLATE

Why people need folate

Folate helps the body to grow and to make healthy red blood cells. The body stores only a little folate in the liver. Unlike iron, folate cannot be reused when a red cell dies. So a person needs to eat folate nearly every day.

Sources of folate

Almost all foods contain some folate, but the foods which contain most are:

- liver and kidney;
- fresh vegetables particularly dark green leaves;

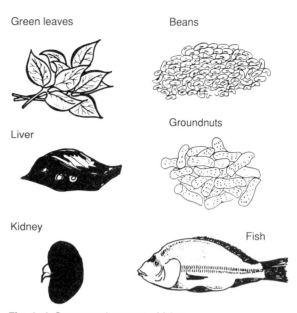

Fig. 4–4 Some good sources of folate.

- fish;
- beans and groundnuts.

Maize and other cereals and roots contain some folate. They are the main source of folate for people who eat large amounts of these foods. Wholegrain cereals give more folate than refined cereals.

Unfortunately, much folate is destroyed when foods are stored or cooked for a long time. To increase the amount of folate in meals people can:

- store and cook the foods for a shorter time (Section 6.9);
- add foods which are rich in folate to meals.

Folate needs

Appendix 2 shows the amount of folate that different people need each day. The people who need most are:

- women, because they lose blood at menstruation;
- pregnant women and women who have just had a baby, because they are making new red blood cells;
- people with sickle cell disease and thalassaemia who have to make red blood cells faster than normal.

4.7 VITAMIN C

Why people need vitamin C

- Vitamin C helps the body to use calcium and other nutrients to build bones and blood vessels.

- Vitamin C helps the body to absorb non-haem iron (Section 4.10).
- Vitamin C helps to destroy free radicals (see Section 17.2).

Important sources of vitamin C

- vegetables, for example green leaves, peppers, tomatoes, pumpkin (provided they are not over-cooked—see Section 6.9);
- fresh fruits, particularly citrus fruits such as oranges, guavas, and berries;
- fresh potatoes, cassava, yams, plantains, and cooking bananas;
- fresh milk, and breast milk.

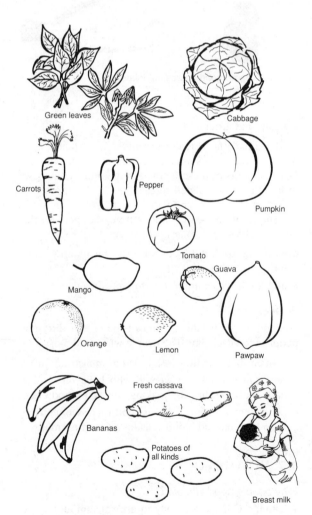

Green leaves
Cabbage
Carrots
Pepper
Pumpkin
Tomato
Guava
Mango
Orange
Lemon
Pawpaw
Bananas
Fresh cassava
Potatoes of all kinds
Breast milk

Fig. 4–5 Some good sources of vitamin C.

Vitamin C dissolves easily in water and is lost when food is cut into pieces, heated, or left standing after cooking.

4.8 VITAMIN D

Vitamin D is sometimes called 'the sun vitamin' because the skin makes vitamin D when the sun shines on it. Most people who live in sunny places have enough vitamin D. The body stores vitamin D in the body, in the liver and storage fat.

Why people need vitamin D

Vitamin D helps the body to absorb and use calcium and phosphorous to build healthy bones and teeth. Vitamin D needs are greatest at times of rapid growth—that is, in infants and young children, adolescents, and pregnant women.

Foods which are sources of vitamin D

- milk, butter, animal ghee, and cheese;
- fatty fish;
- eggs;
- liver;
- foods with added vitamin D—for example, some types of margarine and canned and powdered milks;
- cod-liver oil is rich in vitamin D, but it should not be necessary to buy it.

Sunshine as a source of vitamin D

The best way to get enough vitamin D is to:

- Go outside in the daylight for at least 10 minutes every day (or most days) with the face and arms uncovered (Fig. 19–8).

The person must be outside, because skin cannot make vitamin D from daylight which has come through glass. Even if it is cloudy, there is enough light for the skin to make vitamin D.

4.9 MINERALS

The body needs minerals in small amounts to help chemical processes, and to build tissues and fluids—such as iron for blood and calcium for bone.

We discuss *iron* (see also Chapter 20) and *iodine* (see also Chapter 21) in detail, because lack of these minerals is common and causes serious nutritional disorders. We discuss *fluorine*, *zinc*, *calcium*, *sodium*, and *potassium* briefly, because there may be a lack of them in some places or at certain times.

4.10 IRON

The body uses iron:

- *To make haemoglobin for red cells.* Haemoglobin is the red protein in red blood cells, which contains iron. It carries oxygen from the lungs to the cells. Cells need oxygen to 'burn' starch, sugar, and fat to release energy.

- *To help other cells to function.* There is a small amount of iron in all cells, especially in muscle, which helps chemical processes in the cells.

We need iron from food:

- *to replace worn out red cells.* Each red cell lives for about 4 months. The body reuses some of the iron from the dead cell—but some iron is lost.

- *to replace lost red cells.* Red cells (and iron) are lost from the body when someone bleeds, for example, when women menstruate.

- *to build new tissue especially red cells.* Children need to make more red cells and other tissue in order to grow. Women need to make extra red cells and other tissue when they are pregnant.

The body stores a certain amount of iron, mostly in the liver, spleen, and bone marrow.

Different forms of iron in food

Iron is a difficult nutrient to get from food. Most foods only contain a small amount of iron, and sometimes it is not in a form which passes easily through the gut wall. This means that the body absorbs only a small part of the iron that is in the food, usually between 5 and 15 per cent. The remainder of the iron passes out in the faeces.

The amount of iron that a person absorbs depends on:

- the total amount of iron in the meal;

- the type of iron in the food;

- the other foods in the meal;

- the amount of iron that the person needs.

The total amount of iron in a meal

We absorb a larger amount from meals which contain a lot of iron than from meals which contain little iron, even if only a small proportion of the iron is absorbed.

Example

Meal A contains 20 mg iron.
Meal B contains 10 mg iron.

If the proportion of iron absorbed from each meal is 10 per cent, what is the amount of iron that we absorb from each meal?
[From meal A, we absorb 2 mg; from meal B, we absorb 1 mg.]

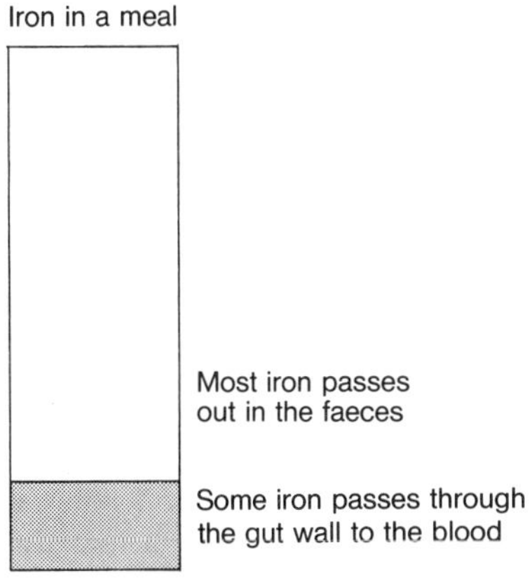

Iron in a meal

Most iron passes
out in the faeces

Some iron passes through
the gut wall to the blood

Fig. 4–6 Only a small proportion of the iron in food is absorbed.

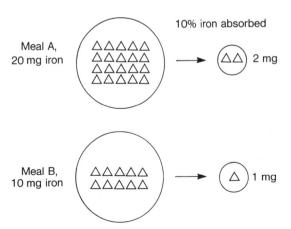

Fig. 4–7 The more iron there is in a meal, the more iron we absorb.

The type of iron in the food

There are three types of iron in food:

- *Haem iron.* Iron in blood and meat from animals, birds, and fish is in a form called haem iron (iron from haemoglobin). Haem iron can pass more easily through the gut wall. We absorb about 15–35 per cent of the haem iron that we eat, (Fig. 4–8).

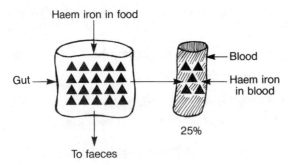

Fig. 4–8 Absorption of haem iron.

- *Non-haem iron.* The iron in plants, eggs, and milk is in a form called non-haem iron. Non-haem iron does not usually pass easily through the gut wall. We may absorb less than 5 per cent of the non-haem iron in cereals, legumes, and eggs, (Fig. 4–9).

  We absorb about 10 per cent of iron from cow's milk. Breast milk is an exception. Babies absorb about 50 per cent of the iron from breast milk, even though it is non-haem iron.

- *Iron added to food.* Manufacturers add iron to certain foods such as wheat flour and bread, infant formula, and some other processed foods. This type of iron is usually absorbed quite well.

Large amounts of iron may get into food or beer from iron cooking pots, or sometimes from dust. Although only a small proportion of this iron is absorbed, the total amount of iron eaten and absorbed may be quite large. Occasionally people absorb so much iron that it causes liver damage.

Other foods in the meal

The other food and drink taken with a meal can increase or decrease the amount of *non-haem* iron that is absorbed, (Fig. 4–10).

Foods which *increase* the absorption of non-haem iron are:

- foods rich in vitamin C (Section 4.7):
  - *fruit*, especially if it also contains citric acid—for example, citrus fruits such as oranges, lemons, and limes;
  - *vegetables*, for example, tomatoes, peppers, pumpkin, provided they are not overcooked.

  So you absorb more iron from a meal of maize and beans if you eat plenty of vegetables or fruit with it.

- foods which contain haem iron (such as liver, meat, chicken, or fish);
- fermented and germinated foods—fermenting and germinating destroys some substances which prevent iron absorption.

  Foods and drinks which *decrease* the absorption of non-haem iron:

- foods which contain *tannin* such as tea and coffee— you absorb less iron from a meal of maize and beans if you drink tea with it;
- wholegrain cereals, for example, wholegrain maize and wholemeal bread—they contain a substance called *phytate* which prevents iron absorption.

However, the other foods in the meal do not increase or decrease the absorption of *haem* iron.

We are not sure if eating green leafy vegetables increases or decreases the amount of iron absorbed. Some green leaves contain useful amounts of iron and vitamin C (if they are not overcooked), but they may also contain anti-nutrients (polyphenols) which decrease iron absorption.

The proportion of non-haem iron absorbed from refined cereal flour may be larger than from wholegrain flour. But refined flour contains less iron, so the total amount absorbed may be almost the same.

The amount of iron that the person needs

A person who has anaemia or low iron stores absorbs more iron from food, (Fig. 4–11). The increased absorption helps, but it may not be enough to prevent iron deficiency. Pregnant women, who have high iron needs, absorb more iron from food than non-pregnant women.

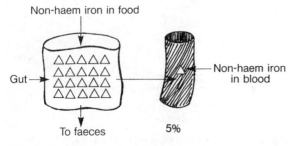

Fig. 4–9 Absorption of non-haem iron.

These *increase* absorption:

- Vitamin C-rich foods

- Meat, chicken fish, liver

- Germinated and fermented foods

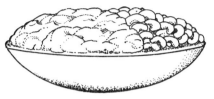

Meal of maize and beans

These *decrease* absorption:

- Tea and coffee

- Wholegrain cereal (wholegrain maize, wholewheat bread)

Fig. 4–10 Absorption of non-haem iron from a meal.

Important sources of iron

Haem iron:

The best sources are liver, kidney, spleen, heart, blood, meat, chicken, and fish.

Non-haem iron:

- *Legumes and cereals* contain useful amounts of iron, but it is the non-haem form. The amount absorbed depends on the other foods in the meal.

- *Dark green leaves* may not be a good source of iron if they contain anti-nutrients which interfere with absorption.

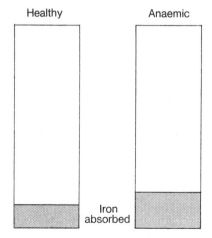

Fig. 4–11 An anaemic person absorbs a higher proportion of the iron in the food than a healthy person.

Iron availability

Figure 4–12 illustrates how, when people eat cereals and legumes with vitamin-C rich foods or with foods which contain haem iron, they absorb more non-haem iron. We say that adding vitamin C or meat or fish increases the *availability* of the iron.

- **Meal 1** in Fig. 4–12 consists of rice and peas only. It contains only non-haem iron. Very little is absorbed, and most of it passes out in the faeces. This is a *low iron availability* meal. About 5 per cent of iron from this kind of meal is absorbed.

- **Meal 2** consists of rice and peas with pumpkin. Pumpkin (if not overcooked) is rich in vitamin C. This time, a little more of the non-haem iron is absorbed. This is a *medium iron availability* meal. About 10 per cent of iron from this kind of meal is absorbed.

- **Meal 3** consists of rice and peas with fish. It contains both non-haem iron and haem iron. The fish provides haem iron which is well absorbed. The fish also increases the amount of non-haem iron which is absorbed. This is a *high iron availability* meal. About 15 per cent of the iron from this kind of meal is absorbed.

Iron needs

The amount of iron that a person needs to *eat* each day depends on the availability of the iron in their food.

Table 4.2 and Appendix 2 show the amount of iron that people need to eat each day if they eat high, medium, or low iron availability meals. They show that:

- Iron needs vary with *age*. Young children have the highest needs per kg body weight, because they are growing and building new blood and other tissues.

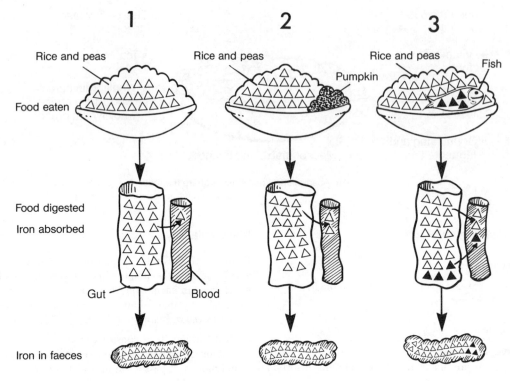

Fig. 4–12 Adding vitamin C-rich foods or food which contains haem iron to a meal increases the availability of non-haem iron.

Adult men and non-menstruating women have the lowest needs.

- Menstruating girls and women need about twice as much iron as men or non-menstruating women, because they lose blood each month.

  The type of contraceptive that a woman uses alters the amount of blood lost, and so alters her iron needs. Women on oral contraceptives have lower iron needs than women using IUDs.
- Pregnant women need extra iron especially in the last trimester when the amount of blood and muscle in the baby and placenta and uterus increases quickly.

The iron needs shown are for healthy people. People who have low iron stores, or who have lost much blood from an injury, childbirth, or an illness such as hookworm need extra iron (see Chapter 20).

Notice that people who have low iron availability meals need to eat twice as much iron as people who eat medium iron availability meals, and three times as much iron as people who eat high iron availability meals—to get the same amount of iron into their bodies.

4.11 IODINE

Why we need iodine

The thyroid gland at the front of the neck uses iodine to make *thyroid hormones*. Thyroid hormones help to control many processes in the body, including:

- the development and function of the brain and nervous system;
- the way the body uses energy and keeps warm;
- growth of children.

Iodine in food

Iodine comes from the soil. If soil contains enough iodine, plant foods which grow on that soil contain enough. Where soil is low in iodine, plant foods which grow there are iodine deficient. Soils low in iodine are found mainly in inland areas, especially where there are high mountains, and also in places where there are frequent floods.

The amount of iodine in foods from animals, birds,

Table 4.2. Daily iron needs (mg) from different diets

Age	Iron availability of diet		
	High	Medium	Low
Children—both sexes			
6–12 months	7	11	21
1–3 years	5	7	13
3–5 years	5	7	14
5–7 years	7	10	19
7–10 years	8	12	23
Boys			
10–12 years	8	12	23
12–14 years	12	18	36
14–16 years	12	18	36
16–18 years	8	11	23
Girls			
10–12 years	8	11	23
12–14 years	13	20	40
14–16 years	13	20	40
16–18 years	16	24	48
(If pregnant see pregnant women)			
Men			
18–60 years	8	11	23
> 60 years	8	11	23
Women			
Childbearing age	16	24	48
Pregnant			
1st trimester	6	9	19
2nd trimester	29	44	88
3rd trimester	42	63	126
Average	26	38	76
Lactating	9	13	26
> 60 years	6	9	19

and fish depends on the iodine in the foods that they eat. For example:

- Meat and milk from cattle which live on iodine-deficient plant foods are low in iodine.
- Fish and other food from the sea are usually rich in iodine, because they get iodine from seawater.

Important sources of iodine include food from the sea and iodized salt (see Chapter 21).

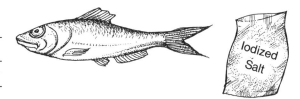

Fig. 4–13 Foods rich in iodine.

Iodine needs

Table 4.3 shows *total* daily iodine needs at different ages. Needs are highest:

- during the growth of infants, children, and adolescents;

  (The needs of children *per kilo body weight* are higher than for adults, though their *total* needs are less.)
- during pregnancy and lactation.

Table 4.3. Iodine needs

Age	Needs (µg/day)
3–6 months	40
6–12 months	50
1–3 years	70
3–7 years	90
7–10 years	120
Adolescents and adults	
Boys and men	150
Girls and women	150
Pregnant	+25
Breastfeeding	+50

4.12 CALCIUM

Bones and teeth are made mainly from protein and calcium. So calcium is a body-building nutrient. Everyone needs some calcium each day, because bone cells slowly wear out and must be replaced and because calcium is used in some body processes. Pregnant and breastfeeding women and growing children need extra calcium because they are making new bone cells or breast milk.

When older women stop menstruating, their bones may lose calcium and become thin and weak. This is called *osteoporosis*. Eating plenty of calcium and being physically active throughout life helps to prevent osteoporosis.

Most foods contain some calcium, and most people eat enough. Vitamin D helps the body to absorb and use calcium.

Good sources of calcium are:

- breast milk;
- milk of all types and foods made from milk such as canned milks, milk powder, soured milk, and cheese;
- small fish containing bones that you eat;
- beans and peas;
- finger millet;
- dark green leaves;
- water from places where there is lime or chalk in the soil ('hard water' which uses a lot of soap).

4.13 FLUORIDE

Fluoride is a mineral that is important for bones and teeth. Unfortunately, too much fluoride is harmful.

The *right* amount of fluoride makes bones and teeth harder and prevents tooth decay (holes in the teeth, caries). But, if a child gets too much fluoride while his teeth are growing, it may replace some of the calcium. This makes bones and teeth weaker. The teeth may develop pits, they may stain brown, and they may break. This is called *fluorosis*.

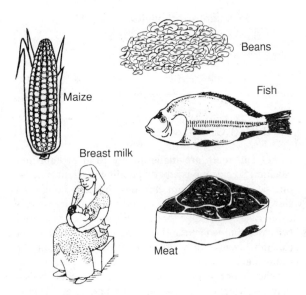

Fig. 4–14 Some good sources of zinc.

People get most of their fluoride from water. In some areas there is very little fluoride in the water, and in other areas there is a lot. People who live in areas with very little fluoride get more caries. But people who live in areas with a lot of fluoride may get fluorosis.

4.14 ZINC

Children need zinc to grow and develop normally. Children and adults need zinc to heal wounds and to fight infections.

Zinc deficiency

People seldom lack zinc by itself. Usually lack of zinc is due to a generally poor diet. The person lacks other nutrients and Calories at the same time. So, for example, if a child is not growing well, it is difficult to know how much this is due to a lack of zinc, and how much it is due to lack of Calories and other nutrients.

Zinc deficiency may cause:

- slow growth;
- slow sexual development in boys;
- slow healing of wounds;
- poor appetite;
- mental changes such as apathy;
- skin changes;
- diarrhoea (especially persistent diarrhoea).

Zinc is an *anti-oxidant* and may be needed to destroy *free radicals* to prevent tissue damage during infection (see Section 17.2).

Zinc needs

People with the highest zinc needs are:

- rapidly growing children;
- pregnant and lactating women.

People at risk of zinc deficiency are:

- growing children, undernourished children;
- pregnant and breastfeeding women;
- old people on poor diets;
- people with sickle cell disease;
- alcoholics (who often eat poor diets).

The body needs about 4–6 mg zinc a day. Most people eat about 9–15 mg a day. The amount of zinc absorbed varies in a similar way to iron.

Important sources of zinc

- Meat, chicken, fish.
- Wholegrain cereals and legumes.
- Breast milk (it contains small amounts which are well absorbed).

4.15 SODIUM AND POTASSIUM

The cells of the body contain potassium, and body fluids contain sodium. The body needs both minerals to work properly.

Normally, when we are well, we get enough sodium and potassium in our food. We only lose a small amount in sweat and urine. But, when people have diarrhoea, they lose sodium and potassium with water in the faeces. They need to eat food or drink fluids which contain enough sodium and potassium to replace what they lose (oral rehydration salts, or ORS, see Section 13.4).

Sodium

There is sodium in most foods. Salt (sodium chloride) is the richest source, so we add extra sodium when we add salt. We can get enough sodium from natural foods but most of us enjoy added salt. Some people eat more salt than they need, because they like the taste. Eating large amounts of salt may increase the risk of high blood pressure in some adults.

Potassium

Most foods are good sources of potassium. Useful sources for people with diarrhoea are:

- fruits, especially bananas, and the water from coconuts;
- vegetables, spinach, pumpkin;
- legumes.

4.16 WATER

Almost every part of the body contains large amounts of water.

- A 50 kg adult contains about 31 litres of water (see Fig. 1–3).
- A 10 kg child contains about 8 litres of water.

We can live without food for a few weeks, but we cannot live without water for more than a few days.

That is why giving drinks is so important when people lose a lot of water, such as during diarrhoea.

Why people need water

- to make body cells and fluids, such as blood, digestive juices, and tears;
- for body processes, such as digestion, which take place in water;
- to keep the lining of the mouth, gut, lungs, and other parts of the body moist and healthy;
- for urine which carries away body waste;
- for sweat to cool the body.

Water needs

An adult needs about 2–3 litres of water a day. People need extra water when:

- they sweat a lot during hot weather, or when they take a lot of exercise;
- they have a fever;
- they lose water because of diarrhoea or vomiting.

A breastfeeding mother may feel more thirsty than usual.

Sources of water

Almost all foods contain some water, especially fresh fruits and vegetables, and roots such as potatoes and fresh cassava.

Dry cereals, and cereal or root flours contain a little water before they are cooked. If they are cooked in water, they absorb a lot of water, which makes them *bulky*. Thin gruels, for example from maize or cassava, contain a lot of water.

Fats and oils contain very little water. Cooking oil, for example, contains almost no water. Food which is cooked in fat or oil contains much less water than food which is cooked in water.

Sugar contains no water.

Breast milk contains plenty of water, so babies less than 6 months old do not need drinks of water or other fluids (Chapter 10).

Table 4.4. Summary of how the body uses nutrients

Starches and sugars	For energy To make storage fat
Fibre	To keep gut healthy To help digestion
Fats	For energy To build cells For storage fat
Proteins	To build cells To make fluids For chemical processes For energy To protect against infection
Minerals	To build cells To make fluids For chemical processes
Vitamins	For chemical processes To protect against infection
Water	For chemical processes For building cells To make fluids

THINGS TO DO

Food demonstrations

You may like to do these exercises on the same day, when you have collected all the foods, because many of the foods in the different demonstrations are the same.

1. Put several different types of local foods on a table. Try to include milk, liver, dark green leaves, a cereal, a legume, egg, fish, and fresh fruit.

   Ask trainees to:

   a. Group together foods which are good sources of vitamin A.
   b. Repeat for the other vitamins.
   c. Make a mixture of foods which provide plenty of all the vitamins.

2. Ask groups of trainees to use food composition tables (Appendix 1) to calculate the following (which are average daily requirements).

   (a) amounts of foods which each provide 500 RE vitamin A;

   (b) amounts of foods which each provide 200 μg folate;
   (c) amounts of foods which each provide 30 mg vitamin C;

3. Put different local foods on a table. Try to include milk, liver, meat, chicken, fish, a cereal, a legume, dark green leaves, and fresh fruit.

   Ask trainees to show:

   (a) which foods contain haem iron;
   (b) which foods are useful sources of non-haem iron;
   (c) which foods help the body to absorb non-haem iron;
   (d) how they could make a medium iron availability meal from plant foods.

4. Ask trainees to make a mixture of foods which provide plenty of all the vitamins and iron.

Class exercises

5. Ask trainees to list the foods that they ate yesterday. Use Appendix 3 to decide which are useful sources of:

   (a) haem iron;
   (b) non-haem iron;
   (c) calcium;
   (d) zinc.

6. Ask trainees to draw labelled pictures of low, medium, and high iron availability meals.

7. Discuss the normal local diet. Decide if commonly eaten meals have low, medium, or high iron availability.

8. Ask trainees to use Table 4.2 to calculate iron needs in a coastal fishing village where the main foods eaten are fish, rice, groundnuts, and vegetables. Sometimes people eat chickens.

   a. What are the daily individual iron needs of the following groups of villagers:
      - children aged 3–5 years [5 mg];
      - boys aged 10–12 years [8 mg];
      - girls aged 16–18 years [16 mg];
      - pregnant women [26 mg].

   b. How much fresh fish flesh would each pregnant woman need to eat each day if she is to get half her iron needs from fish?
      (Half iron needs = 13 mg. Fish flesh = 1.7 mg/100g. So she needs to eat 13/1.7 × 100 = 765g. Will most women eat this amount? [No])

   c. Discuss the problems of pregnant women getting enough iron.

   d. Discuss how much more difficult it is for women on low iron availability diets.

Field visit

9. Ask trainees to visit a canteen or a hospital kitchen in order to look at the meals being prepared. Or, to discuss with the supervisor the meals planned for a week. Decide if the meals are low, medium, or high iron availability. Suggest how the meals could be improved using cheap, locally available foods.

10. Ask trainees to visit local shops to find out which foods, tonics, or toothpastes are fortified with minerals (iron, fluoride, iodine, calcium, etc.) and to report their findings to the class. Discuss whether the fortified foods are likely to help the nutrition of local people and whether they seem to be good value for money.

USEFUL PUBLICATIONS

Davidson, R. and Eastwood, M. A. (1986). *Human nutrition and dietetics* (8th edn). Churchill Livingstone, Edinburgh.

FAO (1988) *Requirements of vitamin A, iron, folate and vitamin B_{12}*, Report of a Joint FAO/WHO Expert Consultation. FAO, Rome.

5 Foods

5.1 TYPES OF FOOD

Food is the source of all nutrients except vitamin D and a few minerals. The amount and type of nutrients in a food depend on:

- the type of food;
- for plant foods, the soil that it grew in;
- for animal foods, the type of food that the animal ate;
- the way in which the food has been processed (for example, milled, dried, canned);
- whether minerals or vitamins have been added to the food during processing (*fortification*);
- the way in which the food is cooked.

A food is an *important source* of a nutrient when it gives us a high proportion of our daily needs for that nutrient. This happens when:

- A food is *rich* in a nutrient. For example, mangoes are rich in vitamin A.
- We eat a *large amount* of a food which contains a moderate amount of the nutrient. For example, for people who eat a lot of maize, maize is an important source of protein.

In this chapter we discuss the main types of food and their nutrient content. Suppose we are in a town somewhere in Africa. Let us see which foods there are in the market and stores.

5.2 STAPLES

A *staple* food is a food which we eat in large amounts and which gives us most of the energy that we need. Usually the staple provides important amounts of protein and other nutrients as well.

Cereals

As we enter the market, we see a man selling cereals. He has wholegrain maize, maize flour, rice, sorghum, and millet. Another important cereal is wheat, which is often made into bread, chapattis, or pasta.

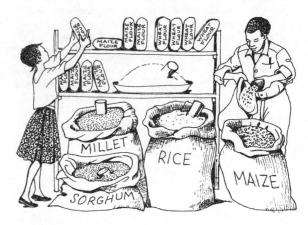

Fig. 5–1 Cereals for sale.

Cereals are the staple food for many people.

Maize is an important staple in many parts of Africa. It is popular because it gives high yields, birds cannot eat the growing cobs, and it is easy to mill. Some maize is eaten fresh ('green') on the cob, some is eaten as whole grains, but most is milled into flour. The nutrients in cereals vary depending on how they are processed (Chapter 6).

Sometimes people mix different cereal flours together. Sometimes they mix them with root flours, such as cassava. This may give a better combination of essential amino acids and other nutrients than that given by a single flour.

Roots and starchy fruits

Nearby, an old woman sells cassava, yams, and round (Irish) and sweet potatoes. These are also important staple foods for many people, especially before the cereal harvest. She also has some plantains and cooking bananas.

Roots like cassava and sweet potatoes are useful because:

- They can grow in poorer soils and need less rain than most cereals.
- The family can harvest them over a period of time, as they need the food. This spreads the workload.

- It is not necessary to mill roots—though people often do mill dry cassava and yams and make them into flour.

- Most roots (except bitter cassava—see Section 7.8) are easy to prepare and cook.

- People can eat the leaves of cassava and sweet potato, which are a useful source of some nutrients.

Nutrients in cereals, starchy roots, and starchy fruits

Figure 5–3 shows the energy and nutrient content of the common staple foods when they are cooked.

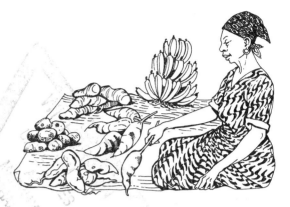

Fig. 5–2 Roots and starchy fruits for sale.

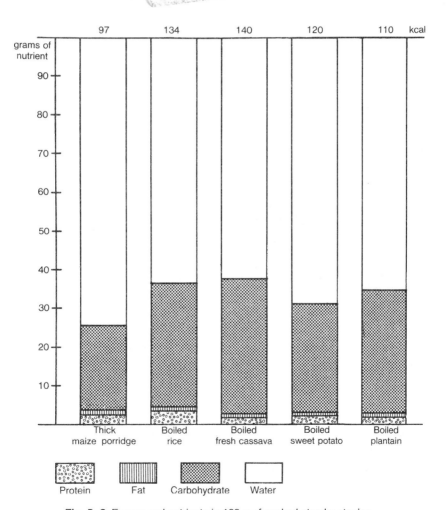

Fig. 5–3 Energy and nutrients in 100 g of cooked starchy staples.

- Cereals and roots are good sources of energy, mainly from starch. They are also useful sources of fibre (especially if they are not highly processed; see Chapter 6).
- Cooked cereals provide protein, iron, and B vitamins. They provide more of these nutrients than cooked roots or plantains.
- Fresh roots and starchy fruits provide useful amounts of vitamin C if they are not cooked too long.
- Yellow sweet potato, yellow maize, and plantains give some vitamin A.

So starchy roots and fruits can be an important source of some vitamins if people eat large amounts of them.

5.3 LEGUMES

The women in the next stall are selling dried *legumes*. The word 'legume' means that the seeds of the plant grow in a pod. Groundnuts and all the different beans, peas, lentils, and grams are legumes. The women in Fig. 5–4 are selling kidney beans, cowpeas, pigeon peas, green grams, groundnuts, and soybeans.

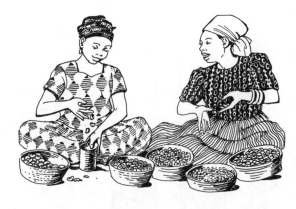

Fig. 5–4 Women selling beans, peas, and groundnuts.

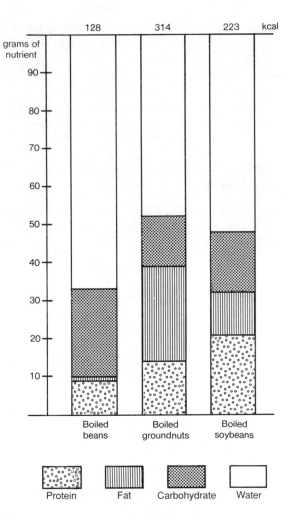

Fig. 5–5 Nutrients in 100 g cooked legumes.

Nutrients in legumes

Figure 5–5 shows the average amounts of different nutrients in boiled beans, groundnuts, and soybeans.

- Beans and peas contain more protein than cereals and starchy roots. People who eat large amounts of legumes get much of their protein from them. If they eat legumes with a cereal, the proteins from the two foods 'help' each other, and make a more complete protein (see Chapter 3). Soybeans contain more protein than other beans, and the protein is more complete.
- Groundnuts and soybeans contain more oil than beans and peas, so they are rich in both energy and protein.
- Legumes also contain iron and other minerals, and B vitamins. The iron is non-haem iron, so the amount absorbed depends on the other foods in the meal (see Section 4.10).
- Most beans and peas contain anti-nutrients (see Section 1.2) which make them difficult to digest. Soaking, or thorough boiling, or letting them start to grow (sprout) removes these anti-nutrients.

5.4 VEGETABLES AND FRUIT

Vegetables

There are many vegetables in this market, because it is the rainy season.

- There are orange vegetables: carrots, pumpkins, and tomatoes.
- There are dark and medium green leaves: pumpkin, cowpea, and sweet potato leaves, amaranthus, spinach, and kale.
- There are also cabbages and onions.

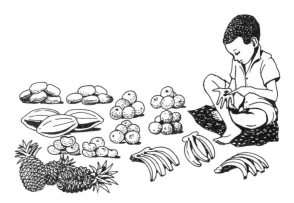

Fig. 5–7 Fruits for sale.

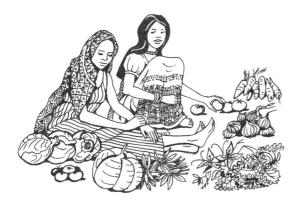

Fig. 5–6 Selling vegetables.

Nutrients in vegetables

- Most vegetables are *not* a good source of energy, because they contain no fat, and only small amounts of protein, starch, and sugar. They are mostly water.
- Vegetables are a good source of soluble fibre (see Section 2.2).
- Most fresh vegetables (even pale green cabbages) are good sources of vitamin C and folate.
- Dark and medium green leaves contain more protein, riboflavin, folate, and vitamin A than most other vegetables. The darker the leaf, the more vitamin A it contains. They contain iron, but it is probably not well absorbed.
- Red and orange vegetables are usually rich in vitamin A.
- Onions are important *flavouring foods* (see Sections 5.9 and 8.4).

If we come back to the market in the dry season, we might find these women selling *dried green vegetables*. These are useful when there are no fresh vegetables,

but some of the vitamins are lost during drying, particularly vitamin C.

Fruits

Here (Fig. 5–7) is a boy selling fruits—mangoes, oranges, tangerines, pawpaws, pineapples, and bananas.

Nutrients in fruits

- Fruits are good sources of sugar which provides some energy.
- Fruits provide soluble fibre.
- Citrus fruits (oranges, tangerines, lemons, limes), guavas, baobab fruits, pawpaws, and mangoes are rich in vitamin C.
- Orange fruits, such as mangoes and pawpaw are rich in vitamin A.
- All fruits contain a lot of water.

5.5 FOODS FROM ANIMALS

Fish

Now we come to the part of the market where they sell fish (Fig. 5–8). This woman is selling fresh and dried fish. Inspect fresh fish carefully to make sure that it is really fresh (Box 7.2).

Nutrients in fish

Fish is a very good source of:

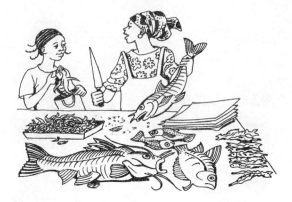

Fig. 5–8 Fresh and dried fish.

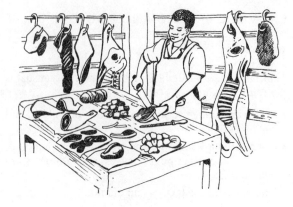

Fig. 5–9 Meat for sale—tasty but expensive.

- complete protein;
- haem iron and other minerals—if bones are eaten, they provide calcium;
- B vitamins.

Also:

- Sea fish is an important source of iodine.
- Fish liver is an excellent source of several vitamins, especially vitamin A.
- Fatty fish (e.g. dagaa) is rich in essential fatty acids.

Dried fish and *smoked fish* contain almost the same nutrients as fresh fish except they contain less water. So the other nutrients are more concentrated. *Salted fish* is similar to dried fish except that it contains more salt.

In the store near the market there is some *canned fish*. Canned fish is clean and safe. It does not need cooking, but it is usually expensive.

Meat and chicken

Next we come to a butcher selling meat, (Fig. 5–9), and nearby is a girl selling chickens (Fig. 5–10). The health authorities try to inspect all the meat sold in the market to make sure that it contains no worm cysts or other infection.

Nutrients in meat and chicken

Meat and chicken are very good sources of:

- complete protein;
- haem iron and zinc;
- B vitamins.

They also provide energy from both protein and fat.

- Meat sometimes has a lot of fat, which is a good source of energy. But it is mostly saturated fat, so it is not rich in essential fatty acids.
- Chicken usually has less fat, and the fat is less saturated.

Sometimes there is a lot of bone and gristle on meat. Bone flavours the water that it is cooked in, but provides few nutrients. So bone and gristle are mostly waste. So the nutrient content of a piece of meat depends on how much is *lean meat* (muscle), how much is fat, and how much is bone and gristle.

Offal

Offal means the other parts of an animal or bird that you can eat—for example, heart, liver, kidneys, blood, and gut. Most offal is rich in the same nutrients as meat, but it is usually cheaper. Blood and bloody offal are excellent sources of haem iron.

The *liver* is a store of many nutrients in animals, birds, and fish. Liver is richer than meat in:

- haem iron;
- vitamin A;
- folate;
- other B vitamins;
- vitamin C;
- vitamin D.

However, because each animal has only one liver and it is sometimes wormy and not fit for sale, good liver sells quickly and can be difficult to get.

Table 5.1. Comparison of nutrients in liver and lean meat

Nutrient	Liver (1 kg)	Lean* meat (1 kg)
Fat	47 g	19 g
Protein	200 g	220 g
Iron	100 mg	46 mg
Vitamin A	15,000 RE	Trace RE
Thiamine	5 mg	2 mg
Riboflavin	30 mg	2.6 mg
Niacin	100 mg	75 mg
Folate	2500 µg	150 µg
Vitamin C	150 mg	0

*No fat on meat.

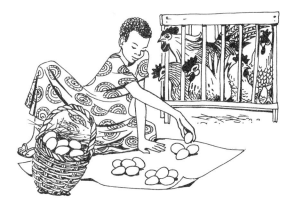

Fig. 5–10 Chickens and eggs.

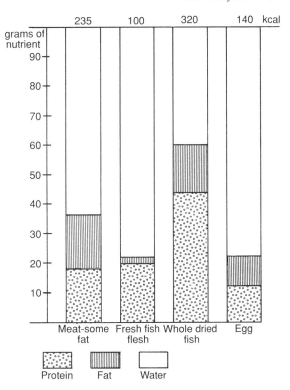

Fig. 5–11 Energy and nutrients in 100 g edible portion of meat, fish, and eggs.

Eggs

The girl selling chickens in Fig. 5–10 also sells eggs. Eggs are rich in:

- complete protein;
- some B vitamins.

The yolk contains some fat, and some non-haem iron which is not well absorbed—so eggs are *not* a good source of iron.

5.6 OILS AND FATS

Next to the market is a small store (Fig. 5–12) which sells many foods including maize oil, margarine, cooking fat, ghee, and butter. Most oils and fats are processed in factories which is one reason why they are expensive.

Nutrients in fats and oils

Figure 5–13 shows that these fats and oils are almost pure fat, and contain almost no other nutrients. Sometimes manufacturers add vitamins A and D to margarine and other fats.

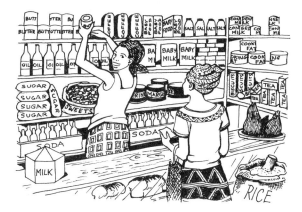

Fig. 5–12 How many different foods can you see in this store?

Vegetable oils

Most vegetable oils, for example, maize, sesame, groundnut, cotton seed, and sunflower oils, are rich in unsaturated and essential fatty acids.

Red palm oil is very rich in vitamin A, if it is not bleached. The fresher the oil, the more vitamin A there is.

Animal fats

Butter and other animal fats contain few essential fatty acids. Butter usually gives small amounts of vitamins A and D. It may contain 15–20 per cent water, so it gives slightly fewer Calories than most other fats.

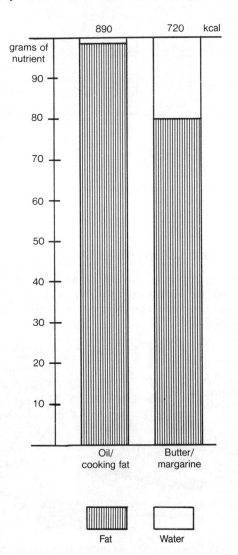

Fig. 5–13 Energy and nutrients in 100 g fats and oils.

Margarine and cooking fat

Margarine and cooking fat are made from vegetable and sometimes fish oils, both of which usually are unsaturated fats, and contain essential fatty acids. However, during processing the fatty acids change, and the oils become harder. Most margarine and cooking fat contain less unsaturated fatty acids, and less essential fatty acids than the oils from which they are made.

Some manufacturers make a soft margarine which contains more of the essential fatty acids. This is called *polyunsaturated margarine*.

Ghee

Ghee is made from butter (or margarine). During processing, the butter is heated to remove water. This makes it keep better. Ghee has the same proportion of essential fatty acids as the butter or margarine from which it was made.

Coconut

In the store are some coconuts which have come from the coast. The water from the inside of the coconut contains some sugar and potassium—the amount depends on how ripe the coconut is. The flesh of a mature coconut:

- is rich in fat, so it is a good source of energy;
- contains some incomplete protein;
- contains few vitamins.

Some people eat coconut flesh as a snack. More often people grate the flesh, and squeeze it in water to make 'milk' or 'cream' to use in cooking. How much protein and fat the coconut milk contains depends on the amount and temperature of the water used to prepare it. Table 5.2 compares the nutrients in cow's milk to those in coconut milk made with one coconut and about ½ litre of hot water.

So coconut milk is *not* a substitute for cow's milk, and it is *not* suitable for young babies. Coconut milk is a good food to add to the family meals, including weaning foods, because it increases the fat and energy of the

Table 5.2. Comparison of nutrients in cow's milk and coconut milk

	Amount in 100 ml		
	Fat (g)	Protein (g)	Vitamins
Cow's milk	4	4 (complete)	Many
Coconut milk	35	5 (incomplete)	Fewer

meal. About 3½ spoonfuls (35 g) of our coconut milk gives about the same energy as 1 spoonful of oil.

5.7 DIFFERENT KINDS OF MILK

The store also sells fresh, canned, and dried milk. The way the milk is processed affects the nutrients in it.

We usually think of milk as a protein-rich food. But milk from cows, camels, and goats contains about equal amounts of fat and protein. Milk from sheep and buffaloes contains *more* fat than protein. Breast milk also contains more fat than protein.

Animal milk is a good source of:

- *Energy from fat and sugar (lactose)*. The fat is saturated and contains few essential fatty acids. (Breast milk contains more unsaturated fats and essential fatty acids.)

- *Complete protein*. It is a good source of protein for older children, but contains too much for young babies.

- *Calcium* (but not iron).

- *Most vitamins*, especially vitamin A and folate.

Fresh milk

Fresh milk should be boiled, if it is not heated or soured or processed (for example, canned). Boiling kills dangerous bacteria and bacteria that sour milk. If the milk is covered in a clean container, it should keep for a day or two. Most fresh milk sold in shops has been heated to kill harmful bacteria. The three main methods of heating milk are:

1. *Pasteurization*. The milk is heated to a temperature below boiling. This kills dangerous bacteria but does not change the taste or destroy nutrients. The milk keeps for a few days if kept clean.

2. *Ultra high temperature—UHT*. The milk is heated to a very high temperature (140–150°C) for a few seconds. This kills all the bacteria so that the milk keeps for several months if it is sealed in clean containers. UHT does not alter the taste very much, or destroy many nutrients.

3. *Sterilization*. The milk is heated above boiling for several minutes. This also kills all the bacteria so that the milk keeps for several months if it is sealed in clean containers. Sterilization changes the taste and destroys many vitamins especially folate.

Homogenized milk is milk which has been specially mixed so that the cream does not come to the top. It does not change the nutrient content.

Skimmed milk is milk from which the fat (cream) has been removed. Most of the vitamin A and D is also removed, because these vitamins are in the fat.

Soured milks

Some people sour milk. When milk sours, harmless bacteria grow in it. This changes some of the lactose into acid, and changes the taste. The other nutrients are not altered. Harmful bacteria cannot breed easily in soured milk, so it keeps longer. *Yoghurt* is a special kind of soured milk.

Cheese is made from soured milk, from which the water is removed. The nutrient content depends on how the cheese is made. Making cheese is a good way of preserving milk.

Canned liquid milks

- *Evaporated milk*. Manufacturing sterilizes the milk, removes part of the water, and sometimes fat, and seals it in cans. This destroys vitamin C and folate, but extra vitamins may be added.

- *Condensed milk*. Manufacturing sterilizes the milk, removes most of the water, and adds a lot of sugar and sometimes vitamins. Sometimes much of the fat is removed (condensed *skimmed* milk). Condensed milk keeps better than other milks when the can is open, because the sugar prevents bacteria from growing. It is very sweet, and it is popular in tea, and sometimes spread on bread. Condensed milk is *very bad* for babies because it contains too much sugar.

Dried milks

- *Whole dried milk*. Drying removes almost all the water leaving a dry powder. Much vitamin C and some B vitamins are lost, but the other nutrients (protein, fat, minerals, and most of the vitamins A and D) remain.

- *Dried skimmed milk—DSM*. Most of the fat and water are removed. Much vitamin C and B vitamins are lost when the milk is dried, and most of the vitamins A and D are removed with the fat. DSM keeps better than whole dried milk, because it con-

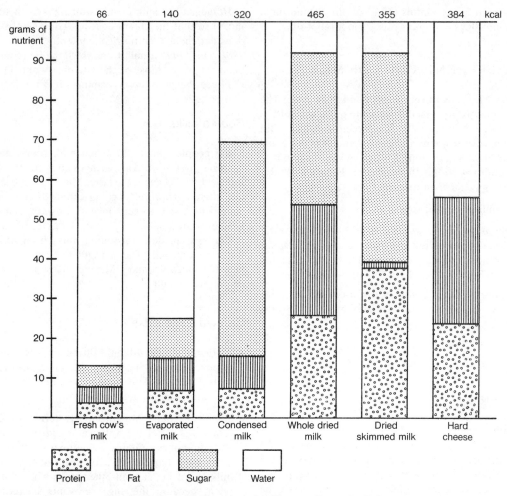

Fig. 5–14 Energy and nutrients in different milks and milk foods.

tains less fat. Usually vitamin A is added to DSM for feeding programmes.

- *Infant formula (baby milks)*. There are many different kinds of formula. Most are made from whole dried milk or skimmed milk, with vegetable oil, sugar, vitamins, and minerals added. Sometimes formula is made from soybean instead of milk. Manufacturers try to make the proportions of nutrients similar to the proportions in breast milk, but many differences remain (see Section 10.3).

Baby foods

On a shelf in the store there are packets of baby cereals. Most of these contain mixtures of milk powder and

cereal flour, with some minerals and vitamins added. These foods can be convenient because they often need little cooking, but they have no other advantage, and they are very expensive (see Section 11.11).

Information on labels

To know exactly what nutrients a particular can or packet contains, you need to read the label. The information about nutrients is usually accurate. However, the information about the suitability of products for babies, and *when* to give them, may be misleading (see Chapter 10).

5.8 SUGAR AND SUGARY FOODS

Sugar

The store sells bags of refined sugar. Sugar is rich in energy—but it contains no other nutrients. Some nutrition workers think that children should not eat sugar because:

- Refined sugar and sugary sweet foods and honey are a cause of tooth decay (see Section 22.11). However, the sugars in fruit and milk and sugar cane are not a problem.
- Eating a lot of sugar and sweet food may cause obesity, and other diseases in later life (Chapter 22).
- A young child who eats sugar, may soon want other sweet foods—such as the sweets and sweet biscuits which are also on sale in this store, and sweet drinks.
- A mother who adds sugar to her child's porridge may not think it is right to add green leaves, groundnuts, or beans as well.

However, sugar is sometimes a useful way to increase the energy concentration of food. For example, if oils and fats are too expensive, and sugar is cheaper; or if a person is sick and sweet foods encourage him to eat.

Glucose

The store also sells glucose. Glucose is an expensive kind of sugar which is also bad for the teeth. The body makes all the glucose it needs from starchy foods which are cheaper and healthier. No one, not even athletes, needs to 'top-up' their energy intake with glucose. Babies do not need and should not have glucose drinks. Glucose is a waste of money.

Sodas

Bottled drinks, or 'sodas' are refreshing and hygienic when you are thirsty, but they are expensive. They are made mainly from sugar, water, flavouring, colouring, and gas and so give only energy. Sodas do not contain vitamins like real fruit juices, and they are bad for the teeth. So it is better to keep them for special occasions.

5.9 OTHER FOODS

Flavouring foods

In the store we find many foods to make meals taste

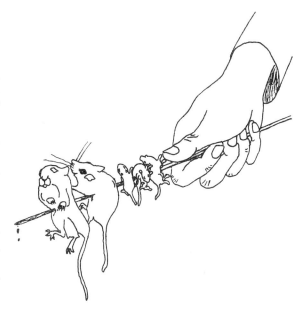

Fig. 5–15 Children often catch mice to eat or sell.

good (see Section 8.4). The most important is salt, but there are many spices including pepper, ginger, cardamom, curry powder, and cloves. In other parts of the market we saw onions and there are also chillies, garlic, and herbs. Most of these foods give few nutrients.

Salt (if it is iodized; see Chapter 21) provides iodine.

Coffee, tea, and cocoa

These drinks are usually made with sugar and milk, and so they give some energy, protein, and vitamins. Coffee and tea may reduce the absorption of non-haem iron from other foods if people drink them with meals.

Wild foods

Wild foods, such as mice, wild birds, and insects and honey, wild fruits, and vegetables, are not sold in this market. However, they are important foods for many people, especially small boys who often collect or catch and eat them.

Beer

Bottled beer contains alcohol (which gives some Calories) and small amounts of B vitamins. Beer helps friends to enjoy themselves, but sometimes people drink too much which can cause quarrels, broken homes, and poverty.

In one country in Africa, the amount spent on bottled beer could buy enough maize to give everyone in the country an extra half a cup of thick maize porridge every day.

Beers brewed at home from sorghum, millet, maize, or plantains usually contain less alcohol but more carbohydrate than bottled beer. They give more Calories as well as some protein, iron, and B vitamins. Also, home-brewed beer is cheaper. Often the beer is brewed and sold by women, so the profit stays in the community and often belongs to women.

THINGS TO DO

For these exercises, trainees need to use the food composition tables (FCT) in Appendix 1 and tables of energy and nutrient needs in Appendix 2.

Classroom exercises

1. Weigh out normal-sized helpings of different foods. Ask trainees to use the FCT to calculate how much fat, or protein, or other nutrients there are in each portion.

2. Ask trainees to list those foods which are a good source of protein. Ask them to use Appendices 1 and 2 to find what weight of each food would supply a man of 20–30 years with enough protein for a day. Repeat for fat, vitamin A, and vitamin C.

3. Ask trainees to find out how much refined maize flour would supply all the energy needed by a 10–12-year-old boy. What other nutrients does this amount of maize flour contain? Repeat for fresh cassava and millet.

Field visits

4. Take trainees to the local market and stores and ask them to:

a. List the important foods for sale.
   Use the list to make a local 'Foods composition table' using your national FCT or Appendix 1.

b. Ask food sellers:
- What amounts and types of food do people buy most?
- How often do most families buy food?
- Which family member usually does the shopping?
- Do people buy different foods at different times of the year?
- Do poor people buy different foods from rich people?

Discuss with trainees what they have learned. How can they use this information when they discuss foods and budgeting with families?

5. Find out which oils and fats are sold in the area. Ask trainees to say which contains most unsaturated fatty acids. Remember that saturated fats are hard at cold temperatures.

6. Ask trainees to collect as many cultivated and wild green leafy vegetables as possible. Use the FCT to discuss what nutrients they contain. Discuss how to cook them and, if possible, prepare some dishes.

USEFUL PUBLICATIONS

CFNI (Caribbean Food and Nutrition Institute) (1985). *Nutrition handbook for community workers.* CFNI, Kingston, Jamaica.

FAO (1982). *Legumes in human nutrition.* FAO, Rome.

FAO (1988). *Traditional food plants*, Food and Nutrition Paper, no. 42. FAO, Rome.

FAO (1989). *Utilization of tropical foods*, Food and Nutrition Papers, no. 47/1 (cereals); 47/2 (roots and tubers); 47/3 (trees); 47/4 (tropical beans); 47/5 (tropical oil seeds); 47/6 (sugars, spices and stimulants). FAO, Rome.

IITA (International Institute for Tropical Agriculture) (1989). Food crops utilization and nutrition—a training manual. [Available from IITA, PMB 5320, Ibadan, Nigeria.]

6 Food processing*

6.1 WHAT FOOD PROCESSING MEANS

Food processing means doing something to a food to:

- preserve it, that is, to:
  - prevent micro-organisms multiplying in the food;
  - stop the action of enzymes which make foods 'become older' and 'go bad';
- remove toxins and other harmful substances;
- make the food easier to handle and store;
- make it easier to prepare and cook;
- make it taste better;
- make it easier to digest;
- replace or add micronutrients;
- extract a more concentrated food such as:
  - fat (from oil seeds, milk, etc.);
  - sugar (from sugar cane and honeycombs);
  - starch (from cassava or cereals).

Many processing methods do several of these things at the same time. This chapter describes:

- drying;
- milling;
- fermenting and souring;
- germinating and malting;
- canning and bottling;
- fortifying;
- cooking.

6.2 NUTRITIONAL EFFECTS OF PROCESSING

Food processing increases the foods available to people throughout the year and reduces the risks of food-borne diseases. Some processing methods alter the amounts of nutrients in foods or the amounts digested or absorbed (see Box 6.1).

---

* This chapter was prepared in consultation with Dr Ruth Oniang'o.

6.3 DRYING

Drying, because it removes water from the food:

- prevents micro-organisms multiplying—for example bacteria, yeasts, moulds. The mould which makes *aflatoxin* (see Section 7.8) cannot grow on properly dried foods;
- prevents enzymes which make foods become old and 'go bad' from working;
- reduces the weight of the food, and makes the food easier to handle.

Families usually dry foods, such as cereals, roots, legumes, fish, meat, or vegetables, outside in the sun or shade. Sometimes they dry food such as meat or fish over smoke, or they salt it before drying.

Some foods, such as milk, are dried quickly at high temperatures in factories. Milk that is dried after the fat is removed (dried skimmed milk) keeps better than whole dried milk which still has fat in it.

The method of drying vegetables and fruits depends on the type of food.

- You may need to peel a food, cut it into small pieces, or cook it briefly in boiling water before you dry it.
- Drying under a polythene cover, through which air can pass, protects foods from rain, dust, and animals.

Drying may destroy much of the vitamin C and folate and some of the vitamin A. Drying in the shade reduces losses of vitamin A.

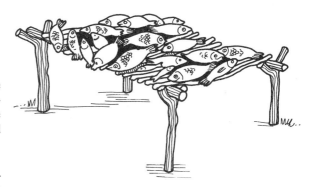

Fig. 6–1 Drying fish.

Box 6.1. How processing alters the nutrient content of foods

Carbohydrate, fats, and protein
- *Milling* may reduce the amount of fat, protein and fibre and increase the proportion of starch.
- *Fermenting* and *malting* alters the proportions of starch and sugar. Fermenting may add alcohol.
- *Bottling* and *canning* may add sugar.
- *Frying* increases the fat content.
- *Cooking* at very high temperatures can spoil fats and proteins.

Vitamin A
- decreases with:
  - drying especially in the sun;
  - boiling for a long time in contact with air (without a lid on the pan);
  - frying for a long time or at high temperatures;
- is increased by fortification.

Thiamine
- decreases when rice is washed.

Riboflavin
- decreases if milk is left in daylight.

Folate
- decreases during:
  - cooking: for example, in green leaves 35 per cent and in potatoes 25 per cent of folate may be lost;
  - storage.

Vitamin C
- decreases in fresh roots, vegetables, and fruits during:
  - storage (but not citrus or baobab fruits);
  - drying;
  - canning and bottling;
  - cooking: for example, 40 per cent of vitamin C in green leaves may be lost. Some vitamin C passes into the water and some is destroyed by heat;
  - reheating.

  or if you:
  - chop them into small pieces;
  - leave them prepared for some time before cooking;
  - leave them cooked for some time before eating them.
- increases when seeds (for example, of legumes) germinate.

Minerals
- *Fortification* may increase the amount. For example, salt fortified with iodine.
- *Fermentation* and *germination* increase the absorption of non-haem iron and other minerals.
- *Milling* may remove some minerals but increase their absorption.

Drying foods reduces the water content and so increases the concentration of other nutrients.
Milling and cooking break down cell walls so that nutrients are digested more easily.

6.4 MILLING

Milling means:

- removing the outer layers of dried cereals or legumes;
- pounding cereals, legumes, and dried roots into flour.

Milling makes foods easier to prepare, eat, and digest. If it removes fat, the flour keeps longer. Methods of milling vary from place to place. For example:

- *At home* people pound soaked or dry food in a pestle and mortar (Fig. 6–2) or grind it between stones (Fig. 6–3).
- *In the community* people mill food in handmills (Fig. 6–4) or hammer mills.
- *Commercially* millers mill large quantities of foods and produce flours and rice of various *extraction rates* (see below).

Milling cereals

- Milling removes the outer inedible layer of the grain. In this form the cereal is called *wholegrain* or *unrefined*. Sometimes this grain is milled into wholegrain flour.
- Then milling may remove the '*germ*' and more of the outside layers from the wholegrain. If the cereal is rice, this is called *polished* rice. Other cereals are usually milled into 'white' or *refined* flour.

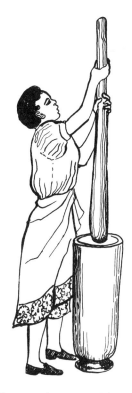

Fig. 6–2 Pounding cereals or roots at home with a pestle and mortar.

Wholegrain flours usually have an *extraction rate* of around 85 per cent. This means that from 100 kg of unmilled cereal, the miller gets 85 kg flour. White flours have an extraction rate of around 70 per cent.

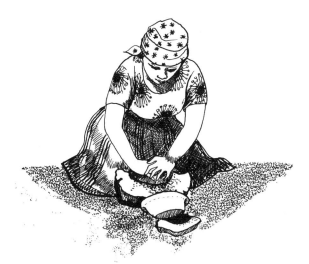

Fig. 6–3 Grinding food at home.

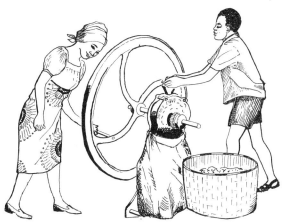

Fig. 6–4 A handmill.

Box 6.2. Wholegrain and refined flours

Wholegrain flour

- Gives more flour from each kilo of grain (the extraction rate is higher)
- Contains more fat, protein, minerals, vitamins, and fibre
- Is easier to produce at home
- Is usually cheaper

Refined flour

- Many people prefer the taste and appearance
- Keeps better because it contains less fat
- Cooks faster and is less bulky when cooked
- More non-haem iron, zinc, and other minerals are absorbed because the flour contains less phytate and fibre

---

Parboiling

Sometimes rice is *parboiled* before milling. Whole rice grains (called *paddy*) are soaked, drained, and steamed. Parboiling slightly cooks the rice and makes the outside of the grain harder. Milled parboiled rice contains more B vitamins and some other nutrients than raw milled rice because:

- Steaming makes the vitamins from the outer layers spread through the rice grain so more remain in the grain after milling.
- Milling may remove less of the vitamin-rich outer layer because the grain is harder.

Milling other foods

Milling roots. First people dry the roots. Or they may soak, ferment, and then dry the roots (for example, cassava). Then they mill the roots into flour.

Milling legumes. Sometimes people mill dried beans and peas into flour. Removing the skins first may improve the absorption of non-haem iron and zinc from the bean flour.

You can mill fat-rich foods like groundnuts into flour or grind them into paste. Grinding breaks the plant cells more so more oil is released so that the paste looks oily.

6.5 FERMENTING

Fermenting changes the taste and nutrient content of foods and helps to preserve them. There are two kinds of fermentation—*sour fermentation* which produces acid and *alcohol fermentation* which produces alcohol.

Sour fermentation

Special harmless bacteria are allowed to multiply in the food before or after cooking. They change some of the starch or sugar to weak acid, which gives the food a sour taste. Fermentation reduces the amount of phytate and increases the absorption of some nutrients (such as non-haem iron and zinc).

Harmful bacteria cannot multiply so easily in sour fermented food, so these foods remain safe to eat for longer than fresh foods.

Examples of sour fermented foods are:

- soured milks, yoghurt, and some cheeses;
- sour fermented flours and porridges. Sour fermented porridges are thinner than plain porridges which contain the same amount of flour and water, so they are easier to eat (see Fig. 6–6 and Section 11.8).

There are many ways to make sour fermented porridges. Box 6.3 describes two of them.

Alcohol fermentation

Micro-organisms called *yeasts* grow in food and change

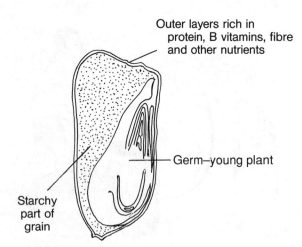

Outer layers rich in protein, B vitamins, fibre and other nutrients

Germ—young plant

Starchy part of grain

Fig. 6–5 A maize grain cut in half.

Box 6.3. Two ways to make sour fermented porridge

Sour fermentation before cooking
1. Prepare fine cereal flour.
2. Mix the flour with water so the mixture is quite liquid.
3. Add a little previously fermented cereal–water mixture to 'start' the fermentation process.
4. Leave to ferment overnight or longer.
5. Keep a little of the fermented mixture to 'start' the next cereal–water mixture.
6. Cook the remainder of the porridge.

Sour fermentation after cooking
1. Prepare thick porridge.
2. Add a spoonful of previously fermented porridge.
3. Leave to ferment. The porridge becomes more sour the longer you leave it.

---

starch and sugar into alcohol and carbon dioxide. In *brewing* yeasts ferment starchy foods such as sorghum, barley, and plantains to make alcoholic drinks such as beer. In *bread-making* yeasts ferment sugar and the carbon dioxide makes the bread rise. The alcohol escapes into the air.

Souring

Sometimes people add an 'acid' food such as lemon or tamarind juice to make porridge sour. The acid alters the taste, makes the porridge thinner and easier to eat, and may improve the absorption of some minerals. It probably does not prevent bacteria from growing, so it may not make the food keep longer.

6.6 GERMINATING AND MALTING

Germinating means making cereal or legume grains start to grow. *Malting* means germinating and then drying the germinated grains.

You can pound malted grains into flour. In Tanzania, malted flour made from sorghum, millet, or maize, is called '*kimea*'. Some people call it '*power flour*', but we think that this is a misleading name. It makes people think that the flour is energy-rich like fat. So we call malted flours 'kimea'.

When cereals or legumes germinate:

- An enzyme called *amylase* forms which breaks starch into smaller molecules so that they absorb and hold less water. This makes porridge thinner and easier for small children to eat (see Fig. 6–6).
- The amount of phytate decreases. So we absorb more iron from kimea porridge than from plain porridge.

Porridge made with kimea is thinner than plain porridge made with the same amount of flour and water. Sometimes kimea porridge is fermented, so it is sour (see Fig. 6–6 and Section 11.8).

6.7 CANNING AND BOTTLING

Bottling and canning preserves foods and may alter the nutrient content and taste. Foods are usually heated or cooked to kill micro-organisms. Sometimes foods such as sugar, salt, acid (e.g. vinegar), or *food additives* (see Section 1.2) are added to help preserve the food. Then it is sealed into cans or bottles.

Canning must be done in a factory. If foods, especially

Box 6.4. One way to make kimea

1. Soak wholegrain cereal grains in water for 12 hours.
2. Spread the soaked grains thinly between wet sacks or leaves and cover them to keep them in the dark.
3. Keep the grains warm and damp for about 2–4 days. During this time, the grains germinate. Wash the grains every 12 hours if possible.
4. Dry the germinated grain and pound into flour. This is *kimea*.
5. Store in a dry container because damp kimea goes mouldy.

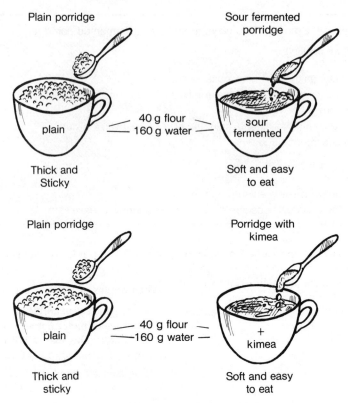

Plain porridge

Sour fermented porridge

plain

— 40 g flour —
— 160 g water —

sour fermented

Thick and Sticky

Soft and easy to eat

Plain porridge

Porridge with kimea

plain

— 40 g flour —
—160 g water —

+
kimea

Thick and sticky

Soft and easy to eat

Fig. 6–6 The differences between plain porridge and sour fermented or 'kimea' porridge which contain the same amount of flour and water.

meat and fish, are not properly canned, they may contain very dangerous bacteria and the toxins which these bacteria make (for example, the bacteria and toxins which cause a disease called *botulism*).

Examples of canned foods are canned meat, fish, butter, cooking fat, legumes, non-leafy vegetables, fruit, and milks. Examples of bottled foods and drinks are jam, tomato sauce, pickles, fruit juices, sodas, and beer (see Fig. 6–7).

6.8 FORTIFICATION

Fortification means adding a micronutrient to a food. Fortification may replace micronutrients lost during processing, or it may add extra micronutrients.

Fortification improves nutrition if people who lack the micronutrient buy and eat the fortified food. The amount of micronutrient in the food must be enough to supplement the diet. But it must not be so much that it causes side-effects, or spoils the taste or appearance of the food.

Examples are salt fortified with iodine and dried skimmed milk and margarine fortified with vitamin A.

6.9 COOKING

Cooking:

- makes many foods taste better and easier to digest;
- destroys micro-organisms in foods;
- destroys enzymes which make foods 'become older' (for example, the enzymes in fruit which eventually makes them overripe);
- destroys some vitamins (see Box 6.1);
- removes anti-nutrients (for example, in cassava and soybeans);
- may add nutrients (for example, frying adds fat).

Box 6.1 described how cooking alters the nutrient content of foods. Box 6.5 lists ways to preserve nutrients during food preparation and cooking.

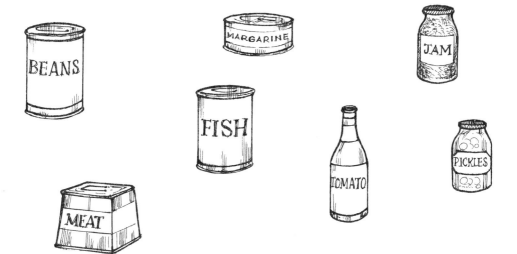

Fig. 6–7 Some canned and bottled foods.

Cooking to remove anti-nutrients

Foods that contain anti-nutrients (see Section 1.2) need to be prepared carefully and cooked (usually in water) to remove the anti-nutrient.

Soybeans

There are many ways to prepare and cook soybeans. One way is:

1. Clean the raw beans and remove broken ones. Broken beans may make a bad smell when soaked or cooked.
2. Boil the beans for 20–30 minutes and drain. Boiling removes the anti-nutrients.
3. If you plan to give the beans to young children, rub the beans under water to remove the skins.

You can pound the partly cooked beans into flour, or grind them into paste and then cook them. Or you can boil the whole beans again until soft.

A good fast way to remove anti-nutrients is to roast soybeans over a fire.

Other beans

The anti-nutrients in other types of beans are removed by boiling, or soaking and boiling, until the beans are soft. Section 7.8 explains how to remove the toxin in cassava.

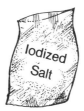 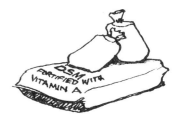

Fig. 6–8 Examples of fortified foods—salt fortified with iodine, and DSM fortified with vitamin A.

THINGS TO DO

Points for discussion

1. Ask trainees to describe the different ways in which their local staple foods are processed. Discuss how these methods affect: taste; appearance; keeping and cooking qualities; and nutrient content.

2. Discuss with trainees how local people store foods in their homes. Should they improve these methods? If so, how?

3. Ask trainees to collect dried foods (e.g. flours, rice, legumes, vegetables, etc.). Discuss the reasons for drying the food. Does drying alter the nutrient content?

Demonstrations

4. Ask a group of trainees to demonstrate how to cook local green leafy vegetables. Discuss afterwards.

Box 6.5. Ways to preserve micronutrients in foods

- Buy foods which look fresh (see Chapter 7) and are undamaged (they keep longer).
- Do not keep fresh foods for too long after buying or harvesting them (vitamins may be lost).
- Be careful not to damage foods when harvesting or storing (damaged foods 'go bad' and lose some nutrients quickly).
- If you dry fruits and vegetables, do it quickly (to preserve vitamin C).
- To dry vitamin A-rich foods, put them in boiling water for a few minutes (to destroy enzymes which make foods go bad) and then dry in the shade (to preserve vitamin A).
- Store fresh foods in cool, well-ventilated places away from sunlight (to keep longer and preserve riboflavin and other vitamins).
- Wash fresh foods just enough to clean them. Do not soak (to preserve vitamin C).
- Wash rice once or twice without rubbing (to preserve thiamine).
- Prepare vegetables just before cooking. Do not cut up more than necessary. Do not soak sliced vegetables (to preserve vitamin C).
- To cook vegetables, put them into boiling water or a stew or soup, place a lid on the pan, and cook until the vegetable is just ready. Do not cook for too long (to preserve vitamins).
- Use the cooking water from vegetables for stews, etc. (so you do not waste vitamin C in cooking water).
- Fry vegetables quickly in oil (to reduce loss of vitamin A).
- Do not keep cooked food too long before eating it (to prevent loss of vitamin C).

---

5. Demonstrate '*kimea*'.
   a. Make or buy some 'kimea'.
   b. Make a big mug of thick porridge with plain flour.
   c. Cool the porridge to body temperature.
   d. Add 1 big spoonful of kimea and stir. The thick porridge becomes thinner.

   Discuss the advantages of this thinner porridge.

6. Demonstrate *sour fermented* porridge.
   a. Prepare a mug of thick porridge using plain flour.
   b. Prepare another mug of porridge using the same amount of fermented flour and the same amount of water.
   c. Ask trainees to examine and taste.

   What are the differences between the two porridges? Discuss the advantages and disadvantages of each.

Field visits

7. Arrange for trainees to visit a local commercial mill to see how cereals are milled.
   a. Ask them to use the food composition tables in Appendix 1 to compare the nutrient content of the different flours produced.
   b. Ask them to find out what happens to the parts of the grain not used for flour.

8. Send trainees to a market, and ask them to identify all the foods which are processed in some way, e.g. dried, canned, fermented, milled, etc.

   Ask them to decide which is the most common form of food processing. Where is it done? (For example, in the home, the community, or in a factory?)

9. Send trainees to local stores to find out which foods are fortified with minerals or vitamins. Then discuss:
   a. Are these micronutrients ones which local people lack?
   b. If so, can these people afford to buy the fortified foods?

USEFUL PUBLICATIONS

Davidson, R. and Eastwood, M. A. (1986). *Human nutrition and dietetics* (8th edn). Churchill Livingstone, Edinburgh.

FAO (1982). *Legumes in human nutrition*. FAO, Rome.

FAO (1989). *Utilization of tropical foods*, Food and Nutrition Papers, no. 47/1 (cereals); 47/2 (roots and tubers); 47/3 (trees); 47/4 (tropical beans); 47/5 (tropical oil seeds); 47/6 (sugars, spices and stimulants). FAO, Rome.

7 Keeping food safe and clean

7.1 SAFE AND UNSAFE FOOD

To keep us healthy the food that we eat and the water that we drink must be clean and safe. It should contain:

- no harmful micro-organisms (bacteria or viruses; or amoebae or giardia);
- no parasites (such as roundworm eggs, tapeworm cysts);
- no toxins (poisons) such as *aflatoxin* or the poison in bitter cassava;
- no harmful chemicals such as pesticides.

Food or water which contains any of these things is *contaminated*. It can make people ill, and it is therefore unsafe to eat or drink. Some kinds of contamination can make a person ill immediately; other kinds make a person sick only after they have eaten or drunk the food or water for many months or years.

Food and water which is unsafe may look dirty or smell bad, and we do not want to eat it. But sometimes it looks clean and smells normal, so that we do not know that it is unsafe.

Many kinds of harmful micro-organisms can contaminate food or water and cause diarrhoea and vomiting, including dysentery, cholera, amoebiasis, and giardiasis. Others can cause typhoid fever and hepatitis. But most micro-organisms are harmless and some are helpful—for example, the micro-organisms in cheese and yoghurt and in sour fermented porridge.

The most important harmful bacteria are:

- bacteria from the gut of people, especially people with diarrhoea;
- bacteria from the guts of animals, especially rats, mice, dogs, chickens, and sometimes cows;
- bacteria which are harmless in small numbers, but which have grown to many millions in food, especially in warm, liquid, cooked food.

Toxins and harmful chemicals can cause diarrhoea and vomiting, paralysis, and even cancer. The toxin in bitter cassava can make iodine deficiency disorders worse (see Section 7.8).

7.2 HOW FOOD AND WATER BECOME CONTAMINATED

Micro-organisms are carried to *food* by:

- hands;
- flies, cockroaches, and other insects;
- rats, mice, chickens, and other animals;
- dirty containers and dishes.

Micro-organisms get into *water* when people or animals defecate or wash in or near drinking water supplies, or when water is carried or stored in contaminated containers.

What happens when micro-organisms reach food

When bacteria reach food, they start to breed. A few bacteria soon produce thousands of new bacteria. The more bacteria there are in a food, the more dangerous it is to a person who eats it.

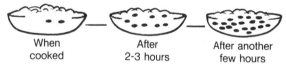

| When cooked | After 2-3 hours | After another few hours |

Fig. 7–1 Bacteria multiplying in food.

Bacteria breed fastest in food which:

- is warm and wet, such as porridge;
- contains animal protein—such as milk, meat, and fish—and in stews and other cooked foods;
- contains *some* sugar such as sweetened porridge (though not in food which is mostly sugar, such as honey, or condensed milk).

Viruses, amoebae, giardia, and worm eggs do not breed on food.

Common reasons why food becomes unsafe

The most important reasons are:

- People prepare food with water which contains human or animal faeces.

65

- People who prepare food do not wash their hands before they touch the food.
- People keep cooked food warm for several hours before they serve it.

Other reasons include:

- People eat raw food, such as fruit, without washing or peeling it.
- People eat food which has fallen on the ground.
- People put cooked food into dirty containers or dishes.
- People keep cold cooked food for a long time before they eat it.
- People do not cover cooked food (in homes, food-stalls, or eating houses).
- There are many flies and other pests around markets or the places where people sell cooked meals.
- Human faeces are left where flies, cockroaches, rats, or pets can reach them.

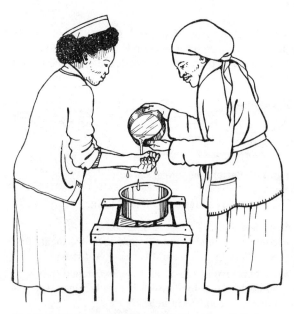

Fig. 7–2 People who prepare food should wash their hands before they touch the food.

7.3 HOW TO PREVENT FOOD CONTAMINATION

First find out from families how they prepare and store food and where they get their water. Visit the water supplies, and watch the way people cook and keep food. This will help you to understand:

- how harmful micro-organisms may be reaching foods or water supplies;
- in which foods harmful bacteria are probably breeding.

When you know how food and water becomes unsafe, you can help families and the community to make them safer. Often the most important things that a nutrition worker can do are to:

- help the community to improve their water supply;
- teach people how to prevent bacteria from reaching food and multiplying in it.

Go through Box 7.1, and the list in Section 7.4. Choose only those things which are appropriate for the people with whom you are working. Discuss these things with people who need to learn about food safety so that they can decide what they can do.

Do not expect people to change too many things at the same time.

7.4 HOW TO KEEP FOOD SAFE

Box 7.1 lists the most important things to do. Here are some other ways:

When buying food

- Buy fresh foods such as milk, fish, and meat on the same day that people will eat them.
- Choose foods which have none of the danger signs in Box 7.2. Buy meat which has been inspected if possible.

When storing food

- Keep fresh food as cool as possible:
  - Put in a clean container and cover with a cloth which is kept damp (the evaporating water cools the cloth and the food).
  - Store in an airy place such as a food safe (see Fig. 7–4) where air can get to it but where flies cannot reach it.
  - Store in a refrigerator.
- Make sure that flours, legumes, and oil seeds are dry, and keep them in a cool dry place protected from mice and other pests.

Box 7.1. The most important ways to keep food safe and clean

- *Eat meals as soon as possible after they are cooked*, so that bacteria do not have time to breed.
- *Use a safe water supply* if possible. If not, boil drinking water for babies for at least 3 minutes. Boil the drinking water for the whole family if there is an epidemic of diarrhoea or cholera in the area.
- *Wash your hands* with soap and water:
  - before you eat or prepare food or feed a child;
  - especially after you pass faeces or clean a baby's bottom or touch animals or soil.
- *Use a toilet and keep it clean*. If small children pass faeces on the ground, put the faeces into the toilet and then wash your hands. Then flies and other pests cannot reach the faeces and get bacteria on their feet.
- *Keep food covered*, especially cooked food and food for children, so that dust cannot fall on it, and flies with bacteria on their feet cannot land on it. Covering with a cloth may allow food to cool more quickly than covering with a plate, so bacteria have less chance to breed (see Figure 7–3).
- *Cook food very well* so that you kill any bacteria or worms in the centre of the food.
- *If you must keep cooked food for another meal*:
  - Cover it and keep it in a cool place.
  - If possible heat the food again just before you eat it. Heat it so that the centre of the food is boiling or very hot.
- *Clean eating and cooking utensils very thoroughly*:
  - Wash utensils thoroughly with soap to remove any food that bacteria could breed in.
  - Dry them on a rack in the sun if possible. The sun kills micro-organisms.
  - Cover the utensils with a cloth if it is dusty.

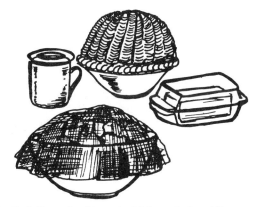

Fig. 7–3 Cover food to protect it from dust and flies.

When preparing food

- Wash fruit (and other food eaten raw) in clean water to remove micro-organisms and worm eggs. Peel it if possible.
- Prepare food on a table so that dust cannot reach it easily.
- Cut meat into small pieces so that it cooks to the middle.
- If cow's milk is not pasteurized or sterilized or soured, boil it.

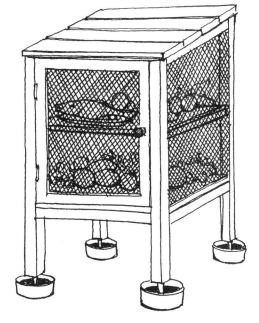

Fig. 7–4 A store for fresh food.

- Do not cough, spit, or scratch your hair or body near to food.
- Do not pick your nose or lick your fingers when you prepare food.

When preparing food for children

- Add milk or egg or sugar to a child's porridge just before you feed it to him, so bacteria have less chance to multiply.
- If you give children powdered milk, mix it into food. Do not mix it with water, or give it from a feeding bottle. Bacteria multiply quickly in liquid milk.

When caring for a sick person

- Wash the dishes and cups that the person uses very carefully.

In the environment

- Bury or burn rubbish at least 20 metres from the house and water supply or put it in covered bins if collected.
- Keep animals and chickens away from the house and places where small children play.
- Add animal faeces to compost. Compost destroys harmful bacteria.

7.5 WHOM TO TEACH ABOUT KEEPING FOOD CLEAN

You may want to teach:

- Schoolchildren.
- Mothers and domestic helpers because they prepare most of the food and feed the babies.
- Kitchen workers in schools, canteens, and eating houses. They prepare or touch food and meals which many people eat. Meals sold in hotels and eating houses may be contaminated if:
  - the food is dirty or bad;
  - the water is contaminated;
  - cooks are not careful about cleanliness;
  - they keep meals overnight and heat them up next day.
- Food-sellers who sell cooked meals and snacks on the street. Food may be contaminated for the same reasons as in eating houses. In the streets, contamination from dust is likely.
- Traders in food shops and markets. Traders may put water on to vegetables to make them look fresh, but if the water contains micro-organisms it contaminates the vegetables. Traders may sell meat or fish which is not fresh.

Public health inspectors are responsible for the safety of canteen and hotel meals, street foods, and foods in markets. You can help them if you teach people who prepare or sell food about food and personal cleanliness. Medical examinations and faecal tests of cooks and food-sellers are not practical or effective in most places.

7.6 TAPEWORMS

Sometimes cattle or pigs eat human faeces which contain tapeworm eggs. The tapeworm larvae develop into cysts in the animal's muscle. If a person eats meat which contains cysts, the tapeworm develops and grows in his gut. Tapeworm eggs pass out with the faeces, and may be eaten by another animal.

People can avoid tapeworm infection if they:

- cook meat very well so that any worm cysts that are in it are killed. Cut meat into small pieces so that it cooks to the middle quicker.
- buy meat which has been inspected. Health inspectors examine animals when they are killed and usually stop the sale of infected meat.

7.7 UNSAFE MILK

Milk from cows may contain harmful bacteria—from the cow itself or from the hands of the person who milked it or from containers that the milk is collected in. These bacteria can cause diarrhoea, tuberculosis, or brucellosis.

Pasteurization or sterilization (see Section 5.7) destroys all the bacteria. If milk is not pasteurized or sterilized, boil it.

7.8 TOXINS AND CHEMICALS

Toxins in mouldy foods

Moulds can grow on cereals and legumes which are not properly dried. One kind of mould makes a toxin called *aflatoxin*, which often contaminates maize, groundnuts, and other starchy foods and legumes.

If people eat a lot of aflatoxin, they may become sick quickly. If people eat food containing aflatoxin for many years they may get liver cancer. Eating aflatoxin makes the body produce many free radicals which may help to cause kwashiorkor (Section 17.2).

How to avoid eating aflatoxins

- Dry legumes and cereals very well and store them in a dry place.

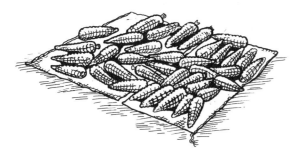

Fig. 7–5 Drying foods properly prevents moulds from growing.

- Advise people not to eat mouldy groundnuts or other food, but to add them to compost.
- Do not give mouldy food to cows or other animals which produce milk. Aflatoxin passes into the milk. Large amounts make some animals sick.

Toxins in cassava

The roots and leaves of *bitter cassava* contain an anti-nutrient called *linamarin*. Linamarin changes to the toxin *cyanide* when the cassava is grated or pounded and the cell walls are broken. To make cassava safe to eat, it is necessary to remove the toxin.

If the toxin stays in the cassava it can:

- cause *acute cyanide toxicity*. The person may die within a few hours. (This usually occurs when a person eats completely unprocessed cassava.);
- cause *paralysis* due to nerve damage;

- make *iodine deficiency disorders*, such as goitre, worse. This only occurs in areas where the diet contains little iodine;
- possibly *interfere with growth* in children.

These effects are worse if a person is undernourished.

Cassava can grow on poor soil, and resist drought. Bitter cassava is less likely to be attacked by pests than sweet cassava. More families grow bitter cassava than formerly. Some families may not know the traditional ways to remove the toxin. Traditional methods are effective, but it is important to do them properly to make the cassava safe. So nutrition workers must learn what is appropriate in the area where they work, so that they can advise families who do not know.

Making bitter cassava safe to eat

Cassava leaves. Boil the leaves in plenty of water until they are well cooked.

Cassava roots. There are many traditional methods which use a combination of processes, including:

- peeling (the concentration of toxin is highest in the peel);
- fermentation combined with grating or pounding to break down the cells and linamarin and allow the cyanide to escape;
- soaking, boiling, or drying to remove the cyanide.

Toxins in other foods

Other foods such as some mushrooms and sea fish may also contain toxins. These toxins are not a big problem

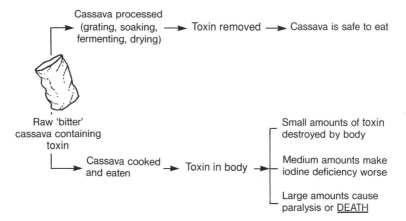

Fig. 7–6 The toxin in cassava.

Box 7.2. Danger signs of unsafe food

These signs warn you that food may contain micro-organisms, dirt, or poisons.

Fresh foods (fish, meat, milk, vegetables, fruit, roots) and cooked meals:

- bad smell;
- unusual taste;
- mould growing on food;
- fish has dull eyes, loose scales, soft flesh, pale gills;
- meat is soft and has a bad colour or smell.

'**Dry foods**' (flour, grain, beans, groundnuts, sugar)
- mouldy or damp.

Oils and fats
- unusual taste.

Cans
- swollen;
- leaking;
- badly dented;
- food looks, smells, or tastes bad or unusual.

Never *eat food from cans like these because they may contain toxins which can kill you.*

---

because the local people usually know which foods are dangerous and how to make them safe. Nutrition workers may need to learn from local people about these toxins.

Harmful chemicals

Many chemicals used in agriculture, such as pesticides and fertilizers, are toxic. They may get into food and water if:

- People use empty chemical containers to store food or water.
- Pesticides are sprayed on to crops just before harvesting.
- Pesticides are used to preserve food during storage.

Sometimes people put chemicals into oil or soda bottles, and someone (usually a child) drinks them by mistake.

To prevent chemicals getting into food or water:

- Do not store chemicals near where people live and eat. Keep them away from children and food.
- Do not put chemicals into bottles normally used for food or drinks.
- Follow the instructions for using the chemicals carefully.

- Wash your hands and body well after you use the chemicals.
- Check with agricultural field workers that the chemicals you use to preserve stored food are safe.
- Wash foods such as fruit, which have been sprayed or mixed with chemicals, in a large amount of water before you use them.
- Burn or bury empty containers so that they cannot be used to store food.

THINGS TO DO

Checking cleanliness

1. *Checklist.* Ask trainees to make a checklist for checking personal cleanliness and food storage and preparation for a school, hospital, market, or food trader. (List only the most important things so the list is short and easy to use regularly.)

2. *Field visit.* Take a small group of trainees to a market or school or hospital kitchen, and ask them to check it for cleanliness. Write down all the things which:

   a. are done well;

   b. could be improved.

Food path for a cooked food

3. With trainees, make a food path for a food like milk, meat, or porridge. Mark on the path the places where bacteria could get into and breed in the food. Discuss the best ways to prevent this.

Example

Porridge path	Porridge cooking $\longrightarrow$	Porridge in mug	$\longrightarrow$	Porridge eaten by child
How porridge may be contaminated	Not cooked long enough to kill germs Cooking pot not properly cleaned	Put in dirty mug Touched by dirty hands	Left long time so germs breed	Fed with dirty hands
How to prevent contamination	Clean utensils properly Cook thoroughly	Wash mug properly Wash hands	Use quickly If not, reheat thoroughly	Wash hands

USEFUL PUBLICATIONS

CFNI (Caribbean Food and Nutrition Institute) (1985). *Nutrition handbook for community workers.* CFNI, Kingston, Jamaica.

Rosling, H. (1988). *Cassava toxicity and food security.* Published for UNICEF by the International Child Health Unit, Uppsala, Sweden.

WHO (1984). *Role of food safety in health and development,* Technical Report Series, no. 705. WHO, Geneva.

8 Preparing meals for the family

8.1 PLANNING MEALS

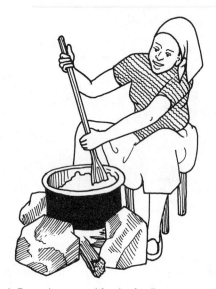

Fig. 8–1 Preparing a meal for the family.

Most women plan and prepare meals every day. If you are a woman, look at the list below and tick the things that you think about when you plan and prepare a meal.

- which foods I have in the store, house, or garden;
- how much money I have to spend on a meal;
- how much different foods cost;
- which foods are in the market;
- which foods and meals my family likes;
- the amounts of each food that I need;
- how long it takes to prepare the meal;
- how much fuel I have and how much I need for the meal;
- which foods are 'good' for the family.

Probably you ticked most of these things.

If you are a man, look at the list and see how many things a woman thinks about before she prepares a good meal. Could you prepare a good meal which your family would enjoy?

If you have plenty of money it is easy to make good mixed meals, but if you are poor it is difficult.

Why we need to plan good mixed meals

We eat because we are hungry. Hunger is a feeling which tells us that we need food. But it only tells us that we need energy, not that we need protein, iron, or other nutrients.

Sometimes people who need food do not feel hungry at all. Sick people and children with diarrhoea often do not want to eat anything, but they need food to recover. During a famine, people may be too weak to feel hungry although they are dying of starvation.

Of course, everyone likes particular *foods*. But the foods that we like may not be the ones that our bodies need. Most children like sweets more than they like dark green leaves.

So, because the body does not tell us what it *needs*, we must learn how to prepare meals which contain enough of the different nutrients. We call a meal which gives enough of all the nutrients a 'balanced meal' or a 'good mixed meal'. Not every meal needs to be balanced, but most of them should be. To know if a meal is balanced or to plan a balanced meal you have to think about two things:

- the mixture of foods;
- the amounts of food.

8.2 HELPING FAMILIES TO HAVE GOOD MIXED MEALS

There are many different foods, and people mix and cook them in many different ways. This book cannot discuss all the meals that people might eat, and it cannot tell you exactly which foods to advise for families in your community.

The best way to help is to learn which foods people in your community use, the amount of different foods that they have, and how they prepare them. Then you can decide if people need to improve their meals. Suggest ways to improve their meals, *only if it is necessary*. And only suggest that a family eats more of a food, or a different kind of food, if you know that they can obtain it.

Discussing with families things that are possible helps them to feel confident that they can improve their diet. Advising them to eat foods that they cannot get may make them anxious and ashamed or angry.

You may want to help people to improve their meals if:

- They ask for help with meal planning.

- Surveys suggest that people's diets lack particular nutrients such as iron or vitamin A.

- You learn that young children eat mainly bulky staple foods, or that many young children are malnourished.

In these situations:

- Discuss with people the foods that they use in meals.

- Decide if they should add other types of foods to their meals.

- Discuss which local foods they could use.

- Discuss how to overcome any problems they may have obtaining, cooking, or using these foods.

Example

An urban family does not eat any dark green or orange vegetables. After talking with the family, you find out that they buy cabbage sometimes. You discuss with them why it would be better to buy dark green leaves and pumpkin. You explain how they can grow some vegetables in cans in the windows.

8.3 THE 'MIXED MEAL GUIDE'

How do you decide if people need to add other foods to their meals? And how do you know what foods to suggest?

The *'mixed meal guide'* (Fig. 8–3) should help you. Many nutritionists now prefer this to the old teaching of the *'three food groups'* (see Box 8.1).

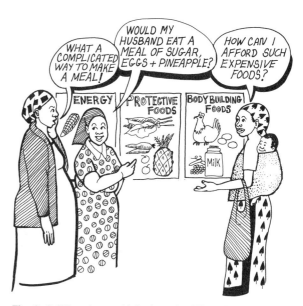

Fig. 8–2 What do you think about the 'Three Food Groups'?

Box 8.1. Why we do not like to teach the three food groups

In the past, health and nutrition workers used the idea of the 'three food groups' (energy foods, body-building foods, and protective foods) when they taught mothers how to plan meals. Now we believe that teaching about food groups is *not* the best way to help families to improve their meals and prevent undernutrition, because:

- **Many foods belong to more than one group.**
  Most foods are *mixtures* of nutrients. Cereals are in the 'energy food' group—but they are an important source of protein and B vitamins as well as starch. Milk is usually in the 'body-building' group, although it contains as much fat as protein, and it contains calcium and several vitamins. Groundnuts also are rich in both energy and protein.
- **People need to eat both starch and fat**.
  Starchy foods and fatty foods are both in the 'energy food' group, so it is not clear that people need both.
- **A meal of one food from each group may not be 'balanced'**.
  The 'three food groups' suggests that you could make a balanced meal from margarine (energy food), cheese (body-building food), and a banana (fruit—a protective food). Or sugar, an egg, and a lemon. But these would be strange meals, and there are several nutrients that they would lack.
- **Important problems are left out**.
  The 'three food groups' only tells you about the *mixture* of food. It does not explain about the *amounts* of food that people need, or about bulky weaning foods, or about feeding children often.
- **Most women do not use the idea of the three groups**.
  Many women know about the 'three food groups' but most admit that they do not follow them, because they often cannot afford to buy the foods, and they do not plan meals in that way.

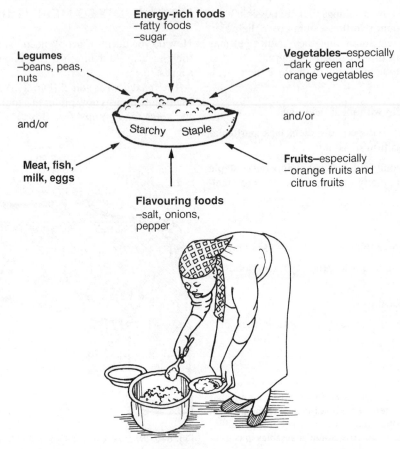

Energy-rich foods
–fatty foods
–sugar

Legumes
–beans, peas,
nuts

Vegetables–especially
–dark green and
orange vegetables

and/or

Starchy   Staple

and/or

**Meat, fish,
milk, eggs**

Fruits–especially
–orange fruits and
citrus fruits

Flavouring foods
–salt, onions,
pepper

Fig. 8–3 The 'mixed meal guide'. The guide shows how you add foods to the staple. Try to add one or more foods from each part of the guide.
From the left: legumes and/or food from animals. *From the right*: fruit and/or vegetables; some energy rich food from above and some flavouring foods from below. *From above*: some energy-rich food. *From below*: some flavouring foods.

You can use the guide:

- to plan meals and menus for institutions or feeding programmes;
- to check that meals contain a good mixture of foods;
- to help people to improve meals.

Do not use the guide when you talk to families—instead talk about foods in the same way as the community.

8.4 THE MIXTURE OF FOODS TO USE

The staple food

The staple is the main part of most meals. For example, thick porridge made from maize, or boiled cassava, or rice. Staples are usually cheap, and they may provide most of the energy, protein, and fibre in a meal, and some vitamins.

Most people do not feel that they have eaten properly if they have not had one of their normal staple foods. If you plan meals for schools, hospitals, and feeding programmes, try to use staples which people like and normally eat. Eating familiar staple foods helps to make sick people or people in refugee camps feel a little better. Some people, especially older schoolchildren, refuse to eat an unfamiliar or low-status staple food even if they are hungry.

However, the staple cannot provide all the nutrients that a person needs—especially a growing child or childbearing woman—because:

- The protein is not complete.
- Starchy foods are bulky.

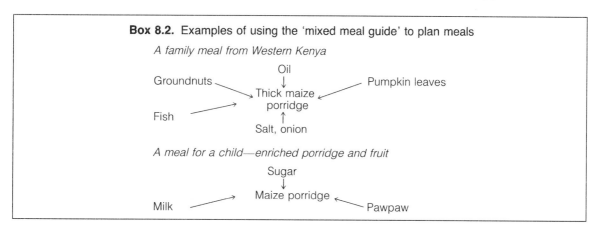

Box 8.2. Examples of using the 'mixed meal guide' to plan meals

Adding foods to the staple

To make a good mixed meal, you need to eat other foods with the staple to:

- provide the nutrients that the staple lacks;
- make the meal less bulky;
- make the meal more tasty and interesting to eat.

People may mix other food with the staple during cooking. They may serve other food separately as a *relish* to eat with the staple. They may eat the other food separately, before or after the main dish (for example, fruit).

Legumes, green and yellow vegetables, and fruit
These are the foods which are most often available. *Legumes* add:

- protein and essential amino acids; they improve the amino acid score (see Chapter 3);
- iron (but it is non-haem iron) and other minerals;
- some starch, fibre, and B vitamins;
- fat (if the legumes are groundnuts or soybeans).

Green and yellow vegetables add:

- vitamin A;
- vitamin C (which helps the absorption of non-haem iron);
- folate;
- fibre.

Fruits add:

- vitamin A (if they are orange);

- vitamin C;
- fibre.

If people eat fruit with or immediately after a meal, the vitamin C increases the absorption of non-haem iron from the meal.

Meals made of staples, legumes, and vegetables or fruit are good mixed meals. They should provide *most* people with *most* of the nutrients that they need. However unless the meal contains a fatty legume, there is little fat, so the energy concentration is low, and the food is bulky. Also, the meal contains no haem iron. So women and children may not get enough energy or iron.

Animal foods and fat-rich foods
To make sure that meals provide enough energy and iron, you need to add animal and fat-rich foods whenever possible. These foods may not be easily available, and they are usually expensive. But people do not need them in very large amounts.

Foods from animals Meat, liver, and other offal, chicken, and fish add:

- complete protein, so a small amount improves the protein value of the meal;
- fat for energy;
- vitamins (especially vitamin A and folate from liver);
- haem iron and zinc.

Milk and eggs add:

- complete protein;
- energy from fat (and from sugar in milk);
- calcium and other minerals and vitamins.

Energy-rich foods Energy-rich foods are foods which:

- are almost pure fat, such as maize oil;

- contain as much fat as carbohydrate or protein, such as groundnuts.

They:

- add energy and reduce bulk;
- add essential fatty acids (especially most vegetable oils; see Section 2.4);
- improve the taste of a meal;
- help the absorption of vitamin A.

Foods which contain large amounts of sugar, such as refined sugar or honey, also add energy to a meal, and may improve the taste.

Flavouring foods

It is important to add these foods, although they do not provide many nutrients (see Section 5.9). They make meals taste good which encourages people to eat more and helps them to get enough nutrients.

8.5 THE AMOUNTS OF FOOD THAT PEOPLE NEED

We saw in Chapters 2 and 3 that women, men, adolescents, children, and old people need different amounts of nutrients. Figure 8–4 shows the amounts of basic low-cost cooked food that different people should eat each day to cover their nutrient needs. To make the diagram simple, we have just used a few foods, but really people should eat a variety of foods each day. *Notice that the amounts of legumes and leaves needed are similar for most people, but the amounts of staple vary a lot.*

Table 8.1 shows the weight of raw foods in the cooked foods in Fig. 8–4.

A USEFUL GENERAL RULE

Give everyone (except babies) different amounts of staple, but the same amount of relish.

8.6 MEALS AND SNACKS

The amount of different foods to prepare for a meal depends on how many people will eat it and who they are. The amount of food each person needs at each meal depends partly on their nutrient needs, and partly on how many meals they eat and the types of foods in each meal.

People do not eat a balanced meal, with the same amounts of nutrients, every time they eat. People also eat *snacks*, that is, small amounts of food and drinks, between main meals—for example, a maize cob or a banana.

Snacks do not usually provide a balanced meal—but they can be a useful source of some nutrients, especially extra energy. Fruits are important snacks, because they provide vitamin C and sometimes vitamin A. Sweets and sodas are common snacks, but they provide mainly sugar.

Figure 8–5 shows how many meals and snacks different members of the family need, to get all the energy and nutrients that they need.

Table 8.1. Weight of raw foods to supply basic daily nutrient needs

Group	Weight (g)				
	Maize flour	Beans	Leaves	Oil	Fruit
Children					
2–3 years	200	100	80	30	
10–12	400	200	100	30	
Men	650	200	110		
Women					
Menstruating	460	150	100		100
Pregnant	500	150	110		100
Lactating	560	200	160		
Old	400	150	100		

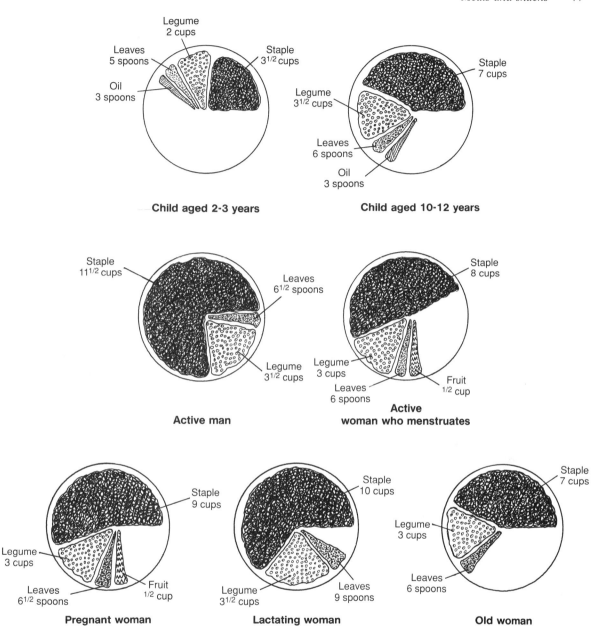

Fig. 8–4 Comparison of amounts of basic cooked foods needed by different people each day.

On this diet menstruating and pregnant women need supplementary iron to cover needs. Fruit is included to increase iron absorption. 1 cup = 200 ml; 1 spoon = 10 ml.

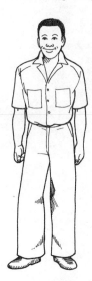

Men

need at least two mixed meals every day and some snacks. They can get enough energy from a few large meals and from bulky foods

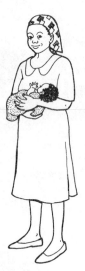

Women

need at least two mixed meals every day and some snacks. If they are pregnant or lactating, they need almost as much food as men—especially if they are also doing hard physical work. They need much more iron and folate than men especially when they are pregnant

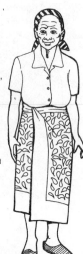

Old people

need at least two and if possible more meals each day as they may not eat much at each meal. They need fewer Calories than younger people, but about the same amount of protein and other nutrients. Women who have stopped menstruating need less iron than childbearing women. Old people may need soft food

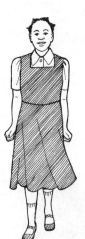

Adolescents

need at least two large mixed meals and some snacks each day. They can eat bulky food. Boys need a lot of Calories. Girls need plenty of iron. Pregnant adolescent girls are still growing so they need more food than pregnant women

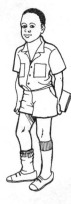

School-age children

need at least two–three mixed meals and some snacks each day

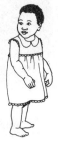

Children: 1–5 years old

need breast milk until they are at least 2 years old. They need at least three mixed meals and two snacks each day. They cannot eat large bulky meals. It is especially important for meals to be clean and not to contain parasites or micro-organisms that could cause diarrhoea or other infection

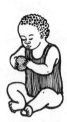

Babies: 6–12 months

need breast milk 8–10 times or more each day. They need small meals, which are not bulky, 3–5 times a day

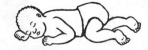

Babies under 6 months

need only breast milk at least 10 times each day

Fig. 8–5 The meals that different members of the family need.

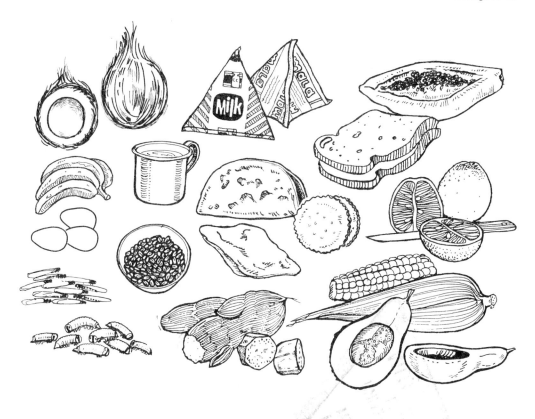

Fig. 8–6 Some good snacks for children and adults.

THINGS TO DO

Calculating foods for meals

1. Ask trainees to use Appendix 1 to calculate how much raw maize flour and dried beans a woman should cook to make a meal which supplies ⅓ of the daily energy and protein needs for a 35-year-old man. (Assume his daily needs are 3000 kcal and 60 g protein.) Discuss the meal. Is it a good mixed meal? What other foods should be added?

Planning meals from available foods

2. Show trainees several local foods (or pictures or names of foods). Then ask them to:
   a. put each food into one of the boxes in the meal plan (i.e. staple, legume, animal, energy-rich, vegetables, fruit, flavouring);
   b. choose 4–5 foods to make a mixed meal for a particular person, e.g. a pregnant woman, an old woman who has no teeth, a young man working as a labourer, a secondary school boy.
   Ask the trainees to explain why they chose each food. Ask for comments on the meal.

3. Put trainees into groups and ask each group to plan a good mixed meal using foods from the local market.

Field visit

4. Ask trainees to visit homes and find out what women and men think is a 'good' meal. After the visit trainees can discuss these meals together. How can nutrition workers use this information to help families plan good mixed meals?

Box 8.3. Snacks

Examples of 'good' snacks
If these are not expensive, they are probably good value for money:

- boiled, pasteurized, sterilized, or soured milks;
- bread—particularly with a fat-rich food such as margarine or groundnut paste;
- bread dipped in soup, milk, or coconut milk;
- mandazi (doughnut), chapatti, bean cakes, biscuits;
- boiled or fried potatoes (e.g. chips), cassava, plantain, yam;
- bananas, avocado, mango, oranges, and other fruits;
- young coconut flesh;
- boiled egg.

For people over 2 years old:
- maize cobs;
- groundnuts;
- small fried fish;
- insects such as locusts, termites, etc.

Examples of 'poor' snacks
These are often poor value for money, or they are bad for the teeth (see Sections 22.10–22.13):

- sodas;
- sweets and lollies;
- ice cream;
- glucose powder and tablets;
- crisps and other similar snack foods.

USEFUL PUBLICATIONS

CFNI (Caribbean Food and Nutrition Institute) (1985). *Nutrition handbook for community workers*. CFNI, Kingston, Jamaica.

Ritchie, J. A. S. (1983). *Nutrition and families*. Macmillan, London.

9 The cost of meals and budgeting

9.1 FINDING OUT ABOUT THE COST OF FOOD

The reason why many people are undernourished is that they do not produce enough food and do not have enough money to buy food.

Sometimes you may be able to help families earn more money, for example, if you promote cash crops or if you support local income-generating projects (see Chapter 23). It is especially helpful for family nutrition if you can help women to increase their income.

Often you can help families to *budget*. To budget means to plan the way in which they spend money, so that they always have enough for food and get the best value for their money. Before you can discuss budgeting and which foods are good value (*'good food buys'*) you need to:

- find out the prices of different foods;
- calculate the costs of different nutrients.

In different places and at different times the cost of food varies. We can only give some general principles and some typical examples to show how to think about costs. Visit different markets and big and small stores and find out the prices of foods. Compare prices in different places, in different quantities, of different brands, and at different times of year.

What you need to find out about prices

1. *The cheapest places to buy food*. Different stores and markets may sell the same food at different prices. For example, the cost of a 250 g can of margarine may be less in a supermarket, and more in a small store or kiosk. Foods may be cheaper near to where they are produced than far away (Fig. 9–2).

2. *Which brands of food are best value for money*. 500 g of Brand A milk powder may cost more than 500 g of Brand B. Usually the cheapest brands are the best value for money, though there may be slight differences in taste and quality.

3. *If it is cheaper to buy foods in larger amounts*. Find out the cost of different quantities of food and work out the cost *per kilogram*. Often large amounts are cheaper per kilogram than smaller amounts. (Two 250 g cans may cost more than one 500 g can; two

1 kg bags of maize may cost more than one 2 kg bag.)

4. *If prices are different at different seasons*. A bunch of spinach may cost more in the dry season than in the rainy season. Fruit may also be cheaper in certain seasons. So foods that are good value at one time of year may not be good value at another time of year.

5. *The difference in cost of buying cooked foods and cooking them at home*. Work out the total cost of preparing a food or a meal at home—including the cost of the food, the fuel, and the labour. Compare this to the cost of ready cooked food.

9.2 THE COSTS OF NUTRIENTS

When you know the prices of foods, you can calculate and compare the costs of the nutrients that they contain. Section 9.4 explains how to do this. For example, you can calculate the cost of 1000 kcal energy or 10 g protein or 10 g fat or 100 RE vitamin A in different foods. Then you can work out which foods are the cheapest sources of energy, protein, and other nutrients.

For example, you can compare:

- the cost of 1000 kcal energy from maize flour, cassava, margarine, oil, and sugar;

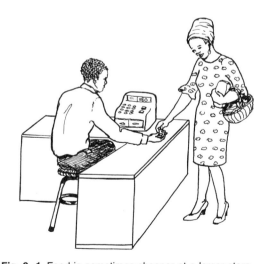

Fig. 9–1 Food is sometimes cheaper at a larger store.

81

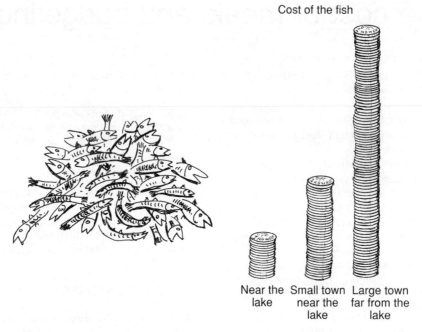

Cost of the fish

Near the lake   Small town near the lake   Large town far from the lake

Fig. 9–2 This kind of fish is cheaper near the lake where it is caught than in town.

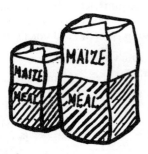

Fig. 9–3 Food may cost less per kilogram if you buy it in larger amounts.

- the cost of 10 g protein from beans and maize;
- the cost of 10 g of protein from a cheap cut of meat and an expensive cut of meat, which has less bone and fat;
- the cost of 100 RE vitamin A in liver and dark green leaves.

It is important to notice that:

- *The cost of foods that contain almost the same nutrients varies*. For example, goat's meat may be cheaper than beef, but it gives the same nutrients. Most types of fish give the same nutrients, but they vary in price. Dried fish may be better value than fresh fish.

- *Foods may contain mixtures of nutrients which make them better value*. For example, liver contains more vitamins and iron than meat (see Table 5.1). So liver may be a better value food than meat, even if it is a more expensive source of protein.

- *Sometimes the cost of 1000 kcal energy from fats or oils is less than the cost from a starchy staple*. Oil may be more expensive per kilogram, but it may be a cheaper source of energy, because the energy in oil is so concentrated.

Knowing the cost of nutrients in different foods helps you to advise families how to choose cheap nutritious foods. It is also important if you are planning meals for a school, hospital, or feeding programme.

Ready-to-eat meals and snacks

Many people in towns buy drinks and snacks and meals from eating houses, canteens, or street food sellers. Find out what these foods and drinks contain and what they cost. Calculate the cost of the main nutrients in the foods. Decide which snacks are good value for money and which are poor value.

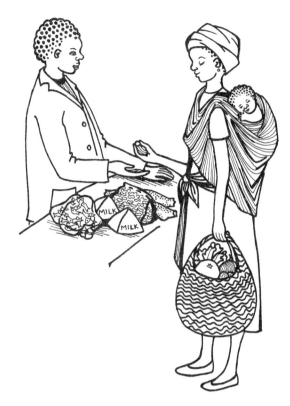

Fig. 9–4 Most women know the cheapest way to feed the family.

9.3 TALKING TO FAMILIES ABOUT BUDGETING AND BUYING FOOD

Many women already know from experience the cheapest way to fill their family's stomachs. They know good value, and they know many ways to prepare good meals on small budgets and many ways to save money.

When you discuss budgeting with women, learn what they do. You may be surprised to find how difficult it would be to feed a family better on the money available. If a woman does something that seems *not* to be economical, try to understand why. There may be a good reason.

However, there may be ways in which you can help some families to budget better. The kinds of families who may need particular help are those who have recently moved from a rural area to a town, or who have been resettled or displaced. They may be used to growing much of their own food, so it is difficult for them to know which are the best foods to buy or where to buy them.

When you know the prices of foods and the costs of nutrients you are ready to discuss which foods are good value. These are some of the questions that you may want to discuss with families.

1. *Can the family buy from cheaper stores?*
   - Are the cheaper stores too far away from their homes?
   - Do these stores sell in quantities that poorer people can afford?
   - Do cheaper stores give credit?

2. *Can the family buy cheaper brands of food?*
   - Is there any advantage to buying the more expensive brand?
   - Does any difference in taste really matter?

3. *Would more expensive foods sometimes give better value for money?*
   - Is it always a good idea to buy cheaper varieties of the same food?
   - Is there more waste in cheaper food—such as cheaper cuts of meat?
   - Is the cost of 10 g protein (or 1000 kcal, or 100 RE of vitamin A, or 10 g fat) also cheaper?
   - Is a more expensive food better value because of the other important nutrients that it contains? (For example, is maize better value than cassava?)
   - Is it wise to buy older, cheaper fruits and vegetables instead of more expensive, fresher ones? There may be more waste and less vitamin C in the older fruit, but this may be balanced by the family being able to buy a larger quantity.

4. *Can the family buy food in larger quantities to save money?*
   - Do they have enough money available to do this, or enough space to store larger amounts of food?
   - Will the family eat all the food before it becomes stale or bad?
   - Would more relatives come for meals if there were extra food in the home?
   - Would neighbours 'borrow' food?
   - Are the shops which sell food in larger quantities further away from home?
   - Could families form a group to buy food 'in bulk' to save money?
   - Who would control and manage the group?

5. *Does the family buy the foods which are the cheapest sources of the various nutrients?*

Do they use these foods already? If not, what is the reason? Maybe they do not know how to prepare them.

6. *Do families (particularly small families) save money if they buy cooked food instead of preparing meals at home?*

   - How much time and fuel do they save?
   - Are the cooked meals safe, clean, and nutritious?

7. *Does the family buy good value or poor value snacks?*

   - Is the cost of nutrients in the snacks high?
   - Do they contain sticky sugar which causes tooth decay?
   - Are there other snacks and drinks which people can buy which are more nutritious?

8. *Does the family know the signs of dangerous, unsafe food?*

   Food which is contaminated with micro-organisms, parasites, poisons, or dangerous chemicals and which can make people ill is very poor value for money. Make sure that the family know the danger signs of unsafe food (see Box 7.2).

Minimum cash needed by families for food

When you help poor families to budget for food it is useful to know approximately the minimum amounts a family must spend to get enough energy, protein, and other nutrients. The amount varies from family to family and place to place.

However, you can estimate from the tables of energy and nutrient needs in Appendix 2 and the food composition tables in Appendix 1 the minimum amounts of basic foods which should provide enough energy and most nutrients for people of different types and ages. We give an example in Section 9.5.

These foods are *not a recommended diet*—they are only to help *you* as a nutrition worker to estimate the minimum amount of cash that a family needs for food each week (see Table 9.2 and Section 9.5).

Box 9.1.   Foods which are always poor value for money

Foods which can make people ill
   - any food which looks or smells bad;
   - food which might contain contaminated water (e.g. diluted fruit juice);
   - foods in which bacteria may have multiplied:
     - moist cooked foods which have been kept warm for several hours (especially meat, fish, milk, eggs, sweetened foods);
   - foods which may contain a toxin:
     - mouldy foods;
     - bitter cassava which has not been properly processed.

Foods which contain a lot of sugar
These foods contain mostly sugar and colouring. They are bad for the teeth and are an expensive way to get Calories. Some may contain vitamins—but it is cheaper to get energy and vitamins from family foods which also supply other nutrients.
   - sodas;
   - bottled 'fruit' juices, such as blackcurrant juice and squashes;
   - sweets, lollies;
   - glucose and glucose drinks.

Other expensive foods which give few nutrients
   - crisps and similar packets of snacks;
   - tonics—it is cheaper to get vitamins from family foods;
   - ice cream.

CASE STUDY: HOW PANDU CHOSE FOOD IN THE MARKET

Pandu is a mother in Africa. Let us follow her around the market that we visited in Chapter 5 and see what she buys, and why she decided to buy that food.

Staples

Pandu passes the store which sells staples without stopping. She has a 25 kg sack of maize flour at home. It is cheaper to buy maize in large bags. The rice is too expensive, though she sometimes buys it for her old mother when she is sick. The roots and starchy fruits look cheap today—they are usually cheaper per kg than the cereals. But Pandu finds that she needs more fresh cassava than maize flour for a family meal. Maize increases so much when it is cooked, so the meal probably costs about the same in the end.

Legumes

Pandu has to decide what relish to give her family with the maize. She stops to look at the different beans. The kidney beans look fresh and of good quality. None of them are wrinkled or mouldy. Pandu decides to buy some. She will get home today in time to soak and cook them, and she has enough fuel.

Vegetables and fruits

Now Pandu comes to the part of the market where they sell fruit and vegetables. Her husband likes beans cooked with tomatoes and onions. She has some onions left. But the tomatoes are rather expensive. The kale seems to be better value at the moment, so she buys that instead. There is none growing at home.

The mangoes are cheap at this time of year too—so she buys a small pile for the children. (The boy lets her have two extra overripe ones for half price.) Her children like mangoes very much, and she heard at the clinic that mangoes help to keep children's eyes healthy.

Foods from animals

Pandu does not stop at the butcher or the egg seller, because she has not got enough money this week and it is not necessary to have both beans and meat.

Last week she bought some of the cheapest cut of meat, but there was a lot of bone and gristle. After cooking, there was only a very small piece of meat for her husband and the older children, and only soup for herself and the youngest child. She prefers to save up and buy a smaller amount of a more expensive cut at the end of the month. Then they can all have some, and it should be better value. If she gets to the market early enough she might buy some liver, but it sells out quickly. She may give her family potatoes or plantain with the meat, to make a change, and they may be a bit cheaper than maize.

Fish

Pandu walks past the fish stall. Her family come from a part of the country where people do not eat fish, and none of them like it.

Oils and fats

Pandu has been careful to keep enough money for some cooking oil and butter.

Oil is expensive per kilogram—but it is only necessary to use a small amount to make a meal taste much better, and Pandu usually buys the cheapest brands. She will buy a bottle of oil. A large can of oil is cheaper per kilo. But Pandu does not have enough money left. She uses oil very carefully, and a bottle will last her a long time. Even if she did buy a large can of oil, her friends would probably borrow some of it when they ran out, so she might not save much money.

She buys a small tin of butter. Bread with a little butter makes a good snack for children, and is cheaper than biscuits.

Milk and bread

Pandu does not buy milk or bread in the market. She buys them at a kiosk nearer her home. She likes to buy some food at the kiosk because the owner is a friend and gives her credit if she needs it. The family like milk in tea. Sometimes she buys condensed milk, because it keeps better.

Sugar

Pandu does not buy sugar either. She has a little left, and she will try to make it last. If she has a lot, the children will eat too much.

So Pandu goes home with beans, kale, mangoes, oil, and butter. Can she make her family a balanced meal, with the maize, onions, milk, and sugar that she has at home? If Pandu were shopping in your town or village, would you advise her to buy any different foods?

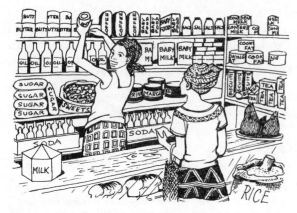

Fig. 9–5 Pandu buying butter in the market.

9.4 HOW TO CALCULATE AND COMPARE THE COST OF ENERGY AND NUTRIENTS IN DIFFERENT FOODS

1. Find out the cost* of 1 kg of the food as it is sold in the store or market (i.e. 1 kg 'as purchased' food). If food is not sold by weight you have to convert measures of foods, such as cans of beans or piles of fruit, into weights using scales or Table A4.4 in Appendix 4.
2. Use Table 9.1 to find out how much of the food provides 1000 kcal. Table 9.1 takes into account any waste in foods when they are purchased.
3. Multiply the weight which provides 1000 kcal by the cost of the food per kg. This is the cost of the amount of food which provides 1000 kcal/kg—in other words, it is the cost of 1000 kcal from that food.
4. Repeat the calculation for other foods, and compare the cost of 1000 kcal from each food.

Table 9.1. Weights of food in kg which contain 1000 kcal, 10 g protein, 10 g fat, or 100 RE vitamin A, calculated from food composition tables in Appendix 1†

Food	Weight of food in kg which contains			
	1000 kcal	10 g protein	10 g fat	100 RE vit A
Bread, white	0.417	0.130	—	—
Maize flour				
Wholegrain	0.289	0.100	—	—
Refined	0.298	0.125	—	—
Maize cob, fresh	0.865	0.285	—	—
Millet flour	0.312	0.179	—	—
Sorghum flour	0.298	0.105	—	—
Rice, polished	0.298	0.143	—	—
Cassava, fresh	0.965	1.126	—	—
Cassava flour	0.292	0.625	—	—
Plantain, fresh	1.166	1.263	—	0.117
Sweet potato, yellow	1.046	0.791	—	0.042
Beans, dried	0.313	0.045	—	—
Soybean, dried	0.247	0.026	0.050	—
Groundnuts, dry	0.175	0.040	0.022	—
Coconut, ripe	0.534	0.579	0.053	—
Carrots	—	—	—	0.012
Dark green leaves	—	—	—	0.023
Medium green leaves	—	—	—	0.042

*For the examples in this section we used the prices of food in Kenya in the early 1990s. Ksh = Kenya shilling.
†Developed with students and staff from AMREF—see Burgess (in press).

Table 9.1. (*contd.*)

Food	Weight of food in kg which contains			
	1000 kcal	10 g protein	10 g fat	100 RE vit A
Light green leaves	—	—	—	0.992
Pumpkin, fresh	—	—	—	0.044
Tomato, fresh	—	—	—	0.141
Avocado	1.667	1.430	0.182	0.227
Orange	—	—	—	0.109
Mango	—	—	—	0.035
Pawpaw	—	—	—	0.068
Sugar/glucose	0.250	—	—	—
Beef some fat	0.426	0.056	0.056	—
Liver	0.741	0.053	0.212	0.007
Chicken	1.066	0.075	0.230	—
Egg	0.812	0.095	0.114	0.057
Fish flesh	0.870	0.045	0.333	—
Fish dried, small (dagaa, kapenta)	0.313	0.023	0.063	—
Cow milk	1.515	0.286	0.270	0.192
Milk powder, whole	0.215	0.038	0.036	0.035
Milk powder, skim (DSM)*	0.282	0.028	—	0.007
Butter/margarine*	0.140	—	0.013	0.014
Lard/cooking fat/oil	0.112	—	0.010	—
Ghee	0.112	—	0.010	0.032
Red palm oil, fresh	0.112	—	0.010	0.002
Sodas	2.222	—	—	—
Beer, commercial	3.333	—	—	—
Baby cereal	0.27	0.17	—	—

—, Food contains little of nutrient or no reliable nutrient values available.
* If fortified with vitamin A.

You can work out more accurate values for Table 9.1 using local food composition tables and 'per cent edible portions' (% EP) using the following formulae.

$$\text{Grams food giving 1000 kcal} = \frac{100\,\text{g} \times 1000\,\text{kcal}}{\text{Calories in 100 g food}} \times \frac{100}{\text{g EP in 100 g food}}.$$

$$\text{Grams of food giving 10 g protein} = \frac{100\,\text{g} \times 10\,\text{g prot}}{\text{g protein in 100 g}} \times \frac{100}{\text{g EP in 100 g food}}.$$

(same formula for 10 g fat)

$$\text{Grams food giving 100 RE vit A} = \frac{100\,\text{g} \times 100\,\text{RE vit A}}{\text{RE vit A in 100 g food}} \times \frac{100}{\text{g EP in 100 g food}}.$$

(1000 g = 1 kg.)

Example
There are 140 kcal in 100 g edible portion of fresh cassava (see Appendix 1).
There are 74 g edible cassava in 100 g unpeeled cassava.
So there are $140 \times \frac{100}{74}$ kcal in 100 g unpeeled cassava.

So there are 1000 kcal in $\frac{100 \times 1000}{140} \times \frac{100}{74}$ g unpeeled cassava

$$= 965\,\text{g cassava or } 0.965\,\text{kg cassava.}$$

Example

To compare the cost of 1000 kcal from maize flour and cassava.

Costs per kilo:

- wholegrain maize flour   5.50 Ksh
- fresh unpeeled cassava   1.00 Ksh

Weight of food which provides 1000 kcal (from Table 9.1):

- maize flour   0.289 kg
- fresh unpeeled cassava   0.965 kg

So the cost of the amount of food which provides 1000 kcal is:

- maize flour = 5.50 × 0.289 = 1.59 Ksh;
- fresh unpeeled cassava = 1.0 × 0.965 = 0.97 Ksh.

So, the cost of 1000 kcal from maize flour is 1.59 Ksh, and the cost of 1000 kcal from unpeeled cassava is 0.97 Ksh.

Example

To compare the cost of 10 g protein from beans and egg.

Cost per kg:

- dry beans   15.00 Ksh
- egg   50.00 Ksh (cost per egg 2 Ksh; weight of one egg 40 g)

Weight of food providing 10 g protein (from Table 9.1):

- dry beans   0.045 kg;
- egg   0.095 kg.

So the cost of the weight of food providing 10 g protein is:

- dry beans   = 15.0 × 0.045 = 0.68 Ksh;
- egg   = 50.0 × 0.095 = 4.75 Ksh.

So, the cost of 10 g protein from beans is 0.68 Ksh and from eggs is 4.75 Ksh.

You may find it more convenient to do these calculations using a table like this.

Food	Cost per kg (Ksh)	Weight containing 1000 kcal (kg)	Cost of 1000 kcal (Ksh)
Maize flour	5.50	0.289	1.59
Unpeeled cassava	1.00	0.965	0.97

9.5 HOW TO ESTIMATE THE MINIMUM COST OF BASIC FOODS FOR A PERSON OR FAMILY FOR A WEEK

1. Use Table 9.2 to find out the minimum amounts of basic foods needed by a particular person for a week (or calculate these yourself using Appendices 1 and 2).
2. Find out the cost per kg of the cheapest locally used cereal (or root flour), legume, dark green leaves, and fat.

Table 9.2. Approximate amounts of foods which cover Calorie, protein, iron, and vitamin A needs for 1 week

	Staple (kg)*	Legume (kg)†	Green leaves (kg)‡	Oil (kg)
Children§				
2–3 years	1.4	0.7	0.7	0.21
5–6 years	2.1	1.1	0.8	0.21
10–12 years	2.8	1.4	1.0	—
Women of childbearing age				
Not pregnant or breastfeeding	3.2	1.1	0.9	—
Pregnant¶	3.5	1.1	1.0	—
Breastfeeding	3.9	1.4	1.4	—
Men and adolescent boys	4.6	1.4	1.0	—
Old people	3.0	1.1	0.9	—

* *Staple* means any kind of dry cereal or root flour.
† *Legumes* means any kind of dry beans, peas, or oil seeds.
‡ *Green leaves* mean *dark* green leaves, not overcooked.
§ Young children need oil or other fat-rich food to make meals less bulky (see Section 11.8).
¶ Pregnant women are unlikely to get enough iron from this diet so they need iron supplements.

Example. Calculating the cost of feeding a person or family for a week

Approximate amounts and cost of basic foods needed per week

For an 11-year-old girl:

	Maize flour	Beans	Spinach	Oil
Amount of food needed (kg)	2.8	1.4	1.0	—
Cost per kilo (Ksh)	5.50	15.0	8.0	
Cost of food for girl (Ksh)	15.40	21.0	8.0	

Total cost of feeding an 11-year-old girl for a week is 44.40 Kshs.

For a family with a pregnant woman, a man, and a 5-year-old boy:

	Maize flour	Beans	Spinach	Oil
Amount of food needed (kg) by:				
Pregnant woman	3.5	1.1	1.0	—
Man	4.6	1.4	1.0	—
5-year-old boy	2.1	1.1	0.8	0.21
Total food for family (kg)	10.2	3.6	2.8	0.21
Cost of food per kilo (Ksh)	5.50	15.0	8.0	25.0
Cost of food for family (Ksh)	56.10	54.0	22.40	5.25

Total cost of feeding family for 1 week is 137.75 Ksh.

3. Multiply the amounts of each food needed by the cost per kg. Add up the costs of each food to find out the total cost of 1 week's food.

4. To find out the cost of feeding a family for a week, work out the cost for each family member and then add these together.

THINGS TO DO

Exercises

1. Ask trainees to compare the costs of nutrients from different local foods using the method described in Section 9.4.

   a. Find out the cost of foods (or ask trainees to find out costs in preparation for the exercise).

   b. If the food is not listed in Table 9.1, use the FCTs in Appendix 1 and the formula in Table 9.1 to calculate the weights of foods which contain 1000 kcal, 10 g protein or fat, or 100 RE vitamin A.
   For example, there are 10 g protein in:

   - 50 g pigeon peas;
   - 625 g cassava flour;
   - 55 g meat.

2. Which is the best buy—fresh fish or dried fish?

   a. Find out the cost and protein content of fresh and dried fish or ask trainees to find out. Remember that:

   - Dried fish has lost most of the water, so the protein and other nutrients are more concentrated.
   - Whole dried fish as purchased contains about 30 per cent protein. Whole fresh fish as purchased contains about 12 per cent protein.

   (To calculate a more accurate value, use the protein content of the particular type of fish from Appendix 1 and local 'per cent edible portions'; see Appendix 4.)

   b. Calculate the cost of 10 g protein in each kind of fish, and decide which is the best value for money.

   c. Discuss other things which affect the value of the food. For example:

   - Dried fish may be easier to buy or to keep.
   - If the fish is eaten whole, it may provide other important nutrients such as vitamin A.

Projects

3. Ask trainees to go to the market to see which foods are available, and then plan meals for a local family.

   a. You can suggest how much money they have to spend, and how many people of different ages live in the family.

   b. Compare the meals planned by different trainees.

   c. Ask trainees to explain why they chose each food, and ask for comments.

4. Ask trainees to find out the prices of different quantities of different types and brands of fats and oils. Calculate and compare together the cost per kilogram of each. Discuss:
   • Which type or brand of fat or oil is best value for money?
   • Is it cheaper to buy in larger quantities? Should we advise families to do this?

5. Ask trainees to visit shops to find out the costs of 500 g of different brands of infant formula.

   a. A 500 g can of powder makes about 3 litres of liquid formula. Compare the costs of one litre of formula and 1 litre fresh milk.

   b. For bottle feeding, a baby needs about forty 500-g cans of formula for the first 6 months. How much will it cost to feed a baby for 6 months on the different brands of formula?

6. Ask trainees to find out the prices per kilogram of green or orange vegetables, and then calculate the cost of 100 RE vitamin A from each. Which is the cheapest source of vitamin A?

USEFUL PUBLICATION

Ritchie, J. A. S. (1983). *Nutrition and families*. Macmillan, London.

10 Breastfeeding

The best food for babies is breast milk. No other milk is as good. Breast milk is all that a baby needs for at least the first 4 months of life. Many babies need nothing but breast milk for 6 months. Breast milk continues to be the main source of nutrients for several more months, and can provide one-third or more of the nutrients that a child needs up to the age of 2 years. It can be a valuable snack for some time longer.

Breastfeeding should continue up to the age of 2 years, or longer if the mother and baby wish. We discuss how to introduce other foods, and stopping breastfeeding in Section 11.16.

10.1 EXCLUSIVE, PARTIAL, AND TOKEN BREASTFEEDING

Exclusive breastfeeding means that the baby has no other food or drink but breast milk—not even a 'dummy' ('pacifier'). If the baby sometimes has small amounts of another food or drink—such as drinks of water or vitamin drops—he is *almost exclusively* breastfed.

Partial breastfeeding means that the baby breastfeeds part of the time, but has some artificial feeds or other drinks or food. Partial breastfeeding is normal from the age of 6 months, when the baby starts to eat weaning foods made from the family food. But artificial feeds are not normally necessary at any age.

Token breastfeeding means that the child still breastfeeds sometimes, but gets only a small amount of breast milk. He gets most of the nutrients that he needs from other food. This is normal in the late stage of weaning (see Chapter 11).

The best and safest way to feed a baby up to the age of 6 months is *exclusive breastfeeding*. Babies do not normally need anything other than breast milk, even in the first few days after they are born. They do not need drinks of water, even in a hot climate. If they are given other drinks or foods, even in small amounts, or if they suck on a 'dummy', some of the advantages of breastfeeding may be lost.

However, partial breastfeeding is better than not breastfeeding at all.

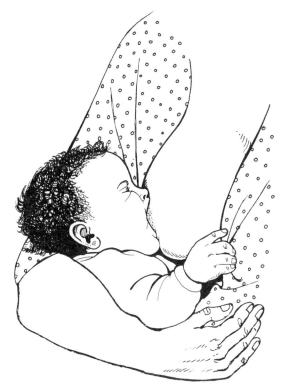

Fig. 10–1 Breast milk is the best food for babies. This baby is suckling in a good position (see Section 10.7) so he is getting the milk easily.

10.2 THE DANGERS OF PARTIAL BREASTFEEDING

Many mothers breastfeed their babies some of the time, but also give the baby some feeds of formula or animal milk, or dilute cereal, tea, juice, or other liquid, usually from a feeding bottle.

- Partially breastfed babies are more likely to become sick and die than exclusively breastfed babies, but less likely than babies who are not breastfed at all.
- When a baby has some artificial feeds, he may suckle less at the breast, and the supply of breast milk will decrease. If he has the artificial feeds from a bottle, he may not suckle properly at the breast. So partial breastfeeding often leads to stopping breastfeeding early.

Box 10.1. The advantages of breastfeeding

Breastmilk

- Contains exactly the nutrients that a baby needs

- Is easily digested and efficiently used by the body

- Protects a baby against infection

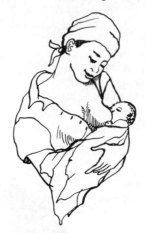

Breastfeeding

- Helps the mother and baby to *bond*

- Helps to delay a new pregnancy

- Costs less than artificial feeding

The dangers of artificial feeding

- The mother and baby may not develop such a close, loving, relationship

- The baby is more likely to become ill with diarrhoea, respiratory, ear, and other infections. Diarrhoea may become persistent (see Section 17.4)

- The baby may get *too little* artificial milk and become malnourished

- The baby is more likely to die than a breastfed baby

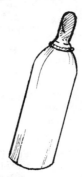

- The baby may develop allergic conditions such as eczema

- The baby may get *too much* artificial milk and become unhealthily overweight

- The mother becomes fertile again and can become pregnant more quickly

- If the baby has drinks of water, glucose water, tea, juice, or other watery feeds, they do not give him many nutrients. But they fill him up and he suckles less at the breast, so he does not get enough breast milk. He may not grow well.
- A few babies get too much milk and become overweight—especially babies who like to suck a lot, and whose parents can afford enough milk.
- The mother is likely to become pregnant again more quickly than if she breastfeeds exclusively.

10.3 WHY BREAST MILK IS A PERFECT FOOD FOR BABIES

Nutrients

Breast milk contains all the nutrients that a baby needs, almost always in exactly the right amounts. Artificial milks (formula, other tinned milks, and animal milks) do not contain the right amounts of all the nutrients.

Scientists keep discovering new differences between breast milk and animal milks. Manufacturers keep changing their formulae, but they can never make an identical product.

The nutrients in breast milk can be more easily digested and absorbed than the nutrients in artificial milks, and they are more efficiently used by the baby's body. A baby needs less breast milk than artificial milk to grow well.

Lactose

Lactose is the special sugar which is found only in milk. It is the only carbohydrate in milk. Lactose provides energy and helps the absorption of calcium. Breast milk contains more lactose than any other milk.

Babies and young children have a special enzyme *lactase* in the intestine to digest lactose. But in the first few months of life babies do not have enough of the enzyme *amylase* needed to digest starch. So it is difficult for very young babies to digest feeds made from cereals.

Fats

Fat is the main source of energy in breast milk and artificial milks, but breast milk contains more poly-unsaturated and essential fatty acids. Feeds made from cereals do not contain enough fat, so they provide too little energy.

The amount of different fatty acids in breast milk depends partly on the mother's diet, and there may be slightly less fat if the mother is severely malnourished.

The fat in human milk is easier to digest because:

- The fatty acids are arranged differently in the tri-glycerides than those in cow's milk (Section 2.4).
- Breast milk contains an enzyme (*lipase*) which helps to digest fat. Animal milks do not contain lipase.

Proteins

The protein in breast milk forms soft curds which are easy to digest. The protein in artificial milk forms thick curds in the baby's stomach which are difficult to digest.

Breast milk contains enough essential amino acids, while artificial milks often do not contain enough. For example, breast milk contains a large amount of the amino acid *taurine* which may be important for growth of the baby's brain. Cow's milk does not contain enough taurine for a baby, and formula manufacturers have to add extra.

Vitamins

Milk from well nourished mothers contains enough vitamins. Their babies do not need extra vitamins. If a mother is undernourished there may be less of some vitamins in her milk—for example, vitamin A. But her milk is still the best food for her baby.

Try to help the mother to improve her diet. If vitamin A deficiency is a problem, give the mother a capsule of vitamin A *before* the baby is 2 months old (Section 19.9). A baby who is artificially fed may need extra vitamins.

Minerals

Breast milk contains the right amount of salt, calcium, and phosphate for a baby. Cow's milk contains too much of these minerals, and they can make a baby ill.

Breast milk and cow's milk both contain about the same amount of iron. But the iron from breast milk is well absorbed, while the iron from cow's milk is not well absorbed.

Breastfed babies do not become anaemic (unless they are low birth weight and lack iron stores), but artificially fed babies may become anaemic. Manufacturers often add extra iron to formula to prevent anaemia, but added iron helps bacteria to grow, and may increase the risk of infection. Breastmilk iron does not help bacteria to grow.

Water

Breast milk contains enough water for a baby. It is not necessary to give a baby extra water, even in a hot dry climate. If a baby is thirsty, he can breastfeed more often.

Artificially fed babies may need extra water, to help them to excrete the extra salts and wasted amino acids in animal milk.

Anti-infective factors

Breast milk contains living anti-infective factors which protect a baby against infection. These are:

- living white blood cells, which help to kill bacteria and viruses;
- antibodies which cover the surface of the gut and prevent micro-organisms getting into the blood; when a mother has an infection, her milk soon contains antibodies against that new infection also;
- other factors, for example, the *bifidus factor* which helps harmless bacteria called *Lactobacillus bifidus* to grow in the baby's gut. *L. bifidus* prevents the growth of more harmful bacteria and gives the faeces of breastfed babies their 'yoghurty' smell.

Breast milk is always safe and clean. It never goes bad in the breasts, even if the mother does not breast-feed for some days. Expressed breast milk remains safe for at least 8 hours, even in a hot climate, and even if it is not in a refrigerator.

Artificial feeds do not contain these living anti-infective factors, so they do not protect babies against infection.

Artificially fed babies suffer from diarrhoea and respiratory, ear, and other infections more often than breastfed babies, *even if the feeds are cleanly prepared and the bottles sterilized.* If feeds are not cleanly prepared, they may be contaminated, and the baby is even more likely to have diarrhoea.

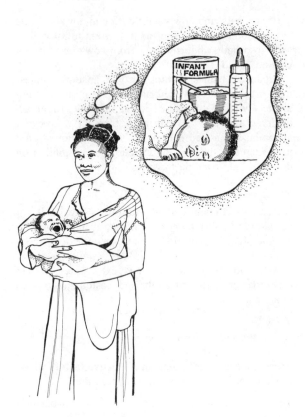

Fig. 10–2 This mother thought that she did not have enough breast milk, and she gave the baby bottle feeds.

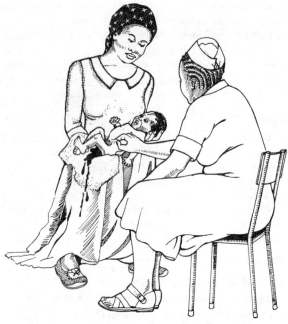

Fig. 10–3 The baby developed diarrhoea and malnutrition.

Growth factors

Breast milk contains *growth factors* which help the baby's intestine to grow and develop so that it is able to digest and absorb other foods.

If a baby has feeds of artificial milk before he can digest it, undigested protein molecules may pass into his blood and cause allergies.

Babies who are given artificial feeds are more likely to develop allergic conditions such as eczema. Exclusive breastfeeding helps to prevent these conditions.

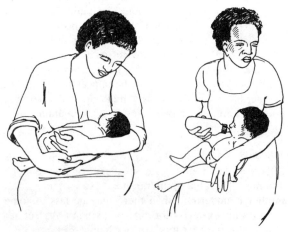

Fig. 10–4 A mother who breastfeeds finds it easier to develop a close loving relationship with her child than a mother who bottle feeds.

10.4 OTHER ADVANTAGES OF BREASTFEEDING

Bonding

A mother who breastfeeds finds it easier to develop a close, loving relationship with her child than a mother who bottle feeds. This close relationship helps the child to develop normally.

If a mother bottle feeds her baby, it is easier to give the baby to someone else to feed or to leave the bottle beside the baby, so that he has to feed himself. The baby then gets less affection and stimulation.

Less bleeding

Breastfeeding makes the uterus contract, which helps to stop bleeding after delivery.

Delaying the next pregnancy

Breastfeeding can be a useful method of family planning, if women know how to use it. The baby must breastfeed frequently during the day and during the night—at least 8–10 times in 24 hours. There should be no interval of more than 6 hours between breastfeeds.

A woman's chances of becoming pregnant are very small (less than 2 per cent) and she need not use another method of family planning if:

- The baby starts suckling within about an hour after delivery.
- The baby is less than 6 months old.
- The mother's periods have not returned.
- The baby is exclusively breastfed.

A woman's chances of becoming pregnant are greater (perhaps 10 per cent) and she should consider using another family planning method if:

- The baby is 6 months old or more.
- She gives the baby any other food or drinks.

However, so long as her periods have not returned, and provided she continues to breastfeed frequently, during the day and during the night, she has *some* protection. This may be helpful if she is unable to use another method.

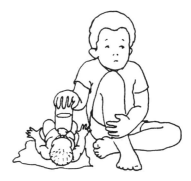

Fig. 10–5 With bottle feeding, it is easier to give the baby to someone else to feed.

If her periods have returned, breastfeeding does not protect her.

Saving money

Artificial feeding is expensive. Buying enough milk to provide a baby with all the nutrients she needs can take a large part of a family's income. For example, in Kenya, formula to feed a 6–10-month-old baby costs about 60 per cent of a labourer's wage.

The cost of breastfeeding is the cost of a few extra nutrients for the mother *plus her time*. If a mother works away from home to earn money, her time is not free. If she stays home to feed the baby, she loses income.

However, many women earn only the minimum wage or below. To feed a baby artificially can cost a

---

CASE HISTORY

Vidah feeds her 10-week-old son on formula. Her husband is a labourer, and he earns Ksh 720 per month. Vidah needs 2 half kilogram tins of formula each week to make up enough bottles, if she follows the instructions on the tin. Often she does not have enough money to buy two tins, and she buys only one tin. If she puts less milk powder in each bottle, she can make one tin last longer—sometimes more than a week. The baby often doesn't finish the feed, and it tastes all right with less milk powder. She has one bottle and one teat, and she rinses it out in cold water and washing powder most mornings. At other times, she just adds more drinking water and a scoop or two of milk powder. Sometimes two bottles of milk last all day.

Last week, the baby vomited twice and then started having diarrhoea. The diarrhoea did not get better, so she took him to the clinic. The nurse gave her some special water and explained how to give it to the baby. The baby weighed 4 kg—only 0.5 kg more than when he was born. The nurse explained that the baby's line on his growth chart was not going up fast enough.

The nurse explained how Vidah should boil the feeding bottle to kill the germs and said that Vidah should put five scoops of powder into every bottle, and give the baby five bottles a day. But Vidah does not have any more money until the end of the month.

On the way home Vidah met a friend, who said that she had heard that it was possible for mothers to start breastfeeding again—even if they had stopped for some time. There was a nurse who helped mothers to breastfeed who lived not far away, and perhaps they could go to see her.

large part of what they earn. If a mother can find a way to breastfeed *and* work or if she can breastfeed at least partially, she can save money. Nutrition workers can help working mothers to breastfeed—many mothers have succeeded (Section 10.17).

10.5 HOW BREAST MILK VARIES

Colostrum

During the first few days after a baby is born, the breasts produce a small amount of yellowish milk called *colostrum*. Colostrum is rich in antibodies, white cells, and growth factor. Some people believe that colostrum is not good for a baby. But it is exactly what a baby needs for the first few feeds to protect him against infection, and to prepare his gut to digest and absorb the mature milk which comes later.

Some people believe that a baby needs other food or drinks at this time. However, babies are born with enough water and nutrients in their bodies for several days. They need nothing but colostrum.

A new mother's breasts feel soft and empty for the first 2 or 3 days. You may need to reassure her that this is normal. If the baby is suckling, the baby is getting all that he needs.

Mature breast milk

After a few days, the breasts start to produce milk in larger quantities, with more fat and other nutrients. The milk has now '*come in*', and the breasts feel full and sometimes hard. The colour of the milk changes from yellowish, to a greyish colour. This is called *mature breast milk*.

Foremilk and hindmilk

Breast milk is not exactly the same throughout a feed.

At the beginning of a feed the milk looks grey and watery. This is *foremilk*. It contains plenty of protein, lactose, vitamins, and minerals, and plenty of water, but not much fat.

Towards the end of a feed, the milk looks much whiter. This is *hindmilk*. It is rich in fat, which provides about half of the energy of a feed. It is important for the baby to have the hindmilk, to get enough energy.

10.6 HOW BREAST MILK IS PRODUCED

Gland tissue in the breast produces milk, which goes along *ducts* or tubes towards the nipple. The milk col-

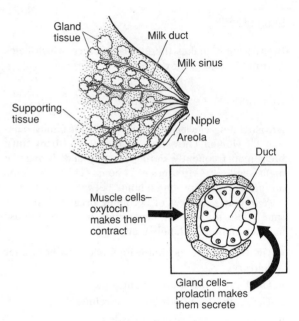

Fig. 10–6 The anatomy of the breast.

lects in *milk sinuses* beneath the *areola*, that is, the dark skin around the nipple.

Prolactin—the milk-screting reflex

When a baby suckles, the mother's body secretes a hormone called *prolactin* which makes the breasts produce milk. This is the *milk-secreting reflex* or the *prolactin reflex*.

It is important to know about this reflex, because it helps you to understand several things about breastfeeding:

- The baby's suckling in the first few days helps the milk to 'come in'.
- If the baby suckles more, the breasts make more milk.
- If the baby suckles less, the breasts make less milk.

If a baby is hungry or thirsty, and he suckles more often and for longer, the mother makes more milk. If a mother wishes to increase her milk supply, she should let the baby suckle more often and for longer for a few days.

If the baby suckles less, because he has other feeds or drinks, or because his mother is away from him for part of the day, or she wants to 'save up' her milk, the breasts will make less milk.

More prolactin is produced during the night, so breastfeeding at night helps to keep up the milk supply.

Oxytocin—the milk ejection reflex

When a baby suckles, the mother's body also secretes a hormone called *oxytocin*. Oxytocin makes muscle cells around the milk glands contract, which makes the milk flow. This is the *oxytocin reflex* or the *milk ejection reflex*, which enables the baby to get the milk.

The oxytocin reflex is affected by how a mother feels. If she has good feelings about her baby, milk flows more easily. If she thinks lovingly about her baby or hears him cry, milk may flow out of her breasts, even without the baby suckling. If she is worried or in pain, milk may not flow well.

Oxytocin also makes the uterus contract, which helps to deliver the placenta and reduce bleeding after childbirth. Contractions during a feed can be quite painful, and you may need to reassure a mother that they are normal, and that they will soon stop.

Why it is important to remove milk from the breast

For a breast to continue to produce milk, it is essential to remove the milk. If milk is not removed, an inhibitor present in the milk reduces and eventually stops milk production. If a baby suckles only from one breast, the other breast stops making milk, even if there is plenty of prolactin.

10.7 HOW A BABY SUCKLES

We use the word *suckle* for the action of breastfeeding. It is different from *sucking* from a bottle. The baby's suckling controls the production and flow of breast milk.

To get breast milk a baby has to take enough of the breast into his mouth. He draws out part of the areola and the breast beneath to form a long 'teat', which contains the milk sinuses (see Fig. 10–9). His tongue presses the milk out of the sinuses. You can sometimes see the long 'teat' for a moment as a baby finishes a feed, before the breast returns to its normal shape.

The nipple forms only part of the 'teat'. The nipple is not what the baby sucks from—it is a marker to show where he should take the breast. The baby can suckle equally well if the nipple looks long or short or flat.

Mothers have to learn how to get a baby to take enough breast into his mouth. Some have no difficulty at all. But other mothers and babies need help at first to get it right—from a midwife or from another experienced woman who knows what to do.

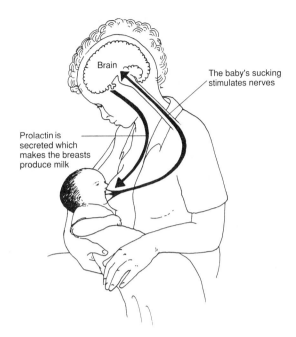

Fig. 10–7 The prolactin reflex.

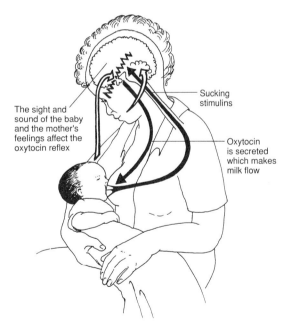

Fig. 10–8 The oxytocin reflex.

If a mother has help early, she can soon overcome any difficulty getting the baby to suckle. If she does not have any help, she may have more serious difficulty, and breastfeeding may fail.

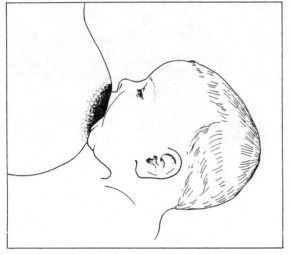

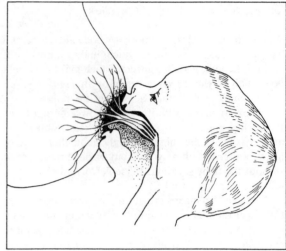

a) Appearance from the outside
The baby is close to the breast with his mouth wide open

b) What is happening inside the baby's mouth
Breast tissue forms a long teat and the baby's tongue presses milk out of the sinuses.

Fig. 10–9 Suckling in a good position.

The mother can sit up or lie down in any position, so long as she is comfortable. The baby can lie beside her, or across the front, or under her arm, so long as he faces the breast and can take enough of the breast into his mouth.

Suckling in a poor position

Sometimes a baby sucks mainly on the nipple—this is called 'nipple sucking'. The baby's tongue cannot press the milk out of the sinuses, so he does not get enough milk. Also, sucking this way is painful, and it damages the nipple skin (see Fig. 10–10). A poor suckling position is the cause of many breastfeeding problems:

- sore and cracked nipples;
- unsatisfied babies, who want to feed very often or for a very long time;
- frustrated babies who fuss at the breast or who refuse to breastfeed;
- mothers who believe that they do not have enough milk;
- babies who fail to grow;
- engorged breasts.

There are two main reasons why a baby may suckle in a poor position:

- The mother is inexperienced, and has no one to help her.
- The baby has been fed from a bottle, either soon after birth, or at any other time. 'Nipple sucking' is often the result of a baby trying to suck from a breast in the same way that he has learned to suck from a bottle.

Finishing a feed

When a baby finishes a feed, he usually comes off the breast by himself. There is usually no need to take him off the breast. It is better to let him continue as long as he wants, so that he gets plenty of energy-rich hind-milk. If a baby has had enough, he looks sleepy and satisfied.

Suckling the other breast

Some babies want to suckle from both breasts at every feed. But some babies may be satisfied after suckling from one breast. A baby may want a little from the second breast, or he may not want any at all.

The mother can let the baby start on her other breast next time, so that he suckles both breasts equally. Then both breasts will continue to make plenty of milk.

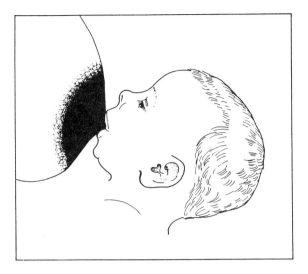

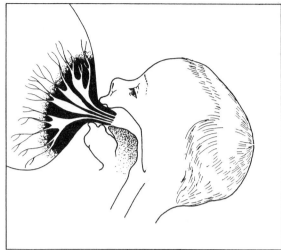

a) Appearance from the outside
The baby is not close to the breast and his mouth is not wide open.

b) What is happening inside the baby's mouth
Only the nipple is in the baby's mouth. His tongue cannot reach the milk sinuses to press out the milk.

Fig. 10–10 Suckling in a poor position.

Box 10.2 Signs of good and poor suckling positions

Signs that a baby is suckling in a good position

- The baby's whole body is facing his mother and is close to her.
- His face is close up to the breast.
- His chin is touching the breast.
- His mouth is wide open.
- His lower lip is curled outwards.
- You see more areola above the upper lip than below the lower lip.
- The baby takes slow deep sucks.
- You can see or hear the baby swallowing.
- His cheeks are round, and not pulled in.
- The baby is relaxed and happy, and satisfied at the end of a feed.
- The mother does not feel any pain.

Signs that a baby is suckling in a poor position

- The baby's body may be turned away from his mother's and not close to her.
- His chin is separated from the breast.
- His mouth looks closed.
- His lips point forwards.
- You can see most of the areola.
- The baby takes many quick, small sucks.
- You do not see or hear the baby swallowing—you may hear smacking sounds as he sucks.
- The baby's cheeks may be pulled in.
- The baby may fuss or refuse to feed because he does not get enough breast milk.
- The mother may feel nipple pain.
- The nipple looks flattened as it comes out of the baby's mouth, and there may be a line across the tip.

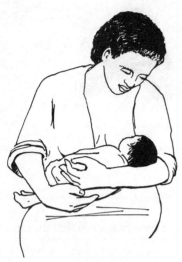

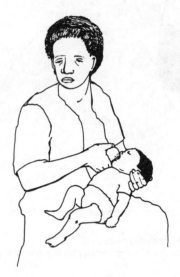

This mother holds the baby close
with his body facing hers. The baby
should get the breast milk easily

The baby has to turn his head
and reach out to suckle. The
mother is holding him as if she is
bottle feeding. This makes it difficult
for the baby to get breast milk

Fig. 10–11 Watch how the mother holds the baby.

10.8 WATCHING A MOTHER BREASTFEED HER BABY

When you see or talk with mothers who have babies, watch how they breastfeed. Notice how the mother holds the baby and how the baby suckles (see Box 10.2). This can help you to understand the kind of help that they may need.

10.9 STARTING BREASTFEEDING

Almost all women can breastfeed if they want to, and if they receive the support and help that they need. Success or failure depends partly on what happens at the time of delivery, and in the first few days.

Early contact between the mother and baby is impor-

tant for both *bonding* and breastfeeding. This means the mother holding her baby quietly and undisturbed immediately after delivery for an hour or so. It may be best if the baby is naked and has skin-to-skin contact with the mother (see Fig. 10–13).

Mothers who have early contact are more likely to breastfeed longer and to behave more affectionately towards their babies. Mothers who do not have early contact are more likely to stop breastfeeding sooner and to behave less affectionately. They are more likely to abandon or abuse their babies.

Breastfeeding soon after delivery is important. Encourage a mother to put her baby to the breast in the first hour. It is not necessary to force the baby to suckle immediately. But most babies show that they are ready to suckle within about an hour. They may be very alert at this time and may suckle strongly. Starting to breast-

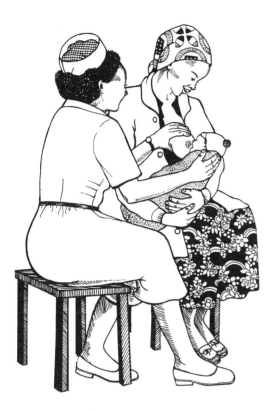

feed soon after delivery helps the milk to 'come in' sooner. The baby gets colostrum, and learns to suckle in a good position more easily. This helps to prevent problems such as engorgement.

Confidence also is necessary for successful breastfeeding. If a woman believes that she can breastfeed, her milk flows better and she is less likely to have problems. She needs to be confident that her body is normal, and that her breasts will produce perfect milk for her baby—whether they are big or small.

A woman who has just had a baby is more sensitive and emotional than normal. This helps her to love and respond to her baby, and to bond with him. But it means that she is easily discouraged, and she easily believes that there is something wrong with her or her breastmilk. For example, if someone says 'Your nipples look a bit flat' or 'Perhaps you don't have enough milk', she may lose confidence and stop breastfeeding.

Women who have breastfed successfully before may have no difficulty believing that they can do it. But a young mother with her first baby or a woman who failed to breastfeed previous babies may find it difficult to believe that she can succeed. These mothers need more experienced women to support and reassure them.

Fig. 10–12 Helping a mother to put her baby on to the breast.

Box 10.3.   Helping a mother to put her baby on to the breast in a good position

If a mother needs help to get her baby to suckle well:

- Let her sit or lie somewhere comfortable, so that she is relaxed. A low seat is usually best.
- Show her how to hold the baby so that:
    - his head and body are in a straight line;
    - his body faces her body and is close to her;
    - his face is facing the breast.
- Show her how to lift her breast with her hand, to offer the whole breast to the baby. She should not pinch the nipple or areola with her fingers, or try to push the nipple into the baby's mouth.
- As you show her, hold the baby at the back of the shoulders—not the back of the head.
- She can touch the baby's lips with the nipple, so that he opens his mouth.
- Wait until the baby's mouth is wide open, and he wants to start feeding. Quickly move the baby well on to the breast.
- Aim the baby's lower lip well below the nipple. This helps to get his chin near the breast.

It is not necessary to hold the breast back from the baby's nose with a finger. He can breathe quite well without that (see Fig. 10–1).

Support for a mother means a kind person who can:

● reassure her that she can breastfeed, and that her milk is perfect and sufficient;

● praise her for what she is doing right;

● explain that what is happening is normal—for example, when there seems to be only a little milk in her breasts during the first few days;

● advise her if she does not know what to do—for example, if she does not know whether she needs to wash her nipples;

● help her if she seems to have a problem—for example, if she cannot get the baby to suckle;

● encourage her to continue if she has any difficulties—such as engorgement.

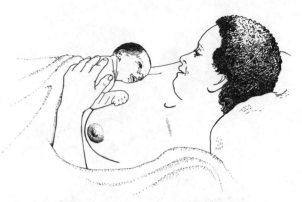

Fig. 10–13 Early contact between mother and baby is important for both bonding and breastfeeding.

Hospital deliveries are safer for both mother and baby in many ways, but they may interfere with breastfeeding. In some hospitals, babies are separated from their mothers after delivery, and may be given bottle feeds. Hospital staff may not know how to help a mother to breastfeed.

Home deliveries usually make breastfeeding easier. Traditional midwives are often skilled at helping mothers to breastfeed. Mother and baby are kept together, and the family is usually supportive. But, unfortunately, some communities do not like to give colostrum. They may give ritual feeds of some other food, and the baby may not be allowed to suckle for a few days. Some modern families may encourage mothers to bottle feed. These practices can interfere with breastfeeding.

So you may be able to improve the start of breastfeeding both in hospitals and in home deliveries.

10.10 CONTINUING BREASTFEEDING

A mother should keep her baby near her and feed him whenever he is hungry during the day and during the night. This is called *unrestricted* or '*demand feeding*'. It is safe for the baby to sleep in the same bed as his mother, provided that neither she nor a partner sleeping with her have drunk too much alcohol or taken drugs.

Most new mothers continue to need support, especially in the first few weeks when they are still learning about breastfeeding and about caring for a baby. Continuous support from one skilled and experienced person is best.

In traditional societies there were plenty of older women around to help and encourage a young mother. Nowadays, many young mothers are left by themselves with no one to help. Help often needs to be nearby, because a woman may be unable to leave the house to go and ask someone. She may be restricted for the first few weeks or she may not feel strong enough.

You can be a valuable source of support at this time, especially if you can visit new mothers in their homes. However, you may not be able to visit as often as the mother needs. But you may know of experienced women or other breastfeeding women in the neighbourhood who would be able to visit or there may be community health workers (CHWs) or traditional birth attendants (TBAs) who could help.

Women's groups can also be an important source of support. You can encourage women's groups to make breastfeeding one of their activities.

In some countries special groups have developed in which breastfeeding mothers help each other. These are called '*direct mother-to-mother*' support groups. If there are several young breastfeeding mothers in your area, you could encourage them to help each other. Perhaps they could meet as a group.

10.11 WHAT YOU CAN DO TO HELP MOTHERS TO BREASTFEED

Before the baby is born

Discuss feeding the baby with each woman before she delivers. Sometimes it is a good idea to get several women together to share their ideas.

● Discuss the advantages of breastfeeding, and the dangers of artificial feeding.

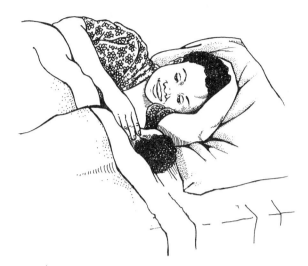

Fig. 10–14 It is usually safe for a baby to sleep in bed with his mother.

- Explain that all women can breastfeed if they want to. The size and shape of the breasts does not matter.
- Ask if they had difficulties feeding a previous baby, and explain how they can succeed this time.
- Advise them to eat extra before the baby is born, so that they have stores of nutrients to make breast milk.
- Explain about colostrum and early feeding, so that they know what to expect when the baby is born.
- Make sure that each woman has someone who has breastfed to support her, for example, her mother or a TBA. If not, try to find another woman or a health worker who can help.
- You may want to explain that there is no need to prepare the nipples—it probably does not help. (If mothers are not concerned about this, say nothing.)

At the time of delivery

Whether the baby is born at home or in hospital, try to make sure that these things happen:

- The mother holds the baby close immediately after delivery, with skin-to-skin contact if that is acceptable.
- She puts the baby to the breast, and lets him try to suckle within about an hour of birth.
- The baby stays with the mother, if possible in the same bed, day and night, from the time of delivery (that is, 'rooming in' or, better still, 'bedding in').
- The mother is given skilled help to make sure that the baby is suckling in a good position at the first real feed, or sometime in the first 24 hours after delivery.
- There is no restriction on the length of feeds. If the baby is suckling in a good position, he will not make the nipples sore. Let him suckle as long as he likes to get the energy-rich hindmilk.
- The mother breastfeeds the baby 'on demand', whenever he seems to want. When breastfeeding is unrestricted:
  - Breast milk 'comes in' sooner.
  - The breasts are less likely to become engorged.
  - Crying is less of a problem.
- The baby is given no other drinks or feeds—and especially not from a bottle. Bottle feeds may make him suckle in a poor position. Milk feeds may cause diarrhoea, infections, and allergies.
- There are no free samples of formula or advertisements for formula in the hospital or health centre. These may confuse mothers and undermine their confidence.
- If the baby is too small or weak to suckle, show the mother how to express her milk and feed it by cup.

When the mother and baby are at home

Try to visit each mother as soon as possible after delivery, especially if she lives alone.

- Congratulate her and admire the baby.
- Ask her how she and the baby are, and how breastfeeding is going. Listen to what she says. Many new mothers are worried about breastfeeding, and they often have minor problems. Encourage them to talk about these and to ask questions.
- Remember that a new mother may be very sensitive, and try to build her confidence. Praise her for all the things that she is doing right.
  - Notice how the mother holds the baby (see Fig. 10–11).
  - If she turns towards the baby, holds him close, and looks at him, these are signs of bonding. Also, it is easier for the baby to suckle efficiently.
  - If she turns away from the baby, and does not hold him close or look at him, there may be a problem. She may be worried or depressed or she may not want the baby. Try to get her to talk about her problems, and if necessary try to get help for her.

Also, holding a baby this way makes it more difficult for him to suckle.

- If the baby is ready for a feed, watch the mother feed him. Make sure that the baby is suckling in a good position and help her to improve the position if necessary.
- Discuss how she feeds the baby. It may help to explain that:
  - Frequent feeding and feeding the baby at night help to keep up her milk supply.
  - It is safe for the baby to sleep in the mother's or parents' bed, if they have not drunk alcohol or taken drugs.
  - The baby may not want both breasts at every feed, or may only want a little from the second side. She can start on the other side next time, so that both breasts continue to make plenty of milk.
- She need not wash her nipples more than once a day, and it is better not to use soap on them. Washing, especially with soap, dries the nipple skin, and they may become sore.
- If it is helpful, show her how to express breastmilk (Section 10.14).

Later visits

Try to see breastfeeding mothers at least once a month, in their homes or in a health centre. Arrange for groups of mothers to discuss breastfeeding together. Try to see all mothers 1–2 weeks after delivery. This is a time when many mothers have difficulties, but it is too soon for their postnatal visit, and they may not come for help.

- Check the baby's weight. Make sure that he has a growth chart, with the birth weight written on it if he was weighed at birth. If the baby is growing well, you can reassure the mother that she has plenty of milk, and this helps to build her confidence.
- Watch the baby breastfeeding:
  - Look at his suckling position.
  - Notice how he finishes the feed—does he look satisfied?
- If the mother has a breastfeeding problem, reassure her and help her to sort it out. For example, she may need to know how to increase her milk supply. See her again a day or two later to find out how she is doing. Many problems are very minor, and reassurance is all that a mother needs.

- Encourage mothers to breastfeed exclusively for at least 4 months, and if possible for 6 months.
  - Explain how this protects the baby against illness; and how it helps to prevent a new pregnancy.
  - Explain how giving other foods before 6 months, especially bottle feeds, may make the mother's breast milk supply decrease.
  - If she is giving other drinks or feeds, suggest that she stops them and breastfeeds more instead.
- Discuss child spacing with families. Explain that a mother needs to consider other methods of family planning, besides breastfeeding, when the baby is 6 months old, or when she starts to give the baby other food, or when she starts her periods.
- If she has to work away from home, help her to breastfeed and work (Section 10.17). Explain about expressing milk to leave for the baby, and about feeding the baby by cup.

10.12 SUSTAINING BREASTFEEDING FOR 2 YEARS

Talk to mothers, fathers, and other family members too.

- Encourage mothers to continue to breastfeed frequently after they start to give the child other food. Explain that breast milk provides most of the nutrients that a baby needs for several more months.
- Encourage them to continue to breastfeed 'on demand' for 2 years or more (see Section 11.15).
  - Explain how breast milk continues to provide valuable nutrients.
  - Explain how breast milk helps to prevent some kinds of diarrhoea up to 3 years of age, and that children who breastfeed are less likely to become seriously ill if they do have diarrhoea.
- Encourage them to continue breastfeeding when the child is sick or recovering from illness (see Section 13.3).
  - Sick children may lose their appetite for other food, but often continue to breastfeed. Explain that breast milk is a nutritious and easy-to-digest food for a sick child.
  - Breastfeeding comforts a sick or unhappy child.
- Encourage parents to leave at least 2–3 years between babies and tell them where they can get advice on family planning. Explain that sexual intercourse does not harm the milk, but it is better for the health

of both mother and child if she does not have another baby until this one is 3 years old.

- Explain that it is important for the mother to eat enough.
  - The body stores that she built up during pregnancy may all be used up after she has breastfed for 6 months.
  - She needs to eat extra for as long as she breastfeeds.

10.13 COMMON WORRIES THAT A MOTHER MAY NEED REASSURANCE ABOUT

Constipation and loose faeces

An exclusively breastfed baby's faeces are usually very soft and have a characteristic 'yoghurty' smell. A baby may pass faeces more than eight times a day, or not at all for up to a week. He may cry, and go red in the face, and pull up his knees when passing the faeces. This is all normal, but you may need to reassure a mother that her baby does not have either diarrhoea or constipation.

A baby who has some artificial feeds may have much more solid faeces, because some of the milk passes through undigested. The faeces smell different, because different bacteria grow in his gut. If a baby passes frequent, watery, faeces, it is more likely to be diarrhoea.

The mother's figure

A mother may worry that breastfeeding will spoil her figure or the shape of her breasts. Explain that breast-feeding helps her to lose the weight that she put on during pregnancy. Having a baby changes the shape of the breasts a little, whether she breastfeeds or not. If she wears a well-fitting bra to support her breasts during breastfeeding, they should not become long.

Small breasts

Some women with small breasts worry that they will not be able to produce enough milk. Reassure them that small breasts can produce just as much milk as large breasts.

10.14 USEFUL TECHNIQUES TO TEACH MOTHERS

How to express breast milk

Most women find it useful at some time to be able to express their milk, for example:

- to leave breast milk for the baby when they are at work;
- if the baby is small or weak or ill and cannot suckle;
- to relieve full or engorged breasts.

With a good technique, they can usually express a cupful or more. If a woman has difficulty expressing milk, it is often because her technique is poor. Some women can express plenty of milk, in very unusual ways. If it works for them, let them do it their way. But if a woman is having difficulty, you may be able to help her to do better.

What to tell a mother to do

- Prepare a clean cup—if possible, pour boiling water into the cup to kill any germs.
- Wash your hands.
- Sit down in a comfortable relaxed position.
- Use one or all of these methods to help the milk to flow
  - Warm the breasts with cloths dipped in warm water.
  - Have the baby on your lap or nearby, so that you can look at him.
  - Massage the breasts gently, or stroke them lightly, or roll your knuckles over them, towards the nipple.
- Place your finger and thumb one each side of the breast behind the nipple, near the edge of the areola (see Fig. 10–16).
- Press in towards the chest wall.

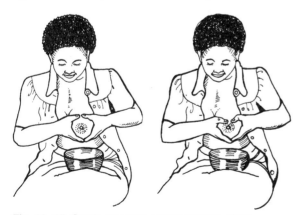

Fig. 10–15 Gentle massage or light stroking of the breasts helps the oxytocin reflex and the flow of breast milk.

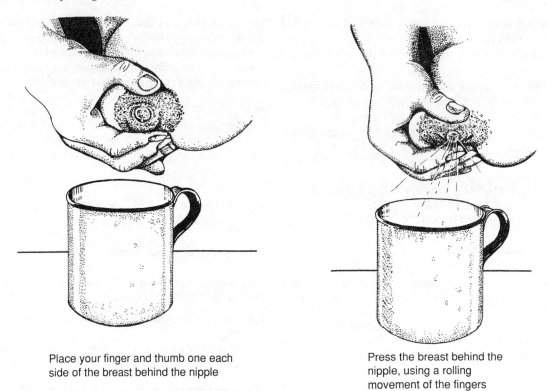

Place your finger and thumb one each
side of the breast behind the nipple

Press the breast behind the
nipple, using a rolling
movement of the fingers

Fig. 10–16 How to express breast milk.

- Press the breast behind the nipple, using a rolling movement of the fingers.
  - Do not move the fingers along the skin, or it will rub and may make the breast sore.
  - Do not pinch the nipple itself—remember, the baby presses the milk out from sinuses beneath the areola.
- Press and squeeze; press and squeeze.
  - The milk may come out in strong streams, or it may trickle out more slowly.
  - It may take a minute or two for the milk to start coming—do not give up!
  - Hold the cup in your other hand to collect the milk.
- Move the finger and thumb round the nipple, to make sure that you empty all parts of the breast.
- Repeat with the other breast.

Praise the mother and give her lots of encouragement if she produces only a small amount at first. She will produce more in time.

Feeding a baby from a cup

If a baby cannot feed from the breast, it is better to give expressed breast milk (EBM) or other milk with a cup than with a bottle. Even very small babies can feed from a cup (Fig. 10–17). Feeding bottles are never necessary.

A cup is much easier to clean, so it is less likely to cause diarrhoea. A cup does not interfere with a baby's suckling. It may be harder work for a baby—especially a very small baby—to suck from a bottle, than it is to breastfeed.

Some mothers like to use a spoon and cup. That is also safe for the baby. But most mothers find it much easier to feed the baby directly from the cup alone. You need less hands that way! It is easiest with a very small cup or glass. Spoon feeding takes longer, and mothers are more likely to give up.

Some people worry that a baby may choke if milk pours into his mouth too fast. But you do not pour the milk in—you just hold the cup to the baby's lips and he sips up the milk with his tongue. Hold the baby half

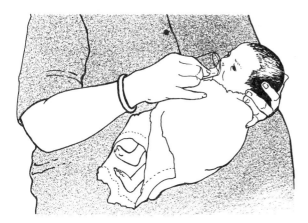

Fig. 10–17 Even very small babies can feed from a small cup or glass.

sitting up—not lying down—so that if milk pours too fast, it spills out of the baby's mouth. If a mother finds this too difficult, she can try with a spoon.

10.15 INCREASING THE MILK SUPPLY AND RELACTATION

You may want to explain to a mother how she can increase her milk supply, for example, after she or the baby has been ill, and the supply has decreased.

If she has stopped breastfeeding altogether, and her breast milk has dried up, suckling can make it flow again. This is called 'relactation'.

If the baby is still breastfeeding, the milk supply increases in a few days. If he has stopped breastfeeding, it may take 1–2 weeks before much milk comes. It is easier if the baby is still young, and if he stopped breastfeeding recently. But relactation can succeed at any time, even with a woman who has not breastfed for years, and who wishes to feed a grandchild. Even a woman who has never been pregnant can produce breast milk if she suckles an adopted baby.

Try to help the mother and baby at home if possible. Occasionally it is better to admit them to hospital for a week or two so that you can give the mother enough help—especially if she may use a bottle at home.

How to help a mother to increase her breast milk or relactate

- Discuss the problem which may have caused a poor breast milk supply, and sort it out if you can. For example, if she started giving the baby bottle feeds, advise her to stop them.

- Try to give her confidence that she can produce breast milk again, or increase her supply. Try to talk to her *twice a day* if possible.

- Make sure that she has enough to eat and drink. Warm drinks may help to give her confidence, but it is the baby's suckling, not the food or the drink, that makes the breast milk come.

- Encourage her to rest more, especially when she feeds the baby.

- She should keep the baby near her and do as much as possible for him herself.

- The most important thing is to *let the baby suckle often*.
  - She should let him suckle whenever he seems interested. Sometimes this is easiest when the baby is sleepy.
  - She can offer him the breast every 2 hours—or at least 10 times in 24 hours.
  - She should keep him with her and breastfeed at night.
  - She should let him suckle longer than before at each breast.

- Make sure that the baby suckles in a good position.

- Try not to give the baby other milk feeds, especially if he is less than 6 months old, and if the mother is still producing breast milk. However, if her breast milk has dried up, other milk feeds may be necessary, while waiting for the breast milk to come back.
  - She should give the other feeds from a cup, not from a bottle.
  - She should not use a 'dummy'.

- To start with, give the baby the full amount of artificial feeds for a baby of his weight (150 ml/kg/day), or the same amount that he has been having before. Each day, reduce the total volume of feed by 30–50 ml.

- If the baby refuses to suckle on an 'empty' breast, the mother may be able to drip the artificial milk down the nipple as the baby suckles. She can drip the milk on to the nipple from a small cup, or a spoon, or a syringe if one is available.

- If a fine tube is available, put one end of the tube along the nipple, and the other end in the cup of milk. The baby then sucks milk through the tube while he suckles at the breast. It is important that the milk does not flow too fast through the tube. If necessary slow the flow—for example, the mother can squeeze the tube between her finger and thumb; or tie

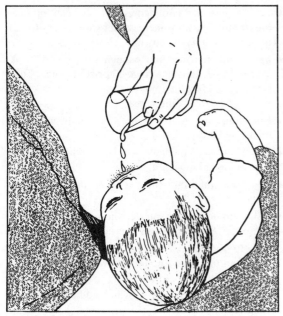

Dripping milk down the nipple as the baby suckles

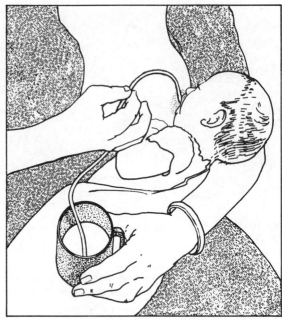

The baby gets milk through a fine tube while suckling at the breast

Fig. 10–18

a knot in it; or hold the cup of milk lower down. Wash the tube carefully between feeds (see Fig. 10–18).

- Weigh the baby regularly and check his urine output to make sure that he is getting enough milk (Section 10.20).

10.16 ARTIFICIAL MILK FEEDS

You may sometimes need to teach a family how to give artificial feeds. For example, if the baby's mother is dead or absent, and if there is no one else who can breastfeed the baby; or to help a mother who works away from home and who has real difficulty expressing enough breast milk.

- Help the family find the cheapest brand of artificial milk.
- Tell them not to use sweetened condensed milk—it contains too much sugar—and not to use dried skimmed milk—it does not contain any fat.

This is what to teach a family about using powdered or fresh milk.

Using powdered milk:
- Follow the instructions on the tin.

- Mix the feed with recently boiled cooled water.

Using fresh cow's milk:
- Boil 2 parts of milk with 1 part of water. Add a level teaspoonful (5 g) of sugar to each cup of feed.

How much milk to give:
- Give a total of 150 ml (3/4 cupful) per day for each kilogram of the baby's weight. Divide the total into 5–6 feeds.

Example
A baby of 6 kg needs 4.5 cups of milk per day. Offer the baby five feeds of 1 cup each.

If the baby does not finish all of a feed at once:

- Keep the feed covered. Do not keep it for more than half a day. Give the left-over milk to an older child to drink.
- Give the feeds by cup—do not use a bottle.
- Wash the utensils thoroughly with soap each time you use them, and leave them in the sun to dry.
- If possible boil utensils or pour boiling water over them.

- Wash your hands before you make the feed or feed the baby.
- Offer the baby extra water to drink, and vitamin drops if available.

10.17 HELPING WOMEN WHO WORK AWAY FROM HOME

Working away from home is a common reason for a woman to feed a baby artificially. Many people are concerned about improving women's working conditions so that they can breastfeed their babies. But improvements will not happen quickly, and many women need support to do the best they can now.

If the work place is near where the family live, the mother may be able to go home during the day to breastfeed, or a helper may be able to bring the baby to her. If the work place is too far, it is best if the mother can take the baby to work with her. But there are often no childcare facilities, and it is often difficult to travel to work with a baby.

However, even when breastfeeding during working hours is not possible, there are ways in which a mother can feed her child partly or completely on breast milk.

How you can help a working mother
- Encourage her to believe that she can work and breastfeed. Many mothers do.
  - It is better for her baby.
  - It can save money.
  - She will feel more satisfied.
- Explain that the she needs to breastfeed exclusively and frequently during her maternity leave to give the baby the benefit of breastfeeding and to build up her milk supply. She should not start giving bottles and formula 'to get the baby used to them'.
- When she starts work, advise her to sleep with her baby so that he breastfeeds at night. This means:
  - He will suckle more at night, and get most of the milk that he needs then.
  - He may sleep more and need less milk during the day.
  - It will help to keep up her supply.
- Teach her to express her breast milk to leave for her baby.
- She can express early in the morning before she goes to work. She should leave enough time to express, and not try to do it in a hurry. She may have to get up

even earlier, which is hard when she already works long hours, but it is only for a few months.
- She can feed the baby after she has expressed. He will be able to get more milk from the breast.
- She should leave the expressed breast milk in a clean covered container, in a cool place.
  - Breast milk will stay fresh and safe for the baby for up to 8 hours, even if she has no refrigerator.
  - If she has a refrigerator, it will stay fresh for the next day too.
  - She should try to leave ½–1 cupful of breast milk for each feed that the baby will need while she is out.
  - She should not boil or reheat the breast milk, because that destroys the anti-infective cells and antibodies.
- If she cannot express enough:
  - Leave ingredients for one or more artificial feeds for the baby to have during the day (see Fig. 10–19).
  - Teach the helper to mix the feed just before she gives it.
- She should teach the helper to feed the baby from a cup (see Fig. 10–20).
  - If the baby cup feeds, he is keen to suckle when the mother is at home. He gets more breast milk and keeps up the supply.
  - If the baby bottle feeds when the mother is at work, the baby may begin to lose interest in suckling at the breast, and her breast milk may decrease.
- She should express her breast milk while she is at work, to prevent engorgement and leaking, and to keep up the supply.
  - If she can take a clean screw-top jar to collect the breast milk, she can bring it back to give the baby later.
  - If she has to throw it away, it does not matter. Her breasts will make plenty more.

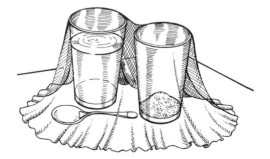

Fig. 10–19 Leave the ingredients for an artificial feed for the helper to mix up just before she feeds the baby.

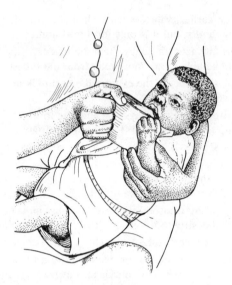

Fig. 10–20 Teach the helper to feed the baby from a cup or jug.

10.18 HELPING SINGLE MOTHERS

Single mothers have great difficulty supporting themselves and caring for their babies, especially if they are young.

Sometimes a young mother's own mother or another relative may care for the baby, and they may need help to do so. There may be no relative who can help, and the mother may need support from other sources. Try to find out what is available in your area, and help the mother to get it. Economic help is usually the most urgent.

Breastfeeding is still the best way to feed the baby, if there is a way to do it. It is often best if the mother and baby can stay together and be supported as a family. Then she can breastfeed at least partially. If another relative takes over the care of the baby, such as an aunt or grandmother, she may be able to relactate to breastfeed him.

If no one is able to breastfeed the baby, artificial feeding by cup is necessary.

How you can help

- Help the mother to find the economic support that she needs, such as a job or joining an income-generating group. Put her in touch with other services which may be able to help, for example with child care.
- Visit the mother, and the person who is caring for the baby. Discuss how to feed the baby, and how to give at least some breastmilk if possible.
- If the baby must have artificial feeds, help the mother or carer to find the cheapest suitable type. Make sure that they understand how to prepare feeds, how much to give the baby, and how to feed him by cup.
- Follow up the mother, baby, and carer as often as you can to make sure that the baby is growing and is well cared for.
- If the baby is not fully breastfed, you may want to advise them to start giving weaning foods when the baby is 4 months old.

10.19 WHEN THE BABY'S MOTHER IS DEAD

- Visit the family to find out what help they need— examine and weigh the baby often.
- Suggest that an aunt, a grandmother, or another woman breastfeeds the baby, especially if he is less than 6 months old. Many women can produce breast milk again if they believe that they can and if the baby suckles often.
- If the person who cares for the baby cannot breastfeed him, help her to find the cheapest good sort of artificial milk and show her how to prepare it and feed it by cup.

10.20 THE PROBLEM OF 'NOT ENOUGH MILK'

Many mothers decide to feed their babies artificially— either partially or completely—because they believe that they do not have enough breast milk.

Almost every woman can produce enough milk for her baby:

- if she wants to;
- if the baby suckles in a good position;
- if the baby suckles frequently.

Many women can produce enough for two babies. Very few women (perhaps less than 1 per cent) really cannot produce enough milk.

Undernourished mothers

Mothers who are undernourished can produce breast milk, provided the baby continues to suckle (see Section 18.5). Their breast milk is still the best food for their babies. Sometimes babies of severely malnourished mothers may stop growing on breast milk alone after 3–4 months of age.

- Try to improve the mother's diet, during pregnancy and after the baby is born.
- Advise the mother to breastfeed frequently.
- Discourage her from giving artificial feeds, especially by bottle.

If the baby is not growing:

- Continue breastfeeding and give supplementary artificial feeds by cup.
- If the baby is 4 months of age, his mother can start giving him weaning foods instead of artificial milk feeds.

Why a mother may think that she does not have enough milk

The baby may seem unsatisfied. For example, he may:

- cry more than the family expects;
- want to feed more often than the mother expects;
- take a long time over feeds;
- fuss at the breast, or refuse to feed;
- suck his fingers;
- take bottle feeds and sleep longer.

The mother may worry, for example, that:

- Her breasts are not full as soon as the baby is born.
- Her breasts feel softer than they did before.
- Breast milk does not drip out as it did before.

What you can do

1. *Decide if the baby is getting enough milk.*
   - Check the baby's weight to see if he is growing (Fig. 10–21). If he is growing at a healthy rate, he is getting enough breast milk. Up to the age of 6 months, a baby should gain at least 500 g each month.
   - Ask the mother if she knows how many times the baby passes urine in a day, or how many wet nappies he has. If the baby passes urine more than six times a day, he is getting enough breast milk (provided he is not having other drinks as well).

If he is not gaining weight or not passing enough urine:

2. *Make sure that the baby is not sick.* A baby who is not growing at a normal rate may be sick.
   - Examine the baby and, if you are worried, ask a more experienced health worker to see him.

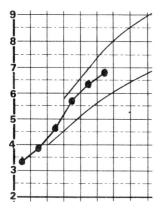

This baby is growing at a healthy rate – he is getting enough breast milk

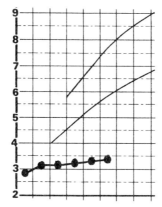

This baby is not growing at a healthy rate – he is not getting enough breast milk

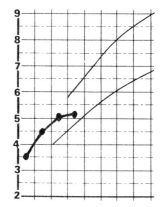

This baby's growth is slowing down – he is not getting enough breast milk

Fig. 10–21 Check the baby's weight to see if he is getting enough breast milk (for more about growth and weighing see Chapter 14).

3. *Check the mother's breastfeeding technique.*
   - The baby may be suckling in a poor position—help the mother to improve it.
   - The baby may not be suckling often enough, for example the mother may be away from the baby by day; or she may not feed him at night.
     - Discuss how she can feed the baby more frequently.
     - Show her how to express breast milk to leave for the baby if she has to be away from him.
   - The baby may not be suckling for long enough at each feed—for example, the mother may be stopping the feed after only a minute or two, or the baby may be too hot and sleepy. Discuss how she can get the baby to suckle for longer. Explain that she should let him finish the first breast first, before she offers the second.
   - The baby may be having some other food or drink—for example, bottle feeds or drinks of water. Find out why. Advise her to stop giving the other feeds, and to breastfeed more. If she has to give other feeds, suggest that she gives them by cup.

4. *Support the mother and give her confidence.* The main problem may be that the mother lacks confidence. There may be no one to tell her that what she notices is normal, and that all that the baby needs is for her to hold him and let him breastfeed again.

   The baby's father or a grandmother may be there, and they may try to help. But they may also think that the mother does not have enough milk. There may be friends and shopkeepers nearby who can tell her how to bottle feed, but no one who can tell her about breastfeeding.
   - Reassure the mother about the things that worry her.
     - Help her to feel that she is doing well, and encourage her to continue breastfeeding.
     - If the baby is gaining weight at a normal rate, reassure her that the baby is getting enough milk.
   - Discuss with the family why the baby may be crying.
     - Crying does not always mean hunger.
     - The baby may need to be held and to suckle more for comfort.
   - Help the mother to find other people in the community who can give her some support—for example, a more experienced breastfeeding woman.

10.21 COMMON BREASTFEEDING PROBLEMS

Engorgement

When the milk first 'comes in' a few days after delivery, the breasts may become very full and hard. Sometimes they feel full of lumps like stones. Usually the milk flows well and, if the baby suckles often, the breasts become softer.

Sometimes the breasts become swollen and painful, and the milk does not flow well. This is called *engorgement* and it is due to too much milk and tissue fluid collecting in the breast. The nipples may be pulled tight, so that it is difficult for the baby to take the breast into his mouth.

Engorgement is most likely if there is a delay before the baby starts to breastfeed. Unrestricted breastfeeding from soon after birth, with the baby suckling in a good position, usually prevents the problem.

To treat engorgement, it is essential to remove the milk.

- Show the mother how to express some of the milk.
- Warming the breasts with warm water may help the milk to flow.
- As soon as the breasts are softer, help her to put the baby on to the breasts in a good position.

After a few days the breasts become soft, even though the milk supply continues to be plentiful. You may need to reassure the mother that she has not 'lost' her milk.

Blocked duct

Sometimes a tender swelling forms in one part of a breast. This is usually because the milk is not getting out of that part of the breast.

- Advise the mother to feed the baby frequently on the side with the swelling.
- Show the mother different positions to hold the baby in while he is suckling—for example, under her arm—to make sure that the milk is removed from all segments.
- While the baby is suckling, the mother can gently massage the swelling towards the nipple.
- She may need to express milk, gently massaging the swollen part. It may help to bathe the breast in warm water.

Mastitis

If engorgement or blocked duct continue for more than a day or two, the breast may be infected, and develop mastitis or an abscess. The breast is very tender and the mother usually feels unwell and has a fever.

- It is essential to remove the milk. If possible the baby should continue feeding. If not, help the mother to express the milk.
- It may be necessary to give an antibiotic. You may need to refer the mother to a health worker who can give an antibiotic or treat an abscess.
- The mother needs to rest. Talk to the family about giving her extra help until she recovers.
- Help the mother to build up her milk again when she is well.

There is no need for the baby to stop breastfeeding because of a breast infection. The bacteria will not make him ill, and most antibiotics are quite safe. However, if the mother is afraid to let the baby feed from the infected breast, express and discard the milk until the breast heals. Continue to feed the baby from the other breast, and let him suckle again from the infected breast as soon as possible.

Sore nipples

If a baby suckles in a poor position, the mother feels pain. There may be nothing to see, or there may be a line across the tip of the nipple at the end of the feed. If the baby continues to suckle in a poor position, he may damage the nipple skin and cause fissures (cracks).

- Help the mother to get the baby to suckle in a better position.

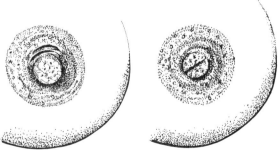

Fissure around the base of the nipple

Fissure across the tip of the nipple

Fig. 10–22 Two kinds of nipple fissure.

- After the baby has fed, she can leave a drop of hindmilk on the nipple, to help healing.
- It may help to dry the nipples in the air.

The pain usually stops as soon as the suckling position improves. If there is a fissure, it heals quickly. It is not usually necessary to rest the breast. Creams and ointments do not help. Some of them make sore nipples worse.

Sore nipples which continue for a long time, or sharp pain which goes deep into the breast may be due to *thrush* infection. The baby may have white patches of thrush in his mouth. If you think that this is the problem, treat the mother and baby with:

- *gentian violet paint*, to both the baby's mouth and mother's nipples;

or

- *nystatin drops* in the baby's mouth, and *nystatin cream* on the nipples.

Flat nipples

Many women have nipples which look 'flat'. But the shape of the nipple does not matter—so long as the baby can stretch the part of the breast beneath the areola to form a 'teat'.

Ask the mother to test the nipple to see if it stretches out easily (see Fig. 10–24). If the nipple does not stretch out easily, the baby may need extra help at first to take enough of the breast into his mouth. Nipples often improve soon after the baby is born, and once he has suckled a few times.

- Reassure the mother that she can breastfeed and that, if she persists, the baby will learn.
- Show her how to get the baby to take enough of the breast into his mouth.
- She can express some milk to soften the breasts, so that they are easier for the baby to take.
- If necessary, she can feed the baby on expressed milk from a cup for a few days until he suckles better.
- Encourage her to go on trying. See her again every day until the baby is suckling well.

10.22 BABIES WITH SPECIAL NEEDS

Low birth weight (LBW) babies

Breast milk is especially important for very small babies. Many can suckle when they weigh about 1600 g

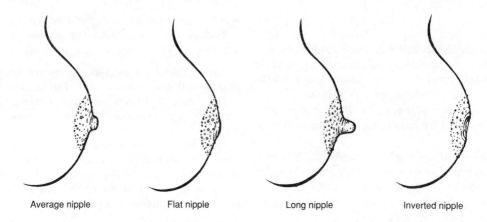

Average nipple   Flat nipple   Long nipple   Inverted nipple

Fig. 10–23 Some different nipple shapes.

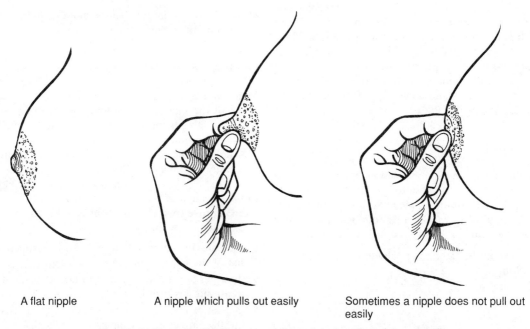

A flat nipple   A nipple which pulls out easily   Sometimes a nipple does not pull out easily

Fig. 10–24 Testing a flat nipple to see if it pulls out easily to form a 'teat'.

(or about 32–34 weeks gestational age); but they may not be able to suckle strongly enough to get all that they need until they weigh about 1800 g (or about 36–37 weeks gestational age, see also Section 16.6).

If a mother delivers prematurely, her breast milk contains more protein than the milk of a mother who delivers at term. Low birth weight (LBW) babies need this extra protein.

- Let the mother be with the baby as much as possible, and let her do all that she can for him.

- It is important to keep the baby warm. A good way to do this, when the baby is well enough, is for the mother to hold the baby next to her body between her breasts (the 'kangaroo method'; see Fig. 10–25).

- Let the baby suckle as soon as he is able. This helps

the mother to produce breast milk, and it helps the milk to flow.

- Until the baby can suckle enough, the mother should express her breast milk and feed it to the baby by cup (see Section 10.14), or by tube.
- LBW babies need to start feeding in the first 6 hours. A mother who has breastfed a previous baby may be able to express colostrum on the first day. If it is a first baby, she may not be able to express much until the second day. The baby may need breast milk from another mother for the first few feeds.
- To keep up her milk supply, the mother needs to express as often as the baby needs to feed—that is, every 2–3 hours by day and night, and at least eight times in 24 hours. If she expresses only once or twice a day, her supply will decrease.

If the baby has to be in hospital, the mother should stay with him. Sometimes this is not possible, and the mother has to try to express her breast milk at home, and take it to her baby. It is very hard to do this, and a mother needs a lot of support and encouragement.

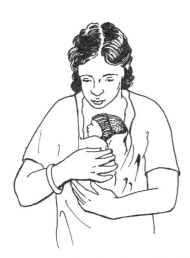

Fig. 10–25 Mothers can keep low birth weight babies warm with their own bodies.

Twins

Most mothers can provide enough breast milk for twins. If the twins are low birth weight, their mother may need to express breast milk for them until they can breastfeed.

Success depends on her family helping her to look after the twins and the rest of her family. Talk to the

Table 10.1.   Volume of milk for LBW babies

Day 1	60 ml/kg body weight	
Day 2	80 ml/kg body weight	
Day 3	100 ml/kg body weight	Divide volume into eight feeds and give one feed every 3 hours
Days 4–7	Increase total by 20 ml/kg each day	
Day 8 onwards	Give 200 ml/kg daily, until baby weighs 1800 g, is breastfeeding, and gaining weight	

With small-for-dates babies, who are not premature, increase the total up to 280 ml/kg/day (see Section 16.7).

family, and explain that the babies will be healthier if they breastfeed. Discuss how the family can help the mother.

Handicapped babies

Mentally handicapped babies need to breastfeed. They may take longer to learn to suckle well, and their mothers may need to express milk and cup feed for a longer time. Give extra help and support to these families.

Sick babies

Sick babies recover sooner if they continue to breastfeed, especially babies with diarrhoea (see Sections 13.3 and 13.4). It is not necessary to stop breastfeeding

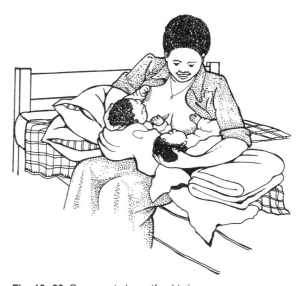

Fig. 10–26 One way to breastfeed twins.

to 'rest' the baby's gut. Sick babies may continue to breastfeed as much or sometimes more than before.

If the baby is able to suckle:

- The mother should offer the breast more often.

If the baby is too weak to suckle:

- Admit the mother and baby to hospital or health centre.
- Show the mother how to express her breast milk. If necessary, give the expressed breast milk (EBM) by tube. When the baby can drink, give the EBM by cup or spoon.
- The mother should express every 3 hours, day and night, to keep up her breast milk supply.
- When the baby can suckle again, his mother can put him to the breast. She should feed the baby more often for a few days until her milk supply builds up, and the baby has regained any weight lost during the illness.

10.23 WHEN THE MOTHER IS SICK

It is not usually necessary for a baby to stop breastfeeding because his mother is sick. The risks of bottle feeding are usually greater than the risks of continuing to breastfeed. Breast milk contains antibodies which protect a baby against most infections that a mother may have.

If a sick woman stops breastfeeding, first her breasts become engorged; then her milk dries up.

Only a very few drugs can harm a baby through the breast milk—for example, anticancer drugs. Most commonly used antibiotics and other drugs are safe.

The main difficulty is that the mother may be too weak to hold and care for the baby for a time. If possible, keep the baby with the mother:

- Continue breastfeeding normally.
- Let somebody stay with her—for example, a relative—to help care for the baby.

If it is not possible to keep the baby with the mother, let her express her breast milk. Let someone else give the milk to the baby by cup. If her EBM cannot be given to her baby, she may have to throw it away. But it helps if she can express to keep up her supply.

If she cannot express her breast milk, or her EBM cannot be given to her baby:

- Let someone feed the baby on EBM from another mother, or on artificial milk by cup.

- Let the baby start to suckle again as soon as the mother is well enough.
- Help the mother to build up her supply again (see Section 10.15).

If the mother has a Caesarean section, the baby can start to suckle as soon as the mother is conscious after the operation—usually in 4–6 hours. The baby can wait until then—he does not need any other drink. Help the mother to find a comfortable position for breastfeeding—lying either on her back or on her side until she is able to sit up.

If she has an ordinary illness such as a cold, or fever, continue breastfeeding as normally as possible.

If she has a chronic illness such as TB or leprosy, breastfeed normally, and make sure that the baby is followed up for signs of infection, and treated if necessary.

If the mother is HIV + (AIDS). Most babies who get AIDS are infected before they are born. The risk of getting AIDS through breast milk is low. In most situations the risk of feeding the baby artificially is greater than the risk of breastfeeding.

Women who are HIV + should breastfeed normally. If babies have EBM from another mother, and there is a possibility of HIV infection, pasteurize or boil the EBM. The HIV virus is easily killed by heat, and pasteurized or boiled EBM is safe.

If she is mentally ill, someone else may have to help her to care for the baby. They can take the baby to her to breastfeed.

If she is in hospital, admit the baby with the mother if possible, and care for them together. It may help if another relative stays with the mother to help care for the baby.

10.24 BREASTFEEDING AND A NEW PREGNANCY

Many women became very worried and stop breastfeeding if they find that they are pregnant again. They believe that breastfeeding harms a child if another baby is on the way.

Some children do become ill and stop growing when their mother becomes pregnant. Some become severely malnourished. But it is usually because they stop breastfeeding suddenly and lose the nutrients from breast milk. Often they are already undernourished before the pregnancy because they have insufficient weaning food, and they do not get enough extra nutrients to replace the breast milk.

Some mothers find that their breasts become tender with a new pregnancy and that breastfeeding is uncomfortable.

Some notice that the supply of breast milk seems to decrease. Towards the end of pregnancy, breast milk becomes more like colostrum again, to be ready for the new baby.

Medically it is not harmful to breastfeed during a new pregnancy. It does not harm either the breastfeeding child, or the unborn baby. Some mothers breastfeed for the whole pregnancy, and then breastfeed both babies together. It does not harm the mother, though she needs to eat enough to provide nutrients and energy for both the babies and herself.

What can you do

Discuss family planning with all parents soon after a baby is born.

- Explain the dangers of having another baby too soon, and the advantages of a well-spaced family.
- Explain how breastfeeding can help to protect against pregnancy, and explain when this protection is not reliable.
- Make sure that mothers get the family planning advice that they need.

If a breastfeeding mother does become pregnant:

- Explain that it is safe to continue breastfeeding, but that she should eat more.

- Discuss why it is dangerous for the child to stop breastfeeding suddenly.
  - Encourage her to continue breastfeeding until the baby is at least 6 months old.
  - If she wants to stop breastfeeding, encourage her to stop gradually and to give the child plenty of other food (see Section 11.16).

10.25 PROMOTING BREASTFEEDING IN THE COMMUNITY

The attitudes of fathers, relatives, friends, and the community can all affect women's decisions about breastfeeding. They may be helpful or unhelpful.

In some places, people think that breastfeeding is normal and important, and most mothers breastfeed successfully. In these places, it is important to *protect* breastfeeding. Make sure that people continue to value it.

In other places people do not understand the importance of breastfeeding, or they may disapprove of breastfeeding in public places. Then it is more difficult for women to breastfeed successfully. Children may not see that breastfeeding is natural and easy, and they are less likely to breastfeed their own children. In these places, it is necessary to *promote* breastfeeding, to encourage people to value it more.

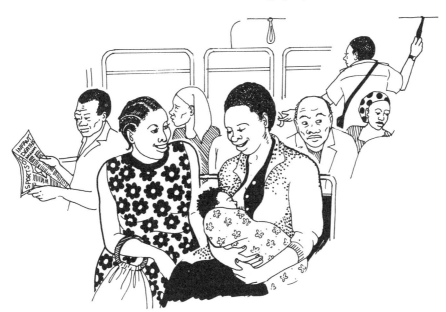

Fig. 10–27 Do people in your community disapprove of breastfeeding in public?

10.26 UNDERSTANDING THE LOCAL SITUATION

Before you can decide how to protect and promote breastfeeding in you area, you need to learn about the local situation—you need to understand both practices and attitudes. First form a general impression. Later, you may think of doing a small survey.

- *Talk to mothers* about how they feed their babies, and their reasons for what they do.
- *Talk to other family members* including fathers, grandmothers, and grandfathers.
- *Talk to other people in the community*, including adolescent boys and girls and people who employ women workers, about their attitudes to breastfeeding.
- *Talk to local traditional birth attendants (TBAs)* and make friends with them. Ask them to explain to you how they help mothers to breastfeed.
- *Visit the hospitals* where mothers in your area deliver their babies. Make friends with the ward staff. Learn their views about breastfeeding, and their practices. You will probably find that they generally favour breastfeeding, and that some of their practices are good, while some are harmful.

    Be very polite and do not criticize. You may not be in a position to influence what happens in hospitals, but it is helpful to understand. Try to share your ideas with the staff, if they are interested.

Try to answer these questions:

- How many mothers breastfeed exclusively for 6 months?
- How many mothers breastfeed for more than 1 and 2 years?
- Do mothers have their babies to hold as soon as they are born?
- Are babies separated from their mothers soon after birth?
- How soon do mothers let babies start to suckle?
- Do mothers like babies to have colostrum?
- How many mothers give formula, glucose, or ritual feeds before they start breastfeeding?
- How many mothers never start to breastfeed?
- How many mothers both breastfeed and bottle feed—especially before the baby is 6 months old
- What are the common reasons for giving bottles or for stopping breastfeeding before 2 years of age?
- How many mothers say that they do not have enough milk?

- What are the common ages for stopping breastfeeding?
- Who influences decisions about breastfeeding?
- What are the common breastfeeding problems?

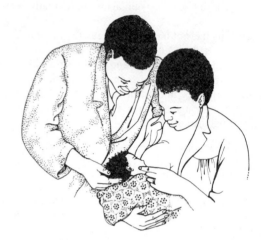

Fig. 10–28 The attitudes of fathers and other family members affect women's success with breastfeeding.

10.27 HOW BELIEFS AND ATTITUDES AFFECT BREASTFEEDING

In many places, people regard breastfeeding as normal, but they have other ideas that can interfere with it. For example:

- *Colostrum is not good for a baby.* This belief may delay the start of breastfeeding, and can lead to many problems.
- *The baby needs more than breast milk.* Sometimes people approve of breastfeeding, but believe that it is not enough by itself, and that babies need something else as well. The baby may get only a small amount of the other food or drink, and may take plenty of breast milk as well. However, he is more likely to get diarrhoea. If a baby cries more than the family expects, they may decide that the baby is hungry, and give some bottle feeds.
- *Breast milk may go bad.* In some communities, people believe that if a mother is ill or if she has not breastfed for a few days, her milk is not good. Or that, if a child becomes ill, it is a sign that the mother's milk is not good. Babies may stop breastfeeding unnecessarily.
- *Breast milk in one breast is bad.* In some communities, many mothers feed babies from one breast only,

because they believe that the milk in the other breast is 'bad' for the baby. Sometimes there was a problem with one breast for example, engorgement or breast infection.

- *Babies should not breastfeed if the mother is pregnant.* In some communities, this is the commonest reason for stopping breastfeeding.

- *Babies should not breastfeed if they are sick or if the mother is sick.* Sometimes babies stop breastfeeding because of minor illnesses.

- *Bottle feeds make a baby fatter and healthier.* Some mothers give babies bottle feeds as well to make them fatter, because they believe that this is healthier. Other members of the family may also encourage the mother to give artificial feeds as well as breastfeeds, to make the baby fat and more healthy.

Some women prefer to bottle feed. They may believe that bottle feeding is better than breastfeeding, or they may simply not want to breastfeed.

- *Following fashion.* Bottle feeding may seem to be the fashionable and prestigious way to feed a baby. Glamorous or important people may bottle feed. A woman's friends may all bottle feed, and for her it may be the 'normal' thing to do.

- *Fear of becoming unattractive to men.* Some women fear that if they breastfeed they will lose their figures, that their breasts will become long, and that men will not find them attractive. This may be a real fear for woman who depend on their bodies or on men for money.

- *Fear of being 'tied'.* Some women do not want to have to stay with the baby all the time to breastfeed—they want to be free to go out with their friends, or to work.

- *Shyness about feeding in public.* Some women are now embarrassed to breastfeed in public places.

What you can do

- Praise mothers who breastfeed.
- Set an example—breastfeed yourself, and do not use a feeding bottle. Make sure that people see how you manage to work and breastfeed.
- Discuss with families—including men—the advantages of breastfeeding, and the importance of exclusive breastfeeding. Discuss how men can encourage women to breastfeed.
- Talk to families about babies crying.
  - It is normal for breastfed babies to want to feed more often than artificially fed babies.

- When a baby who cries a lot is given a bottle feed, she may sleep longer and appear to be more satisfied. This is because artificial milks are more difficult to digest, and stay in the baby's stomach for longer.
  - Many babies continue to cry just as much when they are given a bottle feed. All that many babies need is to be held more and to suckle more. If there really is too little milk, this will increase it.
- Discuss the fatness of babies—that babies can be overweight and it is not a sign of better health.
- Talk to women's groups and ask them to encourage breastfeeding.
  - They can *promote* breastfeeding in the community.
  - They can tell families and young people about its advantages, and encourage women to breastfeed exclusively for 6 months.
  - They can *support* breastfeeding mothers and their families.
- Give up-to-date information to other community workers so that they can promote breastfeeding.
- Discuss with TBAs how they can support breastfeeding. Show them respect, and praise them for their helpful practices. They may be willing to change their unhelpful practices, if you explain the reasons.
- Talk to employers about the importance of breastfeeding. Explain that they can promote breastfeeding if they give their women workers 3–4 months paid maternity leave, nursing breaks, flexible working hours, and day care centres. Women who have healthy babies worry less and may be better employees.
- Include breastfeeding in sex education for boys and girls.
  - Encourage boys to admire women who breastfeed.
  - Explain that a woman who breastfeeds need not lose her figure.
  - Encourage girls not to have a baby before they are ready to accept the demands that a baby makes on its mother.
  - Point out that breastfeeding a healthy baby is much less trouble than bottle feeding and a sick baby.
- Ask famous and important people to support breastfeeding, so that it becomes fashionable.

10.28 COMMERCIAL PROMOTION OF FORMULA

Advertisements for baby formula encourage bottle feeding. These advertisements often suggest to women that they may not have enough milk, and this makes them lose confidence. For example, advertisements say things like

'*Breast milk is best but if you cannot breastfeed or if you do not have enough milk, then our formula is the best substitute.*'

Advertisements make people believe that formula is really very good and that, if they have a problem and if they have to use formula, then their baby will be perfectly healthy. This makes it easy for a young woman to decide that it is safe to use formula. Pretty pictures of babies on tins of formula also encourage women to buy it.

Some manufacturers give free samples of formula to hospitals or to midwives or even to mothers. If a mother is given a free sample, she is more likely to fail to breastfeed.

In 1981, the World Health Organization produced the 'International Code of Marketing of Breast-milk Substitutes'. The aim of the code is to control the promotion and advertising of formula. Many countries have now adopted similar codes. Some have made promotion of formula illegal.

What you can do

- Do not have advertisements or calendars or other materials which show baby milks, bottles, or teats in your office, clinic, or ward.

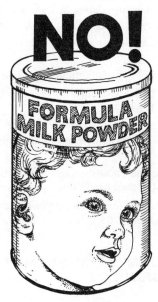

Fig. 10–29 The 'Code' does not allow manufacturers to put pictures of healthy babies on tins of formula.

- Do not have tins of baby milk—even empty tins for another purpose—where families can see them.
- Do not give out free samples of formula to breastfeeding mothers. If you have any, keep them for babies whose mothers are dead or absent, when there is nobody who can breastfeed the baby.
- Do not give out materials on baby care prepared by formula manufacturers.
- If a manufacturer's representative tries to give you free samples, refuse. Explain that you are trying to help mothers to breastfeed, and that formula samples interfere.
- If you see an advertisement for formula, or a calendar from a formula manufacturer on the walls of a health centre or hospital, or a health worker's office, ask the staff to take it down. Explain that advertisements encourage bottle feeding.
- Try to get breastfeeding posters to replace advertisements, so that people have something attractive to put on the wall.
- Learn about the WHO Code, and find out if your country has a similar code, or if there is a group in your country who is working on a code. Tell them if you see any advertisements which the code does not allow. Or, write to IBFAN at one of the addresses in Appendix 6.

THINGS TO DO

Finding out about local practices

1. Help trainees to do a small survey of breastfeeding in the area among families with children aged 0–2 years old.

   a. Find out what percentage of mothers breastfeed exclusively until the babies are 6 months old.

   b. Find out what percentage of mothers give their babies artificial feeds, and how many use feeding bottles, what age they started, and why they decided to do so. How many breastfeed partially? How many mothers give other drinks, such as tea or juice or dilute cereal, before the age of 6 months?

   c. What age do most babies stop breastfeeding? What makes mothers decide to stop?

2. Ask trainees to find out about traditional breastfeeding practices in the area. For example:

   - How long is it traditional to breastfeed for?
   - Do mothers like the baby to have colostrum?

- How long do mothers wait before they start to breastfeed?
- Who helps mothers when they start to breastfeed?
- Are there special foods and drinks for a breastfeeding mother?
- How do they help her?
- Do some people believe that breast milk sometimes 'goes bad' and makes a baby sick?
- Do people believe that the milk is safe if the mother has not fed the baby for a day or two?
- Do mothers breastfeed when another pregnancy has started?
- Is it safe for a woman to breastfeed another woman's baby?
- Does anybody do this? Who can do it? Who cannot?

Discuss which practices are *helpful*, which are *harmful*, and which are *harmless*.

3. Ask trainees to talk to some grandmothers and ask them how they fed their babies. Ask them how things have changed.

4. Ask some TBAs to tell trainees what they think about breastfeeding.

   a. What do they do to help mothers to breastfeed?

   b. What can happen that makes it difficult for a baby to breastfeed?

Exercise on the cost of artificial feeding

5. Ask trainees to visit shops and to talk to shopkeepers to find out which artificial milks and feeding bottles are available in your area.

   a. Which brands of formula are common?

   b. How much does one tin of formula cost?

   c. What other kinds of artificial milk do mothers use for babies?

   d. How much do they cost?

6. Work out how much it costs to feed a baby artificially with different brands of formula. Assume that an average baby needs about 40 half-kilogram tins of formula for the first 6 months of life.

   a. Calculate the *average* cost per month for this amount of formula of different brands. (The actual amount per month is less at the beginning and more as the baby gets bigger.)

   b. Find out how much some people in ordinary jobs earn—for example, the minimum wage, agricultural labourer's wage, a domestic worker's wage.

   c. What proportion of some ordinary wages would it cost to feed a baby on formula?

7. Work out how much it costs to feed a baby for 6 months on other available milks.

   a. *Full cream milk powder*
   Assume that the average baby needs 30 half kilogram tins of full cream milk powder for 6 months. (The amount is less than for formula, because you have to add sugar.)

   b. *Fresh cow's milk*. Assume that an average baby needs 135 litres of milk for the first 6 months of life.

Demonstration

8. Demonstrate how to help a mother put her baby to the breast in a good position. (A doll is useful for this demonstration. If necessary make one out of a plastic bag, paper, or old cloth. You can use a large fruit or vegetable for the head.)

9. Demonstrate how to express breast milk.

   a. Ask trainees to practise the movement on their cheeks or the soft part of their forearm. It may help to draw a 'nipple' on the forearm.

   b. Ask females to practise on their breasts privately later.

10. Look in the market and in people's homes to see if you can find small cups or other utensils that would be useful to feed a small baby.

    a. Demonstrate to trainees how to use these to give EBM to a baby.

    b. Try giving a baby a drink of expressed breast milk from a small cup. Make sure the cup is very clean.

Role play

11. Ask trainees to role play helping mothers in some of the common situations that occur in your area. For example:

    a. a mother of a healthy 3-month-old baby who thinks that she doesn't have enough breast milk, because the baby seems to cry a lot;

    b. a mother who is giving her healthy 2-month-old baby two bottle feeds a day in addition to breastfeeds, because she wants to make the baby fatter;

    c. a nurse who has to start work again after maternity leave;

    d. a mother whose 2-month-old baby has diarrhoea and is not growing well.

12. Ask trainees to role play helping these mothers to put the baby to the breast in a good position:

    a. a young mother who has just had her first baby;

b. a mother who has sore nipples, and whose baby is 1 month old.

Hospital or clinic visit

13. Arrange for trainees to watch some mothers breast-feeding in maternity wards, health centres, or children's wards. They should ask each mother how the baby is and how breastfeeding is going for her. They should watch how the mother feeds the baby, and observe the baby's suckling position.

    Discuss with trainees how the baby is suckling, and point out the signs of a good position. If you think the position could be improved, discuss this with the trainees. (But do not interfere with the mother unless she says that she has a problem.)

14. Arrange for trainees to talk to women in an antenatal clinic to ask them how they plan to feed the baby, and what they feel about breastfeeding.

15. When trainees visit the maternity ward, ask them to observe the routine practices, and to ask the ward staff about practices.

    a. Do the babies have early contact? rooming in? unrestricted feeding?

    b. Do the babies have feeds of formula or glucose? from bottles?

    c. How are low birth weight babies fed?

    d. Do mothers of LBW babies stay in hospital with their babies?

    e. Are there any advertisements for formula or free samples?

16. When trainees visit health centres, clinics, or offices, do they see formula advertisements or free gifts from formula manufacturers?

USEFUL PUBLICATIONS

IBFAN (1990). *Protecting infant health: a health worker's guide to the international code of marketing of breast milk substitutes.* IBFAN, Penang, Malaysia.

Royal College of Midwives (1990). *Successful breastfeeding.* Churchill Livingstone, Edinburgh.

Savage King, F. (1992). *Helping mothers to breastfeed* (revised). AMREF, Nairobi.

WHO/UNICEF (1989). *Promoting, protecting and supporting breastfeeding: the special role of the maternity services. A WHO/UNICEF joint statement.* WHO, Geneva.

11   Starting other foods

11.1 WEANING

Weaning is the process of introducing foods other than breast milk to a child, and gradually increasing the amount, so that eventually the child gets enough energy and nutrients from ordinary family food.

The three stages of weaning

Stage 1. The baby gets almost all nutrients from breast milk but starts other foods. These first foods must be specially prepared so that they are easy for the baby to eat. They are called '*weaning foods*'.

Stage 2. The child continues to get the same amount of breast milk and he gets increasing amounts of other food. The type of food slowly changes from soft weaning foods to the usual family foods.

Stage 3. The child takes slowly decreasing amounts of breast milk and eats increasing amounts of family foods. Weaning is completed when a child gets all her nutrients from family foods.

11.2 WHEN TO START OTHER FOODS

The ages at which children start each stage of weaning varies. Most children should start having other foods at

about 6 months of age. Stage 1 becomes Stage 2 after about a month. Stage 3 should begin and end as late as possible. Many children start to take less breast milk at about 12 months of age and finish breastfeeding completely when they are 2–3 years old or more.

Why 6 months is the best time to start giving other food

By the age of 6 months, many children cannot get enough energy and nutrients from breast milk alone. They have grown to two or more times the size that they were when they were born. They are still growing fast, and becoming more active.

Most babies now *need more energy and nutrients* than breast milk alone can provide. They need other food as well. Some babies may outgrow the supply of breast milk and begin to need other food at about 4 or 5 months.

For some babies, breast milk may be sufficient for more than 6 months. However, it is important that they start other foods at around this time, because after the age of 9 months they are less willing to try new tastes and new foods.

By the age of 6 months a baby's gut can digest most of the foods that the rest of the family eats. Before the age of 4 months, a baby cannot easily digest other foods, for example, starch.

Why it is better not to start weaning foods too early

If a mother gives food before it is necessary:

- The baby is more likely to get diarrhoea, because weaning food is often contaminated.
- The baby may suckle less at the breast, and so the supply of breast milk decreases.
- Because the baby suckles less, the mother is more likely to become fertile again, so she may become pregnant before she is ready.

It is not necessary to give fruit juice or other drinks or water before a baby starts weaning foods. Breast

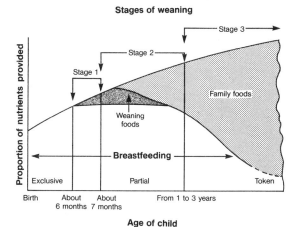

Fig. 11–1 The stages of weaning.

milk normally contains enough vitamins and enough water, even in a hot climate. Even drinks of water reduce the amount of breast milk that a baby takes.

Why it is better not to start weaning foods too late

If a mother does not start to give food until after the age of 6 months:

- The baby may stop gaining weight at a healthy rate, and may become underweight.
- It becomes more difficult to persuade the baby to start eating solid foods at a later age. Babies who do not start to eat other food may want nothing but breast milk or other milk or liquid foods after the age of 1 year. This can cause malnutrition.

11.3 HOW BABIES SHOW THAT THEY ARE READY TO START OTHER FOOD

At about the age of 6 months most babies show from their behaviour that they are ready to start other foods.

- They sit up and reach out for food which their mothers are eating.
- They like to put things into their mouths to feel and taste them—even inedible things like leaves and soil.
- They are interested in new tastes and they are willing to try new food.
- They are able to take food into their mouths and swallow it more easily. Younger babies push solid food out of their mouths with their tongues.
- They may have one or two teeth and they start to chew. Babies often like to try to chew on something hard.
- They may seem really hungry—even though they get plenty of breast milk. (This is *not* the same as a younger baby less than 4 months old crying for comfort, or being unsatisfied with breastfeeding because of inefficient suckling.)

We can also tell that a baby needs more food if his growth slows down, even though he breastfeeds fully and has no infection.

When children become able to chew

A baby starts to chew at about 6 months of age, but she cannot chew effectively at this age.

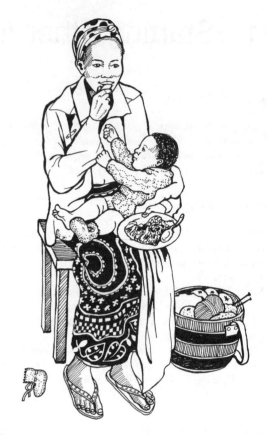

Fig. 11–2 At about 6 months of age a baby sits up and reaches out for food which his mother is eating.

From about 6–9 months of age, food must be semi-liquid or mashed, so that it is soft enough for the baby to eat. From about 9–12 months, a child can chew well enough to eat food which is cut into small pieces. By the time a child is 2 years old, she has all her teeth, and can chew well enough to eat most family food.

11.4 WHY WEANING IS A DANGEROUS TIME

The weaning time—that is, from about 6 months to 3 years—is dangerous for children.

A child may not get enough energy and nutrients if:

- He does not get enough weaning or family food.
- He stops breastfeeding much before the age of 2 years (for example, because his mother is pregnant again).

Children get many infections because:

- Weaning foods and drinks may contain micro-organisms which cause diarrhoea.
- Children crawl about and explore and may touch dirty things and put them in their mouths. They may get diarrhoea or worms as a result.
- They meet more people and other children who may be carrying infections.
- They have lost the immunity which they got from their mothers, but they have not yet fully built up their own immunity.

If they are to grow and remain healthy, children need special care during weaning, to make sure that they eat enough and to prevent and treat infections.

Why children may not get enough energy and nutrients from weaning food

- *Children may not eat often enough.* Some children eat only once or twice a day. Children cannot eat enough in only one or two meals.

- *The food may not contain enough energy or nutrients.* The foods which many families give to young children (especially low-cost weaning foods) have a low concentration of energy and nutrients.

- *Children may not eat enough at each meal.* A poor family may not be able to give enough food at each meal. Young children eat more slowly than older children or adults. If they eat from the same dish as the family, they may only eat a little before all the food is finished.

- *Children may eat little because they are sick.* Infections reduce a child's appetite. Families may not know how to encourage sick children to eat.

11.5 WEANING FOODS

One way in which you can help families with young children is to discuss with them how to wean a child safely, how to prepare good home-made weaning foods, and how to feed a child often enough.

Good weaning foods need to be:
- rich in energy and nutrients;
- clean and safe;
- soft and easy to eat;
- easy for a family to obtain;
- easy to prepare.

It is difficult to achieve all these things together. Foods which are rich in energy and nutrients are often expensive and difficult for families to obtain. Making foods soft and easy for a baby to eat takes time and fuel and may need special utensils.

The children who are most at risk of undernutrition are from poor families, who cannot buy expensive foods. These families may find it difficult to buy enough of any kind of food or fuel or special utensils. They may also be very busy and have little time to prepare special foods several times a day.

Try to find out how a family can most easily prepare good weaning foods from local low-cost foods. Notice how families of healthy children prepare weaning foods—this may give you ideas which you can pass on to other families.

11.6 USING STAPLES FOR WEANING FOODS

The first food that a baby eats is usually a soft or semi-liquid food made from a starchy staple food. If the food is made from a flour we call it a '*porridge*'. The flour may be a cereal flour (such as maize), or a root flour (such as cassava). If the food is made of mashed starchy roots, such as cassava or potato, we call it a '*pap*'.

Porridges and paps are important weaning foods because they are:

- liked by most children;
- soft and easy for a baby to swallow;
- easy to obtain;
- cheap;
- easy to prepare.

But plain porridges and paps are not enough by themselves because they are:

- *not* rich in energy;
- *not* rich in some nutrients.

Why plain porridges and paps are not rich in energy and nutrients

- *The staple may not contain enough of some important nutrients.* For example, roots contain very little protein. Cereals contain more protein, but they may lack some essential amino acids. Most cereals contain little or no vitamin A or C.

- *Porridge may be cooked with a lot of water.* When starch is cooked in water, the starch granules absorb a lot of the water and swell up (see Section 2.1). The swollen granules stick together, which makes the porridge thick and sticky. As the porridge cools, it becomes thicker and stickier, and difficult for a baby to eat. To make the porridge thin and semi-liquid, and easy for a baby to eat, families add a lot of water during cooking. They may add more as the porridge cools.

Families are less likely to add water to root staples, bananas, or plantains, so paps do not usually contain as much water as cereal porridges.

11.7 THE PROBLEM OF BULKY FOODS

You can look at the effects of cooking starch in water in two ways:

1. Adding water makes the food *bigger*, or *bulky*, so that a person has to eat a larger volume of the food to get the energy and nutrients that he needs.
2. Adding water *dilutes* the energy and nutrients, so that each cupful of the food contains more water, and less energy and nutrients.

There is often less energy and nutrients in thin porridge than in milk. For example,

Breast milk contains about 0.75 Calories per ml.
Thin porridge contains about 0.5 Calories per ml.

An adult can eat a large volume of food at one meal. But small children have small stomachs, and it is difficult for them to eat large amounts. They cannot eat much at one meal. So if their food is bulky, they may not get enough energy and nutrients.

How starchy foods differ in their bulkiness

Different starchy foods absorb different amounts of water. Millet absorbs more than maize; maize absorbs more than rice.

Fresh starchy roots such as cassava or potato do not absorb so much water as cereal flours during cooking. However, they already contain a lot of water before they are cooked. So paps are bulky foods too. When starchy roots are baked or fried they may lose water and become less bulky.

Bread and chappatis contain less water than boiled staples. (100 g chappati = 328 kcal; 100 g bread = 240 kcal; 100 g thick maize porridge = 100 kcal.)

Boiled beans and peas are also bulky, because they contain starch which absorbs water. But beans and peas are not as bulky as most cereals or roots because they contain less starch and more protein.

11.8 HOW TO OVERCOME THE PROBLEM OF BULKY WEANING FOODS

To enable young children to get enough energy and nutrients from bulky foods, there are three things that families can do:

- *feed children often*;
- *enrich the bulky food*;
- *change the starch so the porridge is thinner*.

Feeding children often

To get enough energy and nutrients, a young child needs to eat about five small meals a day, as well as breastfeeding. Figure 11–3 explains why.

The bowl at the bottom of the picture shows the amount of thick maize porridge that a child needs to eat to get enough energy in a day if he eats nothing else. We assume that the child needs 1000 Calories per day, and that the food contains 1 Calorie per ml. So the bowl contains 1000 ml of porridge.

In the mugs on the left, the porridge is divided into three portions for a child to have three meals during the day. Each mug contains more than 330 ml (equal to more than 1.5 cups). In the cups on the right, the porridge is divided in five portions, for a child to have five meals during the day. Each cup contains 200 ml.

Look at the drawing of a child's stomach. How much porridge could it hold? You can see that the child could eat one of the 200 ml pieces, but not a 330 ml piece.

So to get enough Calories from food like thick maize porridge the child needs to eat five times a day, not three times a day.

Families may not have time, fuel, or money to cook and feed children often. Many families have few utensils, so each meal means having to wash up too. But if they prepare enough food at one time for the whole day, there is time for bacteria to breed in the food and cause diarrhoea.

However, you can suggest that the family prepares food for the child 2–3 times each day, and divides the meal into two. The child can eat the first half of the

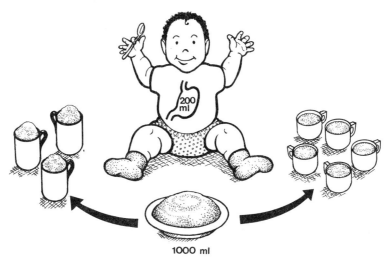

Fig. 11–3 Why small children need to eat often.

meal as soon as it is cooked, and the other half 2–3 hours later. Foods keep safely for 2–3 hours if they are covered and put in a cool place. *Or* the family can give the child a snack between meals which does not need to be freshly cooked (for example, a banana or some bread). *Or* you can suggest that the family prepares fermented porridges which keep longer (see below).

Enriching the bulky food

To enrich a bulky food means to add food which is energy-rich or food which is nutrient-rich, or both. Porridge or pap which has energy-rich or nutrient-rich food added to it is called *enriched porridge* or *enriched pap*.

Adding oil or fat

For example, margarine, butter, ghee, or oil may be added. It is only necessary to add a small amount such as one spoonful to a child's meal. Add oil to the staple before cooking to prevent the food tasting oily.

Adding fat or oil to a bulky food increases the energy concentration of the food in two ways:

1. The oil contains many Calories, so it adds energy to the food without increasing its volume.
2. The oil makes thick porridge softer and easier to eat, so it is not necessary to add so much water.

Frying food. Another way in which families can add oil is to *fry* the food. Many children like potatoes or cassava or left-over stiff porridge or rice fried in oil. Cooking food in oil instead of in water, makes two things happen:

1. The heat drives some water out of the food, so that it becomes less bulky.
2. Some of the oil enters the food and so increases the energy concentration of the food.

Adding a protein-rich food

For example:

- Add mashed beans, peas, or lentils.
- Add egg. Children can eat eggs when they are 6 months old. Mix raw egg into porridge when it is almost cooked, and cook for 3 minutes.
- Add mashed fish to a pap.
- Mix pounded dried fish with cereal or root flour and cook together.
- Mix together cereal and bean flours and use the mixture to make porridge. A good mixture is 2–3 parts cereal flour to 1 part legume.

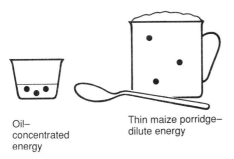

Oil-
concentrated
energy

Thin maize porridge-
dilute energy

Fig. 11–4 Energy concentration of oil and thin porridge (one dot = 100 kcal).

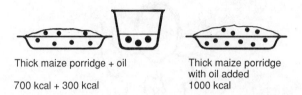

Thick maize porridge + oil

700 kcal + 300 kcal

Thick maize porridge
with oil added
1000 kcal

Fig. 11–5 Energy concentration of thick porridge with and without oil added (one dot = 100 kcal). The porridge with added oil is almost the same size as the porridge without oil, but it contains more energy. The energy is more concentrated.

Families can add the protein-rich food to a bulky starchy food such as plain porridge, or to porridge which is also enriched with an energy food. *Or* they can feed the child mashed beans, peas, lentils, or an egg separately but at the same meal.

Adding a food that is rich in both energy and nutrients

A good way to enrich porridge is to add an energy-rich food that also contains other nutrients.

For example add:

- paste made from groundnuts, simsim, or other oil seeds;
- mashed bambara nuts;
- skinned well-cooked mashed soybeans.

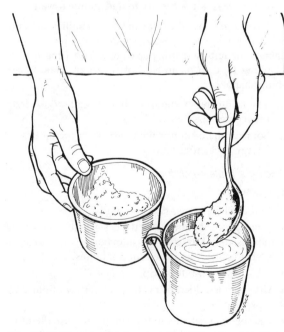

Fig. 11–6 Mix groundnut paste into porridge to add both energy and nutrients.

Or replace some of the water for cooking the porridge with:

- fresh whole milk or soured milk;
- coconut milk or cream.

Or add groundnut or soybean flour to a cereal flour, or to a cereal bean flour. A good mixture is 4 parts cereal and 1 part groundnut.

Adding foods that are rich in micronutrients

To make sure that a young child gets enough folate and vitamins A and C, and to increase the absorption of iron and zinc, families should give some of the following foods each day. They can either mix the foods with an enriched porridge or pap, or give them separately.

- mashed dark green vegetables;
- mashed orange vegetables such as pumpkin or carrots;
- mashed tomatoes;
- mashed orange fruits such as pawpaw or mango;
- juice of orange or lemon.

Changing the starch so the porridge is thinner

There are three ways to change starch so that it absorbs or holds less water when it is cooked. The processes are cheap, but many families are not familiar with them.

Making soured or fermented porridge

'Soured' porridge can mean:

- a sour fermented porridge—some of the starch changes to acid so the porridge tastes sour;
- porridge with a *sour food*, such as lemon or tamarind juice, added.

Sour fermented porridge (see Section 6.5). Souring breaks the starch granules, and changes the starch so that it either absorbs less water (if fermentation is before cooking) or holds less water (if fermentation is after cooking).

Sick people, old people, and breastfeeding mothers often eat soured porridge. Unfortunately, nutrition workers have ignored these foods until recently.

In many areas it is traditional to make sour fermented porridge from cereals or root flours, such as sorghum, millet, maize, or cassava flours.

The advantages of sour fermented porridge as a weaning food are:

- *It is more difficult for harmful bacteria to grow in it.* Sour fermented porridge keeps safely for 2–3 days, even in warm weather. It is less likely to give a child diarrhoea than ordinary porridge which is kept. A mother can make enough to last 2–3 days. Her children can eat it several times a day, but she does not need to cook each time.

- *It is thinner and easier for a baby to eat than plain porridge.* The starch does not thicken as it cools, so it is not necessary to add as much water to make the porridge soft. So you can make sour fermented porridge with more flour in each cupful. Each cup then contains more energy and nutrients than plain porridge.

- *The absorption of iron is increased.* The absorption of non-haem iron, zinc, and some other minerals is better from soured than from ordinary porridge.

- *Children may prefer the taste.* Some children prefer the 'sour' taste of fermented porridge, and so they eat more. Some mothers report that sick children prefer sour porridge.

Porridge made with sour food (see Section 6.5).
- The sour lemon or tamarind juice may make the porridge thinner and easier to eat.
- Children, especially sick children, may prefer the taste.

Using germinated cereal flour—or 'kimea'
(see Section 6.6).

There are two ways to use kimea:

1. *Use kimea instead of plain flour to make porridge.* As it cooks, the kimea absorbs less water than plain flour. Kimea porridge is thinner than plain porridge made with the same amount of flour and water, so it is easier for the baby to eat.

2. *Add a little kimea to warm, plain thick porridge.* The enzyme (amylase) in the kimea partly digests some of the cooked starch. The starch releases some of the water absorbed during cooking, and the porridge becomes thinner and more liquid. The por-

ridge stays thin and semi-liquid even when it is cold. Children can eat more of the thin porridge than of the thick porridge, so they get more energy and nutrients.

Toast cereals and legumes

If you toast cereals and legumes before you make them into flour, they absorb less water when you cook them, so the porridge is less bulky. Toasted flour also keeps longer (see example in Box 11.1).

11.9 FEEDING YOUNG CHILDREN FAMILY FOODS

Another way to help families is to discuss with them how to prepare good meals for young children from the family foods. This is usually cheaper than buying special foods, and it introduces the child at an early age to the tastes of family foods.

Encourage families to give several different foods at each meal, including some green or orange vegetables or fruit. Either mix these with the other food, or give them separately (see Fig. 8–3, p. 74).

How to prepare family foods for young children

These are some ideas for you to discuss with families

- Mash the staple food with a little sauce from the family stew to make it soft—but do not use a very spicy sauce—or mash the food with a little milk, coconut, cream, ghee, or margarine. The sauce, milk, or fat enriches the food and makes it soft for the child to eat. For example:
  - Mash 2 spoons of thick maize porridge with 2 spoons of sauce;
  - Mash 2 spoons of potato with 1 small spoon of margarine or 2 spoons of milk.
- Mash or mix the staple food with mashed or pounded groundnut, sim-sim, skinned beans, peas, or lentils to make it soft and to enrich it with other nutrients.
- Cut well-cooked meat, chicken, liver, or other organs into very small pieces.
- Remove the bones from fish, and mix the fish flesh into the staple, sauce, or stew. *Or* cook pounded dried fish with sauce and mix with staple.
- Dip bread or chappatis into sauces or stews. Or mix pieces of bread and chappati with beans, groundnuts, or vegetables.

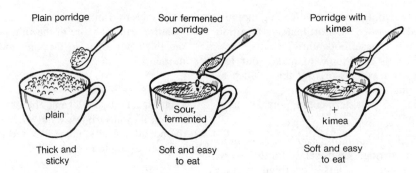

Fig. 11–7 Sour fermented porridge and porridge with added kimea is thinner and easier to eat than thick porridge.

- Take beans or other legumes from a stew, and skin and mash them.
- Mash cooked eggs or cut them into small pieces. Add small amounts of margarine or ghee if available. Give by itself or mix with the staple.
- Mash cooked vegetables or cut them into small pieces. Give different kinds of vegetable—especially dark and medium green leaves and orange vegetables such as pumpkin and carrot. Cook them for as short a time as possible. If the child does not like a vegetable, mix a little with the staple food. Gradually increase the amount of vegetable in the mixture.
- Mash or chop fruit, or make juice. For example:
  - make an orange juice drink (but do not add water which may be contaminated); *or*
  - add lemon juice to porridge or other food; *or*
  - mash or chop mangoes, pawpaw, banana, avocado, pineapple, or other fruit.
- Mix some of the family food into mashed fruits and vegetables such as bananas, pawpaw, or pumpkin.

Box 11.1.   Toasted cereal and legume flour

How to prepare the flour
1. Take 4 parts cleaned cereal grains (e.g. maize, millet, sorghum, rice, wheat) and 1 part cleaned legume (e.g. beans, peas, groundnuts).
2. Toast the damp legumes lightly. To do this, heat them in a large pan over a low fire for 15–30 minutes.
3. Toast the cereal grains too.
4. Pound the cereal grains and legumes together to make flour.
5. Sieve the flour, and pound the coarse part again. Or mill the legume and cereal together or separately in a hand mill.
6. Make sure that the flour is dry and store it in a tightly closed strong polythene bag or airtight can.
   - If the flour contains a fatty food like groundnuts or simsim, it keeps for about 1 month.
   - If there is no fatty food, and the flour remains dry, it keeps for about 4 months.

Note. One kilogram cereal with 250 g legume makes enough flour to provide about 15 portions of porridge each containing about 300 Calories and 10 g protein.

How to make porridge from the flour
Thin porridge
Use 3 heaped large spoons of toasted flour (55 g) and 2 cups of water (400 ml). This provides about 200 Calories and 6 g protein.

Thick porridge
Use 4 heaped large spoons of toasted flour (83 g) and 2 cups of water (400 ml). This provides about 300 Calories and 10 g protein.
   These amounts are enough for 1–2 meals depending on the child's age and appetite.

Box 11.2. Preparing other foods to enrich weaning foods

How to remove the skins from legumes (beans or peas)
1. Soak legumes in water for 4–6 hours and rub off the skins.

2. Toast the legumes over a slow fire. Break the skins with a grinding stone or pestle and mortar; then winnow.

How to prepare groundnuts for small children
1. Toast the groundnuts and pound them into flour. Add the flour to porridge, stew, mashed bananas, etc. The flour does not need to be cooked.

or

2. Fry or roast the groundnuts. Grind into groundnut butter or paste. Add the paste to porridge, or stew, or spread it on bread, on cold potato or cassava.

or

3. Pound raw groundnuts and cook with flour to make porridge, or add to a stew.

How to prepare fish meal for young children
Pound dried fish into a flour and sieve it to remove sharp pieces of bone. Do not keep longer than 1–2 days. Small dried fish are easy to pound.

How to use pounded fish
Cook the pounded fish with flour to make porridge. If you like, add lemon juice to the cooked porridge to prevent a strong smell of fish. *Or* cook the pounded fish with sauce from the family pot for 5–10 minutes to make sure that any germs are killed.

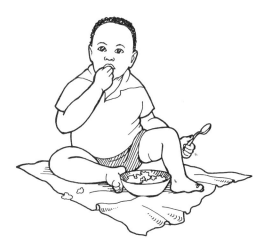

Fig. 11–8 Feeding young children on family foods is usually cheaper than buying special foods.

11.10 GOOD SNACKS FOR YOUNG CHILDREN

One way in which a family can increase the number of times that a child eats is to give her snacks between main meals. Snacks may not give a good mixture of nutrients. Some snacks contain mostly energy. So they should not *replace* main meals.

There are some suggestions for useful snacks for older children in Box 12.1 page 149. Here are some snacks that are suitable for young children. Add other favourite good-value snacks from your area, such as:

- fresh boiled, pasteurized, or soured milk;
- pieces of boiled cassava, plantain, or other 'left-over' staple; these can be mashed with milk, coconut cream, or margarine to make them soft and more energy-rich;
- bread dipped in boiled or soured milk, coconut cream, stew, or fruit juice to make it soft;
- bread, chappatis, or biscuits spread with groundnut or simsim paste, or butter, or margarine or honey;
- doughnuts (mandazi), biscuits, or beancakes;
- chopped or mashed fruits such as banana, pawpaw, orange, mango, avocado.

11.11 COMMERCIAL WEANING FOODS

Commercial weaning foods are foods prepared in factories for young children. Examples are packets of

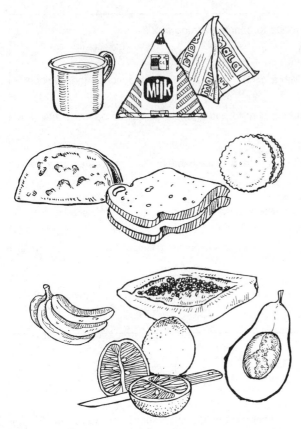

Fig. 11—9 Good snacks for weaning-age children.

special cereals or cans or jars of sieved vegetables, sweet foods, or whole 'meals'.

The *advantages* of commercial foods are:

- They are quick and easy to prepare, and may not need cooking.
- They are clean and safe—at least until the packet or can is opened.
- Most babies like them.
- Some commercial cereal-based foods contain a good mixture of nutrients. They are not as bulky as plain porridge.

The *disadvantages* are:

- They are very expensive. They are too expensive for many families—especially those who are likely to have malnourished children. For example:

    The cost of 1000 Calories in a commercial food can be over six times the cost of 1000 Calories in a home-made weaning food.

Even commercial weaning foods which are subsidized may be too expensive, and they may not reach the families who need them most.

- The label often recommends giving them before the baby is 4 months old. This is too early, and may interfere with breastfeeding, as well as having all the other disadvantages of giving weaning foods too early.
- Cereals may need only cold water to prepare them, so the food is not cooked. If the water is contaminated, it may make the child sick.
- Some foods such as strained vegetables, are not rich in some important nutrients.
- These foods may not always be available if they are imported.

These foods may be a useful 'convenience' food occasionally for families who can afford them. But they should not replace home-made weaning foods.

Misleading advertisements for baby foods

Commercial weaning foods are often advertised in a way which suggests that they have some special advantages for babies, or that babies need them before 4 months of age. This kind of advertising makes some families believe that, to feed their children in the best way, they ought to buy these foods, and give them very early.

This kind of misleading advertising is now discouraged in many countries. You need to understand clearly the disadvantages of commercial foods. You may need to reassure families (especially in towns) that it is not necessary to buy expensive baby foods to feed their children in the best way. Help them to make weaning foods from ordinary family food which are as good or better than commercial foods.

Drinks for babies

Glucose drinks

Cans or packets of glucose *should never be used* to make drinks for babies. The reasons are:

- Giving any sort of drink to a baby under 4–6 months reduces his appetite and interferes with breastfeeding, and it may cause diarrhoea.
- The family may put the glucose drink in a bottle. Bottle feeding interferes with suckling and may also cause diarrhoea.

- Glucose is an expensive kind of sugar. Glucose gives only energy. It is much better for a child to get energy from foods such as breast milk and porridge which also give other nutrients.
- Sometimes vitamins are added to glucose—such as vitamin D. But children can get vitamins in a cheaper, better way from their food. Most children get plenty of vitamin D from sunlight which is free.
- Glucose is a sugar so it is bad for children's teeth. Sweet drinks are an important cause of tooth decay in baby teeth, especially when given by bottle.
- Babies who have glucose drinks may become 'addicted' to sweet foods, and so they may be at risk of tooth decay all their lives.

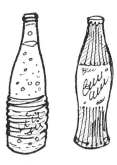

Fig. 11–10 Sodas and bottled soft drinks are made mainly of sugar, water, colouring, and flavouring. They should not be given to young children.

Fruit juices and bottled sodas and other soft drinks

Blackcurrant and other bottled fruit juices are also *not* good for children. These juices contain sugar, a little fruit juice, and sometimes extra vitamin C as well as food additives to preserve and colour them. They are very expensive and bad for the teeth. Children can get all the nutrients that are in these juices from fresh fruits and other foods which are much cheaper. Sometimes the drink has to be diluted with water; the water may be contaminated.

11.12 FEEDING BABIES AT ABOUT 6 MONTHS

This is the time when a baby is learning to take foods other than breast milk.

Advise the family to:

- Start giving other foods at about 6 months of age. They can start at 4–5 months if the baby shows that he really needs it. But it is not necessary to give weaning foods at 4 months to get the baby 'used' to them.
- Give 1–2 spoonfuls of soft porridge or pap once or twice a day. It is best to give the food after the baby has breastfed, or between breastfeeds, so that the baby continues to suckle as much as possible. If the baby has food before a breastfeed, she may suckle less at the breast.
- As soon as the baby is eating porridge or pap, start another food. For example, start mashed fruit or vegetable, either with the porridge or at another time of day.
- Use a spoon or a cup to feed the baby. Never use a bottle. Bottles are difficult to keep clean, and they interfere with suckling at the breast (see Section 10.14).
- Let the mother feed new foods to the baby herself. Then the baby feels safe and happy. When the baby is eating well, someone else can help to feed him.
- Continue breastfeeding whenever the baby seems to want to. This should be at least 10 times in 24 hours.

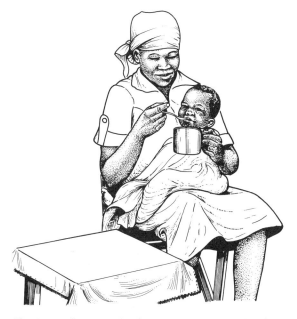

Fig. 11–11 Start weaning foods at around 6 months of age.

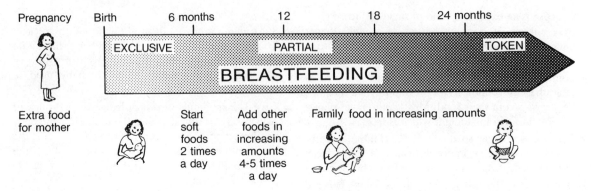

Fig. 11-12 Feeding young children at different ages.

11.13 FEEDING BABIES FROM 6-12 MONTHS

At this time the baby's energy and nutrient needs increase quickly.

Advise the family to:

- Continue to breastfeed as often as before. Breast milk continues to be the main food, and the baby has weaning foods *in addition*. Weaning foods should not replace breast milk.
- Give *enriched porridge*. As soon as the baby is used to plain porridge, add other foods to enrich it.
- Give mashed *fruit* or *vegetable* or undiluted fruit juice, or add lemon juice to the porridge, to make sure that he gets enough vitamin C. Give dark green or orange vegetables, pawpaw, or mango to make sure that he gets enough vitamin A.
- Start to give food from the *family meals*. Try a little of any suitable soft food that you are cooking for the family.
- When he starts wanting to *chew*, give him something hard to chew on—but make sure that it is clean and safe.

- Slowly increase:
  - the amount of food;
  - the number of meals each day;
  - the different sorts of food.

Build up the amount so that by the age of 1 year, a child is eating other food about 4–5 times a day.

11.14 FEEDING CHILDREN FROM 1-3 YEARS

This is the time when foods other than breast milk become the main source of energy and nutrients.

Advise the family to:

- Continue to breastfeed including at night. Now the child has breast milk in addition to other foods—instead of the other way round as before. Breastfeeds should not replace other meals.
- Give the child other food about five times a day. For example, give two family meals, one meal of enriched porridge, and two snacks a day.

Box 11.3.   Some important points about introducing new foods

If the baby refuses a new food or spits it out:
- Leave it for a few days and then try again. *or*
- Mix the food with another food that the baby likes. *or*
- Squeeze a little breast milk over the food so that it smells like breast milk.

If the food seems to make the baby sick:
- Leave it for a few days and then try again.
- If the food makes the baby sick again, stop giving it until the baby is older. (A few babies are allergic to some foods.)

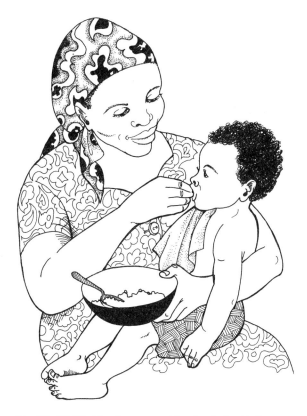

Fig. 11–13 Start to give some of the family food between 6 and 12 months.

- Give the child some of all the family foods. Give staple with beans, peas, groundnuts, and vegetables—and meat, fish, egg, and milk if available.

11.15 SUSTAINING BREASTFEEDING

Encourage mothers to continue to breastfeed for at least 2 years, and for longer if mother and child both wish (see Section 10.12).

- Breast milk can provide one-third or more of the energy, protein, and iron, and most of the vitamins A and C that a child needs between 1 and 2 years of age. It can provide valuable nutrients that the family food may lack. It may prevent malnutrition in children for whom it is difficult to get enough nutrients from family foods.

- Breast milk can continue to provide nutrients after the age of 2 years. However, by the age of 3 years, a child is usually having only a few short breastfeeds by day or at night. This is *token* breastfeeding. Breast milk now provides only a small part of the nutrients that the child needs, but it can be a useful snack and can comfort the child.

- Breastfeeding continues to protect against some infections up to about 3 years of age and is an important source of nourishment and comfort for a sick child.

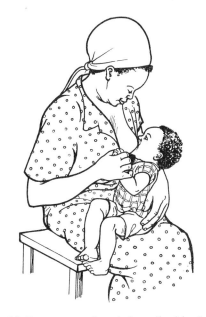

Fig. 11–14 Encourage mothers to breastfeed for 2 years or longer.

Box 11.4.   Example of a 1–3 year old child's menu for a day

Early morning	Breastfeed
Breakfast	Enriched porridge–fruit
Midmorning	Breastfeed and left-over porridge
Lunch	Potato and vegetable stew from family pot
Afternoon	Breastfeed and mashed left-over potato
Early evening	Thick cereal porridge, beans, and sauce from family meal
Late evening	Breastfeed
Night	Breastfeed

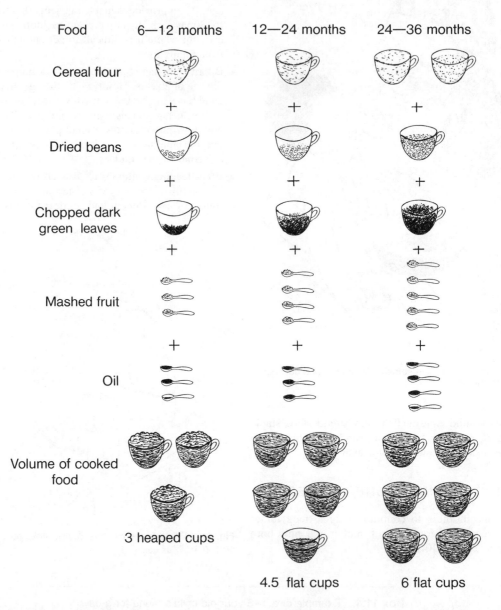

Fig. 11–15 Approximate amounts of food needed by young children each day if they eat mainly enriched porridge. This figure is based on the quantities in Table 11.1. You may need to remeasure the amounts using local foods, local cooking methods, and local measures. In this figure: 1 cup = 1 ordinary teacup = 200 ml; 1 spoon = 1 eating ('desert') spoon = 10 ml.

Table 11.1. Example of daily amounts of food needed by young children.* Remember that children need to eat a variety of foods. This table is *not* a diet to recommend, but it gives *you* an idea of the quantities a child needs

	Age of child (months)		
	6–12	12–24	24–36
Frequency of feeding			
Breastfeeds	10 or more	Frequent	Fewer
Meals/snacks	4–5	4–5	4–5
Amounts of food per day			
Cereal flour (g)	60	110	200
(ml)	100	180	340
+			
Dry legume† (g)	30	50	100
(ml)	40	63	125
+			
Raw dark green (g)	30	40	50
leaves—chopped (ml)	90	130	160
+			
Fruit (pawpaw) (g)	30	40	50
mashed (ml)	30	40	50
+			
Oil‡ (g)	20	25	30
(ml)	23	28	35
Approximate volume of cooked food (ml)§	625	880	1200
% energy needs from food (rest from breast milk)	50	66	100
Energy (kcal)	503	794	1320
Protein (g)	14	23	44
Fat (g)	21	27	33
Iron (mg)	6	10	17
Vitamin A (RE)	177	275	400
Vitamin C (mg)	31	45	66

One level cup (teacup) = 200 ml; one level spoon (eating/dessert) = 10 ml.

* A big child may need more than these amounts, and a small child less. The appetite of a *healthy* child is also a useful guide to the amounts of food that she needs. To check that the child is eating enough, weigh her regularly.
† Some or all legumes could be replaced by slightly smaller amounts of chopped meat, fish, egg, or milk.
‡ Oil can be replaced by fats or by the amount of a fatty food such as meat or nuts which supplies this amount of oil.
§ Volume of these amounts of food assuming that:

- For a 6–12 month old child all cereal is made into soft porridge (containing 0.5 kcal/g).
- For 12–24 months half the flour is made into soft porridge and half into stiff porridge (containing 1 kcal/g).
- For 24–36 months all flour is made into stiff porridge.

11.16 STOPPING BREASTFEEDING

When the child decides to stop

Some children lose interest in breastfeeding and stop by themselves between 12 and 18 months. If this happens it can be difficult to make the child continue. The most important thing to do is to make sure that the child gets enough other food, so that she continues to grow at a healthy rate. Many children do not lose interest in breastfeeding until the age of about 4 years.

When the mother decides to stop

There is no medical reason to stop breastfeeding at any particular time, but mothers often decide that they cannot continue beyond 2 or 3 years.

If a mother decides to stop breastfeeding, encourage her to stop *slowly*. In some communities it is the custom to stop breastfeeding suddenly. Sometimes the child has had only a little weaning food in addition to breast milk before this time. Now, he is expected to change suddenly to family food. Sometimes the family sends the child away from the mother, so that he cannot demand to breastfeed. Stopping breastfeeding suddenly in this way can make a child unhappy. Some children refuse to eat other foods, and they become malnourished and ill.

How to stop breastfeeding slowly
Advise the mother to:

- Make sure that the child is eating other foods five times a day.
- If necessary, increase the amount of food and the number of meals that the child has.
- Increase the length of time between breastfeeds, so that the number of breastfeeds decreases. For example, at first, she might stop giving any breastfeeds during the morning; after a week or two, she might also stop giving breastfeeds during the afternoon.
- For that part of the day, avoid situations which make the child think of breastfeeding—for example, having the child on her lap if she sits down to eat or to have a drink. If the child is old enough to understand, she may be able to explain that he can breastfeed later, but now is not the time.
- Give the child plenty of breastfeeds at other times.
- Give the child extra loving attention, and make him feel close to her in other ways.
- Advise her not to push the child away from the breast when he tries to breastfeed. This may make the child feel anxious and unhappy.
- Stop the night breastfeeds last of all.

Box 11.5. Giving a child his own plate of food

A child needs his own plate, spoon, and cup for his meals for two reasons.

1. To learn to feed himself. Advise the family to encourage a baby to feed himself as soon as he wants to—usually at about 9 months of age. He will not feed himself efficiently at first. The mother should help to make sure that the baby gets most of the food, and that not too much is spilled.

2. So that he gets enough food. Small children eat more slowly other children and adults. If they feed themselves from the family dish, the food may all be finished before a young child has had enough. The mother or someone else must help the child.

   Discuss how it can help to give a young child all the food that he needs on his own plate; to give him plenty of time to eat; to encourage him to finish it; and to make sure that he has had enough.

11.17 CHILDREN WHO 'REFUSE' TO EAT SOLID FOOD

'Refusing' to eat is an important problem. One of the ways in which you can prevent malnutrition is to help families to avoid or overcome this problem.

- *The child may be ill*. She may have lost her appetite because of an infection, or worms, or she may have a sore mouth or throat. The family should take the child for treatment.

- *The child may be unhappy*. For example, the mother may be sick or away, or she may have a new baby. The child needs extra love and attention, especially during meals.

- *The child may be teething*. Give her something clean and hard to chew on—such as a spoon.

Sometimes families worry because their child of 1–2 years *never* seems to want solid food. Some children seem to want only to breastfeed, or to take other fluids, for example, from a feeding bottle. Sometimes these children fail to grow at a healthy rate and they become malnourished.

Some people used to think that children refuse to eat solid food because they have breastfed for 'too long'. Some mothers and some health workers believe that the only way to get the child to eat more is to stop breastfeeding.

But the refusal is *not* caused by breastfeeding. It is due to the way in which the family introduces weaning foods. For example, it may happen if the family:

- starts to give weaning foods after 9 months of age;

- tries to force the child to eat solids, or food that she does not like, so that meal times become unpleasant for the child;

- continues to allow the child to breastfeed just before or during family meals;

- gives the child a lot of sweet snacks and drinks;

- gives weaning foods such as porridge from a feeding bottle.

Sometimes, it follows an illness, during which a child stops eating food.

To help to avoid refusal of food

- Encourage families to start giving babies suitable weaning foods at the appropriate time.

- Encourage families to watch children's appetites; and to give a child lots of love and encourage her to eat if she is sick, or unhappy, or if the mother has a new baby.

- Advise families strongly *not* to give the child bottle feeds or a dummy as a substitute for breastfeeding, or to help 'wean' the child, and not to give thin porridge from a bottle.

How you can help if the problem does arise

Ask the family how they feed the child. This may give you some ideas about what they could do differently. Help the mother to find a way to encourage the child to eat more family food without stopping breastfeeding suddenly. Discuss with her all the ideas in Section 11.16 for slowly reducing the number of times the child breastfeeds. Suggest some of these ways to encourage the child to eat more:

- Make sure that the child is hungry at meal times, that he has been active for some time, and has not just had a snack or sweet drink. However, the child should not be too tired and sleepy.

- Give him food that he likes, which is not too spicy.

- Avoid forcing a child to eat, or urging him too much. If he refuses a meal, take the food away, cover it, and offer it again 1–2 hours later. Do not offer other foods or drinks during this time. If it is safe to keep the food longer, offer it at the next meal. Give more attention when the child does eat than when he refuses.

- Do not breastfeed the child during family meals, and do not let him have a breastfeed instead of a meal. Let the child eat with other children, or let someone else other than the mother hold the child at meal times.

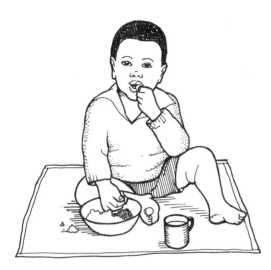

Fig. 11–16 Give a child his own plate of food.

- Avoid breastfeeding the child a short time before offering other food. It may spoil his appetite. (This is the opposite of what you may want to advise before the age of 1 year, when breast milk is the main food.)

11.18 FEEDING YOUNG CHILDREN AGED 3–5 YEARS

At this age, many children have stopped breastfeeding, so they must get all the nutrients that they need from other foods. However, a child's appetite increases, and she eats faster, so she can eat more at each meal. Her food needs for each kilogram of her weight are less. So she does not need to eat as often as a younger child.

Discuss with families how they can:
- Make sure that their children eat at least three times a day.
- Pay attention to children during meals, to make sure that they eat enough.
- Make sure that children get plenty of energy-rich and nutrient-rich foods from the family meals. A child may not be able to eat a very large helping of the staple food, but she needs plenty of the other foods which are rich in protein and micronutrients. In particular she needs plenty of vitamin A, and plenty of

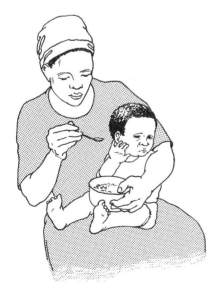

Fig. 11–17 Sometimes a child 'refuses' to eat solid food.

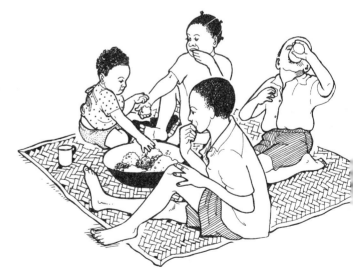

Fig. 11–18 Make sure that young children get their fair share of food.

iron and vitamin C to prevent anaemia. She also needs some oil or fat.

- Give good snacks to children (see Section 11.10 and Box 12.1), and avoid snacks which are not good value for money (Box 9.1).

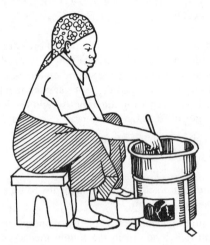

Fig. 11–19 Cook a young child's food thoroughly to kill dangerous micro-organisms.

Bacteria breed in food which sticks to plates and bowls.

- *Cook porridge thoroughly to kill as many micro-organisms as possible.* They should not add water which may be contaminated to porridge as it cools.

- *Add protein-rich foods to porridge a short time before feeding the child.* Bacteria multiply faster in protein-rich and sweetened porridge than in plain porridge. Adding protein or sugar a long time before the child eats the porridge gives bacteria a better chance to multiply

Teach a helper who prepares food or who feeds the child how to keep food clean and safe.

Sometimes you may suggest that families prepare sour fermented porridge which they can keep safely for 2–3 days (see Sections 6.5 and 11.8). But, if they prepare porridge without souring, advise them also:

- *To prepare the food at least twice a day.*

- *Not to keep the porridge or other weaning foods overnight.* This is especially important if the weather is warm. It may be safe to keep food overnight if the weather is cold.

11.19 KEEPING WEANING FOODS CLEAN AND SAFE

Infection from food and water is one of the main causes of diarrhoea in young children. An important way to prevent diarrhoea is to prevent contamination of weaning foods. Chapter 7 describes the most important ways to keep all the family food clean and safe. With weaning foods, families need to take extra care, because young children easily become sick.

Advise families to
- *Wash hands*
  - before preparing the food;
  - before feeding a young child;
  - after using the toilet;
  - after cleaning a young child's bottom;
  - after clearing up children's faeces.

- *Wash the child's hands too.*

- *Boil water for the child to drink* (unless the water comes from a safe source).

- *Clean the plate or bowl for the child's food carefully.*

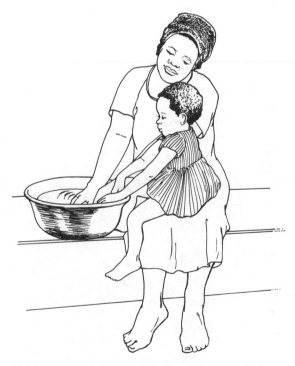

Fig. 11–20 Wash hands before feeding a young child.

THINGS TO DO

Class exercises

1. Ask trainees to use the food composition tables in Appendix 1 to calculate the amounts of local vitamin-rich foods which give 20 mg vitamin C or 300 RE vitamin A. These are approximately the amounts that a young child needs each day. Ask them to find out:

   a. How much do these amounts of food cost?

   b. Which local food is the richest source of vitamin A?

   c. Which is the cheapest source of vitamin A?

2. Give each trainee details of a child (e.g. Sammy is 1 year old and breastfeeding) and ask her to write down how she would feed him over 1 day using local low-cost foods. She should write down when she would feed the child, which foods, and how to prepare them.

3. Ask trainees to collect information about the foods and meals eaten by young children in the area. Calculate and compare the nutrient value, costs, time of preparations, and amount of fuel used for different meals.

4. Ask trainees to collect information on the snacks that people buy for young children.

   a. Find out which nutrients and how much sugar they contain.

   b. Try to find out if the snacks are prepared and stored in a clean way.

   c. Calculate the cost of 1000 kcal from each snack (see Section 9.4).

   d. Discuss which snacks are 'good buys'.

Discussion

5. Ask the class to discuss how they would advise parents about making enriched porridge or pap. Discuss how the advice may vary from place to place.

Food preparation in class

6. Prepare some enriched porridges and paps together. Discuss which recipes are practical and acceptable.

7. Ask trainees to prepare beans, soybeans, or ground-nuts so that a small child can eat and digest them easily.

Food demonstration

8. Show why young children need to eat five times a day. Make thick porridge with 300 g cereal flour or cereal legume flour. This amount gives a 12-month-old child enough energy for one day (about 1000 kcal).

   a. Divide the porridge into three equal parts. Ask trainees: 'Could a 12-month-old child easily eat one part for a meal?'

   b. Put the porridge together again and then divide it into five equal parts. Ask trainees: 'Could the child easily eat one of these parts at a meal?'

   c. Discuss how practical it is to advise parents to feed children frequently.

9. Prepare sour fermented porridge. You need to plan this over several days. Ask trainees whether people in their area use this. Discuss the advantages and disadvantages of sour fermented porridge, and whether or not to encourage it.

10. Show how oil or fat makes porridge thinner and easier to eat. Make 2 cups of porridge.

    • For the first cup, cook 35 g flour with water to make about 200 ml (1 full teacup) of porridge.

    • For the second cup, cook 35 g flour with the same amount of water plus 1 big spoonful oil (10 ml) to make about 200 ml porridge.

    Examine both cups of porridge when they are cool. Notice that the porridge in the first cup is thick and sticky, but the porridge in the second cup is softer and easier for a child to eat.
    Which cup gives the most energy? (The first cup gives about 120 kcal, the second cup gives about 120 + 90 kcal = 210 kcal.)
    Which cup do you think that a child would prefer? (Porridge in the second cup is softer and easier to eat, and should taste better. Most children prefer it.)
    (See TALC Slide set WFE, Slide 10. See Appendix 6 for full reference.)

11. Put suitable amounts of raw foods on plates, or ask students to do this and then discuss the meals. Ask trainees to work out the cost of one or more of the meals.

Demonstration or exercise—preparing a good mixed meal for Sunny

Figure 11–21 shows an example of how to prepare a good mixed meal for a girl of 2 years, called Sunny. You can use this example as the basis of a demonstration or exercise.

It may be useful to copy the diagrams on to a board, or large sheets, or overhead transparencies. You could make separate drawings to use like a flipchart; or you could make one drawing and one diagram and add foods or nutrients to it in different colours during the different stages of the discussion.

Sunny's meal

Sunny has stopped breastfeeding. She eats three meals a day and two snacks between meals. Each meal should provide ¼–⅓ of her daily energy and nutrient needs.

Figure 11–21(a) shows Sunny's plate for her midday meal, and the nutrients that she needs to eat at this meal.

What can her mother put in the plate to make a good mixed meal for her?

The staple food

She puts ¾ cup of thick maize porridge in the plate. Figure 11–21(b) shows the amounts of Calories, protein, iron, vitamin A, and vitamin C that the porridge gives.

A legume

She adds ⅓ cup of mashed peas. Figure 11–21(c) shows the nutrient needs that the porridge and peas cover.

Vegetables and fruit

She adds 2 spoons of cooked spinach and half an orange. Figure 11–21(d) shows how many of Sunny's nutrients needs are covered by the porridge, peas, spinach, and orange.

Look at the amount of food on Sunny's plate. There is already a little more than 1 cupful of food. (150 ml porridge + 66 ml peas + 20 ml spinach = 236 ml food.) Sunny cannot eat much more than this, but the meal does not give her enough Calories. What can her mother do?

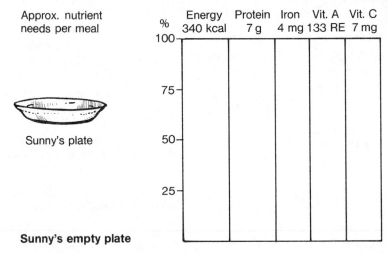

Sunny's empty plate

Fig. 11–21(a) shows Sunny's plate for her midday meal, and the nutrients that she needs to eat at this meal.

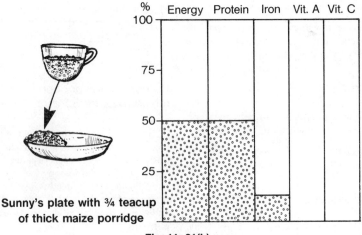

Sunny's plate with ¾ teacup of thick maize porridge

Fig. 11–21(b).

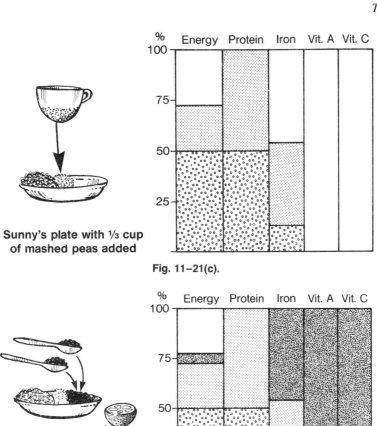

Sunny's plate with ⅓ cup of mashed peas added

Fig. 11–21(c).

Sunny's plate with 2 big spoonfuls of spinach added and half an orange

Fig. 11–21(d).

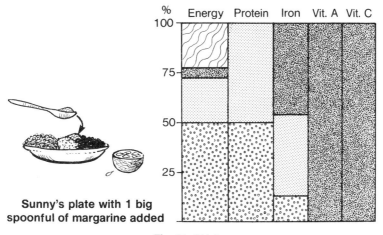

Sunny's plate with 1 big spoonful of margarine added

Fig. 11–21(e).

She can add an *energy-rich food* which adds energy without increasing the size of the meal very much. She adds 1 spoonful of margarine. Figure 11–21(e) shows that the meal now covers all Sunny's energy and nutrient needs.

If Sunny's mother cannot afford oil, margarine, or another type of fat, she could use groundnuts or other sorts of oil seed or coconut.

If the family has enough money, or keeps animals, Sunny's mother can add some food from animals, such as a glass of milk, or an egg, or a small piece of meat or liver or fish.

USEFUL PUBLICATIONS

Alnwick, D., Moses, S., and Schmidt, O. G. (ed.) (1988). *Improving young child feeding in Eastern and Southern Africa*. International Development Research Centre, Ottawa.

Oniang'o, R. K. (1988). *Feeding the child*. Heinemann, Nairobi.

WFPHA (1984). *Program activities for improving weaning practices*. UNICEF, New York.

12 Feeding older children and adults

12.1 NUTRIENT NEEDS OF SCHOOL-AGE CHILDREN

School-age children need to eat good mixed meals so that they grow properly and have plenty of energy to work, play, and learn. Girls need to eat well so that, when they are women, they are well nourished and have healthy babies.

School-age children do not usually develop severe malnutrition unless there is a famine. This is because:

- Children between the ages of 5 and 11 years grow more slowly than younger children.
- Their stomachs are bigger so they can eat more food at one meal.
- They have become resistant to many of the common infections.
- They can ask for food when they are hungry, and they can eat fast enough to get a share of the family meal.
- They visit relatives and neighbours, who may give them snacks.
- Boys, and sometimes girls, collect and eat fruits, insects, and other wild foods.
- Girls may eat when they help to cook the family meal.

However, many school-age children from poorer homes eat poor meals and they may be undernourished in the following ways.

- *They may have been undernourished when younger or be eating poor diets now.* These children are shorter and thinner than well fed children. They may become tired quicker. They may be ill more often.

- *They may be hungry.* They may not have much food in the morning or at midday so they are often hungry. This is sometimes called *short-term hunger*. Hungry children cannot study well or work hard, and they do not want to play like other children.

- *They may be anaemic.* Many school-age children are anaemic. Adolescent girls are at greatest risk of anaemia because they menstruate and lose iron in the blood each month. Anaemic children tire quickly and have difficulty learning (see Chapter 20).

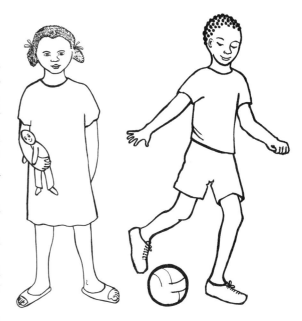

Fig. 12–1 School-age children need good meals.

- *They may lack iodine.* In some places children lack iodine. These children may not be able to learn as quickly as normal and they may develop goitre (see Chapter 21).

12.2 SCHOOL-AGE CHILDREN AT SPECIAL RISK OF UNDERNUTRITION

There are many groups of older children who are especially likely to eat poor meals and to be hungry and undernourished. You may need to give them or their families special help and advice. Children who are at special risk are those who:

- come from poor families—for example, children of unemployed parents, one-parent families, or children who work on large tea or other commercial estates;
- have a mother or father who is dead, sick, mentally ill, very young, or alcoholic;
- look after themselves because their families have

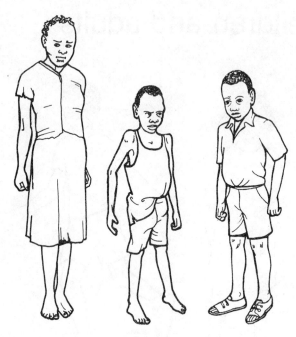

Fig. 12–2 Some school-age children are undernourished.

abandoned them or because they have run away from home;

● live in areas where there are food shortages or where iodine deficiency is a problem;

● are refugees or displaced people;

● are mentally or physically disabled;

● have heavy wormloads (see Section 16.12);

● are at boarding schools where the food is poor;

● eat a lot of low-value snacks such as sweets and sodas. (Often these are children who live in towns and whose parents are away all day.)

12.3 THE FOOD NEEDS OF SCHOOL-AGE CHILDREN

School-age children need two to three good mixed meals each day. Healthy children, especially adolescent boys, are often hungry, and they need snacks between meals (see Box 12.1).

Food in the morning

Children need breakfast before they go to school or to work. A cup of tea is not enough. A good breakfast is especially important if children have to walk a long way, or if they do not eat much in the middle of the day.

Porridge makes a good breakfast, especially if it contains milk, groundnuts, egg, margarine or oil.

Often children eat food in the morning which is left over from the previous day. Left-over food tastes better and is safer if it is heated so that the middle is boiling hot. If the food is fried it gives the children more energy for the day ahead.

Sometimes it is difficult for mothers to cook before children leave home. These children can eat cold food like bread or bananas or cold cooked foods like maize porridge, cassava, or plantain. If possible, parents should add other types of food such as groundnuts, cooked beans, margarine, egg, milk, or fruit.

Food in the middle of the day

Children need food in the middle of the day; otherwise they are too hungry to work or study well in the afternoon. A midday meal is especially important for children who eat only a small, simple breakfast.

If possible, the midday meal should contain two or three different foods. However, some food is better than no food, and all children should have something to eat in the middle of the day, even if it is only cold maize porridge.

Carrying food from home

A child who goes to work or school can take some food from home. Find out which local foods make good-value, easy-to-carry meals or snacks. Whenever possible, the food which the child takes should include a staple, some protein-rich food, and some vegetables or fruit.

For example:

● *Starchy foods*. Bread, maize cob, mandazi (doughnut), chappati, maize porridge, cold cassava, sweet potato, or plantain.

● *Other foods*
  ● Soybeans, groundnuts, groundnut paste, fish, boiled egg, samosa, or milk;
    and
  ● Tomato, carrot, pumpkin, pawpaw, avocado, banana, orange, or mango.

Buying food from food-sellers

Sometimes parents give money to their children to buy food. But children may buy foods such as sweets or

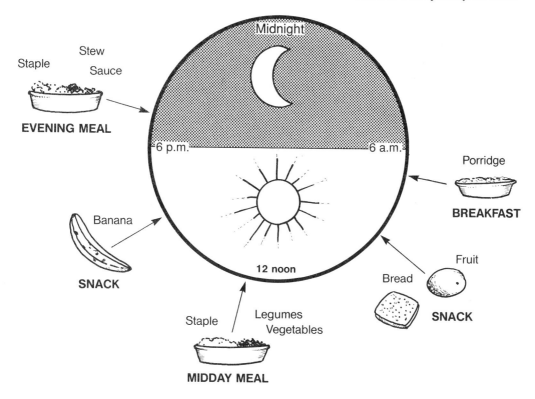

Fig. 12–3 A school-age child needs 3 meals and at least 2 snacks each day.

sodas which are not good value. Sometimes the only meals that they can buy are not nutritious or clean. Parents should teach children which foods are best value for money (see Chapter 9).

Meals at school

If children are lucky, their schools or employers provide meals in the middle of the day. These meals should contain plenty of the staple food, especially if the children are hungry adolescents. Meals should also include some beans, peas, or groundnuts (or meat or fish) and some fresh vegetables or fruit (see Chapter 30).

Food in the evening

The evening meal may be the only hot meal that older children eat. It should be a good mixed meal. Girls and boys must have their share of all the foods in the meal. The family should serve the meal before the children are tired and sleepy.

12.4 CHILDREN WITH SPECIAL FOOD NEEDS

Some children have higher nutrient needs than others. Discuss with families how they can make sure that these children have the extra food that they need.

- *Adolescents who are growing fast.* Between the ages of 11 and 16 years children grow very quickly. This is called the *adolescent growth spurt.* It is the time when children change into young men and women. Children of this age need extra food. If they say that they are hungry they are not being greedy.

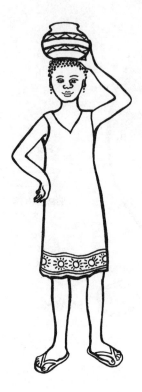
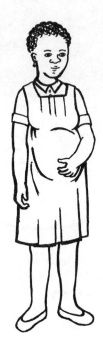
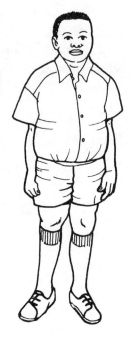

Fig. 12–4 Girls need meals which provide plenty of iron.

Fig. 12–5 Pregnant adolescent girls are often undernourished.

Fig. 12–6 Some children are obese.

- *Girls who menstruate.* Girls need meals which provide plenty of iron.

- *Girls who become pregnant.* Girls grow and develop until they are about 15–17 years old. Some girls are pregnant or already mothers by this age. They need extra food of all kinds, especially foods which provide iron. If they do not eat enough, they may become thin and anaemic. Their babies may have a low birth weight (see Chapter 18).

Other children with special needs are obese children. The children of rich families may become too fat if they eat a lot of sugary or fatty foods and if they take little exercise (see Section 22.6). You may need to advise them about eating more fruit and vegetables and less energy-rich foods.

12.5 FOOD NEEDS OF ADULTS

All adults need:

- good mixed meals so that they get a balanced mixture of nutrients, including fibre;
- enough food to give enough energy and nutrients;
- clean safe meals and water so that they do not become sick.

12.6 SPECIAL NUTRIENT NEEDS OF WOMEN

Table 12.1 compares the nutrient needs of men and women of the same weight. The figures for all men's needs are called 100 per cent. If women's needs are the same as men's the figure for them is also 100. If women

---

Box 12.1. Snacks for school-age children

Examples of good snacks
These snacks are often good value for money:

- boiled, pasteurized, or soured milks;
- bread or chappati especially with an energy-rich food such as margarine or groundnut paste or simsim paste;
- doughnut (mandazi), bean cakes, biscuits;
- boiled or fried cassava, plantain, yam, or potato (e.g. chips);
- boiled or roasted maize cobs;
- bananas, pawpaw, avocado, mango, oranges, and other fruits;
- coconut flesh;
- boiled egg;
- cooked groundnuts, soybeans, and other oil seeds;
- small fried fish;
- insects such as locusts, termites, etc.;
- sugar cane.

Examples of poor snacks
These are often poor value for money and they are bad for the teeth—keep them for special treats.

- sodas;
- sweets and lollies;
- ice-cream;
- glucose powder and tablets;
- crisps and other similar snack foods.

---

need less, the figure for them is smaller; if women need more, the figure for them is larger.

Notice that women may need less energy than men. But women need *at least the same amounts of the other nutrients*. They need more iron—especially when they are pregnant. Their needs for the other nutrients also

Table 12.1. Comparison of the nutrient needs of men and women of the same weight. Women's needs are given as a percentage of men's needs*

Nutrient	Men	Women		
		Menstruating	Pregnant	Lactating
Energy	100	79	83	97
Protein	100	100	113	138
Vitamin A	100	100	118	167
Folate	100	100	226	161
Iodine	100	100	117	133
Iron	100	236	380	131

* These values were calculated for men and women weighing 60 kg. If women weigh less than men (as they often do) they need a lower percentage of energy and nutrients.

increase during pregnancy and lactation. This is why anaemia, iodine deficiency, and other deficiency diseases are more common among women than among men.

Some women need as much energy as their husbands because they do more agricultural and other heavy work in addition to housework. Women often work longer hours than men. Some women are undernourished because they eat less than they need in order to feed their families better.

Husbands and families should realize that all women, not only pregnant women, have special nutrient needs.

12.7 MEALS FOR WOMEN

A rough guide is that women should eat at least the same amount of sauce, relish, stew, and snacks as men, and as much staple as they want. In particular, they should have foods rich in haem iron, like meat, fish, and liver, when these foods are available, as well as vitamin C rich foods to increase iron absorption, and foods rich in folate and vitamin A.

Women who eat good mixed meals usually feel well.

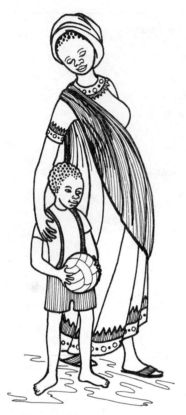

Fig. 12–7 Energy and nutrient needs increase during pregnancy. This mother and her school-age son both need good mixed meals.

They have plenty of energy and stores of nutrients for when they become pregnant.

During pregnancy

Pregnant women need extra energy and nutrients, especially in the last trimester of pregnancy, because:

- Their bodies must build the new baby and placenta.
- The amount of blood in their bodies increases.
- They need to store fat, vitamin A, and other nutrients so that they can make breast milk.

Pregnant women are able to absorb more iron and other nutrients than normal. But they still need to eat extra.

Nutrient needs do not increase much until the last trimester. But it may be difficult for many women to suddenly increase their food intake. So a woman should increase the amount that she eats as soon as she knows that she is pregnant.

Pregnant women who are well nourished or overweight need to make sure that they eat enough foods that provide iron and vitamins, such as fresh fruit, vegetables, and meat or fish, but they need not increase their energy intake much.

Adolescent girls who become pregnant have very high nutrient needs because they are still growing. They need special care and plenty of good food.

While breastfeeding

Energy and nutrients to make breast milk come partly from the woman's food, and partly from the stores that she built up before and during pregnancy. Good stores are more important for making breast milk than eating more food after the baby is born.

A breastfeeding mother needs about 500 kcal and 18–21 g protein extra each day (Sections 2.11 and 3.5). She needs to eat foods which provide vitamins A and C, which may be low in breast milk if she does not get enough. She needs to eat foods which provide iron, to help her to build up her iron stores again.

A well-nourished woman should return to her pre-pregnant body weight by about 4–6 months after delivery. However, if she eats a lot of extra food at this time she may not use up the fat stores, so she may not lose the extra weight. Some women become obese at this time.

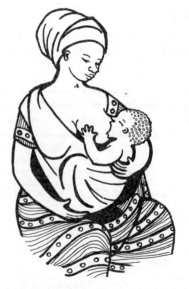

Fig. 12–8 Lactating women need extra energy and nutrients.

How to help to improve meals for women

Find out about the nutritional status of women in your area, and about the meals that people eat. You need to know:

- How much and which sorts of foods women and girls eat.
- Whether some women need better meals.
- Which groups of women need help most.
- Any customs which encourage women to have good meals, especially when they are pregnant or have just given birth.

Some suggestions for improving meals that might be useful:

- Eat more vitamin C rich foods such as fruit, raw tomato, or carrot with a meal to increase iron absorption.
- Eat a little extra meat, fish, chicken, and especially liver when possible to increase the haem iron in the meal.
- Eat more dark green or orange vegetables, or orange fruits to get more vitamin A.
- Eat snacks such as cold cooked staple between meals when pregnant or lactating to get more energy.
- Encourage the belief that women need to eat more when they are pregnant. This is not being greedy and will not make the new baby too big.

12.8 MEN'S NUTRITION NEEDS

Men need more Calories than women if they are doing similar work (see Chapter 2). They need the same amount of protein for each kilo of weight. But men do not usually show signs of undernutrition because:

- They do not have the extra nutrient needs that women have for menstruation, pregnancy, and breastfeeding. Their iron needs are much lower than women's.
- Most men have good appetites and so can easily eat enough bulky foods to get all the Calories and nutrients that they need.
- They often get the biggest share of the family meal.
- They have more opportunity and money to buy meals and snacks outside the home.

However, it is important for men to eat good mixed meals and to stay healthy because they are often the family's main wage earner, or they provide an important part of the labour which produces the family food. Men who do not eat enough or who are anaemic cannot work so hard. They may earn less or produce less food. They easily become sick.

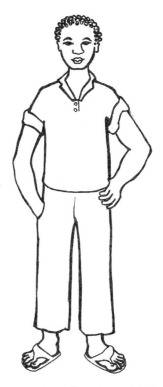

Fig. 12–9 Men are not usually undernourished.

Nutrition problems of men

- Men may become undernourished if the family has very little food. In some places there may be certain times of the year, such as the hungry season, when men are at risk of undernutrition.
- They may become undernourished if they are chronically sick.
- Migrant male workers who live alone may not eat enough. They may be poorly paid, and they may send much of their money home. They may drink alcohol instead of eating a meal. They may need advice about which foods are good value, and how to prepare cheap, good meals.
- An increasing number of richer middle-aged men develop coronary heart disease, stroke, or other dis-

orders of overnutrition (see Chapter 22). Some of these men die or are disabled so they cannot support their families.

Meals for men

Men do not need energy-rich foods as much as children, or iron-rich foods as much as women. Men do need plenty of legumes, staple foods, vegetables, and fruits to give them fibre, which helps to protect them from some of the disorders of overnutrition.

The best way to prevent men from becoming undernourished is to help improve family food supplies, and to give advice on buying and preparing food to men who live alone. Some men need advice to help them reduce the amount of alcohol that they drink.

12.9 SPECIAL NEEDS OF OLD PEOPLE

Good food helps old people to stay healthy and active for longer, and to resist infections. As people grow older they are usually less active, and need less energy. But they still need plenty of protein, minerals (especially calcium), vitamins, and fibre. The iron needs of women decrease when they stop menstruating.

Table 12.2 compares the average energy and nutrient needs of women aged 30 and women aged 65 years of similar weights. The table shows that old people need less staple foods, fat, and sugar than younger adults, but that they should have their fair share of legumes, milk, eggs, vegetables, and fruit. They need to eat enough fibre to prevent constipation. They need less haem iron, so they do not need meat, fish, or liver as much as younger women and children. This is important if there is not much of these foods available.

Table 12.2. Energy and nutrient needs of women aged 30 and 65 years

	Woman aged 30 years	Woman aged 65 years
Body weight (kg)	50	50
Energy (kcal)	2140	1830
Protein (g)	48	48
Iron (mg)	48	19
Vitamin A (RE)	500	500
Vitamin C (mg)	30	30

Old people may prefer foods which are soft and easy to eat and swallow, especially if they lack teeth. For example, they may like milk, eggs, thin porridge, mashed beans and groundnuts, thick soup, boiled vegetables, and mashed or soft fruits. Most old people cannot eat large meals, and prefer to eat smaller meals or snacks several times a day.

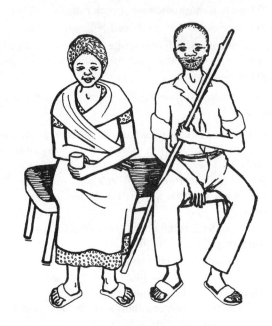

Fig. 12–10 Some old people do not eat well.

Why some old people do not eat well

Many old people are well fed because they live with their families who respect and care for them. But some old people are undernourished. They are thin, anaemic, and may lack nutrients such as vitamin A. Some are obese, or have heart disease or diabetes. Some are alcoholic. Old people may be 'at risk' of undernutrition if:

- They or their families cannot afford to buy the good foods that they need.
- They have to care for or support many grandchildren.
- They live alone and have no relatives to help them and care for them.
- They live in 'Homes' which do not provide good meals.
- They have lost their teeth, and find it difficult to eat foods which need to be chewed.

As families break up and the younger people move away from home there are more old people who live alone. Undernutrition may become a big problem in the future. Old people who live alone:

- are often poor;
- may be lonely and miserable so that they do not want to eat;
- may have poor sight, or be sick, disabled, or mentally confused, and so find it difficult to grow food, to shop for food, to cook food, or to eat it. If they are sick they may not want to eat;
- if the old person is a man, he may not know how to prepare and cook food;
- if the old person is a woman, she may not be interested in preparing meals for herself, when she does not have a family to care for.

12.10 HOW TO HELP OLD PEOPLE

You might be able to:

- Discuss with old people meals that they can prepare and eat easily, and that are good value for money.
- Teach relatives and others who care for old people about the special food needs of the old.
- Advise relatives who send money home to arrange for someone to help old people to buy and prepare good meals.
- Encourage school-age children and adolescents to respect and learn from old people, and to help them to cultivate, shop, and cook. Old people feel happier and better if they feel respected and useful.
- Encourage community workers to help old people. For example, they might make regular home visits to old people who live alone, or arrange for someone to help them grow or cook food.
- Encourage income-earning activities that help old people to earn money and to feel useful—or that raise money to help old people or produce nutritious foods for them.
- Help old people to get treatment for illnesses, for dental problems, and for disabilities.
- Help to plan suitable good mixed meals for hospitals and homes where old people live.
- Encourage old people to take as much exercise as they can, because this helps to keep them healthy and active.
- Give support to old people who have to care for grandchildren.

Meals for old people

Advise people who care for old people:

- If old people have a poor appetite, give them small, frequent, nutritious meals which are easy to eat.
- Give soft foods if they have teeth missing or if their mouths are sore. Foods used to feed children during the weaning period are often suitable for old people with poor appetites or no teeth—for example, sour fermented porridge (see Section 6.5).
- Make sure that the food is prepared in a safe, clean way. Infections are more serious in old people than in younger adults.
- Give plenty of safe, clean drinks.

THINGS TO DO

Classroom exercises

1. Ask groups of trainees to use the 'mixed meal guide' in Section 8.3 to plan a good breakfast or lunch for a 10-year-old boy.

   a. Weigh or estimate the weight of each food (see Appendix 4, Table A4.4).

   b. Then use the method described in Appendix Section A4.4 and the food composition tables in Appendix 1 to calculate the energy, protein, and vitamin A content of the meal.

   c. Use the values in Appendix 2, Table A2.1 to check that the meal provides at least $\frac{1}{3}$ of the Calories, protein, and vitamin A needs of 10-year-old boys.

   d. Work out the cost of the meal using local prices for each food (see Chapter 9).

2. Choose two or three local staple foods. Ask trainees to calculate the amounts which would give the extra energy needed by an active, well nourished pregnant woman (i.e. 200 kcal).

   For example, there are 320 kcal in 100 g finger millet flour (see Appendix 1). So there are 200 kcal in 100/320 × 200 g = 63 g millet flour. Let trainees measure this amount of staple.

Group work

3. Ask groups of trainees to plan and if possible prepare a meal for an old man who has no teeth.

4. Ask trainees to find out from young men who live alone

what they eat. Share and discuss this information. What useful nutrition advice would they give to men like these?

Field visits

5. Visit a school and find out which foods the children eat for breakfast and at school. Discuss with teachers and students ways to improve these meals if necessary.

6. Watch children buy food from food sellers. Find out how the sellers prepare these foods and how much they cost. Discuss which foods are good value, and how you could help the food seller to improve the nutritive value and cleanness of the foods.

7. Take trainees to visit some old people at their homes or in an old people's home or hospital and ask them which their favourite foods are. Are they given these foods? Can they get them if they live at home?

USEFUL PUBLICATIONS

Horwitz, A., MacFadyen, D. M., Munro, H., Scrimshaw, N. S., Steen, B., and Williams, T. F. (ed.) (1989). *Nutrition in the elderly*. Published for WHO by Oxford University Press, Oxford.

Pollitt, E. (1990). *Malnutrition and infection in the classroom*. UNESCO, Paris.

13 Feeding sick people, especially children

3.1 WHY SICK PEOPLE NEED FOOD

During infections the body uses as many Calories and nutrients as normal. The need for some nutrients may increase; for example, the body may use more energy if there is fever. Micronutrients such as vitamin A and zinc that help to destroy free radicals (see Section 17.2) may be particularly important.

But during infections the body often gets less energy and nutrients than it uses. This is because:

• People who are ill often eat less than usual.
• The gut may absorb less nutrients, particularly during diarrhoea. For example, during diarrhoea, the gut may absorb less fat than normal.

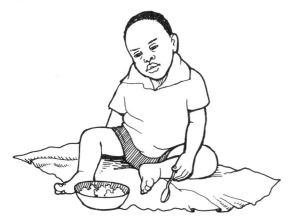

Fig. 13–1 A sick child may have a poor appetite.

If the body does not get enough food it breaks down its own fat and muscle to supply the nutrients that it needs. This is why people often lose weight when they are ill and look thin. Children may stop growing.

After the body overcomes an infection, it tries to rebuild the muscles and fat which were broken down and to regain the weight that it lost. Often during recovery a person eats and absorbs more food than normal. A child, especially if he is given extra food, may regain weight very fast. This is called *catch-up growth* (see Sections 15.8 and 17.14). Catch-up growth

also occurs after a child has been treated for worms (see Section 16.12).

Most of this chapter is about feeding sick children, because young children are sick more often than adults. However, the main points apply to people of all ages—the most important one is that everyone needs food when they are ill.

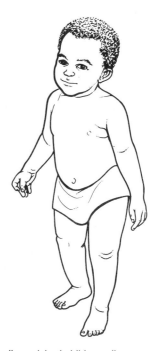

Fig. 13–2 A well nourished child usually recovers quickly.

• *Children who are well nourished* when they get an infection are likely to lose less weight, and they usually recover quickly.

• *Children who are already malnourished* when they get an infection are likely to lose more weight and to take longer to recover.

• *All children* recover more quickly and lose less weight if they are helped to eat when they are ill.

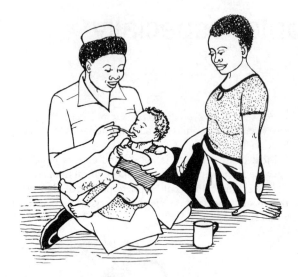

Fig. 13–3 A malnourished child who becomes sick may take a long time to recover.

13.2 WHY A SICK CHILD MAY NOT EAT ENOUGH

The child may have a poor appetite

When a child is ill, especially with fever, diarrhoea, or vomiting, he may not feel hungry. A sore mouth or throat may make it painful to eat. A blocked nose or problems with breathing (for example, with pneumonia) may make it difficult to eat. So a sick child may refuse to eat food which his mother offers him.

Most families know that, if a child is ill for a long time, he becomes thin and that, if a child is often ill, he may become thinner and thinner. Most parents are very worried when their children do not eat and they become thin. But often they feel helpless, because they think that there is nothing that they can do. Parents often regard a good appetite as a sign of good health in a child, and they may regard a poor appetite as a sign of poor health. But they may not see how the poor appetite is helping to cause the poor health.

The family may offer the child less food

It can be very difficult to feed an ill child who has lost his appetite. The mother or other carer may try to feed the child a bit, but they soon give up. Some families believe that it is harmful to feed a sick child, especially if he has diarrhoea. They may see that when a child with diarrhoea eats or drinks, he passes more faeces. So they think that food makes diarrhoea worse.

Some parents do not know that a sick child needs to eat. They may not know that, if they can persuade a sick child to eat more, they may help the child to recover and prevent him from becoming thin. Parents who do know that sick children need food may not know how to encourage them to eat.

The family may offer the child more dilute food

Families may make special soft, thin foods to encourage sick children to eat. For example, they may add water to make thinner porridge than the child normally eats. As a result, they give the sick child more dilute food, which contains less energy and nutrients than usual.

So changing the *type* of food also reduces the amount of energy and nutrients that a child eats. This may be more important than reducing the *amount* of food that they offer.

13.3 WHAT FAMILIES NEED TO KNOW ABOUT FEEDING SICK CHILDREN

- Well nourished children can fight infections better than undernourished children (see Section 16.3).
- Sick children who eat some food can fight infection better than sick children who eat almost nothing.
- When a child is ill, it is important to encourage him to eat, even if he does not want to.
- Sick children need food with enough energy and nutrients—not watery, dilute food.
- As soon as a child starts to recover from an illness and his appetite improves, he needs extra food to make up for the meals that he did not eat when he was ill.
- It is important to watch the child's growth line as he recovers. He should grow faster than usual at this time. He needs extra food until he weighs more than before he was sick.

Helping families to feed sick children

Find out what families do already. Many women know a lot about feeding sick children. They know which foods sick children like and how to persuade children to eat. Give women an opportunity to discuss these things. Encourage them to learn from each other's experiences, and learn from them yourself. They may have some good ideas which you can build on.

Discuss which foods a sick child can eat. A child who is ill may only be able to eat a small amount of food at

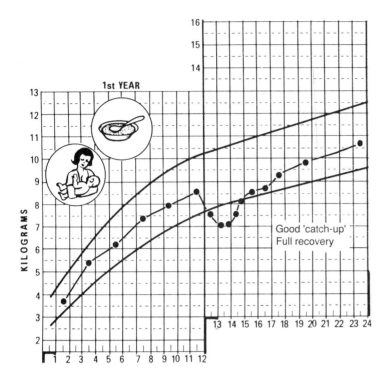

Fig. 13–4 A growth line showing 'catch-up' growth and full recovery (see also Sections 15.9, 17.9, and 17.14).

each meal. He may not be able to eat solid foods, such as thick porridge, or fatty or fried foods, or spicy foods. You may be able to help the family to think of foods which they can prepare quickly and easily, which are both nutrient-rich and easy for the child to eat.

The most important thing is to get a child to eat as much as possible of **something**.

These are some ideas to discuss with families.

Continue to breastfeed

If a child still breastfeeds, encourage the mother to continue. Breast milk is an excellent nutrient-rich, easy-to-digest food for sick children, and suckling comforts a sick, unhappy child. Even if a child has lost his appetite for other food, he may continue to breastfeed as much or even more than before. Encourage mothers to breastfeed more during recovery—more breast milk means more catch-up growth.

If breastfeeding was partial, or token before the illness, and the child now suckles more than before, the mother's breast milk may increase. (Some women notice slight engorgement when this happens.)

If the child has already stopped breastfeeding he may be willing to start again. This is easiest if he is less than 6 months old and stopped a short time ago, but it is worth trying at any time. Encourage the mother to offer her breast for comfort. If the child suckles, the mother is likely to find after a few days that she has milk again.

If a baby is too weak to suckle, show the mother how to express her breast milk and feed it to the baby from a small cup, or with a cup and spoon. Breast milk helps the baby to recover, and expressing it helps to keep up the supply (see Section 10.14).

Feed the child more often than usual

If a child has a poor appetite, he can eat only a little at a time. Usually the best way to help a child to eat more is to feed him more often—every 2–3 hours, or more often if he will take it.

Choose a food that the child likes and can eat easily

Find out what the child likes and what foods are available. Often, the foods need to be thin and smooth, so that the child does not have to chew them. Many sick children prefer liquid food, so they may like milk, or porridge or pap with milk or sugar, or soup. If families give the child vegetables, they should mash them very well.

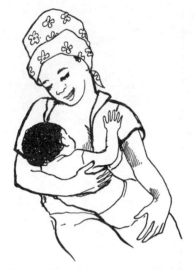

Fig. 13–5 Breast milk is an excellent food for sick children.

Most sick children prefer food with a mild or sweet taste, so the food should not be too salty or spicy. However, some may prefer a familiar strong taste. Children may like bananas, or potatoes mashed up, or bread with milk or sauce from the family meal, or bread mashed into milk or sauce. Some families may make sour fermented porridge for sick people (see Section 6.5).

Make sure that the food contains all the nutrients the child needs

It is important not to make the child's food too watery and dilute. When parents make soft or liquid foods, they should not add too much water. They can soften the food with milk or sauce or a little oil if possible.

- *If the child is ill for several days*, the family should try to vary the food. They can mash and soften some of the foods from the family meal. If possible, they should include mashed fruits (such as pawpaw) or vegetables (such as carrots, pumpkins, or green leaves) that are rich in vitamins A and C.

- *If the child has measles*, vitamin A is especially important. In areas where vitamin A deficiency is a problem, children with measles or severe diarrhoea or other infection may be given high-dose vitamin A capsules as part of the treatment (see Sections 19.8 and 19.9).

- *If the child has persistent diarrhoea*, he needs foods

rich in vitamin A, folate, iron, and zinc (see Section 13.4).

- *If the child has malaria*, he needs foods which are rich in folic acid.

- *If the child has hookworm*, he needs foods rich in iron and vitamin C, because he may be anaemic.

Encourage the child to eat but do not force him

Sometimes families *force* a child to take food. This is dangerous. Forcing food into a child's mouth may make him vomit, or the food may go down his trachea and choke him.

It takes a lot of patience and time to persuade a sick child to eat, but it is worth it. *How* the child is fed can make a lot of difference. If the child has fever, offer food when his temperature is lower, for example, after a dose of paracetamol or in the morning.

It can be helpful if the mother or other carer:

- offers food when the child is alert, rather than sleepy;

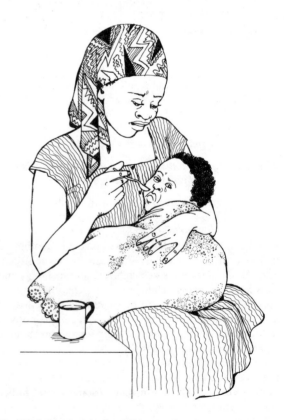

Fig. 13–6 Encourage the child to eat but do not force him.

Box 13.1. Signs of dehydration in children with diarrhoea

These are signs that the child's body has become dry because of loss of water in the diarrhoea faeces:

- thirst greater than normal;
- urine dark, small amount;
- dry mouth;
- sunken eyes;
- sunken soft spot on the top of the head (fontanelle);
- a fold of skin goes back slowly;
- unwell, sleepy, or irritable;
- fast, deep breathing.

The child needs more fluids and needs *oral rehydration solution* or fluids by injection (see Box 13.3).

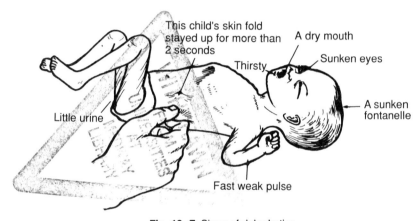

Fig. 13–7 Signs of dehydration.

- washes the child first to make him feel more comfortable;
- cleans his mouth so that eating is more comfortable;
- clears his nose so that he can breathe more easily;
- holds the child in a comforting position on her lap (or on the father, grandmother, or favourite older child's lap);
- makes feeding into a game with a toy or pet animal;
- feeds the child at the same time that other children eat.

13.4 FEEDING CHILDREN WITH DIARRHOEA AND VOMITING

Advice for the family if a child has diarrhoea

Give the child extra to drink

Children with diarrhoea lose a lot of water and may become *dehydrated* (Box 13.1). They also lose sodium

and potassium. Extra drinks can prevent dehydration. They also help a child's appetite to return faster, so the child loses less weight.

The type of drink to recommend depends on what is available, what the community already knows, and what the child normally drinks. Most fluids are helpful, especially if the child also has food. It is important that drinks do not replace food. Possible drinks include:

- *Food-based fluids* such as soups, and drinks made from staples. These are especially suitable if the community already knows and uses this kind of fluid. If possible, the fluid should contain a little salt. If the fluid does not normally contain salt, you may be able to teach the family to add some (see Box 13.2).

- *Salt and sugar water.* You may want to recommend this if families have salt and sugar and can prepare the mixture safely (see Box 13.2).

Box 13.2. Fluids for children with diarrhoea to prevent dehydration

There are many ways to make drinks for children with diarrhoea. Here we give some basic recipes only. If possible, find the recipe that has been worked out for your country, using local measures that people find easy to use.

Salt and sugar water
To 5 cups (1 litre) of clean drinking water add:
    8 level teaspoons of sugar (18 g);
    1 level teaspoon* of salt (3.0 g).

Or

To 1 glass of clean drinking water add:
    scoop of sugar in hand;
    pinch of salt.

Food-based fluids
1. To 5.5 cups (1.1 litre) of water add ½ cup (50–60 g) cereal flour (rice, maize, millet, wheat, or sorghum)
   Or add 1 cup (200 g) mashed boiled potato to 5 cups (1 litre) of water.

2. Boil until the mixture bubbles.

3. Take off the fire and leave to cool.

4. Add one level teaspoonful of salt (3.0 g).

The mixture is then ready to give to a child with diarrhoea. Remember this is a *drink* to replace *water*. It is not a food.
The child needs to eat food as well as the solution.
The amount of faeces that the child passes may decrease sooner with food-based fluids than with salt and sugar water.

How much fluid to give
Give the same amount as for oral rehydration solution in Box 13.3.

* Note: 'Level teaspoon' measures must be really level—take extra salt or sugar off and flatten with a knife. Adding too much salt or sugar can be dangerous.

- *Plain water.* This can be effective if the child also eats some food which can provide some salt and other nutrients.

- *Other drinks.* Fruit juice, coconut water, tea, and sodas all provide water. Fruit juice and coconut water provide potassium.

Continue to breastfeed

Advise the mother to breastfeed the child frequently—at least every 3 hours or more often. Some mothers think that they should stop breastfeeding a child with diarrhoea. In the past, health workers sometimes advised mothers to stop breastfeeding. But now we know that this advice was wrong, and that it is important to continue. Breast milk helps the gut to heal, and it helps the child to recover from diarrhoea more quickly. Breastfeeding is often the easiest way to give a child water and nutrients.

Artificially fed babies

Babies who are artificially fed are at special risk from diarrhoea, for a number of reasons (see Section 10.3).

If the baby is less than 6 months old, advise the family to:
- Continue to feed the baby at least 3-hourly.
- Dilute the animal milk or formula with an equal amount of water for 2 days.
- Return to full strength feeds again after 2 days. (Make sure that they normally give the correct amount of artificial feeds in the correct strength; see Section 10.16.)

Artificial feeds may make diarrhoea worse. This sometimes happens because damage to the gut makes it difficult for the baby to digest the lactose in animal milk. In this case, either:

- Suggest that the family give soured or fermented milks (such as yoghurt), which contain less lactose.

Box 13.3. Oral rehydration solution (ORS)

ORS is the fluid usually used to treat dehydration. You can make ORS from packets of *oral rehydration salts* which contain a special mixture of glucose and sodium and potassium salts. Mix the contents of the packet with a certain volume of clean drinking water (usually a litre, but check the instructions on the packet). The glucose helps the absorption of the sodium, potassium, and water. If you do not have ORS packets, make oral rehydration solution this way:

Salt/sugar	Amount for 1-litre solution (g)	Volume in small 5- or 10-ml syringe (ml)†	Note
Sodium chloride* (common salt)	3.5	3	You cannot make ORS without this
Glucose	20	30	You cannot make ORS
or			without
Sucrose (common sugar)	40	50	one of these
Trisodium citrate dihydrate	2.9	3	You can make ORS without
or			these but
sodium bicarbonate	2.5	3	it is better if you have
Potassium chloride	1.5	1.5	one or more of them

How much fluid to give
After each loose stool give:

- to children less than 2 years old: ¼–½ cup or glass (50–100 ml);
- to children of 2 to 10 years old: ½–1 cup or glass (100–200 ml).

Give more fluid than this if the child is thirsty and does not vomit. If the child vomits, wait 10 minutes; then continue giving the fluids more slowly—for example, one spoonful every 3 minutes.

- For children over 10 years old and adults, give as much as they want.

Reference: WHO (1990).

* For very young infants and severely malnourished children, a solution containing less sodium chloride may be advisable—see Section 17.8.
† The volume of different salts and sugars varies according to how it is made and stored. Therefore the above volume measurement is not always accurate, and you should check it locally. Use a precision scale, for example in a local pharmacy, to weigh the correct amount of each salt and sugar that you will use. Then measure the volume of that amount of the salt or sugar in a syringe. Check the volume again when you use a new supplier.

---

or

- Ask mothers of young babies if they would be willing to start breastfeeding again (see Section 10.15). Difficulty digesting lactose in breast milk is rarely a problem.

If the baby is more than 6 months old, he should be taking weaning foods. It is not necessary at this age to dilute artificial feeds during diarrhoea. To reduce the risk of the diarrhoea becoming persistent, mix the animal milk or formula with cereal or other staple food.

Continue to feed the child as normally as possible

The family should give the child small, frequent, soft, easy-to-eat, nutritious meals (see Chapter 11 and Section 13.3). Meals should not be too dilute, they should not contain too much fibre, and they should not contain a lot of sugar which can make diarrhoea worse. It is important for children to have food as well as fluids during diarrhoea because:

- Food helps the body to absorb fluids. Plain water is only effective if the child also has some food to provide salt, and other nutrients to help absorption of salt and water.

- Foods can provide potassium which home-based fluids may lack. Most fruits and vegetables are good sources of potassium—especially banana, spinach, avocado, and pumpkin.
- Food helps the gut to recover more quickly. If a child starves during diarrhoea ('resting the gut'), the gut is damaged *more*, and takes longer to recover.
- Nutrients such as vitamin A and zinc may help the gut to recover more quickly.

If a child with diarrhoea eats, the amount of faeces may at first seem to increase. This is not because the food makes the illness worse—it is because *some* of the food is not absorbed. However, much of the food is absorbed and, the more the child eats, the more nutrients the body can use. Usually, if the child continues to eat, the amount of faeces decreases *sooner*.

Advice if diarrhoea persists

In some children diarrhoea continues for more than 14 days. This is called *persistent diarrhoea*, and it is commonest in children who are artificially fed. Children with persistent diarrhoea often have poor appetites, and are likely to become malnourished.

Advise the family to mix the animal milk or formula with starchy porridge or to give soured or fermented milk, so that the concentration of lactose in the food is less.

If diarrhoea continues, the child may need food without milk. Help the family to make soft, easy-to-eat porridge, enriched with protein (such as legumes, or if possible meat, chicken, or fish), a little oil (if possible, vegetable oil which is easy to digest), and foods which provide vitamin A, folate, iron, and zinc (see Appendix 3). Children with persistent diarrhoea often lack these micronutrients. Give supplements if available (see Section 17.12).

Advice if a child vomits

- Stop giving food for 4–6 hours.
- Give small drinks only—for example, give about 2 spoonfuls (10 ml) every 10 minutes.
- If the child has not vomited after 4–6 hours, give a small feed—for example, ¼ cup (30 ml) of milk or porridge.
- If the child keeps this down, try another small feed after about 2 hours.
- Increase the amount of food as the child is able to keep it down.

- If the child vomits again, return to smaller amounts of food, or to drinks.
- If the child continues to vomit every time that he eats or drinks or if he has signs of dehydration (Box 13.1), the family should take him to a health centre quickly. The child may need fluids by injection.

If a child is vomiting because of whooping cough, try to feed him again soon after he has vomited. He is more likely to keep the food down if it is given straight away.

13.5 FEEDING A CHILD DURING RECOVERY FROM ILLNESS

When children start to recover from infections, they are hungrier than usual. It is important for them to have extra food at this time, especially if they did not eat much during the illness.

Giving more food enables their growth to 'catch-up'. If they do not eat extra food immediately after an infection, or after treatment for worms, they miss the chance to 'catch-up'. Each time they are ill, they become more underweight. So they need extra food until they have regained lost weight and are growing at a healthy rate.

When they are ill, they may use up their stores of vitamin A, iron, and other nutrients. They need good mixed meals to fill up their stores again. Discuss with families the different ways in which they can give a child extra food at this time. They may be able to:

- Feed the child an *extra meal* or nutritious snack every day until he weighs more than he did before the illness began.
- Feed the child *extra food* at each meal. If the child's appetite is good, he can get the extra food that he needs by eating larger meals.
- Feed the child foods which are *extra rich* in energy and nutrients—for example meat, fish, liver, eggs, milk, margarine, oil. Even poor parents may be willing to buy some of these foods for a short time, if they know that the child needs them.

Babies should suckle more often, which gives them more breast milk, and also helps to build up their mothers' supply.

After acute diarrhoea, a child usually needs an extra meal a day for about a week. After persistent diarrhoea, the child needs an extra meal a day for at least a month.

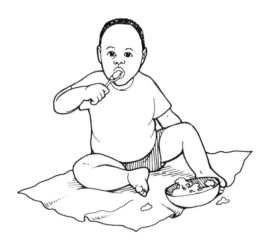

Fig. 13–8 A child recovering from an illness is often hungrier than usual.

13.6 SICK OLDER CHILDREN, ADULTS, AND OLD PEOPLE

People of all ages need food when they are sick but, like children, they usually do not want to eat much. Some of the ways to help sick people to eat enough are to:

- *Offer foods which the person likes and can easily eat.* Sick people may find it easier to eat food which is thin and smooth, or liquid. When we are ill, we often prefer a more childish sort of food than when we are well.

- *Give small meals more often than usual.* People may not be able to eat as much food at each meal when they are ill, as when they are well. Old people's appetites may not return as quickly as children's appetites as they recover from an illness. They may need frequent small meals for longer.

- *Make sure that people who are ill have good mixed meals.* Make sure that the person's meals contain all the nutrients that he or she needs. The best way to do this is to try to give a lot of different foods in the meals, including legumes, vegetables, fruits, and foods from animals sometimes. This is especially important for a person who may be ill for a long time, and for people with illnesses from which they will not recover.

- *Give meals which supply plenty of iron and folate.* Old people, women, and growing children easily become anaemic, so they need foods rich in folate and iron added to their food.

13.7 PEOPLE WITH HIV INFECTION AND AIDS

Children and adults with AIDS may have many illnesses, and they may become very thin and wasted. This is partly because the AIDS virus infects the gut, causing diarrhoea, and partly because AIDS patients have many other infections, which reduce their appetites.

In the early stages of HIV infection, before AIDS develops, eating good mixed meals may help a person to stay well for longer. This stage may last a number of years. Breastfeeding a baby with HIV may prevent other infections, so that he survives longer.

When an adult or child with HIV starts to become ill with AIDS, good feeding may help them to feel better and to recover for a time. It may help them to resist the other infections which make AIDS worse. Good feeding cannot prevent AIDS or wasting, but it may slow down the illness. There is no special food which has been proved to cure HIV or AIDS.

Nutrition workers can help to keep AIDS patients as well as possible for as long as possible. Give families the support and help that you can, and encourage them to give people with HIV good mixed meals, and to feed AIDS patients in the same way as any other sick person.

THINGS TO DO

Practical exercises and discussion

1. Prepare a food-based fluid for a child with diarrhoea.

2. Plan a good mixed meal for a sick old person, with locally available foods. Discuss whether the meal is rich in folate and iron.

Field visit

3. Arrange for trainees to talk to some parents of sick children in a hospital or health centre about how they have fed the child during the illness.

   a. They should ask what kind of food they give the child, and why, how much the child eats, and how often they feed the child.

   b. If possible, they should watch the child feeding.

   c. If the child is young enough to breastfeed, ask if the mother is still breastfeeding him and if he is feeding as much or more or less than before.

USEFUL PUBLICATIONS

Aga Khan University (1990). *Cereal based oral rehydration therapy for diarrhoea*. Aga Khan Foundation, Geneva and International Child Health Foundation, Columbia, Missouri.

Jelliffe, D. B. and Jelliffe, E. F. P. (1989). *Dietary management of young children with acute diarrhoea*. Published by WHO in collaboration with UNICEF, Geneva.

14 Growth and development

14.1 CHILDREN'S SIZE AND GROWTH

Figure 14–1 shows a child called Wambui who is 3 years old and healthy. Figure 14–2 shows the same child from when she was born until she was 2 years old.

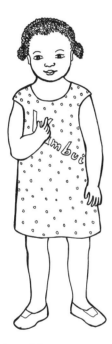

Fig. 14–1 Wambui aged 3 years.

At each age Wambui is *bigger* than she was before. She is taller and broader and her limbs are thicker. As a result of being bigger she is *heavier*. This increase in size and weight is called *growth*.

Healthy, well nourished children grow at approximately the same *rate*. Therefore the rate at which a child grows is a good sign of the child's health and nutrition. A child who is growing at the normal healthy rate is almost certainly well nourished. A child who is not growing at the normal healthy rate is probably not well nourished.

Signs that a child is growing at the normal rate

Parents know that their children are growing because they see them:

- become taller;
- become fatter;
- become heavier to carry;
- grow out of their clothes.

However, parents may not know if a child is growing at the normal healthy rate, and they need help to find out.

Nutrition workers do not live with the children, and so do not see how the children are growing. But you need to know, so that you can help the parents to keep the child healthy and well nourished.

The only way for parents and nutrition workers to be certain about how a child is growing, is to *measure the child regularly*. In some situations we measure children's heights or lengths to find out how tall they are; in other situations we measure the thickness of children's arms to find out how fat they are.

But in most situations the best way to find out if a child is growing normally is to *weigh* her. A child's weight is made up of both height and fatness, and can show growth more clearly.

If a child is gaining weight at a healthy rate, you can reassure her parents that she is growing well. If a child is not gaining weight at a healthy rate, you and her parents find out quickly. Often it is easier to help a child who has not gained weight for a short time, than it is to help a child who has not gained weight for a long time.

Other signs of health and good nutrition in children

Parents know other signs, besides growth, which show that a child is healthy. They see that their child:

- has shining skin, strong shining hair, and bright eyes;
- has a good appetite;
- is active and playful.

A child with these signs is likely to be healthy and well nourished, and growing at a normal rate.

165

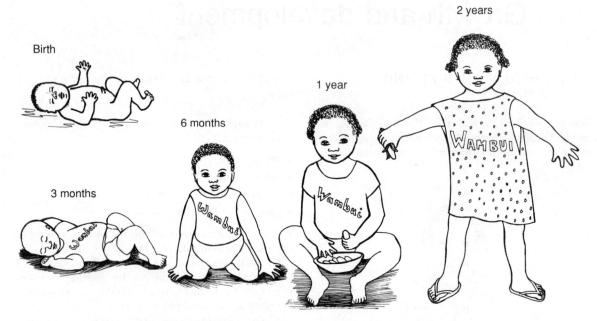

Fig. 14–2 Wambui at different ages from birth to 2 years.

A poor appetite, or decreased activity, are often the first signs that a child is not healthy and not well nourished. These signs can occur before the child stops gaining weight. Mothers notice changes in their children's appetites and activity, but they may not mention them to health or nutrition workers. Always ask about appetite and activity when you see a child. So the signs that parents see, and weighing, are both useful ways to know that a child is growing and healthy.

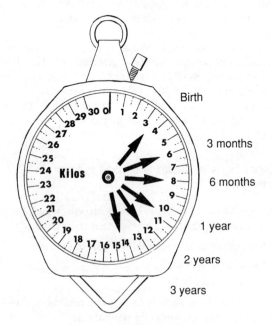

Fig. 14–3 Wambui's weights at different ages.

14.2 DEVELOPMENT

A well-nourished child is full of energy. She is interested in the world around her, so she wants to learn, and she enjoys playing. A playful child stimulates her mother and other members of the family to talk, play, and do things with her. Play is not just fun, to entertain a child while she waits to grow up. Play helps children to learn and develop normally.

However, even well nourished children vary in how clever they are—just as they vary in how tall they are. We must be careful not to teach mothers that giving a child more or better food can make her more clever. That is quite different from knowing that a well nourished child has the best chance of developing normally.

As Wambui grew in size, she became able to do new things. She started to smile, to hold up her head, to sit, to look around her, to crawl, to stand, to walk, and to run. She learned to talk and to feed and dress herself.

She began to play, to explore, and to ask questions. She became attached to her parents, learned to recognize strangers and to play with other children. She learned what it feels like to be happy, jealous, and angry.

All normal, healthy, children become able to do these things, and to have new emotions, in more or less the same order, and at roughly the same ages. This is what we call *child development*. Normal development is another sign that a child is well nourished. The stages of development that it is useful to remember are given in Section 14.10.

What a young child needs to grow and develop normally

A young child has the best chance of growing and developing normally if she has:

- a loving caring family;
- a clean safe home;
- enough good food and safe water;
- encouragement and opportunities to play and learn;
- protection from infection and accidents;
- health care when sick.

Nutrition workers should know that children need all these things, and should try to help families to provide them.

14.3 VARIATION IN HEIGHT AND WEIGHT

Figure 14–5 shows seven 3-year-old children. They are all healthy and well nourished. But they are not all exactly the same height—some are taller than Wambui, and some are shorter.

Their different heights show that healthy children vary in size. But they do not vary very much. They vary within a certain *range*. So there is a range of healthy heights for 3-year-olds. Boys and girls are almost the same size at this age.

Children also vary in how much they weigh, and there is a range of healthy weights for children of each age. For example, almost all healthy 3-year-old children weigh between 11 and 18 kg.

So it is not possible to say exactly how tall or how heavy a child should be. But we can say what the *middle* or *median* height and weight is for healthy children of each age. In Fig. 14–5, Wambui's height is the middle or median height of the group.

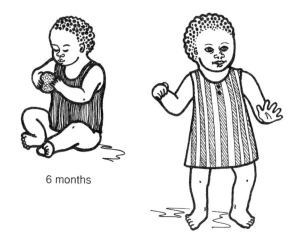

6 months

1 year

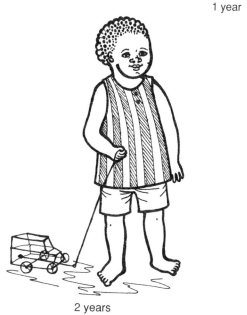

2 years

Fig. 14–4 As children grow, they also develop and become able to do new things.

The *median* weight of healthy, well nourished 36-month-old children is 14.3 kg. The median height and weight at each age are usually called the *reference height for age* and the *reference weight for age*.

14.4 GROWTH CHARTS

When you weigh children, you want to know how their weights compared with the reference weight and the

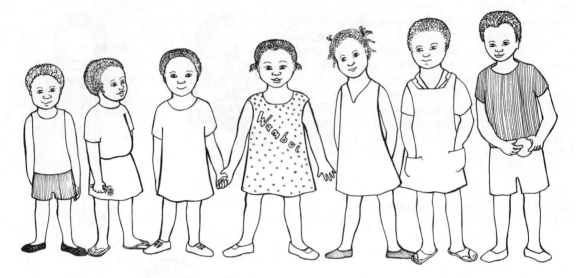

Fig. 14–5 A group of healthy 3-year-olds. Wambui is in the middle. Healthy children of the same age vary in size.

range of weights for healthy children of the same ages.

It is impossible to remember the reference weights and the range of weights for healthy children of all ages. It is not easy always to use a table of reference values. Instead, we use charts which have reference weight-for-age curves drawn on them. These charts are called *growth charts*. There are many different kinds of growth chart, which are similar in principle but which vary in detail.

All growth charts have a weight-for-age graph printed on one side. The graph is divided into 5 years, for the first 5 years of the child's life. Some charts are for only the first 3 years.

The *boxes* along the bottom of the graph and the *columns* above them are each for 1 month of the child's life. The first box and column on the left are for the month in which the child was born. The *straight lines* going across the chart are for weight, and the numbers up the left-hand side show how many kilograms each line is for.

There are two *weight-for-age curves* on the chart in Fig. 14–6. The upper of these two curves shows the median or reference weights-for-age. This is the *reference curve*. The lower curve shows the lower end of the range of healthy weights.

Some charts have more than two weight-for-age curves on them. Figure 14–7 shows a chart with a weight-for-age curve *above* the reference curve. This 'topmost' curve shows the upper end of the range of healthy weights. There is another weight-for-age curve

below the lower curve. This shows weights that are 60 per cent of the reference weights.

In some countries, charts are now in use which have more than three or four weight-for-age curves on them. Some charts have coloured bands.

14.5 THE REFERENCE WEIGHTS AND THE RANGE OF HEALTHY WEIGHTS

Figure 14–8 shows a chart with the reference curve and the lower curve from Fig. 14–6. The topmost curve above the reference curve is shown as a dotted line. The weights of 100 healthy children have been plotted on the chart.

If you count the dots, you will find that there are 50 above the reference curve, and 50 below it. This is because the reference curve is the *median* or middle value of the healthy weights at each age. The reference curve is also called the **50th centile**, because the weights of 50 out of every 100 children in a healthy community are *below* it.

Notice that the weights are scattered all over the chart, but there are more of them *near* the reference curve than there are far away. So the weight dots of *most* healthy children are *near* the reference curve, either above or below it.

Some of the healthy children have weights which are near the lower curve. Count the number of weight dots

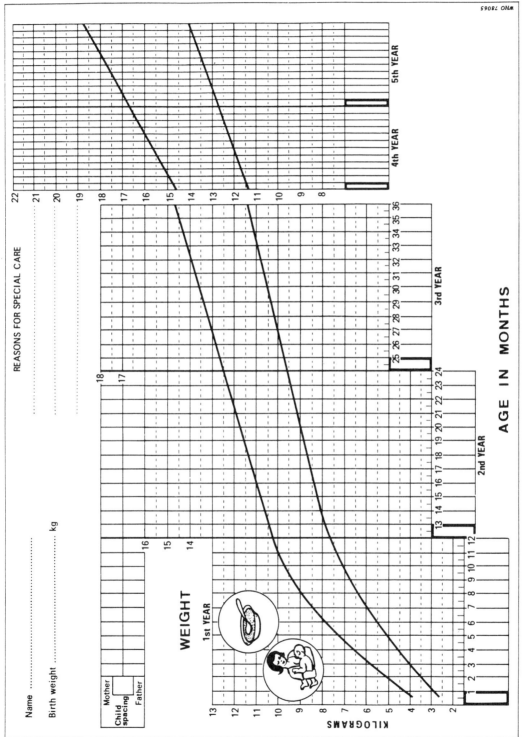

Fig. 14–6 Growth chart developed by the World Health Organization (WHO). The upper reference curve on the growth chart is the median for boys and the lower line is the 3rd centile for girls. The 3rd centile curve is slightly below 80 per cent of the reference curve. In some weight charts the 80 per cent curve is used instead.

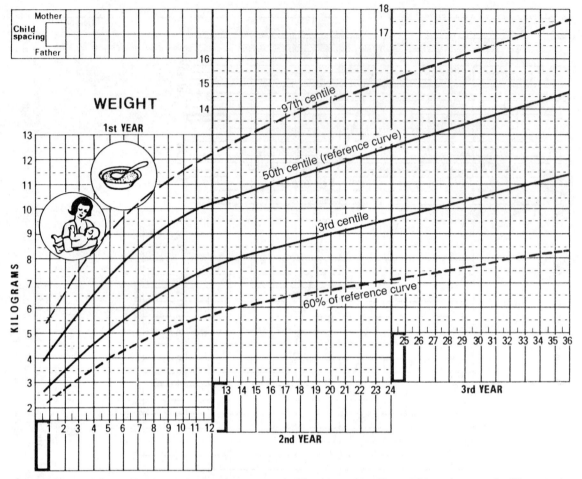

Fig. 14–7 Growth chart with a curve showing the upper end of the range of healthy weights and a curve for 60 per cent of the reference weights.

below the lower curve. There are only three. So there are a *few* healthy children with weights below the lower curve, but not many. The lower curve is also called the **3rd centile**, because the weights of three out of every 100 healthy children are below it. However, notice that even the three dots which are below the lower curve are not very far below it. No healthy child's weight is below the 60 per cent curve.

Some of the healthy children have weights which are near the topmost curve. Count the weight dots which are *above* the topmost curve. There are only three. So there are a *few* healthy children with weights above the topmost curve, but not many. Almost all children have weights below this curve. The topmost curve is also called the **97th centile**, because 97 out of every 100 healthy children have weights which are *below* it.

So the 50th centile curve shows the *reference* or *median* weights. The 97th centile and the 3rd centile show the top and bottom of the *range* of healthy weights. Any child whose weight falls between the 3rd and the 97th centile is *within the normal range*. A child whose weight is above the 97th centile, or below the 3rd centile is said to be *outside the normal range*. The weights of a few healthy children are outside the normal range, but they are very few, and their weights are not far outside the range.

Children with weights above the reference curve

Most growth charts do not have a 97th centile line—the upper curve is the *reference* curve. Remember that the

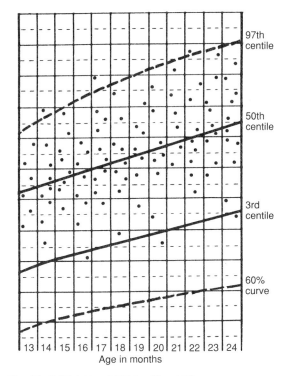

Fig. 14–8 Weights of 100 healthy children.

weights of 50 out of every 100 healthy children are *above* the reference curve. This means that in a healthy community you *expect* to find that half of the children weigh more than the reference or median value. So do not think that any child whose weight is above the reference curve is overweight. Only children whose weights are above the 97th centile curve are likely to be overweight.

If a 97th centile curve is not drawn, you can tell where it should be, because it is the same distance above the reference line as the 3rd centile is below.

14.6 HOW THE REFERENCE CURVE SHOWS GROWTH

The reference weight-for-age curve shows how, as children become older, they become heavier. The slope or shape of the curve shows the *rate* at which healthy children's weights increase at different ages. Boys and girls grow at the same rate in early childhood.

If you weigh a child regularly, plot the weights on a chart, and join the dots with a line, you make a *growth* *line* for that child. The *shape* of a healthy child's growth line should be similar to the *shape* of the reference curve. The child's weight should increase at about the same rate as the reference curve.

However, as we explained in Section 14.3, healthy children of the same age vary in *size*, so different children's growth lines vary in their *position* on the chart. Some children's growth lines are above the reference curve, some are below the reference curve. Most healthy children have growth lines above the 3rd centile, but three out of every 100 children have growth lines a little below the 3rd centile.

The *growth rates* of healthy *large* children and healthy *small* children of the *same age* are about the same. In other words, they gain about the same weight each month. For example, between 12 and 23 months of age all healthy children gain about 200 g each month. This is a healthy growth rate for large and small children of this age.

But the growth rates of younger children are faster. For example, during the first 6 months of life, a healthy child gains at least 500 g each month. So the reference curves rise more steeply in the first year of life. This gives the reference curve a special shape which is important when we need to decide if a child is growing fast enough.

Irregularity of individual children's growth curves

Most children's growth lines are not as smooth and regular as the reference curve. Sometimes the child's line rises a little faster for a time; sometimes it rises more slowly for a month or two. But the overall shape of a healthy child's growth line should be nearly the same as the shape of the reference curve.

14.7 HOW A GROWTH CHART SHOWS WHETHER A CHILD IS WELL NOURISHED OR NOT

What do you know if there is only one dot on a child's chart?

If you weigh a child once, you can plot the weight on the child's chart. This one dot tells you about a child's *size*, but it does not tell you if the child is growing.

One dot can tell you if a child's weight is within the normal range, and it can tell you about his *probable* health and nutrition now. But it cannot tell you for certain if he is healthy and well nourished or not, because healthy children vary so much in weight.

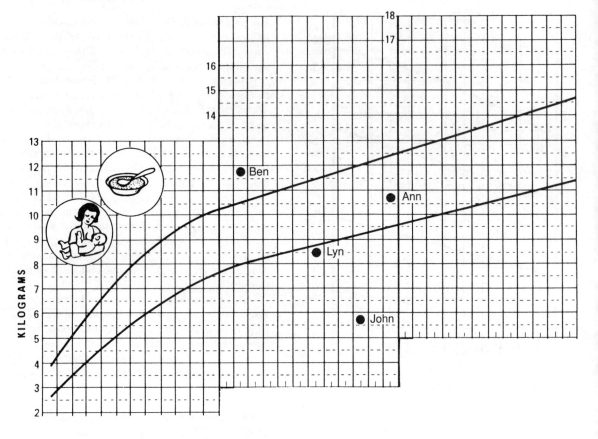

Fig. 14–9 Growth chart showing single weights of four children.

- *The weight dot may be ABOVE the reference curve.* Ben's weight (Fig. 14–9) is above the reference weight for age. Ben is probably well nourished, but you cannot be sure. He could be a large child who has stopped growing.

- *The weight dot may be BETWEEN the reference curve and the 3rd centile.* Ann's weight (Fig. 14–9) is within the healthy range. Ann is probably well nourished—but you cannot be sure.

- *The weight dot may be a LITTLE BELOW the 3rd centile.* Lyn's weight (Fig. 14–9) is a little below the normal range for healthy children. We call a child whose weight is below the normal range *underweight*. Lyn *may* be small and growing at a healthy rate. However, most children whose weights are below the lower curve are not getting enough nutrients and are undernourished.

- *The dot may be FAR BELOW the 3rd centile.* John's weight (Fig. 14–9) is definitely too low, and John is almost certainly undernourished.

What do you know if there are several weight dots on a child's chart?

Several weight dots tell you about a child's *growth*. You can make a growth line for the child, which you can compare to the reference weight-for-age curve. You can see whether or not the weight is increasing, and whether the child is growing at a healthy rate.

If a child is growing at a healthy rate, then his parents, and the health and nutrition workers, know that he is well nourished. If a child is not growing at a healthy rate, then his parents and the health workers know that he is *not* well nourished.

So weighing a child several times tells you much more about his health and nutrition than weighing him once.

We call weighing a child regularly and plotting his growth line on a growth chart *'monitoring'* the child's growth.

14.8 DIFFERENT SHAPES OF GROWTH LINE

Healthy growth

In Fig. 14–10(a) Sam's and Sally's weights are both increasing at a healthy rate. Their growth lines are rising at the same rate as the reference curve. Sam and Sally are both well nourished.

Healthy growth below the 3rd centile

In Fig. 14–10(b) Susan's weights are below the 3rd centile. Susan was born small and, like all low birth weight babies, she is at greater risk of sickness than a larger child and may need special care (see Chapter 16). But Susan is growing well. Her growth line shows that she is as healthy and well nourished as she can be.

Slow growth

Figure 14–11 shows how Mary's, Martin's, and Meg's weights are increasing. But their growth lines are rising more slowly than the reference curve. This is called *growth faltering*. This is a warning sign that the children may be undernourished—especially Meg who is also underweight.

Flat growth line

Figure 14–12 shows how Jose's and Jane's weights have not increased at all for about a year. John's weight has not increased for 6 months. Their growth lines are flat. Jane's curve has already crossed the 3rd centile curve.

John, Jane, and Jose have stopped growing. They all have *growth failure*, and they are undernourished. This is particularly serious for John and Jane who are underweight, and who are at greater risk than larger children.

Losing weight

In Fig. 14–13 you can see that Emma, Ewan, and Eddy have all stopped growing and are losing weight. They are all undernourished, and losing weight usually means that the child is ill with an infection. This is particularly serious for Eddy who is also small and for Ewan whose weight has fallen below the 3rd centile.

Fast weight gain

Sometimes a child's growth line rises faster than the reference weight-for-age curve. In Fig. 14–14 Ewan is gaining weight fast because he is recovering from undernutrition and illness. Fast weight gain is a good sign of recovery. It is called 'catch-up growth' (see Section 15.8). Lena's fast weight gain is a sign that she may be becoming overweight, because of over-nutrition.

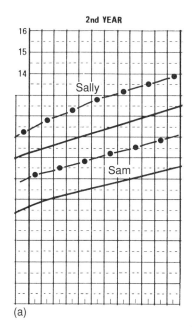

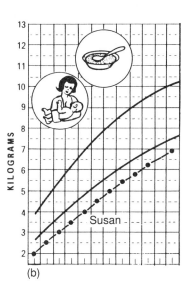

Fig. 14–10 (a) Sam and Sally's growth lines; (b) Susan's growth-line.

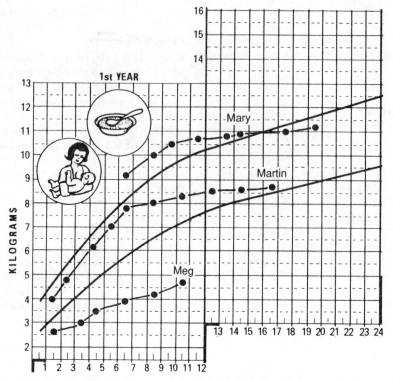

Fig. 14–11 The growth lines of Mary, Martin, and Meg.

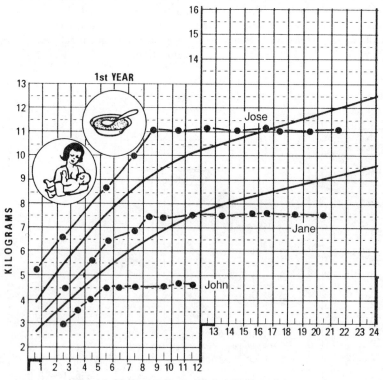

Fig. 14–12 Growth lines of John, Jane, and Jose.

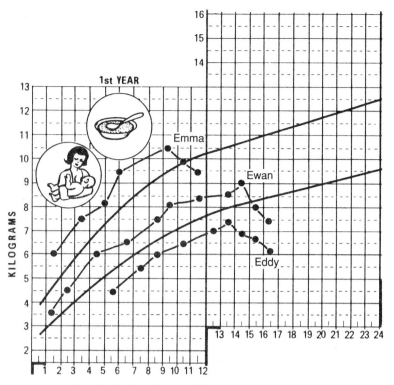

Fig. 14–13 Growth lines of Emma, Ewan, and Eddy.

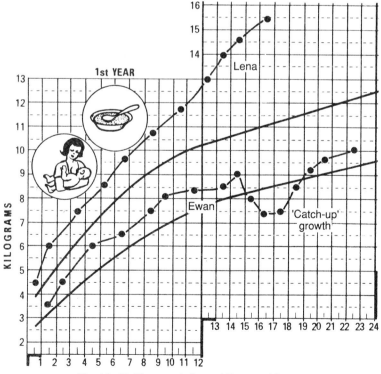

Fig. 14–14 The growth lines of Ewan and Lena.

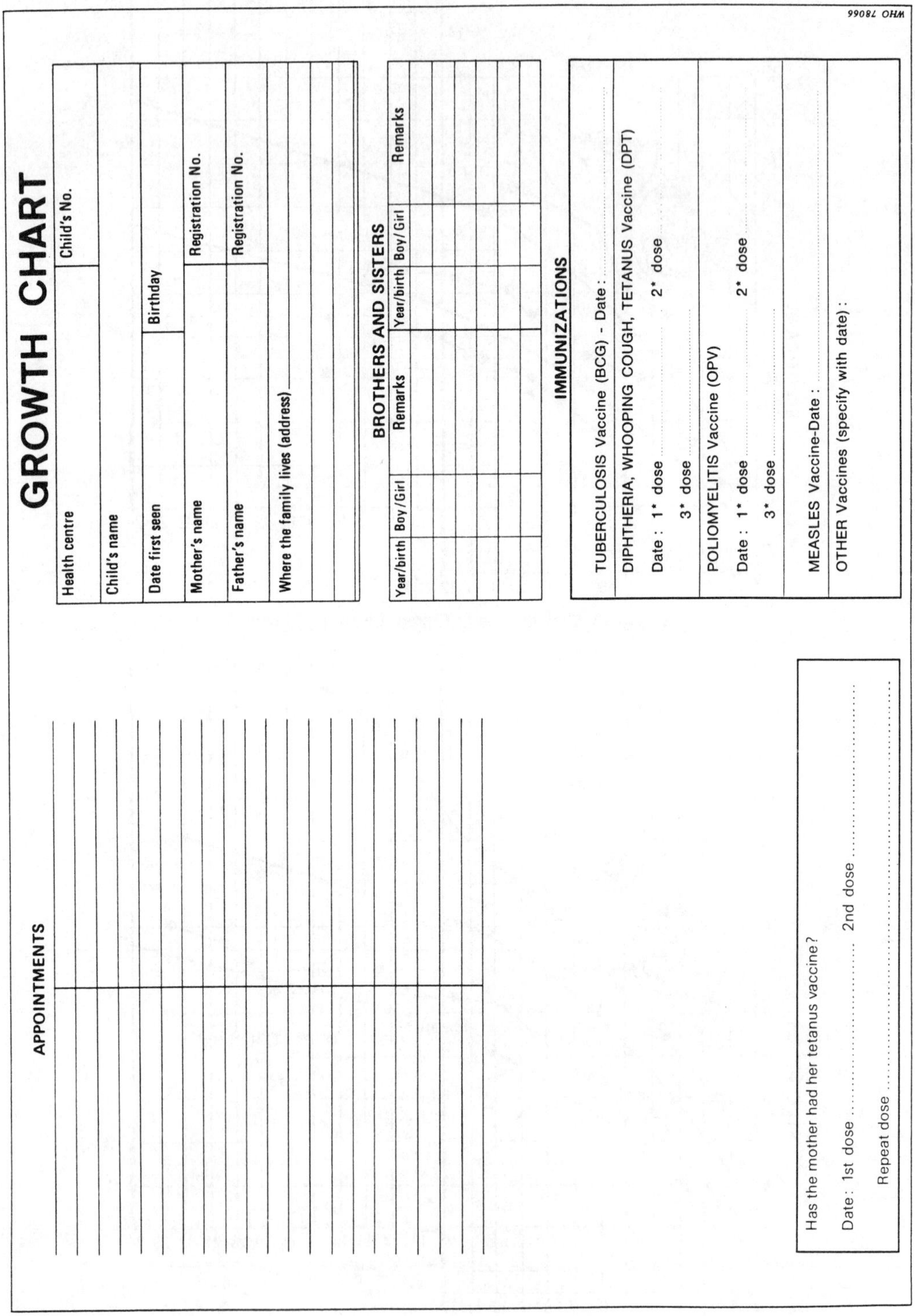

GROWTH CHART

Health centre	Child's No.
Child's name	
Date first seen	Birthday
Mother's name	Registration No.
Father's name	Registration No.
Where the family lives (address)	

BROTHERS AND SISTERS

Year/birth	Boy/Girl	Remarks	Year/birth	Boy/Girl	Remarks

IMMUNIZATIONS

TUBERCULOSIS Vaccine (BCG) - Date : ....

DIPHTHERIA, WHOOPING COUGH, TETANUS Vaccine (DPT)

Date : 1* dose .... 2* dose ....

3* dose ....

POLIOMYELITIS Vaccine (OPV)

Date : 1* dose .... 2* dose ....

3* dose ....

MEASLES Vaccine-Date : ....

OTHER Vaccines (specify with date) :

APPOINTMENTS

Has the mother had her tetanus vaccine?

Date: 1st dose .... 2nd dose ....

Repeat dose ....

WHO 78066

Fig. 14–15 The back of the WHO growth chart.

14.9 FILLING IN A GROWTH CHART

Fill in the back of the chart

On the back of the growth chart are spaces to fill in details of

- the child (such as name and date of birth);
- the family (such as address and details of other children);
- immunizations of the child and mother;
- appointments to attend the clinic, for example, for treatment.

Fill in details of the child and family the first time that you see the child, and fill in details of immunizations and appointments as they occur.

Make a *calendar* for the child

The purpose of the calendar is to save you working out how old a child at each visit and to prevent mistakes if you or the family work the age out differently at different visits. Families may not be able to tell you a child's exact age in months, but they often know when a child was born, or they have a record of the birth from hospital.

Figure 14–16 shows how to fill in the calendar in four steps:

1. Write the month and year of the child's birth in the first thick lined or shaded box. Add the day if you know it.

2. Write the birth month in all the other thick-lined boxes—remembering to increase the year each time.

3. Now fill in all the other boxes with the correct month. Always use the first 2–3 letters for the month. Do not use numbers, as they may be confused with ages. If you fill in all the birthday months first, you notice if you have left out a month.

4. Write the correct new year with each 'January'.

It is worth taking a few minutes to make the calendar the first time that you see the child. Then the chart is ready to use each time someone weighs the child. The small numbers at the bottom of the months columns tell you the child's age in months.

Plot the child's weight on the chart

Each time you weigh the child:

- Find the column for the present month in this year.
- Move up the column until you meet the weight line for the number of kilograms that the child weighs. Make a dot.
- Join the dot to the dot for the previous weighing.

If the child did not come in the previous few months:

- Leave those columns empty. Draw the line straight across the 'empty' month columns.

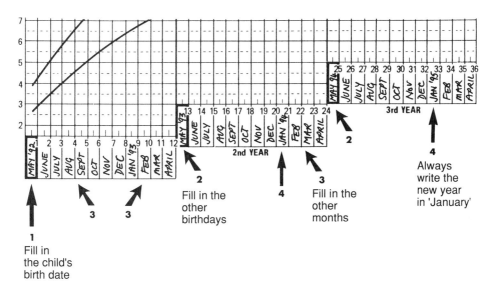

Fig. 14–16 Filling in the calendar on a growth chart.

If a child does not weigh an exact number of kilograms:

- If a child weighs something and a half kilograms (say 7.5 or 8.5 kilograms) put his weight dot on the *half kilogram line.*
- If a child's weight is between a whole and a half kilogram, for example, he might weigh 10.1 or 9.8 kilograms; put the dot *between* the kilogram line and the half-kilogram line (see Fig. 14–17(a)).

If a child comes to be weighed more than once in a month. Some mothers like to bring their children to the clinic more than once a month.

- If the child is not sick, and if his weight is the same each time, it is not necessary to record the weight twice.
- If the child is sick, or if his weight increases or decreases between visits, then you may want to record his weight both times.

   Put the dot for the *first visit* early in the month on the left side of the column (see Fig. 14–1(b)). Put the dot for the *later visit* on the right side of the month column.

When you weigh children at the beginning of a month, put all their weights on the left of the weight column. Then, if they come again before the end of the month, you have space to record another weight.

14.10 IF YOU DO NOT KNOW A CHILD'S DATE OF BIRTH

If a child was born at home, his family may not have a record of the date. But you can still use a growth chart for the child.

- Estimate the child's birth month as nearly as you can.
- Keep to that month—do not change it.
- Make a calendar using that month as his birth month.
- Use this calendar to record his weights.
- Then his growth line will be the right shape on his chart.

The line may not be in *exactly* the right place, but that is not as important as the shape.

Estimating a child's birth month

If the baby is less than 3 months old
Most mothers who bring their babies for the first im-

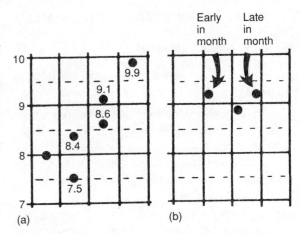

Fig. 14–17 (a) Where to put the dot if a child does not weigh an exact number of kilos; (b) where to put the dot when you weigh a child early or late in the month.

munization can remember the month of the child's birth with a little questioning.

If the child is older

You should be able to estimate the age of most children under 3 years old to within about 3 months. This is near enough to give a child a useful growth line. The younger a child is, the more accurately you can estimate his month of birth.

   With a little questioning, the mother may be able to remember the season when the child was born. It may also help you to look at the child's development and teeth. Children vary a lot, but these may give you an approximate idea of a child's age.

Looking at the child's development
The most useful stages of development to remember are these:

- 6–8 weeks—the baby begins to smile.
- 3 months—he can control his head.
- 6 months—he can sit up with help.
- 9 months—he can sit up without help.
- 12 months—he can pull himself up to stand.
- 15 months—he can walk.

   Some children walk before they are 12 months old, and a few do not walk until they are 18 months old. Another problem is that a child who is not growing, may develop more slowly than a child who is growing well. A child who stops growing may also stop walking, even though he could walk before. Some children develop more slowly for other reasons.

However, a mother often knows if her child is developing more slowly than normal. She compares him to other children who were born at the same time; or with what she remembers about her other children.

Looking at the child's teeth

Most children have their first tooth when they are about 6 months old. From that age until they are about 2 years old, they grow approximately one new tooth every month. So, if you count how many teeth a child has and then add 6, this is the child's approximate age in months.

But some perfectly healthy normal children have no teeth until they are 1 year old. Other children start to have teeth when they are 3 months old. And, if a child is not growing, his teeth may come through later. However, if a child has 20 or 22 teeth, then he is almost certainly at least 2 years old.

14.11 SOME COMMON MISTAKES WITH GROWTH CHARTS

Writing 'January' instead of the child's birth month in the first box

In Fig. 14–18, the child was born in November. The health worker put 'January' in the first thick box, so November is in the box for when he was 10 months old. The health worker thought that he was very underweight. Really, the child is a healthy weight for his age.

Writing the month in which the child was first weighed instead of his birth month in the first box

Julius was born in June, but he lived a long way from the health centre. His mother did not bring him to be weighed until December when he was 6 months old. Figure 14–19 shows how the health worker put 'December' in the first thick box. When she weighed Julius, she was very surprised to find his weight so far above the upper curve.

Remember—*The first box is for the child's birth month.*

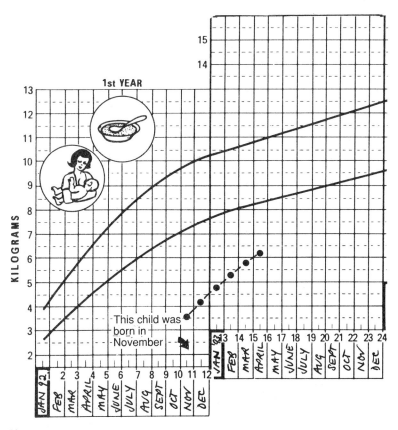

Fig. 14–18 Writing 'January' instead of the child's birth month in the first column.

Missing out months

It is easy to miss a month as you write them all in the boxes. To avoid this, first write the birth month in *all* the thick boxes.

Writing the months as numbers

If you put numbers instead of names for the months, it is easy to think that the numbers are ages. The child might be 9 months old in December, but you might put the dot in the column for September which is 'month 9'.

Not leaving a space between the dots if the child is not weighed for a few months

Andi's mother brought him to be weighed regularly until he was about 9 months old. After that she did not come so often. She did not bring Andi from April 1992 until November 1992. The health worker was very busy and did not check the calendar. Figure 14–20 shows how she put the weight for November in the column for May, next to Andi's previous weighing. He weighed 7.7 kg. The weight dot was above the lower line, so she thought that Andi was a healthy weight for his age. If she had put the weight dot in the correct column—for November—she would have seen that Andi was underweight and not growing.

Not using the calendar—trying to estimate the child's age each time

A mother may say that her child was '1 year old' in June and '2 years old' in August. This may be true, but you cannot use age in years to fill in a growth chart. If you try to work out a child's age at each visit, you may do it differently on different days: for example, in January, you might decide that the child is 17 months old, and then in February that the child is 22 months old. This makes the growth curve the wrong shape.

Recording a child's weight in the wrong year

Mahmoud was last weighed in September 1992, when he was 16 months old and weighed 9.4 kg. He seemed quite well, and only had common illnesses. His mother

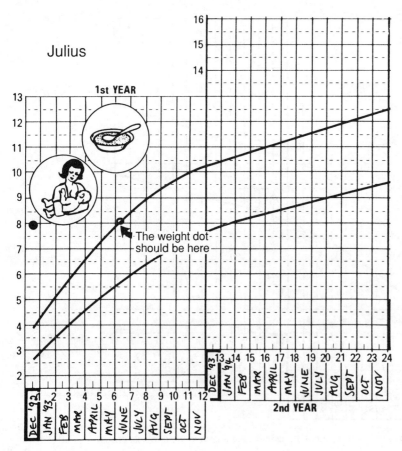

Fig. 14–19 Writing the month in which the child was first weighed instead of his birth month in the first box.

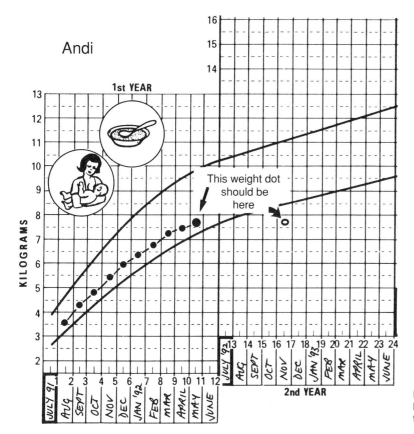

Andi

This weight dot should be here

Fig. 14–20 Not leaving a space between the dots if you do not weigh the child for some months.

was too busy to bring him to be weighed again, until November 1993. He then weighed 9.6 kg.

Figure 14–21 shows how the health worker put his weight dot in the column for November *1992*. She thought that Mahmoud was growing well. If she had put the dot in the correct column, for November 1993, she would have seen that he had become underweight, and was not growing well.

Remember to write the new year every January and write the year in every thick-lined box where you write the birth month. Then it is easier to record a child's weight in the column for the right year.

Putting a weight dot the wrong side of the kilogram line

Mandi was 8 months old, and weighed 7.5 kg. This is a healthy weight for a child of 8 months. By mistake, the health worker put the dot half a kilo *below* the 7.0 kg line, on the line for 6.5 kg. The health worker thought that Mandi was underweight, and she was very worried.

14.12 SCALES FOR WEIGHING CHILDREN

Spring scales

Inside is a spring which is attached to a needle. The weight of the child stretches the spring, and moves the needle. The needle points to a number on a dial which shows the weight of the child.

Different types include:

- *Bathroom scales.* These are not accurate enough to weigh young children.

- *Hanging scales* (Fig. 14–22). These are more accurate, and very suitable for weighing children. They are cheap and easily portable for home visits. There is a hook at the top of the scale, which you hang on a beam in a house or on a tree. Some people manage to hold the scales up with their hands—this depends on how heavy the child is. There is another hook below the scale from which you hang the child, in a small seat, a basket, his own carrying cloth, or a pair of pants.

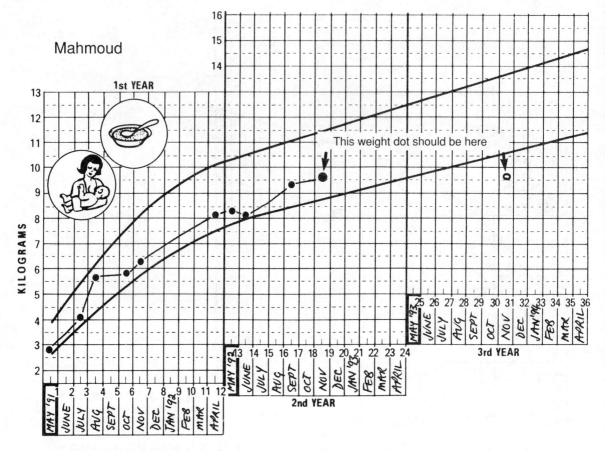

Fig. 14–21 Recording a child's weight in the wrong year.

- *Direct recording scale.* This is a newly developed scale which is simple but accurate. The scale hangs from a tree or beam, and the child hangs on the scale, stretching a spring. The child's growth chart is inserted into the scale. A pointer on the spring indicates on the growth chart where the child's weight dot should be. Family members can mark the chart themselves, and so become more involved in the weighing process. (For more information write to TALC; see Appendix 6.6).

'Beam balance' scales

There may be a tray where the child sits or stands; or a place to hang from, like the 'hanging scales'. There is an arm or beam along which you move a weight, until it balances the weight of the child, and the arm stays freely in the horizontal position. There is a scale along the arm, and the position of the weight along the scale shows the weight of the child.

Checking the scales

To make sure that your weighing is accurate, you must check your scales regularly.

- Every time, before you weigh a child, 'zero' the scales (Fig. 14–25).
  - With *spring scales*, with the weighing pants, basket, or seat in place, but no child, check that the needle points to 'zero'. If the needle does not point to zero, adjust it. There should be a screw on the scales to make the adjustment.
  - With *beam balance scales*, make sure that the arm swings freely when the weights are at the 'zero' mark. There should be a screw on the arm which you can adjust if necessary.

Remember to 'zero' scales every time you weigh a child.

- Every week you should weigh 2–3 standard known weights (e.g. weighing 5, 10, and 15 kg) on the scale

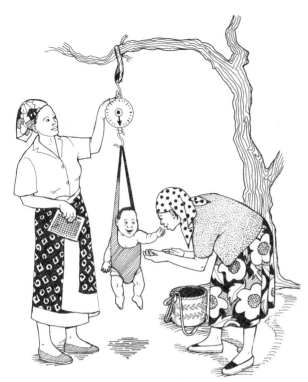

Fig. 14–22 The correct way to weigh a young child on hanging spring scales.

to make sure that it is still accurate. You can use things of a standard weight—such as a bag of maize flour. Or you can weigh 2–3 large stones of about 5–15 kg on some accurate scales (for example in a shop). Label them with their exact weights, and then use them to check your scales.

14.13 HOW TO WEIGH A CHILD

Putting the child on to the scales

It is important to put a child on to a scale carefully and gently. You do not want the experience to be frightening and unpleasant for him. Also, a child who is frightened may move about so much that you cannot read his weight on the scale. The problem can arise with any kind of scale. It is usually *how* we do the weighing, not the kind of scale we use, which upsets a child.

Undressing a child to be weighed

It is more accurate to weigh a child without any clothes and shoes on, or with just a light pair of pants. If he has clothes and shoes on, they add to his weight. However, sometimes it is too cold, or local customs do not allow a child to be weighed naked, or undressing frightens the child.

You can always remove a child's shoes. But if you feel that you have to weigh a child with his clothes, try to weigh him with the same kind of clothes every time—for example, shorts and a light shirt. Then the clothes add about the same amount to his weight each time, so you can still measure how much weight he has gained.

You can make a note on the weight chart about the clothes worn if it helps you to remember, so that you can weigh the child in the same clothes each time. Ask the mother to try to bring him in the same kind of clothes next time.

To prevent the child from becoming frightened

- Do not have the scales too high. It is easiest for you to read the scale if it is at your eye level—but, if necessary, you can bend down to read it.
- Let the child's mother do as much as possible herself. Do not take the child away from her.
- Explain to the mother what you want her to do.
- Let her put the child into the pants or basket, or on to the tray, and let her stay as near to the child as possible.
- You can weigh a very small baby, who is too small to sit up, in his carrying cloth, (see Fig. 14–23).
- Hang the pants or carrying cloth on to the hook of the spring scale with the mother still holding the child.
- Let the mother hold the child in position on the scale, until he is quiet and you are almost ready to read his weight.
- When you are ready, ask the mother to open her arms, so that she is not touching the child. However, she should stay near. If she moves away, the child may be more frightened. If the child holds on to his mother, she should gently remove his hands, hold them for a moment, and then let go of them.
- She should just let go of the child for a short time while you read the weight. Then she can hold him and pick him up again.

If you practise weighing children in this way, you will find that most children do not cry.

Reading the weight from the scale

On most scales you can read the weight to the nearest 100 g. It is easier to remember the weight if you say it out loud. This helps the mother to remember it too. As soon as you have read the weight, ask the mother to remove the child from the scales. Record the weight

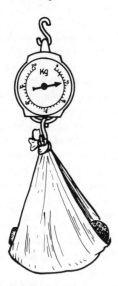

Fig. 14–23 Hanging a baby on the scales in a carrying cloth.

quickly before you forget it. If you can't record it immediately on the chart, write it on the mother's hand.

14.14 SOME COMMON PROBLEMS WITH WEIGHING SCALES

The scales do not measure weights accurately

If the scales are inaccurate, the child's weight will be wrong. He may seem to lose weight or gain weight when he does not.

The scales are not 'zeroed'

If the scales do not read 'zero' before you weigh the child, adjust them. If you do not adjust them, the child's weight will be inaccurate. For example, the empty scales read 1.0 kg. You put an 8-month-old child in the scales, and they read 7.0 kg. You think that the child's weight is within the healthy range. But the child's real weight is $7.0 - 1.0\,kg = 6.0\,kg$, which is underweight.

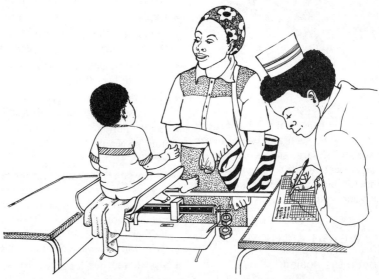

Fig. 14–24 Weighing a child on beam balance scales.

Box 14.1.   How to prevent some common mistakes in weighing children

- Make a complete calendar when you weigh the child the first time.
- Check your scales with known weights at least every week (see Section 14.12).
- 'Zero' the scales every time you use them.
- If a child's weight changes in a way that you do not expect:
  - Weigh him again.
  - Zero the scales, and if possible check them.
  - Make sure that you have put the weight dot in the correct place.

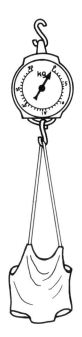

Fig. 14–25 'Zero' the scales every time you use them.

14.15 GROWTH IN HEIGHT

One way to assess children's nutrition is to measure their *height*, but this is not a very useful way to monitor a child's growth.

Rate of growth in height

Measuring the rate at which children increase in height is not a good way to monitor individual children's growth because:

- It is difficult to measure accurately, and it can take a long time in a small child who does not want to lie down or stand up straight.
- Height changes slowly. It may take 6 months before you can be sure that a child's height has increased. So it takes a long time to find out that a child's height has *not* increased, and that the child is not growing.

   Parents and health workers want to know more quickly than that if a child is not growing so that they can do something about it sooner.

- If a child is undernourished, he may lose weight, but he does not become shorter. So if you only measure height, you do not find out that a child has lost weight.

Stunting

If a child is undernourished, his growth in height slows down. A child who is undernourished for a long time is shorter than he should be. We can compare a child's height to the reference height-for-age of healthy children in the same way that we compared weights. Notice that we need to know a child's age to make this comparison.

A child whose height is below the 3rd centile for her age is *stunted*. If the child becomes well nourished, her activity and her immunity to infection may improve. However, her height will only increase slowly. It may be a long time before she catches up the growth in height that she missed. If she continues to be undernourished, she may never catch up the missed growth.

A short child weighs less than a tall child of the same age. If a child is very short, her weight may be below the 3rd centile on the growth chart, because of the shortness. Stunting is an important cause of low weight in children.

A child who has a low weight because of stunting may be well nourished and growing well *now*. The stunting may be because of undernutrition in the past.

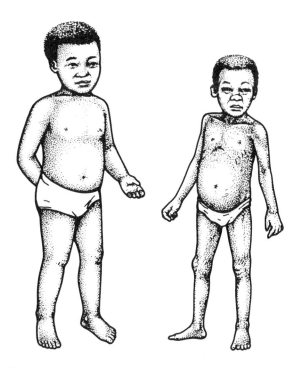

Fig. 14–26 A healthy child and a child of the same age who is stunted because he has been undernourished for a long time.

Why stunting is important

During childhood stunted children are more likely to have infections and to die. Because they have had a period of undernutrition, they may have learned less than well nourished children.

Adult men and women who are stunted may be less strong and not able to earn as much as people who are not stunted. Adult women who are stunted are more likely to have problems with childbirth. Their babies may be smaller and more likely to die or to be undernourished.

How measuring stunting is useful

Although we cannot use height to measure growth, height-for-age is useful when we want to:

- *Assess the nutrition of a population.* For example, when we do a survey of a community. People's heights tell us if they have been or are undernourished. It helps us to find which families or areas are most undernourished.

- *Measure changes in the nutrition situation of a community.* It tells us whether, over a period of time, the nutrition situation is improving or getting worse. This is useful for planners who have to decide how to use funds and other resources, and for people who evaluate the effects of development projects.

14.16 THINNESS AND FATNESS

Another way to find out if a child is well nourished is to measure how thin or how fat the child is. Every mother knows the difference between a thin child and a fat child. Children vary in how thin or fat they are, just as they vary in their height and weight.

A child who is thin but healthy grows and develops normally, and always looks thin in the same way. We use different words such as 'lean' for this healthy kind of thinness. Lean children are not *very* thin.

Children become thin when they are undernourished and they become thin if they are sick. Becoming thin is a sign that a child is not healthy. This unhealthy thinness is called *wasting*. It shows that the child has not only stopped growing, but has probably also lost weight. Children who are wasted look thinner than children who are naturally lean. They look 'skinny'.

Wasting is a sign that a child is undernourished and not growing *now*. The child has a problem that it may be possible to do something about. If the parents can improve the child's nutrition, the child can recover from wasting more quickly than from stunting.

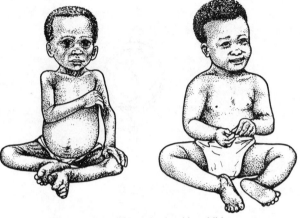

Fig. 14–27 A wasted child and a healthy child.

There are two ways to measure thinness in children:

1. You can measure the child's *weight-for-height*.
2. You can measure the child's *arm circumference*.

Both measures have these advantages:

- *You do not need to know the child's exact age.*

- *You do not need to know previous weights or heights.*

- *The measure is not affected by stunting.*

How measuring thinness is useful

Measuring thinness enables health and nutrition workers to find out quickly if a child is undernourished. This is useful:

- For *screening groups of children* when resources for helping them are limited (for example, in feeding programmes).

- For *assessing the nutrition situation of a community* in an emergency situation.

- For *assessing individual children* whom you have not seen before, when a child does not have a growth chart or previous weights, so that it is difficult to be sure whether the child is growing or not. For example:
  - when visiting a family, village or area for the first time;
  - when a family has come to a clinic or hospital for the first time with a child who is ill.

Measuring thinness during and after a period of illness can help to show that a child is recovering and becoming fatter.

Why measuring thinness is not useful for monitoring growth

In healthy children, changes in arm circumference and weight-for-height occur too slowly to be useful for monitoring growth. Weighing a child regularly is better for growth monitoring, because a child's weight is determined by both height and fatness, and changes occur more quickly.

14.17 MEASURING WEIGHT-FOR-HEIGHT

Figure 14–28 shows Wambui again in another group of seven healthy children. This time, instead of grouping her with children of the same *age*, we have grouped her with children of the same *height*. Some are older than Wambui; some are younger. We do not know the exact age of any of the other children. Their age does not matter.

The weights of these children are all different. Some are fatter, and some are thinner. But they are not *very different*. The weights of children of the same height *vary* within a *range*—in the same way that the weights of a group of children of the same age vary within a certain range.

A child whose weight-for-height is below the 3rd centile, is wasted and undernourished.

Why it is difficult to measure weight-for-height

Measuring a child's height can take time, and it can be difficult to do accurately. You also have to weigh the child, which takes more time. Then you have to look the weight-for-height up in a complex table. The whole procedure can take a long time, and it can be difficult to interpret the measurements. The method is very useful for research, and it is useful for in-patient care of severely malnourished children (see Chapter 17), but it is not very useful for growth monitoring. The extra time is better spent in talking to families.

The weight-for-height or 'thinness' chart

There is a special chart called the *weight-for-height* chart which helps to overcome these problems, and which makes the measurement easier.

The chart is on a large sheet of paper which you pin to the wall. Along the bottom of the chart are weights in kilograms, increasing from left to right. Up the side of the chart are numbers for children's height in cm.

There are three curved bands going across the chart. You can get coloured charts, or you can get black and white charts and colour them yourself.

How to measure a child with the thinness chart

1. Weigh the child.
2. Stand the child with his or her back against the chart (Fig. 14–29(1)) at the place where it shows the

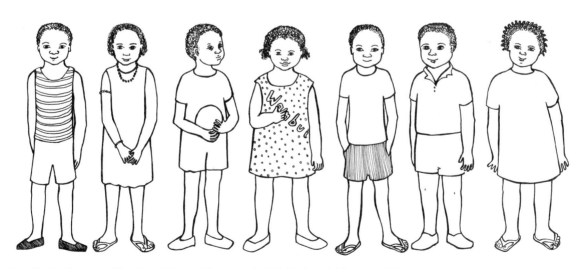

Fig. 14–28 A group of healthy children of the same height. Their weights vary a little.

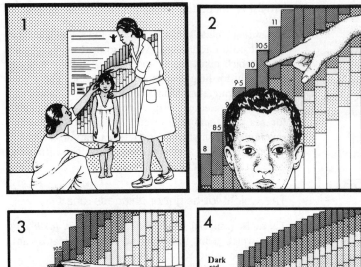

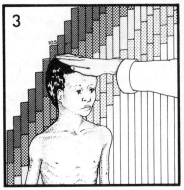

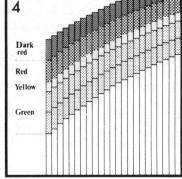

Fig. 14–29 Using the 'weight-for-height' or 'thinness' chart. Reference weight-for-height: dark red, 60–70 per cent; red, 70–80 per cent; yellow, 80–90 per cent; green, 90–110 per cent. (Charts available from TALC; see Appendix 6.)

child's weight. The middle of the child's head must be under his weight (Fig. 14–29(2)).

3. Make sure that the child's heels are flat on the ground and his legs straight, the child's shoulders must be against the chart.

4. Hold a piece of stiff card, or your hand, level on the top of the child's head, and see where it touches the chart. This shows where the top of the child's head reaches (Fig. 14–29(3)).

5. Decide if the child is well-nourished or <u>not</u>:

   a. If the top of the child's head reaches only the *lower* (or green) band, his weight is more than 90 per cent reference weight-for-height. He (or she) is well nourished and not thin (Fig. 14–29(4)).

   b. If the child reaches the *top* (or red) band, his weight is less than 80 per cent reference weight-for-height. He is very thin and malnourished.

   c. If the child reaches the *middle* (or yellow) band, his weight is between 80 and 90 per cent weight-for-height. He or she is moderately malnourished.

14.18 MEASURING THE MID-UPPER ARM CIRCUMFERENCE OR 'MUAC'

A thin child has thin arms, and a fat child has fat arms. The arm circumference is smaller in thin children, and larger in fat children. You measure round the middle of the upper arm, so the complete name is the *mid-upper arm circumference* or MUAC.

Between the ages of 1 and 5 years, the muscles of a healthy well nourished child's arm grow larger, but the fat that the child had as a baby becomes less. So if a child is growing in a healthy way, her arm circumference does not increase very much.

However, if a child is growing slowly, or losing weight, her muscles do not become larger, and the arm circumference is smaller than normal.

The arm circumference chart

Figure 14–31 shows an *arm circumference-for-age chart*. The reference line on the chart rises very steeply in the first year, but from the age of 1 to 5 years it rises very slowly. So, between the ages of 1 and 5, there is really only one reference value—which is 16.5 cm.

Below the reference line, there are two straight lines, which show 'cut-off' points for children of all ages between 1 and 5 years. One 'cut-off' line is at the 13.5 cm level, one is at the 12.5 cm level.

For children below the age of 1 year, measuring arm circumference is not very useful. It is difficult to measure accurately, and you have to know the exact age of the child. But for ages 1 to 5 years it can be very useful, because the exact age of the child does not matter.

- Any child who has an arm circumference below 12.5 cm is very thin and severely undernourished.
- Any child who has an arm circumference between 12.5 and 13.5 cm is moderately thin and moderately undernourished.

In different countries, or in different populations, a different 'cut-off' point may be used, but the idea is the same.

How to measure arm circumference

You can use:

- a tape measure (Fig. 14–30);
- a Shakir strip (Fig. 14–32);
- an insertion tape (Fig. 14–35);
- your fingers (see Fig. 14–36 in 'Things to do').

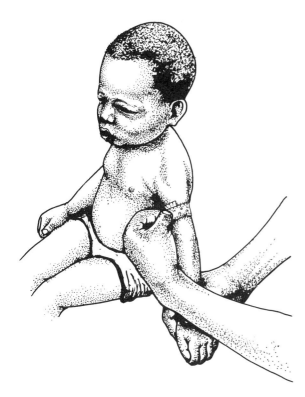

Fig. 14–30 Measuring arm circumference with a tape measure.

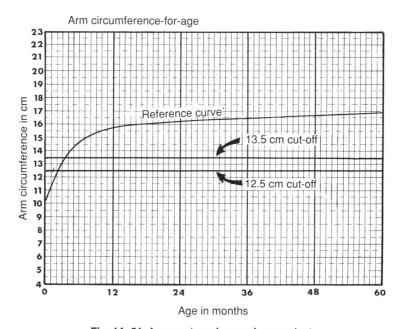

Fig. 14–31 An arm circumference-for-age chart.

A *tape measure* must be of a non-stretch material. Cut it to 30 cm.

A *Shakir strip* you can make out of any strong material that does not stretch or tear easily, such as:

- old X-ray film;
- strips cut from plastic bottles (when empty, they are thinner than they look) or any other thick plastic;
- strong thin card.

Cut a piece of the material about 25 cm long and 1 cm wide. Mark it with coloured pens or crayons. Mark '0' near one end. Measure and mark at 12.5 cm and 13.5 cm from the zero. If you wish you can:

- colour the area between the two marks *yellow*;
- colour part of the strip above 13.5 *green*;
- colour part of the strip below 12.5 cm *red*.

An *insertion tape* is a special kind of tape measure made from non-stretch, non-tear tape, which has lengths in millimetres printed on it. There is a slit at '0' through which you insert the other end of the tape, and a window through which you read the figures for the measure of the arm circumference.

Deciding if a child is between 1 and 5 years old

Measuring the arm circumference is only useful if the child is between 1 and 5 years old. A child is probably over the age of 1 year if:

- he can stand or walk, or has done so in the past;
- he has more than six teeth.

A child is less than 5 years old if:

- when he puts his hand over his head, he cannot touch the ear on the other side.

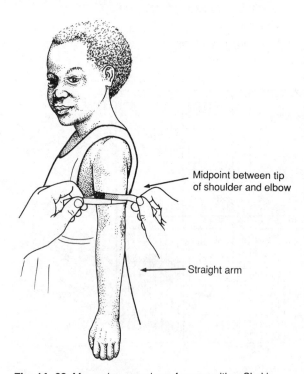

Fig. 14–32 Measuring arm circumference with a Shakir strip.

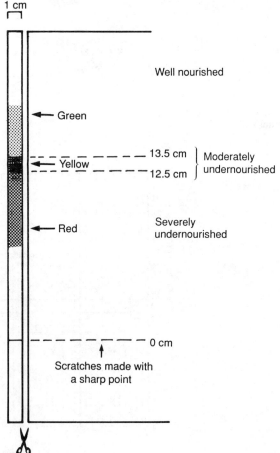

Fig. 14–33 A Shakir strip.

Box 14.2. How to measure a child's arm circumference with a tape or strip

1. The parent can hold the child on their lap.

2. Take the child's left arm, and hold it straight.

3. Find the midpoint of the upper arm between the point of the shoulder and the point of the elbow.

4. Put the end of the tape, or strip, with the '0' mark on the midpoint of the upper arm.

5. Put the tape or strip around the arm so that it fits closely, but not so tight that it makes folds in the skin.

6. Note the reading where the '0' cm mark meets the tape. This is the child's arm circumference.

7. If you are using an insertion tape, read the number which shows most completely in the wide window.

8. Write down the measurement, and decide if it is above or below the cut-off point.

9. If you are using a coloured strip:
   - if '0' meets the green part, the child is not wasted;
   - if '0' meets yellow, the child is moderately wasted;
   - if '0' meets red, the child is severely wasted.

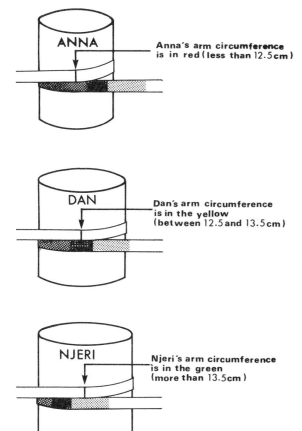

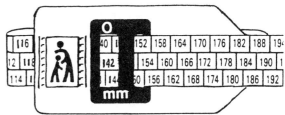

Fig. 14–35 An insertion tape. (Available from TALC; see Appendix 6.)

Fig. 14–34 How a Shakir strip shows if a child is wasted or not.

THINGS TO DO

For several of these exercises trainees need blank growth charts. Try to get these from your local health centre or Ministry of Health.

Or photocopy a blank chart, or copy Fig. 14–6 of this book. You may need to put trainees in groups so that they can share the charts, and ask them to write in pencil so that they can rub out and use them again.

Or make photocopies of a few blank growth charts on overhead transparencies (acetates). While you project them, draw children's growth lines on them. Use water-soluble pens; you can then wash and use the charts again.

Or make large copies of the chart (some countries already have these), and pin them on a board. Fill them in with a pencil so that you can rub out.

Or use a flannelgraph available from TALC (see Appendix 6). You can ask trainees to help you fill in the charts, and then you can use the charts to practise interpretation.

Practise finding birth dates

Use these examples, or make up your own, to give trainees practice at finding children's birth dates.

1. It is July 1993, and it is the beginning of the cold season, which usually lasts about 2 months. The following children come to your health centre. Their mothers are not sure exactly when they were born. Choose an approximate birth month and year for them.

   a. A small baby who cannot hold up his head or sit up, and who has no teeth. His mother thinks that he is about 3–4 months old.

   b. A child who is just beginning to stand up, but he cannot yet walk. His mother thinks that he was born near the end of the cold season last year. He has three lower and two upper teeth.

   c. A child who can walk. His mother has just had another baby. The older child learned to walk just before his mother found out that she was expecting another baby. He has 14 teeth.

Weighing and measuring children

2. Arrange for trainees to visit a local health centre or child care centre to practise weighing and measuring children. If the children have growth charts, the trainees should look at them, and decide if the children are growing well. Discuss findings in class afterwards. (Be careful not to criticize or to discuss any mistakes in front of the families.)

Understanding growth charts

Ask trainees to do the following exercises, to make sure that they understand growth charts.

3. What is the reference weight for children of:

   a. 1 year and 8 months;

   b. 2 years and 4 months;

   c. 3 years and 10 months?

4. Are these children underweight or not (are their weights above or below the 3rd centile)?

   a. a child of 9 months weighing 8 kg;

   b. a child of 20 months weighing 11 kg;

   c. a child of 11 months weighing 6 kg;

   d. a child of 15 months weighing 8 kg;

   e. a child of 18 months weighing 10 kg;

   f. a child of 27 months weighing 9 kg.

Practise filling in growth charts

Give trainees growth charts to practise filling in, As they work check to see if they are doing it correctly. Afterwards, discuss what the examples demonstrate.

5. Make calendars for:

   a. Nandi born March 1993;

   b. Amon born September 1992.

6. Make a growth line for Nandi. (This illustrates leaving spaces on months when a child does not come to be weighed.)

   ● She weighed 3 kg when she was born.
   ● In April 1993 she weighed 4 kg.
   ● In May 1993 she weighed 5 kg.
   ● In July 1993 she weighed 6 kg.
   ● In September 1993 she weighed 7 kg.
   ● In November 1993 she weighed 9 kg.

7. Make a growth line for Amon. (This illustrates putting dots in different positions for fractions of a kilogram, and different times in the month.)

   ● He weighed 3.5 kg when he was born.
   ● In October 1992 he weighed 4.5 kg.
   ● November 1992: 5.0 kg.
   ● December 1992: 5.5 kg.
   ● January 1993: 6.0 kg.
   ● March 1993: 6.7 kg.
   ● May 1993: 7.4 kg.
   ● July 1993: 8.2 kg.
   ● September 1993: 8.9 kg.
   ● October 1993: 9.1 kg.
   ● November 1993: 9.3 kg.
   ● 5 January 1994: 9.5 kg.
   ● 30 January 1994: 9.6 kg.
   ● 3 March 1994: 9.8 kg.
   ● 29 March 1994: 9.9 kg.

8. Make a growth line for Buri, born in July 1993. (This illustrates the need to leave spaces, and not to put the first weighing in the first column.)

   ● October 1993: 5.0 kg.
   ● January 1994: 7.0 kg.
   ● May 1994: 8.5 kg.
   ● August 1994: 9.0 kg.
   ● November 1995: 9.5 kg.

9. Draw growth lines for the children in the following table. (You can give dates instead of ages, so that trainees practise using the calendar at the same time.)

Age (months)	Weight (kg)	Age (months)	Weight (kg)	Age (months)	Weight (kg)	Age (months)	Weight (kg)
Tunu		**Purwa**		**Wegwa**		**Sinto**	
1	4.0	1	4.9	Birth	4.2	Birth	2.3
2	4.5	2	5.7	2	5.2	1	2.9
3	5.1	3	6.3	4	5.5	3	3.8
4	5.6	4	7.3	5	5.8	4	4.3
5	6.2	6	8.7	7	5.8	5	4.7
6	6.9	8	9.4	8	5.7	7	5.6
7	7.7	10	9.6	10	5.9	8	6.3
10	8.8	12	9.7	12	5.9	9	6.7
11	9.4	14	9.6			11	7.2
14	9.8						
Leo		**Shameem**		**Mandi**		**Budi**	
Birth	3.7	1	3.9	Birth	4.0	Birth	3.5
1	3.7	3	4.9	1	5.1	1	4.4
2	4.3	4	5.5	2	6.2	2	5.2
3	4.4	6	6.5	3	7.3	4	6.4
4	4.5	8	7.4	4	8.2	5	7.3
5	4.7	9	7.6	6	9.2	6	8.7
6	4.8	11	7.8	7	9.8	8	11.2
7	4.9	12	7.6	9	10.7	10	12.3
9	5.8	13	7.2	11	11.3	12	13.4
10	6.6	14	6.4	13	11.8	14	14.0
11	6.9	15	7.0	16	12.9		
13	7.3	17	7.9	18	13.4		
15	7.7	18	8.5	20	13.5		
18	8.3			27	14.8		
24	9.0			31	15.5		

Practise interpreting growth lines

Ask trainees to study some growth charts and to decide if the children are growing well or not.

You can examine charts of real children at a local health centre (you may be able to copy some good examples). Or copy any of the charts in Chapters 14 and 15 and interpret them together.

Or you can discuss the growth lines the trainees have plotted for Tunu and the other children in Exercise 9, using the questions that we give below. (In the 'Things to do' section at the end of Chapter 15 we suggest that trainees discuss or role play how they would advise the families of some of these children.)

10. Growth chart—Tunu.

 a. Are her recent weight dots in the healthy range? (yes)
 b. Is her growth line rising, flat, or falling? (rising)
 c. Is her growth line the same shape as the healthy lines? (yes)
 d. Did Tunu grow well in the past? (yes)
 e. Is Tunu growing well now? (yes)
 f. Is Tunu healthy? (Yes, she is growing normally. She is healthy.)

11. Growth chart—Purwa.

 a. Are her recent weight dots in the healthy range? (yes)
 b. Is her growth line rising, flat, or falling? (flat)
 c. Is her growth line the same shape as the reference curve? (No—her growth line is getting nearer to the 3rd centile.)
 d. Did Purwa grow well in the past? (Yes until she was 8 months old.)
 e. Is Purwa growing well now? Is she healthy? (No she is not growing well now—she is not healthy.)

Purwa's growth line shows that, even if a child's weight is above the 3rd centile curve, she may not be growing well. Purwa grew well in the first 8 months of life, but then something went wrong and she stopped growing. It may take a long time before her growth line falls below the 3rd centile, so it may be a long time before she is underweight.

This shows how monitoring growth can tell you that a child is not growing a long time before you find that she has become underweight.

12. Growth chart—Wegwa.

 a. Are his recent weight dots in the healthy range? (No—his weight dots are below the 3rd centile curve—he is underweight.)

b. Is his growth line rising, flat, or falling? (flat)

c. Is his growth line the same shape as the reference curve? (No—it is falling further and further below the reference curve.)

d. Did Wegwa grow well in the past? (He grew well for the first 2 months of life, but not since then. He had a good birth weight.)

e. Is Wegwa growing well now? Is he healthy? (No—he is not growing well, so he is not healthy.)

Wegwa's growth line shows how a child may become underweight if he does not grow well from soon after birth.

13. Growth chart—Sinto.

a. Are her recent weight dots in the healthy range? (No—she is underweight.)

b. Is her growth line rising, flat, or falling? (rising)

c. Is her growth line the same shape as the reference curves? (Yes—her line is below the 3rd centile but the same shape.)

d. Did Sinto grow well in the past? (She has grown well since she was born, but she was born small.)

e. Is Sinto growing well now? Is she healthy? (Yes—she is growing well, and she is healthy but small.)

Sinto's story shows that a child may be underweight but growing well. She is small because she was born small. This is a kind of stunting (see Section 16.7).

14. Growth chart—Leo.

a. Are his recent weight dots in the healthy range? (No—he is underweight.)

b. Is his growth line rising or falling? (rising)

c. Is his growth line the same shape as the reference curves? (Yes, it is now.)

d. Did Leo grow well in the past? (He had a good birth weight, but he did not grow well for the first 7 months of life.)

e. Is he growing well now? (Yes, he is healthy now.)

Leo's story shows that a child may be underweight because he did not grow well in the past, even if he is healthy and growing at a healthy rate now.

15. Growth chart—Shameem.

a. Are the recent weight dots in the healthy range? (No, below it.)

b. Is her growth line rising, falling, or flat? (rising)

c. Is her growth line the same shape as the reference curve? (No, it is rising faster than the 3rd centile curve.)

d. Did Shameem grow well in the past? (She grew well until the age of about 10 months; then she did not grow well for 4 months and she became underweight.)

e. Is she growing well now? (Yes, faster than normal.)

Shameem is recovering from a time of poor growth and weight loss. This is 'catch-up growth' (see Section 15.8).

16. Growth chart—Mandi.

a. Are her recent weight dots in the healthy range? (Yes, they are above the reference curve, and below the 97th centile.)

b. Is her growth line rising, flat, or falling? (rising)

c. Is her growth line the same shape as the reference curve? (yes)

d. Did she grow well in the past? (Yes, and she was born big, 4 kg.)

e. Is she growing well now? (Yes, normally and healthily.)

Many healthy children have weights which are above the reference curve. The reference curve is the *average* (or 50th centile) for healthy children, so about half of all normal children's growth curves should be above it.

17. Growth curve—Budi.

a. Are his recent weight dots in the healthy range? (No, they are a long way above it.)

b. Is his growth line rising, flat, or falling? (rising)

c. Is it the same shape as the reference curve? (No, it rises faster.)

d. Did Budi grow well in the past? (Yes, and he weighed 3.5 kg at birth.)

e. Is Budi growing normally now? (He is growing faster than normal. He may be becoming unhealthily overweight.)

Budi's growth line is above the 50th centile, and it is rising faster than the reference curve. He is becoming overweight.

Demonstrate how to use the 'thinness chart'

'Weight-for-height' or 'thinness' charts are available from TALC (for address see Appendix 6).

18. To demonstrate the chart, you can use real children or 'models'. Make life-size drawings of thin and fat children of different heights and weights. Or cut thin and fat sticks of different heights and label with different weights.

Make and use arm circumference strips

19. Ask each trainee to make an arm circumference strip (see Fig. 14–33) and to practise using it. Use old X-ray

film, a plastic bottle, or strong card. Let them practise using the strips on local children. Or make model arms from sticks or rolls of newspaper.

Demonstrate how to use your finger and thumb to measure arm circumference

20. Ask each trainee to calibrate her own finger and thumb (see Box 14.3).

Box 14.3.   Measuring arm circumference with your finger and thumb

First you need to know the size of the circle that your finger and thumb make (this is '*calibrating*' your finger and thumb).

1. Take some thick sticks that are about as thick as children's arms, or make some rolls of cardboard or newspaper that are about the same size. Measure the circumference of the sticks or rolls with a tape, and find one that is about 12.5 cm, and one that is about 13.5 cm—and some larger and some smaller ones.

2. Put your finger and thumb around the sticks, as in Fig. 14–36. Hold the stick tightly, and find out where the nail of your first finger meets your thumb.

3. Learn the position of the nail on your thumb for a stick of 12.5 cm and for a stick of 13.5 cm. The places should be 1 cm apart. If you like, learn some other places, such as 15 cm, or 11 cm.

To measure a child's arm circumference:

1. Hold the child's left arm straight, and put your finger and thumb around the middle of the upper arm.

2. Find where the nail of your first finger meets your thumb.

3. Decide if the nail meets the thumb inside the 12.5 place; outside the 13.5 place; or between 12.5 and 13.5. Then you know if the child is severely wasted or probably not wasted or moderately wasted.

Another way to do this is first to measure some children, and then to let trainees 'measure' their finger and thumb on some children's arms.

For useful training materials on growth monitoring and promotion see Appendix 6.

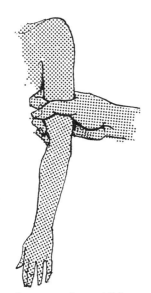

Practise measuring a child's arm.

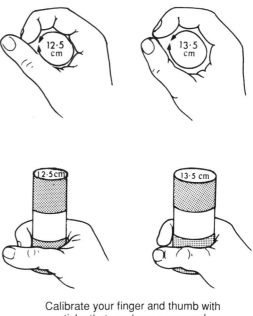

Calibrate your finger and thumb with sticks that you have measured.

Fig. 14–36 Learning how to measure arm circumference with your finger and thumb.

USEFUL PUBLICATIONS

Beaton, G., Kelly, A., Kevany, J., Martorell, R., and Mason, J. (1990). *Appropriate uses of anthropometric indices in children*, ACC/SCN Nutrition Policy Discussion Paper, no. 7. ACC/SCN, Geneva.

Children in the Tropics (1989). Nutritional status: interpretation of indicators. *Children in the Tropics*, Vols 181–2.

Ritchie, J. A. S. (1983). *Nutrition and families*. Macmillan, Basingstoke.

15 Using growth charts to help families

Nutrition workers are often responsible for planning and organizing growth monitoring programmes. You may do the growth monitoring yourself, or you may train or supervise other people, including community health workers, to do it.

15.1 PLANNING GROWTH MONITORING

Growth monitoring should start at or as soon as possible after birth and continue until the child is no longer at risk of undernutrition. For many children this is at about 3–4 years of age.

Give each child a growth chart when he is born, and if possible record the birth weight on it. If a child was born at home, give him a chart the first time you weigh him.

The parents should keep the growth chart, and bring it whenever the child comes for weighing, treatment, or immunization. This may be at a health centre, an outreach clinic, a village community centre, or at home.

Different countries have different guidelines about how often to weigh children, and up to what age. Some countries ask children to come for weighing about once a month until they have had all their immunizations, and every 2–3 months after that time. Children over 2–3 years are less at risk of undernutrition (if they have grown well up to that age), and may come less frequently. Children who are ill, or small, or who are not growing well may need to come more frequently.

15.2 WHAT TO DO THE FIRST TIME THAT YOU WEIGH A CHILD

Introduce yourself to the mother or father or other family member and the child. Register the child as required where you work.

Show the parent the chart, and explain what it is for, and what it means. If you explain the chart carefully, the mother is more likely to be interested in weighing the child, in keeping the chart carefully, and in talking about how she feeds him.

- Spend as much time as you can asking the mother about the child and her family.
  - Find out about the other children, how old they are, if they are healthy or ill or have died.
  - Talking with the mother helps you to know if the family has any special problems and whether the child needs special care.
  - Be careful not to embarrass the mother. If you are friendly, she is more likely to bring her children for weighing regularly.
- Fill in on the chart details about the child and family.
  - Make sure that you have the complete name of the child.
  - Find out the date of birth as accurately as possible.
  - Fill in the birth order by finding out how many older children the mother has.
  - Fill in details about sisters and brothers.
- Also on the first visit, make the child's own calendar at the bottom of the growth chart (see Fig. 14–16).
- Record any 'Reason for special care' (Box 15.1).
- Register the family in your 'follow-up register' if the child is undernourished or at risk of undernutrition. Then if they do not return when you expect them, you can try to visit them at home.

15.3 WHAT TO DO AT EACH VISIT

The order in which you do these things may vary according to how your health centre is organized. Different people may register and weigh the child, and advise the family. The order here may be best if it is possible.

1. Greet the child and parent (or relative), and ask how they are.

2. If the child is sick, or has been sick since the last visit, find out details of the illness.

3. Ask how the child is feeding.

4. Ask to see the child's growth chart. If you have

Box 15.1. Reasons for special care

In the child:

- low birth weight (less than 2.5 kg);
- twin;
- born less than 24 months after previous child;
- disabled (mental handicap, heart problem, cleft palate);
- chronic sickness (e.g. HIV infection).

In the family:

- more than five children in the family;
- other children in the family malnourished or have died;
- only one parent, or no parents;
- mother lives alone with children;
- family very poor;
- mother mentally or physically ill;
- mother is adolescent.

There are many other reasons why a child needs special care; these are just a few of them. Make your own list, and add here important reasons which we have not included.

---

seen the child before, the growth chart will remind you about her, and about what you thought. If you have not seen the child before, she may have a growth chart from somewhere else. This will tell you several things about the child, and you need not ask all the same questions again.

5. Record on the chart any immunizations that are given. If necessary, record the immunizations in your register.

6. Weigh the child (see Section 14.13).

7. Plot the weight on the growth chart, and join the dot up to previous dots.

8. Examine the growth chart. Look at today's weight, and look at the child's growth line.

9. Decide how the child is growing. If this is the first visit, you can only decide if the weight is inside or outside the range of healthy weights. If this is the second or later visit, you can decide whether or not the child is growing at a healthy rate. Explain the growth line to the mother.

10. Discuss what you find with the mother. Some workers find that immediately after weighing the child is the best time to discuss how to feed and care for the child (see Section 15.5). Praise the mother for what she is doing right—there is always

something. Ask if she has any questions, and try to answer them.

11. Write on the growth chart, in the column for the month when they happen, important events in the child's life including:

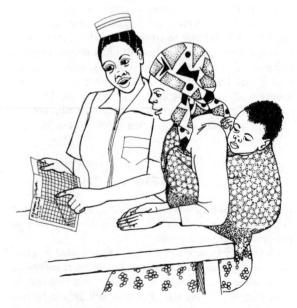

Fig. 15–1 Discuss the child's growth line with the mother.

- starting weaning foods or artificial feeding;
- stopping breastfeeding;
- illnesses.

Knowing when these events occurred helps you to understand the reasons for poor weight gain, and to give appropriate advice.

12. Explain when to return, write the date on the growth chart or card, and show the mother where you have written it.

13. Record the child's visit as necessary.

15.4 WHAT TO LOOK FOR IN THE CHILD'S GROWTH LINE

- *Is the child's weight outside the normal range?* Is it below the 3rd centile or above the 97th centile? (If you have no 97th centile, are the dots further above the reference line than the 3rd centile is below it?)
- *If the weight is below the 3rd centile, is it far below?* (For example, below the 60 per cent curve.)
- *Is the child's growth line rising, flat, or falling?*
- *If the growth line is rising, is it the same shape as the reference line?* Is the child's growth line rising faster or slower than the reference curve, or at the same rate?

If the child has been weighed for a number of months, you also need to ask yourself:

- *How has the child's growth line changed?*

A child's growth line may not always be the same. The child may grow well for a long time, and then grow poorly. Or, the child may grow poorly for a long time, and then start to grow better. So you must look at the child's *past* growth and *present* growth.

If the growth has changed, is it better or worse? If it is better, praise and encourage the mother. If it is worse, notice when the change began, and try to find out what caused it. What happened at that time which may have caused the change? For example:

- Did the child stop breastfeeding?
- Was the child ill?
- Did a change occur in the family's life?

15.5 WHAT TO DISCUSS WITH THE CHILD'S FAMILY

Usually you can talk with the mother or relative who brought the child for weighing. But if you weigh the child at or near his home, you may be able to meet with other family members too.

If the child is growing at a healthy rate

The growth lines in Fig. 15–2 are the same shape as the reference curve. These children are all growing at a healthy rate.

- Explain to each family that their child is gaining weight well. Show them how their child's growth line shows this.
- Ask them how the child is feeding. Praise them for all the good things that they are doing.
- If they are not feeding the child in the best way, discuss this with them. For example (Chart 1), they may have started giving the baby drinks or weaning foods before the age of 4–6 months, or they may be giving some bottle feeds. Explain the problems that feeding a child this way may cause, and discuss what else they could do.
- In many cases there will be no need to give any new advice, but it is a good idea always to find something useful to discuss, so that the family feel that the visit was worthwhile. Check that they know how to go on feeding and caring for the child. Give advice which is suitable for the child's age.

For example:

- If the baby is breastfeeding and less than 6 months old (as in Chart 1), encourage the mother to continue exclusive breastfeeding and not to introduce other food or drinks before the baby really needs them—if possible not before the baby is 6 months old.
- It may be an appropriate time to discuss family planning, and to ask if the parents would like help with that.
- If the mother has to go back to work soon, discuss how she can continue to give the baby breast milk (Section 10.17).
- Make sure that mother and child have received all their immunizations.
- If the baby is already 6 months old (as in Chart 2), encourage the mother to give other food as well, but remind her of the value of continuing to breastfeed the baby both day and night.
- If the child has started weaning foods, discuss how to enrich the child's porridge, and how to give food from the family meal.
- When the child starts weaning foods, he is at greater

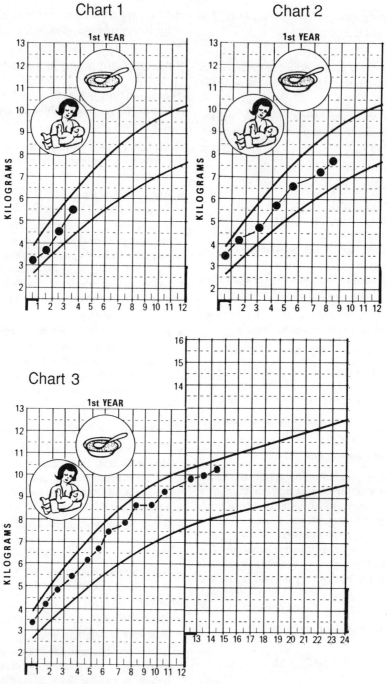

Fig. 15–2 What would it be useful to discuss with the parents of these children?

risk of infection. Explain about the importance of giving drinks to children with diarrhoea (see Section 13.4) and about the importance of foods rich in vitamin A (see Section 19.1).

• If the child is over 1 year old (as in Chart 3), discuss giving the child food from the family meal. Ask if the child is beginning to feed himself yet, and discuss how the family can help him to learn. Ask if the child has his own plate, and discuss ways to make sure that the child gets his fair share of food.

If the child's growth line is below the 3rd centile

The growth line in Fig. 15–3 is of a baby who was born small but who has grown well. Low birth weight (LBW) babies need special care because they are at greater risk from infections than babies who are born larger. LBW babies have small stores of fat, iron, and vitamin A and they can become undernourished very quickly if they do not eat enough or if they are sick. They may fail to gain weight if they are not kept warm enough. If they are always wrapped up and never exposed to the sun, they may develop vitamin D deficiency (see Section 19.15).

- Encourage the mother to continue breastfeeding as long as possible (see Chapter 10).
- Try to see the baby more often than you would see a larger baby. Make sure that any infections are treated promptly, and that the baby has adequate weaning foods at the appropriate time.

- Explain to the mother that it is important to keep small babies warm, but that she should not cover the baby completely all the time. The baby needs some sunlight on his skin to get vitamin D.

If the child is gaining weight too slowly or not at all

The growth line in Fig. 15–4 is rising, but it is not rising as fast as the reference curve. The baby's growth is slowing down, or *faltering*. He has gained less than 500 g a month for 2 months.

The growth line in Fig. 15–5 is flat. The baby has not gained weight for 4 months. She has stopped growing. She has *growth failure*.

A child who has a growth line like either of these is not eating enough. Try to find out why.

- Ask the mother (or other relative) how she feeds the child.

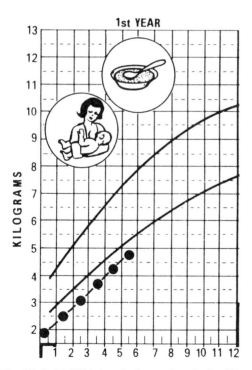

Fig. 15–3 A LBW baby who is growing at a healthy rate. What would it be useful to discuss with the family?

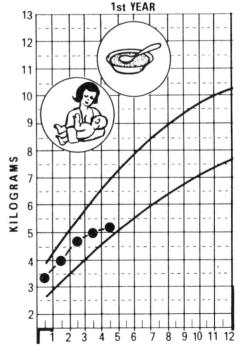

Fig. 15–4 This baby's growth is slowing down. What would it be useful to discuss with his parents?

- Ask how many times the child *breastfeeds* each day. Is the mother away from the child for much of the day? Does she sleep with the child and breastfeed at night?
- Ask if the child has any breast milk *substitutes*, such as bottle feeds, or other drinks, even drinks of water. (It is particularly important to ask about breast milk and breast milk substitutes for the baby in Fig. 15–4, who should still be exclusively breastfed.)
- Ask about the *food* that the child eats. *How many meals* or *snacks* does the child eat each day? What *kind* of food does the child eat? (Bulky or enriched?) Try to get some idea about the *amount* of the food.
- Ask *how the child eats a meal*. Does she feed herself, or does someone help her? Does she share a plate with other children, or does she have her own plate?
- Ask if the child's *appetite* is good or poor.
- Ask if the *family has any problems* which make it difficult for them to give the child enough food. (It

is particularly important to ask about foods for the child in Fig. 15–5, who should be eating weaning foods now.)

- Ask if the child is *sick*.
  - Does she have symptoms such as diarrhoea, cough, or fever?
  - Examine the child to see if there are any *signs* of sickness such as fever, or skin rashes, or sores in the mouth, or discharging ears.
  - You may need to consider if the mother might be HIV+.
- Ask if anything has happened that may have made the child *unhappy*. For example, has the mother stopped breastfeeding because of a new pregnancy? Has the mother or father gone away?

15.6 GROWTH FAILURE AT DIFFERENT AGES

Before the age of 6 months

Up to the age of 6 months, a baby should gain at least 500 g each month. Not growing well for a period of 1 month can be a serious sign at this age (as in Fig. 15–4). The commonest cause is *lack of breast milk*.

The mother may be away from the baby for much of the day, so that the baby is not breastfeeding often enough. Or there may be a problem with how she breastfeeds (see Section 10.20). The mother may be feeding the baby with a bottle containing formula or watery porridge, or she may be giving drinks of water or glucose water, tea, or fruit juice, or she may have started to give weaning foods too early.

Giving anything other than breast milk at this time—even water—can make the baby suckle less at the breast, and grow more slowly. Also, it may cause diarrhoea.

How to help the family

- Encourage the mother to breastfeed the baby exclusively for at least 4 months and if possible for 6 months. The baby does not need water, or glucose water, even in hot weather.
- Make sure that the baby is suckling in a good position.
- Advise the mother to breastfeed more often by day and at night, (see Section 10.15), and to breastfeed for longer with each feed.
- Help a mother who works away from home to breastfeed more (see Section 10.17).

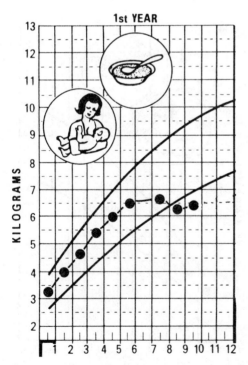

Fig. 15–5 This baby has not gained weight for 4 months. What would it be useful to discuss with her parents?

- Make sure that the child is treated for any infections. Refer the child for help if necessary.
- If you have done all this and the baby is still not gaining weight well after 1 more month:
  - If the baby is still less than 4 months old—refer to a health centre or hospital.
  - If the baby is now 4 months old—consider starting weaning foods.

From 6–12 months

Not gaining weight well for 1 month may not be such a serious sign at this age as it is in a younger baby. However, not gaining for 2–3 months may be serious (Fig. 15–5).

The commonest reasons for poor growth between 6 and 12 months are:

- insufficient or bulky weaning foods;
- frequent or severe infections

If the mother also *stops breastfeeding*, it can make the child's nutrition worse.

How to help the family

- Encourage the mother to continue breastfeeding, day and night.
- Help her to find ways to give the child more food (Box 15–2).
- Help her to prevent infections and encourage the family to seek treatment early if the child is ill. Help her to feed and care for the child while he is sick and recovering.

- If the child is still not gaining weight after another 1–2 months, talk to the family again and find out what the mother feels the problem is. Maybe she has not been able to follow your advice. Maybe she has other problems that you did not learn about before. Try to help her to find some other way to feed the child more.
- If there seems to be no reason for the growth failure, or if the child is ill, refer him to a more specialized health worker.

After the age of 1 year

Growth naturally slows down at this age. Failure to gain weight for 1 month is not usually important, if the child seems well and has gained at a healthy rate before. Failure to gain weight for 3 months may be the beginning of a problem.

The commonest reasons for growth failure at this age are:

- insufficient food;
- frequent or severe infections.

If the mother stops breastfeeding, it can make the situation worse.

How to help the family

- Encourage the mother to continue breastfeeding until the child is 2 years old, and longer if she likes.
- Help her to find ways to give the child more food (Box 15.2). The child should now be eating mainly foods from the family meals.
- Help her to prevent infections and encourage the family to seek treatment early if the child is ill. Help

---

Box 15.2. How to feed a child more

These are some of the ways in which a family can give a child more to eat.

- Feed the child more often—five times a day if possible.
  - Give three meals of family food a day.
  - Give two or more nutritious snacks between meals.
- Give the child more food at each meal.
- Give more energy- and nutrient-rich foods.
- Give the child her own plate of food when eating with other children.
- Feed the child during illnesses.
- Give extra food when the child is recovering from illness:
  - an extra meal a day; extra food at each meal;
  - extra energy- and nutrient-rich food.

them to feed and care for the child while he is sick and recovering.

- Follow up the child. If he is still not gaining weight after another 2 months, talk to the family again, and try to find out what the problem is.

15.7 CHILDREN WHO ARE LOSING WEIGHT

Figure 15–6 shows the growth lines of three children who are losing weight. Loss of weight is a dangerous sign. It shows that the child is suddenly under-nourished. It most often happens when a child is ill with an infection.

If the child had a flat growth line previously, or if the child's line is below the 3rd centile, like Paul, loss of weight may be serious. If the child has been growing well before the weight loss, and her growth line is above the 50th centile, like Pam, then the sign is less serious. Loss of weight is more serious in a baby aged less than 6 months, like Pearl, than in an older child.

How to help the family

- Try to find out why the child has lost weight. Take a history and ask particularly about symptoms of infection and loss of appetite. Consider whether the mother may be HIV+.
- Make sure that the child is treated for any infection. Refer the child if necessary.
- Discuss how to feed a sick child (see Chapter 13), including breastfeeding.
- Explain how important it is to feed the child extra food when his appetite recovers and he is willing to eat again.
- Follow the child up frequently (at least every week) until he is gaining weight well. Make sure that his growth line rises faster than the reference line until he regains the lost weight and is growing at a healthy rate again.

15.8 REGAINING LOST WEIGHT

The growth charts in Fig. 15–7 show two children who lost weight, but who are now gaining weight again.

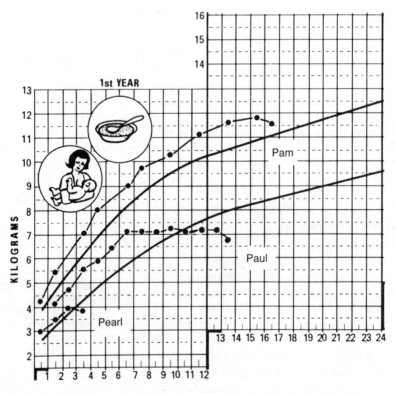

Fig. 15–6 The growth lines of three children who have lost weight. What would it be useful to discuss with their families?

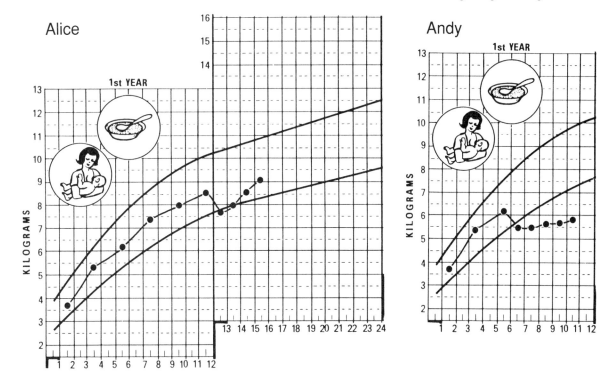

Fig. 15–7 The growth lines of Andy and Alice who have been ill. Who has good 'catch-up' growth?

Good 'catch-up growth'

Alice's growth line is rising faster than the reference curve. She is growing faster than normal. Her growth line has returned to about the same position above the 3rd centile as when she was growing well.

This fast growth is an important sign of recovery from undernutrition. It is called *'catch-up growth'*, because the child is catching up the growth that she missed. Children are usually hungrier than normal during recovery. They need extra food to grow faster than normal.

What it may be useful to discuss with the family

- Praise the parents for feeding the child well, and for giving the extra food that the child needed during that time.
- Encourage them to continue feeding the child a good mixed diet. Explain that the child may not continue to want extra food once she has regained the lost weight. Reassure them that this is normal.
- Encourage them to continue bringing the child for weighing, to make sure that she continues to grow in a healthy way.

Poor 'catch-up' growth

Andy's growth line is rising, but it is rising more slowly than the reference line, and it is getting further below the 3rd centile. He is not showing 'catch-up growth' and is not recovering from the period of undernutrition. If he misses the chance to 'catch-up' now, he may not be able to 'catch-up' later. Each time he is ill, he is likely to become more underweight. He is at risk of continuing to be undernourished.

How to help the family

- Try to find out why the child is not gaining weight fast enough.
  - Is the family unable to give the child extra food?
  - Is the child's appetite still poor?
  - Is the child still sick with an infection?
  - Is there any sign that the child is being abused (maltreated)?
- Consider whether the child could be infected with HIV.
- Make sure that the child is treated or referred as necessary.

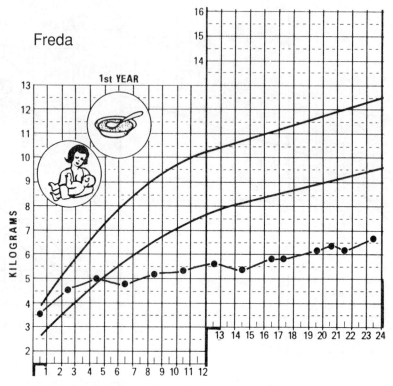

Fig. 15–8 The growth line of a child who has been undernourished for a long time.

- Help the family to find a way to feed the child more.
- Follow up the child frequently (at least every week) until his growth improves.

Prolonged period of slow growth

Figure 15–8 shows the growth chart of Freda who has not grown well for a long time. Freda was a normal size at birth, but now has a weight below the 3rd centile. She is growing slowly, but her growth line is not getting much nearer the reference curve.

Freda is small because she was undernourished and failed to grow for a long time. Now she is small because she is short or stunted (see Section 14.15). She is at greater risk from infections than a large child who has always grown at a healthy rate.

If she eats more she may become more active, and her immunity to infections should increase. She may slowly catch up some of the missed growth. But her weight will not increase as quickly as the Alice in Fig. 15–7, and she is likely to remain short.

What it may be useful to discuss with the family

- Explain that the child is small because she was ill in the past, and that she will not become big or gain weight very fast.
- Explain that if she can eat more now she should become stronger and improve slowly.
- Help them to find ways to feed the child more. A small child may only be able to eat small meals. So it is important to give her more meals each day, and to enrich her food.
- Follow up the child regularly.

15.9 GAINING WEIGHT FASTER THAN THE REFERENCE CURVES

Figure 15–9 shows a baby and a child whose weights are above the reference curve, and who are both gaining weight much faster than the reference curve. Their growth lines are crossing the 97th centile.

If you do not have a 97th centile line, you should be able to see if a child's weight is further above the

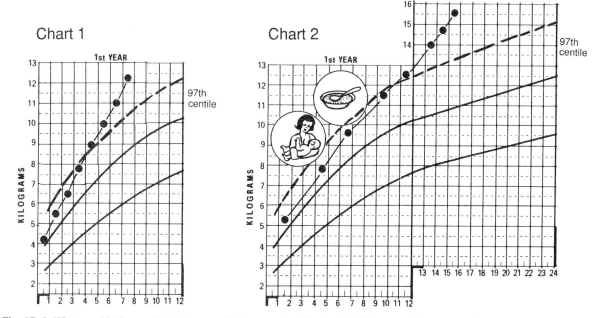

Fig. 15–9 What would it be useful to discuss with the parents of the baby in Chart 1 and the child in Chart 2?

reference line than the 3rd centile line is below it. These children are growing too fast and they are becoming overweight, which can be unhealthy (see Section 22.6).

What it may be useful to discuss with the families

- Ask what milk the child is having. If the child is bottle fed, she may be getting *too much* milk. Discuss how the family can give less. If the mother is breast-feeding, she should not try to give less. The child will outgrow the supply of breast milk.

- Ask what other food the child is having. Suggest that the family give her meals with less fat and sugary foods, but plenty of protein and micronutrients.

- If a baby is overweight and about 6 months old, the family should not delay starting to give weaning foods. They can give small meals without added fat or sugar until growth slows down.

- Examine the child and refer if you are worried about her.

- Ask the family to bring her back for weighing soon.

Box 15.3. Children at special risk from undernutrition

- A child who has lost weight;
- A child with an acute infection especially if the growth line is flat or falling or the last weight was below the 3rd centile;
- A child with HIV infection;
- A child who has just lost a parent, especially the mother;
- A child aged less than 6 months who is not gaining weight at the same rate as the reference line;
- A child aged less than 12 months who has not gained weight for 1 month especially if the weight is below the 3rd centile;
- A child who has not gained weight for 3 months especially if the weight is below the 3rd centile.

Box 15.4.   Useful indicators of serious growth failure

- Newborn babies—low birth weight;
- Babies 0–6 months—gain of less than 500 g in a month;
- Aged 6–12 months—no weight gain for 2 months;
- Aged 12–60 months—no weight gain for 3 months, especially if weight below 3rd centile;
- A falling growth line;
- Weight 2 kg or more below the 3rd centile at any age.

THINGS TO DO

Role play and discussion

1. Ask trainees to role play a nurse or a community health worker explaining growth lines to a child's mother or family, and discussing how to care for the child.

   You can use the children in the 'Things to do' section of Chapter 14 as examples. Different 'mothers' can have children with the different growth charts that trainees filled in. Or copy the growth charts in Chapter 14 or 15. Or copy growth lines from children in a health centre, or make them up.

USEFUL PUBLICATIONS

WFPHA (1985). *Growth monitoring of preschool children: practical considerations for primary health care projects.* UNICEF, New York.

WHO (1986). *The growth chart—a tool for use in infant and child health care.* WHO, Geneva.

16 Undernutrition in children

A child who does not eat enough to cover his nutrient needs is *undernourished*. Undernourished children develop *growth failure* and may become *malnourished*.

Many undernourished children lack energy, protein, and other nutrients. They develop *protein–energy malnutrition* or *PEM*. When the word 'malnutrition' is used, it usually means PEM.

Some children lack just one micronutrient, or they lack one micronutrient more than other nutrients. For example, they have *vitamin A deficiency* or *iron deficiency*. We discuss these *specific deficiencies* in other chapters.

16.1 PROTEIN–ENERGY MALNUTRITION

Protein–energy malnutrition causes a range of conditions, which differ in their signs and severity.

A child may be:

- failing to grow;
- underweight;
- stunted;

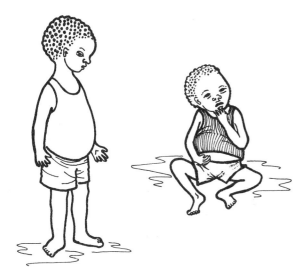

Fig. 16–1 A moderately malnourished child and a severely malnourished child.

but may appear normal.

A child may look:

- thin;
- severely wasted—with *marasmus*;
- oedematous—with *kwashiorkor* (see Section 17.2).

One condition may change into another as a child's food intake changes, or as he develops or recovers from infections.

The different conditions result from an insufficient intake of energy, protein, and micronutrients to cover the child's needs and from infection. Although the term 'PEM' is used, lack of micronutrients, such as zinc, vitamin A, and iron, are partly responsible for the signs.

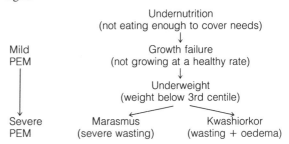

Fig. 16–2 Different stages of protein–energy malnutrition (PEM).

16.2 THE EFFECTS OF UNDERNUTRITION

If a child is undernourished:

- She does not grow as well as she could (Chapter 14).
- She has less energy to do things and to learn.
- She has less resistance and immunity against infections.

Lack of energy

An undernourished child does not have much energy. She does not want to play. She sleeps more. She may be quiet and 'good', or miserable, but she is less interested in the world around her. This lack of interest is sometimes called *apathy*. The child does not explore or dis-

---

Box 16.1. Different words for malnutrition

There are many terms used for different kinds of malnutrition, which can be confusing. In this book we use terms in the following ways:

- *Nutritional disorder* to mean any kind of disorder caused by eating too little or too much of one or more different nutrients.
- *Undernutrition* and *undernourished* to mean insufficient intake of food to cover energy and nutrient needs.
- *Overnutrition* to mean excess intake of energy and nutrients.
- *Malnutrition* and *malnourished* to mean the effects on the body of not eating enough food. These effects are often made worse by infection. (In some other books, malnutrition is also used to mean the effects of eating too much.)
- *Protein–energy malnutrition* or *PEM* to mean the kind of malnutrition which results from insufficient intake of energy, protein, and other nutrients.
- *Specific nutrient deficiency* to mean a condition which is due to lack of only one micronutrient, such as iron deficiency.

Different terms for protein–energy malnutrition
Sometimes people use the term 'protein–energy deficiency', or PED, to make it clear that they mean *under*nutrition, and not *over*nutrition.
Because there is usually a greater lack of energy than of protein, some people use the term '*energy* protein deficiency'.
Children who lack energy and protein, usually also lack other nutrients, such as iron, zinc, and vitamin A, which are partly responsible for growth failure and other signs. Because of this, we like the term 'energy *nutrient* deficiency'. Some workers have suggested '*multinutrient* deficiency'.
All these terms refer to the same condition, but in this book we use the term *protein–energy malnutrition* or *PEM*. Although it is in some ways unsatisfactory, it is still the most widely used and understood.

---

cover things. So she does not learn and develop as quickly as a well nourished child. A child who is undernourished when she is in school finds it difficult to learn.

Many children are mildly undernourished, or undernourished for a short time. If their nutrition improves, their development usually catches up. But their development may not catch up completely if the undernutrition:

- is severe;
- continues for a long time;
- occurs when the child is under 6 months old.

The child may appear normal, but may not achieve as much as he could have.

Undernourished children usually lack both food and stimulating play with adults and other children. Their development catches up fastest if they have both improved nutrition *and* more stimulating play.

Reduced resistance and immunity against infection

Infection means harmful *micro-organisms*, such as bacteria or viruses, or parasites such as *Giardia* or malaria, multiplying in the body and making the person ill. Roundworms and other worms also cause infections.

There are micro-organisms around us all the time, and they often get on to our skin, and into our mouths and gut and respiratory tract. Most micro-organisms do not infect us or make us seriously ill. We are protected by:

- resistance of healthy tissues to infection;
- immunity provided by the *immune system*—white blood cells and antibodies.

If a child is healthy, it is more difficult for micro-organisms to get into her tissues and multiply. If micro-organisms do get into the tissues and multiply, the immune system can usually fight and overcome the infection before it causes serious illness. The child may be ill for a short time, but quickly recovers.

If a child is undernourished, she has difficulty both resisting and fighting infection. So infections can make an undernourished child ill more easily than a well nourished child.

All children get many infections—especially between the ages of 6 months and 3 years. Some infections, such as coughs and colds, malaria, and measles, are equally common in well nourished and undernourished children, but an undernourished child may become more ill, and may take longer to recover than a well nourished child. Other infections, such as diarrhoea and pneumonia, are both commoner and more severe in undernourished children.

Undernourished children often come from poor families, with crowded houses and poor hygiene, so they are exposed to more infections.

16.3 HOW MALNUTRITION AND INFECTION MAKE EACH OTHER WORSE

How malnutrition makes infections worse

- *Micro-organisms are more likely to get into the child's body.* The skin and the cells lining the gut and respiratory tract are less healthy and less able to resist the infection. Vitamin A deficiency may be particularly important. So the child is more likely to be infected.

- *It is easier for micro-organisms to multiply in the body.* The immune system is less able to fight infection than it is in a healthy child. The white blood cells are the part of the immune system which is most affected. The body can still make antibodies, and immunization (for example, against measles) is usually effective even in malnourished children.

A malnourished child may not respond to infections normally. For example, there may be no fever. If the child has a skin infection, there may be no redness or swelling. Fever, redness, and swelling are signs that the body is responding to and fighting infection normally. As a result, in malnourished children:

- *The infection is more likely to become serious.* For example, a cold or cough is more likely to develop into pneumonia. Pneumonia is more likely to become severe.

- *The child is more likely to die.* A malnourished child is more likely than a well nourished child to die, for example, from diarrhoea, pneumonia, or measles.

- *Recovery may take longer.* The body is less able to repair damaged tissues, such as the lining of the gut or the respiratory tract. So, for example, diarrhoea is more likely to become persistent. An ear infection is more likely to continue for a long time, to recur, or to become chronic.

How infections interfere with a child's nutrition

- *Infections reduce the child's appetite.* A child who is ill is less hungry than normal and eats less. If a child normally eats bulky food, it is difficult to get enough nutrients even when he has a good appetite. If the child has a poor appetite, it can become impossible.

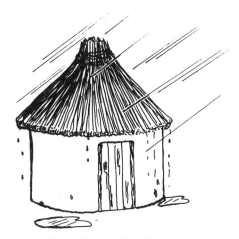

A well nourished child is like this house and can resist infection as the house resists rain.

Fig. 16–3 Two houses.

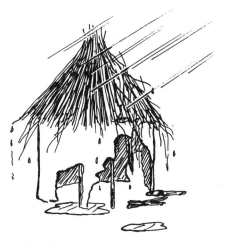

A malnourished child is like this house. The child cannot resist infection; the house cannot stand up in the rain because the ants have eaten all the poles.

- *Some infections make eating difficult.* If the child has a sore mouth, or a blocked nose, or if breathing is difficult, eating becomes more difficult. The child may only be able to take liquid foods. The family may make liquid foods which are very dilute and watery. This reduces the child's intake of nutrients even more.

- *Some infections reduce the absorption of nutrients from the gut.* During diarrhoea, the cells which line the gut may be damaged, and may not be able to absorb as many nutrients as when the child is well—for example, the absorption of fat may decrease. In some infections, nutrients are lost from the gut. If a child is malnourished, the gut takes longer to recover and to start absorbing nutrients normally than if the child is well nourished.

- *Infection increases the need for nutrients.* For example, during fever, the body uses more energy. A child with measles needs more vitamin A. A child with malaria needs more folate.

- *Infection causes breakdown of muscle and fat.* If the body does not get enough food, it breaks down its own tissues to provide the nutrients that it needs. The child loses weight, becomes thin, and stops growing.

During serious infections, such as measles, whooping cough, tuberculosis (TB), severe diarrhoea, pneumonia, and malaria, children lose a lot of weight, so it is easy to see that these infections cause malnutrition. But mild infections, such as mild diarrhoea, coughs and colds, otitis media (ear infection), stomatitis (mouth sores), scabies and worms, can also cause undernutrition, especially if a child has these mild illnesses often.

Figure 16–4 is a calendar for 30 days in a typical young child's life. The child is Esther, and she is 1 year old. The smiling faces show the days on which Esther was well, and eating normally. The sad faces show the days on which she was ill and did not eat much.

Esther was ill on 10 out of the 30 days. So she was ill on one day out of every three. The illnesses themselves were not serious. But, on the days she was ill, Esther did not want to eat much. If a child does not eat much for one day in every three, it greatly reduces the total amount of food that she eats.

The downward spiral of malnutrition and infection

So infection causes undernutrition, because it reduces food intake, but increases the body's need for nutri-

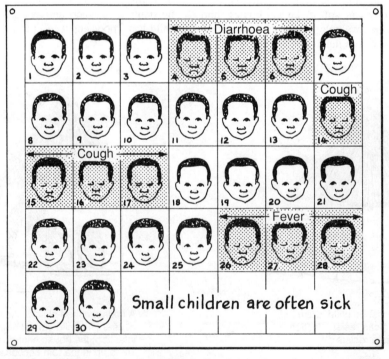

Fig. 16–4 A calendar for a month in Esther's life, showing how often a young child is ill.

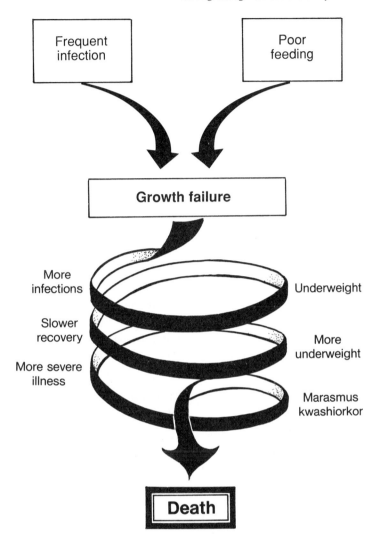

Fig. 16–5 The downward spiral of malnutrition and infection.

ents. If a child does not eat much during an illness, and does not eat enough during recovery to regain the weight she has lost, she becomes malnourished.

Children who have frequent illnesses may not have time to regain the weight that they lose with one illness before the next illness reduces their appetite again. Children who are undernourished may have illnesses which are more severe, and from which they take longer to recover. This leads to them becoming malnourished. This is the *downward spiral of malnutrition and infection* which causes protein–energy malnutrition or death in many children.

16.4 RECOGNIZING MALNUTRITION BEFORE IT BECOMES SEVERE

If you recognize malnutrition early, you can treat it more easily. You can save the child much suffering and the parents much worry. If a malnourished child continues to eat less food than her body needs, she will become worse. She may become seriously ill from infections, or severely malnourished, or both.

If you recognize malnutrition early, before the child is seriously ill, the family can probably treat her at home. When malnutrition has become severe, treat-

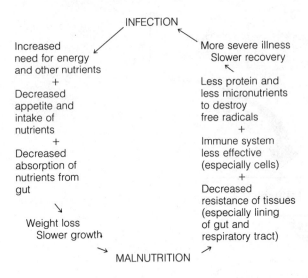

Fig. 16–6 How infection and malnutrition make each other worse.

ment is more difficult, and it is less likely to succeed. The child usually needs to be in hospital, which makes treatment more expensive.

- *Ask about the child's activity.* Often the first sign of malnutrition in a child is that she is less active and plays less. You may not be able to see this, but a mother notices if her child is quiet and not playing as much as other children. Remember to ask mothers about their child's activity.

- *Find out if the child is growing.* The child's mother may be aware that the child is not growing. She may be aware that the child does not need a larger size of clothes, or that the child's beads are not becoming tighter as they should. Ask her if she has noticed this.

    You can see poor growth most easily in the child's growth chart (see Chapters 14 and 15). Look for *flattening of the child's growth line*. A child may fail to gain weight for 6 months or more before she begins to look thin.

- *Look at the child.* Does the child look thin? The child's mother is usually aware of thinness. She may point out that the child's clothes do not fit so well.

16.5 UNDERNUTRITION IN CHILDREN OF DIFFERENT AGES

There are three ways in which a child gets nutrients:

- through the placenta before birth;
- from breast milk;
- from weaning foods and family foods.

A problem with any of these sources of nutrients can cause undernutrition which leads to growth failure. For example:

- if the mother is undernourished;
- if the baby lacks breast milk;
- if the child does not eat enough weaning foods or family foods.

16.6 GROWTH FAILURE BEFORE BIRTH

If a baby does not grow well before he is born, he is small at birth. If a baby weighs less than 2.5 kg at birth he is *low birth weight* or 'LBW'.

LBW babies are more likely to die than larger babies, particularly from pneumonia and other infections. The greatest risk is with babies who weigh less than 2 kg at birth. LBW babies are more likely to die, not only during the newborn period, but also throughout the first 4 years of life, and maybe even longer. They have low stores of nutrients, such as fat, iron, and vitamin A, so they are more likely than larger babies to become severely malnourished.

Babies may be LBW because they are born too early. A baby who is born before 38 weeks of pregnancy is called *premature*. Premature babies have special problems, especially with feeding, because they are not ready to be born. They may need special care in hospital. Babies born before about 32 weeks need to be tube fed.

Babies may be LBW because of growth failure during pregnancy. They may be born at the normal time, but they are *small-for-dates*. Some babies fail to grow throughout pregnancy, so that they are *stunted*, with a low length for age. Some fail to grow only during the last few weeks of pregnancy, so that they are *wasted*, with a low weight for length.

Some babies have growth failure *and* they are premature. Their most serious problem is usually their prematurity.

Causes of low birth weight

The causes of prematurity are not fully understood. Here we discuss the causes of growth failure before birth.

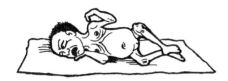

Fig. 16—7 A low birth weight baby.

- *Undernutrition of the mother.* One of the most important causes of low birth weight is that the mother is undernourished, and she cannot supply enough nutrients to the baby (see Chapter 18).

- *Young age of the mother.* Adolescent girls are more likely than adult women to have small babies, because they are still growing themselves, and have large nutrient needs (see Chapter 18).

- *Malaria.* If the mother has malaria, it may harm the placenta, and prevent nutrients from getting to the baby. It also causes anaemia in the mother. In endemic areas, malaria is an important cause of low birth weight. Some health programmes recommend that women take antimalarial drugs during pregnancy.

- *Congenital problems.* A baby who is born with a *congenital abnormality* (such as a cleft palate or Down's syndrome), and a baby who has an infection before birth, such as *congenital syphilis*, may also be LBW, because they have not grown normally before birth. These babies may have an abnormal appearance, or may look ill in other ways, besides being small. If possible, refer them to a more specialized health worker.

- *Other causes.* If a mother drinks a lot of alcohol or smokes when she is pregnant, or if she has toxaemia of pregnancy, it may make the baby smaller. Possibly, if a woman has to work very hard throughout pregnancy, her baby may be smaller, but we do not yet know enough about this.

16.7 DIFFERENT KINDS OF GROWTH FAILURE BEFORE BIRTH

Wasting

Babies may be undernourished during the last trimester of pregnancy if:

- the mother is undernourished before or during pregnancy;

- she is stunted because of undernutrition in childhood;

- she has malaria, or toxaemia of pregnancy;

- it is a twin pregnancy.

These babies:

- look thin, because they have not built up much fat;

- are wasted with a low weight-for-length;

- may become anaemic because they lack iron stores;

- are more likely to become cold than larger babies, because they lack fat to keep them warm;

- are more likely to get hypoglycaemia (low blood sugar) soon after birth, because they lack stores of carbohydrate;

- are at greater risk of infections such as pneumonia.

If these babies get enough breast milk, they can grow very fast soon after birth, and show 'catch-up' growth. They may reach a weight within the normal range for their age in 6–9 months. If they do not get enough breast milk, they may continue to be underweight.

Undernutrition, especially severe malnutrition, both before birth and soon after birth, may have serious effects on the development of a child's brain.

LBW babies may need to be cup fed at first, because they may be too weak to suckle effectively. But they can often feed themselves fully from the breast earlier than a premature baby of the same weight.

What you can do

- Encourage the mother to express breast milk for the baby, and show her how to do it effectively (see Section 10.14).

- Help the mother to feed her baby from a cup, and to let the baby start suckling as soon as he is able.

- Make sure that 'wasted' babies get the extra breast milk that they need. They can take more breast milk than a premature baby of the same weight (see Section 10.22 and Table 10.1).

Stunting

Babies may fail to grow throughout pregnancy if they have:

- a congenital abnormality;

- a congenital infection.

Other babies who appear normal may also fall into this group.

These LBW babies are *stunted*, with a low length or height-for-age.

● They are small, but they do not look wasted.
● They have a normal weight for their length.

They will always be small for their age, even if they have plenty of breast milk. They do not show 'catch-up' growth, and may remain short as adults.

If a LBW baby is well, and gaining weight, and you are sure that she is getting enough breast milk, but she is not showing very fast 'catch-up' growth, it may be because she is stunted.

16.8 UNDERNUTRITION IN BABIES AGED 0–6 MONTHS

Most babies grow well during the first 6 months of life, if they are exclusively breastfed. Almost every mother can produce enough breast milk if she breastfeeds frequently, whenever the baby seems hungry, and if she gives the baby no other food or drink.

Breastfeeding protects the baby against infections. Exclusively breastfed babies have few infections and recover quickly from any that they do have. So undernutrition before the age of 6 months is uncommon in an exclusively breastfed baby.

Lack of breast milk

Malnutrition often occurs because a baby does not get enough breast milk.

Many families cannot afford to buy enough formula or milk to make artificial feeds. They may dilute the milk with too much water, to make it last longer. Or they may give the baby thin cereal porridge instead of milk. They may only make up two or three bottles in a day, and feed them to the baby in small amounts.

Instructions on tins of formula or powdered milk may not be clear; they may be in a language that the mother does not know or she may be unable to read. So some mothers have no means of knowing how to make up feeds correctly. Some mothers give too little milk; a few mothers give too much.

Poor families who lack water and fuel find it difficult to clean and sterilize feeding bottles and teats. Bottles are often contaminated. Bacteria grow in the milk and give the baby diarrhoea. If the family leaves the bottle

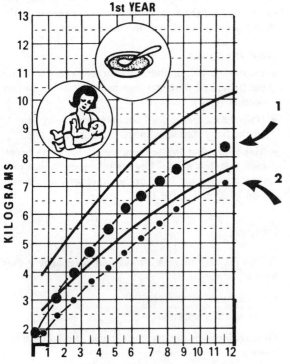

1 This LBW baby showed 'catch-up' growth for about 6 months

2 This LBW baby remains small but grows at a healthy rate

Fig. 16–8 Two growth lines of LBW babies.
1. This LBW baby showed 'catch-up' growth for about 6 months and her weight is within the normal range. She was *wasted*.
2. This LBW baby did not show 'catch-up' growth. She is growing at a healthy rate but remains small. She is *stunted*.
It may be difficult to tell at birth how a LBW baby will grow.

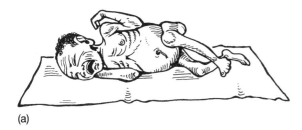

(a)

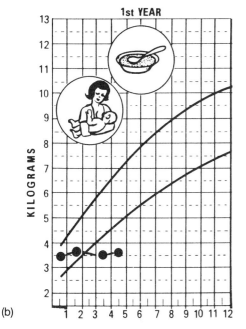

(b)

Fig. 16–9 (a) A baby who lacks breast milk.
(b) His growth chart.

animal milk, the baby may get enough energy and protein. However, animal milk and formula may not contain the right mixture of all nutrients for a baby.

Even if the mother can sterilize the feeding bottle properly, the baby is still more likely to get infections, because he lacks the protection that breast milk provides.

Partial breastfeeding is safer than complete artificial feeding. The baby gets *some* nutrients and *some* protection against infection from breast milk. But a baby who has even a few bottle feeds or other drinks gets less breast milk, and more infections than a baby who is breastfeeding exclusively. So partial breastfeeding can also cause malnutrition.

- Encourage mothers to breastfeed exclusively for 6 months.
- Make sure that working mothers know how to express breast milk to leave for their babies (see Sections 10.14 and 10.17).
- Encourage people who care for babies to feed them from a cup and not from a bottle (see Section 10.14).

> **Lack of breast milk often causes growth failure in the first 6 months of life and severe malnutrition in the first year.**

of milk in the warm and feeds it to the baby slowly, the bacteria have plenty of time to multiply.

Diarrhoea is much commoner in bottle fed babies than in breastfed babies, and it may become persistent (see Section 13.4). Other infections such as pneumonia are also more common and more serious in bottle fed babies. So babies who lack breast milk may become malnourished for two reasons:

1. They may not get enough energy and nutrients.

2. They have more infections.

Their growth lines become flat in the first 6 months of life. They may become severely malnourished in the first year (Fig. 16–9).

If the family can afford to buy enough formula or

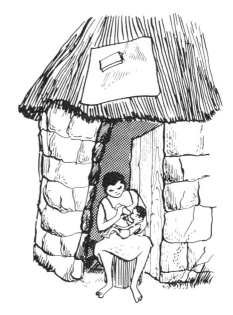

Fig. 16–10 Bottle feeding causes malnutrition in the first year of life.

16.9 UNDERNUTRITION IN BABIES AGED 6–12 MONTHS

The risk of undernutrition increases when babies reach the age of 6 months. From the age of 6 months, babies need both weaning foods *and* breast milk. Some babies do not get enough weaning food. Some stop breastfeeding early.

From this age, babies are also more exposed to infection. They start to eat other food, which may be contaminated and which may cause diarrhoea. They start to crawl on the floor, and they start to put things in their mouths which may also be contaminated. By 6 months of age, the protective antibodies which they got from their mothers through the placenta are finished. Babies are more likely to become ill with infections such as measles.

So between the ages of 6 months and a year babies get more infections, but they may not get enough energy and nutrients. They may stop growing and their growth lines become flat. Children who continue to fail to grow, may be severely malnourished in the second year of life.

> **Lack of weaning food often causes growth failure in the second 6 months of life and severe malnutrition in the second year.**

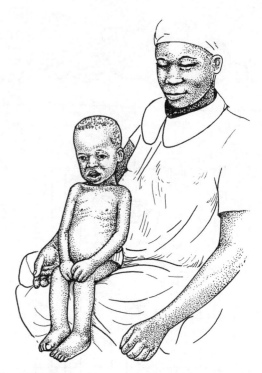

Fig. 16–11 Malnutrition is most common in children aged 1–3 years.

16.10 UNDERNUTRITION IN CHILDREN AGED 1–3 YEARS

The risk of malnutrition continues to be high in children of 1–3 years old. Often growth failure began earlier, in the first year of life.

Children aged 1–3 years may not get enough energy and nutrients because:

- They may not eat often enough.
- The food that they eat is not rich in energy and nutrients.
- They are more active and need more energy.
- They are exposed to more infections, which reduce their appetites.

Children who stop breastfeeding need to eat extra food to replace breast milk. If the food is bulky or dilute it is difficult for them to eat enough extra food. A child may eat more food than before; but if it is more dilute than breast milk, the total amount of energy and nutrients that the child gets may decrease, (see Section 11.7).

Children who do not eat enough stop growing. Their growth lines become flat and may fall below the 3rd centile.

16.11 UNDERNUTRITION FROM 3–5 YEARS OF AGE

After the age of 3 years, children are at less risk of undernutrition. By the age of 3 years, most children can feed themselves. They can eat the same food as adults. Bulky foods are less of a problem. They should have built up some immunity to common infections. However, children can be malnourished at this age if:

- They were malnourished previously, and they have not fully recovered—like the girl in Fig. 16–12 (see Section 18.1).
- They have a severe infection—for example, malaria or pneumonia, or a chronic infection such as tuberculosis (TB) or AIDS.
- There is a severe food shortage.
- There is a severe problem in the family which affects the child's appetite—for example, the mother dies, or the child is neglected or abused.

Older children are also more at risk than breastfeeding babies from variations in the food supply; for example,

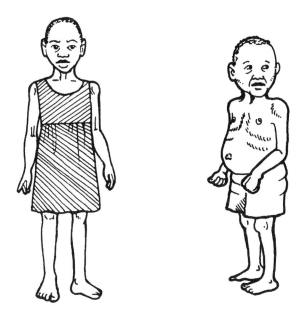

Fig. 16–12 Children aged 3–5 years may be malnourished and stunted.

if there is a seasonal shortage of green vegetables, they may lack vitamin A.

If a child is undernourished, her growth line may be flat or falling. But weight gain at this age is slower than in younger children, so it can be more difficult to tell if a child is growing or not from her weight gain.

A child's weight-for-age may be outside the normal range because she was malnourished in the past, and is now stunted. To find out if a child aged 3 years or more is malnourished now, you can measure her weight-for-height (see Section 14.17).

16.12 WORM INFECTION AND NUTRITION

Worm infections can cause or contribute to under-nutrition and poor growth—especially *roundworm* or *Ascaris*, and *hookworm*. Both types of infection can cause:

- poor appetite, which decreases a child's food intake;
- poor digestion and absorption of nutrients—for example, fat;
- increased loss of nutrients from the gut—for example, protein and iron.

The result may be:

- protein–energy malnutrition;

- anaemia, particularly with hookworm;
- deficiency of other micronutrients, such as vitamin A;

which leads to:

- reduced energy;
- decreased ability to work;
- poor school performance in children.

Roundworms

These are large and like earthworms. When a child passes a roundworm, you can easily see it. An infected child passes roundworm eggs in the faeces, which stay in the soil for many months. Other children become infected when they eat something, or when they suck their fingers or some other object, which is contaminated with soil.

Worms may cause coughs as their larvae pass through the lungs, stomach pain, diarrhoea, difficulty sleeping, and other symptoms. If a child has many worms, they may block the child's gut and make him seriously ill.

Worm infections can be difficult to diagnose because most of the symptoms also occur in other illnesses. You can only be sure that a child has roundworms if he passes a worm, or if you can see eggs in the child's faeces with a microscope.

Hookworm

Hookworms are very small and difficult to see. An infected person passes eggs in the faeces, which hatch in the soil and then enter another person through the skin. The worms hold on to the wall of the intestine, and feed on the person's blood. This causes anaemia, which can be very severe (see Chapter 20).

You should suspect hookworm infection if a person is very anaemic. But you can only be sure that hookworm is the cause of the anaemia if you can see hookworm eggs in the person's faeces with a microscope.

16.13 PREVENTING AND TREATING WORM INFECTION

In areas where worm infection is common, people may have several infections at the same time—roundworm, hookworm, and others. To prevent worm infections, you should help communities to improve water and

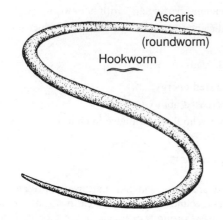

Relative sizes of different common worms.

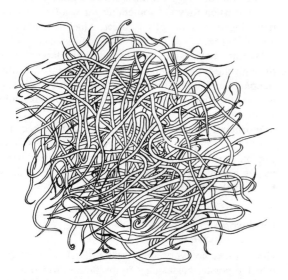

Children may have many worms like this.

Fig. 16–13 Worms.

sanitation, hygiene and living standards. But this may take a long time.

Meantime, it may help to '*deworm*' people regularly—especially children. They may be infected again but, if everybody has less worms, they pass fewer eggs. The environment is less contaminated, and the risk of infection is less.

If children have fewer worms, they grow better, they feel better, they become stronger, and they do better in school. Families usually want their children to have treatment for worms. They may be more interested in their children's growth after treatment than they were before. One problem can be that deworming is so

popular that you run out of drugs. So make sure that you have enough before you start.

There are several modern drugs which are effective against both roundworm and hookworm and other worms, and which are safe. For example:

- *Mebendazole* tablets 100 mg twice a day for 3 days;
- *Albendazole* tablets 400 mg single dose.

Which drug health workers use in an area, whom they give it to, and how often they give it depend on which worms are common, which drugs are available, and the decisions of the local programme organizers. For example, you may give a deworming drug to:

- all children regularly, every few months;
- children who have passed worms;
- people with symptoms such as abdominal pain or anaemia which may be due to worms.

THINGS TO DO

Class exercise and discussion

1. Ask trainees to look at the growth charts from Chapters 14 and 15 and the 'Things to do' section of Chapter 14 which show poor growth at different ages—for example: Figs 14–11, 14–12, 14–13, and Fig. 15–5, 15–6, and 15–8. Discuss the causes of undernutrition in each case.

2. Make a list with trainees of the infections which are important causes of malnutrition in local children. Discuss how these may lead to malnutrition.

Field visit

Arrange for trainees to visit a health centre, to talk to families who bring children for treatment, for example, for diarrhoea, coughs, or fever.

3. Ask trainees to talk to the families and ask:

   a. how they think the children are growing;

   b. how the children are fed.

4. They should also find out about the children's weights and look at their growth charts.

5. They can also talk to the families to find out if they understand the children's charts.

6. Trainees should make a note of their observations to discuss in class afterwards.

   a. How many children did they find who were underweight? How many children had poor growth? What were the ages of the children? How were they fed?

b. Did they see any growth lines of children with infections? What did they observe? How were the children fed?

c. What did the families say about the children's growth and health?

USEFUL PUBLICATIONS

Children in the Tropics (1990). Immunity and nutrition. *Children in the Tropics*, Vol. 189.

Tomkins, A. and Watson, F. (1989). *Malnutrition and infection: a review*, ACC/SCN Nutrition Policy Discussion Paper, no. 5. ACC/SCN, Geneva.

17 Severe protein–energy malnutrition

A child who continues to be undernourished and to have many infections, is likely to develop one of the three main types of severe protein–energy malnutrition (PEM):

- marasmus;
- kwashiorkor;
- marasmic kwashiorkor (a mixture of the other two).

Persistent growth failure and PEM is common in children with AIDS.

17.1 MARASMUS

Marasmus is the result of a child having a very low intake of energy and nutrients. It often follows severe illness or a period of frequent infections. Marasmus usually occurs in the first 2 years of life, but it can occur at any age, particularly during famines.

Signs of marasmus in children

- *Extremely low weight.* The child's weight is usually less than 60 per cent of the reference weight. This means that her recent growth line falls a long way below the 3rd centile.

- *Extreme wasting.* This is the most characteristic sign of marasmus. The child has lost much of her fat and muscle, so her body looks very thin, and her arms and legs look like sticks. The child's arm circumference is often 10 or 11 cm or even lower. She has a low weight-for-height.

- *An 'old person's face'.* The child's face is wasted, and the skin may be in folds. She often looks anxious and worried, so she looks like a very old person.

- *'Pot belly'.* The child's abdomen sticks out, because the muscles of the abdominal wall are wasted and weak.

- *Irritability and fretfulness.* The child suffers and is very miserable, and cries and complains a lot.

- *Hunger.* The child may eat hungrily when you give her some food, if she does not have an infection.

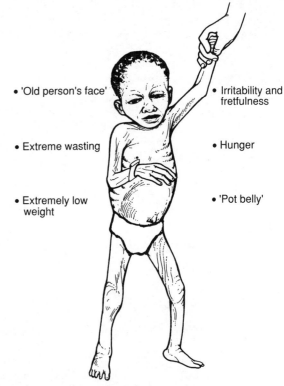

- 'Old person's face'
- Extreme wasting
- Extremely low weight
- Irritability and fretfulness
- Hunger
- 'Pot belly'

Fig. 17–1 A child with marasmus. Marasmic children are easy to recognize.

17.2 KWASHIORKOR

Kwashiorkor is more complicated. It is commonest in children aged 1–3 years, but it can occur in older or younger children. Figures 17–2 and 16–11 show children with kwashiorkor.

Causes of kwashiorkor

Kwashiorkor is mainly due to lack of energy and nutrients. But there are other factors also that cause

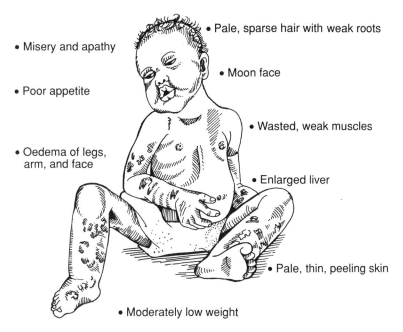

- Misery and apathy
- Poor appetite
- Oedema of legs, arm, and face
- Pale, sparse hair with weak roots
- Moon face
- Wasted, weak muscles
- Enlarged liver
- Pale, thin, peeling skin
- Moderately low weight

Fig. 17–2 A child with kwashiorkor.

some children to develop kwashiorkor, while other children on the same diet develop marasmus. We do not yet fully understand what causes the difference.

An important recent explanation is that there is an imbalance between the production and removal of *free radicals*. Free radicals are highly reactive molecules (usually oxygen—'superoxides'), which are produced during infections and which can damage body tissues. In healthy people, free radicals are destroyed by *antioxidants*—such as vitamin A and zinc. Protein also helps to remove them.

In children, large numbers of free radicals may be produced during infections such as measles. Free radicals may also be produced when a child eats food which contains the poison *aflatoxin* (see Section 7.8). Sometimes children with kwashiorkor have more aflatoxin in their livers than healthy children or children with marasmus. A child who is also undernourished, may lack the micronutrients which remove the free radicals. The free radicals can build up enough to damage the tissues. This damage causes oedema, fatty enlargement of the liver, pale skin and hair, and possibly diarrhoea.

Signs of kwashiorkor

The signs of kwashiorkor may appear very quickly, often when a child has an infection, or stops breastfeeding suddenly. But usually the child has been undernourished and growing poorly for some time before the signs appear.

- *Oedema of the legs and arms and face.* Oedema is swelling due to fluid in the tissues. If you press the swelling gently, you make a small pit in the skin. You see oedema first in the legs, and then in the arms and face as the child's condition becomes worse. If she is lying down, you may find oedema on her back. Oedema may come and go fairly quickly when a child's nutrition suddenly becomes worse or better. Oedema is the main sign which distinguishes kwashiorkor from marasmas.

- *Moon face.* The child's face becomes rounder than usual, and may even look fat. This may be partly due to oedema, but it is also due to other changes in how the child's body works.

- *Moderately low weight.* A child with kwashiorkor is not usually so severely underweight as a child with marasmus. Most children with kwashiorkor have weights below the 3rd centile, but they are not usually below 60 per cent of the reference weight-for-age. Their weight-for-height is also low, but not as low as in marasmus. Some children with kwashiorkor have weights that are above the 3rd centile. Some of the weight is due to oedema fluid.

- *Wasted muscles.* A child with kwashiorkor does not lose all the fat under her skin so she does not look as thin as a child with marasmus. However, a child with kwashiorkor does lose muscle. You can see the muscle wasting most clearly over her shoulders, where there is less fat and no oedema. Oedema sometimes makes a child appear fat. The arm circumference is reduced, but not so much as in a child with marasmus.

- *Weak muscles.* Sometimes a child is unable to walk or sit up. Her abdomen sticks out ('pot belly') because the muscles of her abdominal wall are weak.

- *Misery and apathy.* A child with kwashiorkor looks unhappy. If she is disturbed, she may cry miserably. If she is undisturbed, she is *apathetic*—that is, she lacks interest in the world around her. She just sits or lies in her mother's arms, sometimes moaning, and she shows no interest in life. She does not want to play, or walk, or crawl about.

- *Poor appetite.* The child may not want to eat, so it may be difficult to persuade her to take food. This is different from the hunger that children with marasmus often show.

- *Pale, thin, peeling skin.* The child's skin becomes paler than usual, though some parts may become darker. The skin becomes thin, and may peel off. This is called a 'flaking paint rash' because it looks like old paint. Sores may develop. The skin of her legs and the back of her hands peels first, but also the skin of her buttocks and back may become sore.

- *Pale, sparse hair with weak roots.* The child's hair becomes *sparse*—that is, there are fewer hairs. They may be straighter than normal. You can easily pull out some hairs without hurting the child, because the roots are weak. The hair is often pale, and parents may notice this. However, children may have pale hair for other reasons, so it does not necessarily mean that the child has kwashiorkor.

- *Enlarged liver.* The child's liver becomes full of fat, which makes it larger. You can feel the enlarged liver in the upper right side of the child's abdomen.

The oedema, the fatty liver, and the pale skin and hair may all be due to tissue damage by free radicals.

17.3 MARASMIC KWASHIORKOR

Some children have signs of both marasmus and kwashiorkor at the same time.

Signs of marasmic kwashiorkor

- *Extremely low weight.* The child looks extremely thin and wasted. Her weight is usually less than 60 per cent of the reference weight. This means that her recent growth line is a long way below the 3rd centile. She has a very low weight-for-height.

- *Oedema.* The child has mild oedema of her legs, and sometimes of her arms and face.

- *Other signs.* The child may have any of the other signs of kwashiorkor or marasmus—a thin or moon face; weak hair; skin changes; and misery.

17.4 DANGERS AND COMPLICATIONS OF MARASMUS AND KWASHIORKOR

Risk of death

Children with severe protein–energy malnutrition are likely to die. They need careful treatment, usually in hospital, at least for a time. Even after treatment with special foods and drugs, some of them die. Children who recover may relapse and become malnourished again, and die later. Children with AIDS are almost certain to die.

Problem of sickness

Children with severe malnutrition are ill. They feel miserable and they may be in pain. Their frequent illnesses give the family a lot of worry and expense.

Complications

There are several complications of severe malnutrition, which can make treatment difficult.

Diarrhoea

Malnourished children may have *acute diarrhoea*, due to the same types of infection that all children may get, such as viruses, bacteria, and *Giardia*.

In malnourished children, diarrhoea is often *persistent*. Persistent diarrhoea starts like acute diarrhoea, but continues for more than 2 weeks. *Chronic diarrhoea* is also common. Chronic diarrhoea starts slowly, but continues for a long time, and keeps recurring.

Persistent and chronic diarrhoea are partly the result of undernutrition. The gut wall becomes thin and damaged. It takes longer to recover from infection, and does not digest and absorb food properly. Nutrients are

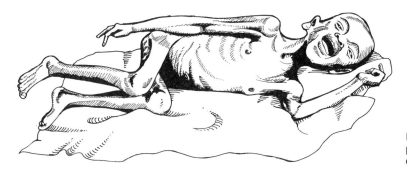

Fig. 17–3 Children with severe protein–energy malnutrition may have diarrhoea and other complications.

lost in the diarrhoea, which makes undernutrition worse.

Diarrhoea in malnourished children is also partly due to *bacterial overgrowth*. The normally harmless bacteria that live in a child's lower gut spread to her upper gut and stomach where they can cause damage and make her ill.

Dehydration

Malnourished children with diarrhoea may become dehydrated. This increases the risk of death, and requires urgent treatment. Usually the best way to treat them is with oral rehydration fluids (see Sections 13.4 and 17.8). A child with kwashiorkor who is dehydrated may lose her oedema, which reappears when she is rehydrated.

Infections

Most severely malnourished children have an infection, for example, otitis media, pneumonia, a urinary tract infection, or septicaemia. However, the signs of infection may not be present, because the body does not respond to infection normally. The infection may be serious, but it can easily be missed, and it can be difficult to diagnose. For example, the child may have pneumonia, but may not have fever or fast breathing.

Hypoglycaemia (low blood sugar)

A severely malnourished child's blood sugar may fall very low. Untreated, prolonged hypoglycaemia can cause severe brain damage and death. Hypoglycaemia is an important sign of infection. Hypoglycaemia may also cause hypothermia.

Hypothermia (low body temperature)

A child who is severely malnourished easily becomes too cold, and may develop hypothermia—that is, a body temperature below 35.5 °C. This is an important cause of death. Malnourished children develop hypothermia because they lack nutrients to burn to keep the body warm. A child's temperature is most likely to fall:

- If she has hypoglycaemia, so that very little glucose gets to her cells to burn for energy.
- When the room temperature is low, for example at night, and she needs extra energy to warm her body.
- During infection, when the body also uses extra energy. Her body temperature may fall instead of rising. (So hypothermia is another sign of infection in these children.)

Anorexia (loss of appetite)

Severely malnourished children may not want to eat, which makes it difficult to feed them. This is commonest with children who have kwashiorkor or marasmic kwashiorkor.

Anaemia

Most severely malnourished children are anaemic due to iron deficiency and sometimes folate deficiency. They may also have anaemia due to other, non-nutritional causes, such as malaria and hookworm. However, iron can produce free radicals, so treatment with iron should not be given until the child begins to recover (see Section 17.12). Good feeding may treat the anaemia sufficiently, so that iron therapy is not needed.

Other nutritional deficiencies

Children with PEM may also have deficiencies of other nutrients, particularly minerals such as zinc, and vitamin A. This may be part of the reason for their low resistance to infection and may contribute to problems such as diarrhoea, skin changes, and poor growth. Vitamin A deficiency can cause sudden and severe damage to their eyes (see Chapter 19).

Long-term problems

Children who recover from severe PEM may be stunted. They may have permanent mental disabilities, especially if they were malnourished during the first 6 months of life.

17.5 MANAGEMENT OF SEVERE MALNUTRITION IN CHILDREN

The management of marasmus, kwashiorkor, and marasmic kwashiorkor is the same. However, children with kwashiorkor are the most difficult to start towards recovery.

Because of the dangers and complications described in Section 17.4, it is usually necessary for a severely malnourished child to have treatment as an in-patient in a hospital or health centre. Sometimes you can treat less seriously ill children at home, or change to home management after the early phase of treatment.

Discuss the child's condition with the family. If you think that in-patient care is necessary, explain the reasons. If it would be difficult to refer or admit the child or the family is unwilling, and if you think that home-based care is possible, discuss whether they would be able to give the child appropriate food and other care at home.

Box 17.1 lists the main criteria for deciding whether a child needs in-patient care, or can be treated at home. One of the most important is *appetite*. If a child is not eating well, then in-patient care is essential.

The aims of treatment

The aims of treatment should be for the child to:

- recover from any infections and complications;
- regain lost weight so that her weight-for-height returns to the normal range (see Appendix 5, Tables A5.4 and A5.5);
- grow at a healthy rate (see Chapter 14).

Box 17.1.   How to decide about in-patient treatment or home treatment of severely malnourished children

A child needs in-patient treatment in hospital or other health facility if:

- She is less than 12 months old; *or*
- She is not eating well; *or*
- She is vomiting; *or*
- She is weak or apathetic; *or*
- She has widespread oedema; *or*
- She is dehydrated, or has severe or chronic diarrhoea, severe anaemia, peeling skin, xerophthalmia, or suspected TB; *or*
- Suitable food or care is not available at home; *or*
- Her home is far from the health facility.

It may be possible to treat a child at home if:

- She is aged 12 months or older; *and*
- She is able to eat enough; *and*
- She is alert; *and*
- If she has oedema, it is only on the feet; *and*
- She has no dehydration, severe or chronic diarrhoea, fast or difficult breathing, severe anaemia, peeling skin, xerophthalmia, suspected TB; *and*
- Food is available; *and*
- Her family are caring and well-motivated; *and*
- Antibiotic and other treatment can be given properly; *and*
- Progress, especially during the first 2 weeks, can be closely supervised (e.g. you can see the child every day).

Approach to treatment

Treatment of severely undernourished children is urgent and needs to start immediately. Treatment needs to be:

1. *Medical* (see Section 17.8):
   - Treatment of dehydration;
   - Treatment of infections (with antibiotics);
   - Keeping the body at a normal temperature.
2. *Dietary* (see Sections 17.9–17.11):
   - Feeding:
     - Early recovery—usually with a milk mixture;
     - Catch-up growth—high energy feeds;
     - Return to good mixed meals using family food.
   - Vitamin and mineral supplements (see Section 17.12).
3. *Social and emotional* (see Section 17.15):
   - Comfort, affection, and mental stimulation for the child;
   - Support and sympathy for her family;
   - Help with the family's social problems.
   - Counselling for AIDS if necessary.
4. *Educational* (see Sections 17.16 and 17.17):
   - Show the family how to feed the child.
   - Talk with the family about children's food needs.
   - Encourage mothers to learn from each other in the ward.

17.6 LEARNING ABOUT A CHILD AND HER FAMILY

Before you can treat a child or help the family, you need to know about the child and her illness and the family. There are many things that it may be helpful to understand, but you cannot learn them all at once. Some things are important to know straight away, to enable you to start treatment. Some things you will learn slowly as you spend time talking with the family and get to know each other. As they learn to trust you, they will tell you more.

How to take a 'history' from a family

- When you first meet the family, greet them kindly, introduce yourself, and start to make friends with them. Make sure that you know and use the mother's or other carer's name and the child's name.

- As you talk with the mother or other family member, you will have a 'list' of questions in your mind of the things that you need to know. You may not always have time to ask them all, and you do not have to ask things in a special order. But the 'list' helps you to remember and to organize your thoughts.

- Let the family tell you what they think is important first, and listen carefully to what they have to say. Even if you do not agree, do not say so, and do not argue. You are trying to learn what *they* think, and how *they* feel.

What you need to know straight away

- What the child's illness is. Let the family tell you about the child's problem, and why they think she is ill, in their own way;
- the child's age;
- how long the child has been ill, and how it started;
- the child's symptoms now, such as cough and fever, diarrhoea and vomiting, twitching, or convulsions;
- the child's previous weights, and previous illnesses, if known. Ask to see her growth chart, or any other medical records that may show her weights, and any illnesses that she has had. This gives you very important information, and may save you from asking a lot of questions;
- which immunizations the child has had;
- what food the child eats—breast milk, artificial milk, weaning foods, or family foods. It may also help to ask *exactly* what she ate *yesterday*.
- if the family has a particular crisis at the moment, that they may need help with.

Examining the child

1. Look for signs of:
   - marasmus (Section 17.1) or kwashiorkor (Section 17.2);
   - dehydration (Section 13.4);
   - infection (see Section 17.4);
   - other nutritional disorders, such as anaemia (Section 20.4) and xerophthalmia (Box 19.1, Section 19.5);
   - any other problem, such as congenital abnormality or injury, or HIV infection.

2. Count the child's respiratory rate (for signs of pneumonia, and to help assess dehydration) and her pulse rate.

3. Check her temperature for fever or for hypothermia (hypothermia is more dangerous).

4. If you suspect hypoglycaemia, check her blood sugar (see Section 17.8).

5. Weigh the child. If she has a growth chart plot the weight on it, and compare with earlier weights. If she has no growth chart, start one for her. Notice where her present weight is compared with the reference curve. As well as a growth chart, she will also need a simpler in-patient weight chart to follow recovery in hospital (see Section 17.14).

Starting treatment

Admit the child to the ward, and start the most urgent treatment—such as rehydrating or warming her, treating hypoglycaemia, giving the first dose of antibiotics (see Section 17.8), and treating vitamin A deficiency (see Sections 17.12 and 19.8).

17.7 WHAT IT IS USEFUL TO LEARN LATER

Later, spend more time with her mother and try to find out more. Try to talk to her privately, or quietly, so that you do not embarrass her in front of others in the ward. You may need to talk to other members of the family, as well as the mother, to learn some things. Remember that you are trying to understand the family's situation in order to help them. You are not 'finding out' what they have 'done wrong' in order to 'tell them what they ought to do'!

- Ask in a sensitive, sympathetic way. Be careful not to sound critical. For example, ask: 'How many times each day do you usually feed Lucy?' and *not*: 'Do you only feed her once a day?'

- Try to ask questions that need a complete answer, to encourage the family to talk. Try not to suggest answers, or to ask questions to which they can just answer 'yes' or 'no'—this does not help you or the family. For example, ask: 'Tell me how you make porridge for Lucy.' and *not*: 'Do you mix beans in her porridge?'

About the child

These are things that may help you to treat the child and understand the reasons for her malnutrition.

- Has she had any serious infections such as measles or whooping cough, diarrhoea, pneumonia, or ear infections? When were these illnesses? Does she have any chronic or recurring problems—such as chronic cough or chronic discharging ear?

- Is she at risk from AIDS? If so, you may wish to counsel the family, and test the mother's blood.

- Does she have any congenital problem—such as a heart problem, deafness, or mental handicap? Or any disability, such as paralysis or blindness?

- How much did she weigh at birth? Were there any problems with the birth?

- Is or was she breastfed, exclusively, partially, or not at all? How much time is the mother away from the baby during the day? Does the mother breastfeed at night? When did breastfeeding stop and why?

- When did the child start any other feeds, such as milk or formula, and why? What kind of other feed does she have? How often does she have it, how much each time, and how is it given (by cup, or from a feeding bottle)?

- When did the child start other foods, such as weaning and family foods? What did she normally eat during a day before the illness began? What is she eating now?

It may help to ask about a child's meals on a day when she was well, and again when she is ill.

About the family

These are things that enable you to learn about the family's resources and to help the family care for the child at home after she recovers.

- Where do they live?

- Who lives with the child, and who cares for her? If the child is not with her parents, why is this so? Is she left with a brother or sister when her mother is working?

- How do the family earn their living? Does the family earn enough to buy food and essentials for all the family? If not, how much money is available? (This is sensitive information—many families are unwilling to talk about it, but it can help you to advise them about budgeting. They may tell you more later, or you may have to guess.)

  Try to decide if the family is very poor, and if other people in the family are undernourished. The appearance of the family may help—are their clothes very

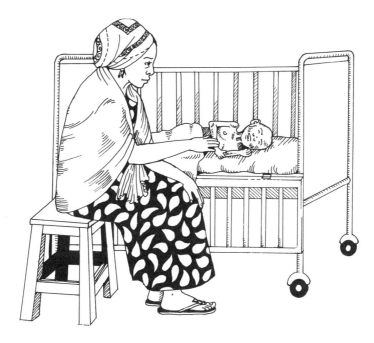

Fig. 17–4 A severely malnourished child usually needs in-patient treatment.

poor? Are they very thin? The size and type of the house may also indicate if the family are poor.

- Do the family have any land on which they grow food? What do they grow?

- Do the mother or father or other carers have any special problems such as chronic sickness, disability, mental illness, or alcoholism? Or special social problems such as unemployment, homelessness, or imprisonment?

- How many other children are there in the family? What were the intervals between their births? Are any of them sick? Have any died? Why did they die?

- Is the mother pregnant again now? This may be obvious from the mother's appearance or she may tell you as part of the answer to other questions—for example, about why the child stopped breastfeeding. She may be shy about it if it is early in the pregnancy and she is not sure, so ask tactfully.

- Has there been any traumatic event in the family recently—such as the death of a parent, or a change of the child's carer or home?

- Does the family have problems with hygiene? For example, can they get plenty of clean water? Do they have a toilet? Do they have to share with other families? The appearance of the family may tell you something about the hygiene in the home, and if they are able to prepare clean safe meals.

When you understand the family and their situation, you will be in a better position to try to help them to find ways to care for the child better.

Families of severely undernourished children are often in a serious crisis. To help the child, you need to help the whole family. You may need to ask social workers or community leaders to help the family.

17.8 MEDICAL TREATMENT

Dehydration

- Rehydrate the child with oral rehydration solution (ORS) (see Box 13.3). Do not give intravenous fluids unless she is in shock.

For severely malnourished children, the sodium in standard ORS is often too concentrated. A more dilute solution is better.

- If you are making ORS from packets, add 50 per cent more water. For example, instead of adding 1 litre of water to a packet of salts, add 1.5 litres.

- If you are making your own oral rehydration solution, use 1.8 g sodium chloride per litre, instead of 3.5 g.

In the first 4–6 hours:

- Give 50–100 ml ORS per kg body weight. Then reassess.

If the child is still dehydrated:

- Continue at this rate for a further 4–6 hours.

If she continues to have much watery diarrhoea, and she is at risk of dehydration:

- Continue to give 100 ml/kg body weight per day to keep the child hydrated, in addition to milk feeds.
- Continue breastfeeding throughout.
- Record the child's breathing and pulse rates, and how often she passes urine. Try to estimate the losses from diarrhoea and vomiting. This will help you to assess how much ORS to give.

Signs of too much fluid are:

- breathing becoming faster;
- pulse rate becoming faster;
- puffy eyes.

Signs of too little fluid are:

- passing little urine;
- breathing and pulse becoming faster;
- loss of body weight.

(Fast breathing may also be a sign of pneumonia.)

- As soon as the child is rehydrated (Box 13.1) start milk feeds (see Section 17.10). This should be done within 24 hours of admission.

Infections

Treat all severely malnourished children with antibiotics. They may have a serious infection even if they have no fever.

- If you know or suspect the cause of infection, give the appropriate antibiotic, in the standard therapeutic dose.
- If there are no clear signs of infection, give:

  1. **Benzylpenicillin** by intramuscular (i.m.) injection: 50 000 units per kg body weight/day divided into four 6-hourly doses, for 5–10 days. So give child aged 0–2 months, or <5 kg weight, 200 000 units/day;
  aged 2–11 months, or 6–9 kg, 400 000 units/day;
  aged 12 months to 5 years, or 10–19 kg, 800 000 units/day;

  and

  2. **Gentamycin**: 5 mg/kg/day (2.5 mg/kg/dose twice daily) by intramuscular injection for 5–10 days (for a child with low urine output, reduce the dose by half).

If gentamycin is not available alternatives are:

- **ampicillin**, 125 mg or 250 mg per dose four times daily orally or 12.5 mg/kg per dose four times daily i.m. or intravenously (i.v.) for 5–10 days.
- **amoxycillin**, 62.5 mg or 125 mg per dose three times daily orally or 15 mg/kg per dose three times daily i.m. or i.v. for 5–10 days;
- **chloramphenicol**, 25 mg/kg per dose four times daily (half the dose in very young infants) for 5–10 days;

and (especially if you suspect bacterial overgrowth, e.g. if diarrhoea is persistent or chronic; the abdomen is swollen with gas; weight gain is unsatisfactory despite feeding)

3. **Metronidazole**: 100–200 mg per dose two times daily for 5–10 days. If necessary, repeat the course. The dose can be given intravenously if the child is severely ill or vomiting the oral dose;

and

4. Specific treatment for tuberculosis (if TB suspected);

5. Specific treatment for malaria (if malaria common in the area);

and (if you suspect intestinal helminths)

6. **Mebendazole** 100 mg twice daily for 3 days.

Body temperature

Hypothermia

If a child develops hypothermia (body temperature below 35.5 °C—see Section 17.4):

- Make sure that treatment with antibiotics for infections is adequate.
- Feed her frequently day *and* night.
- Keep her warm.

How to keep a malnourished child warm:

- Dress her in warm clothes, including a cover for her head.
- Cover her with a blanket when she is in bed.
- Let her sleep with her mother. The mother's warm body keeps the child warm.
- Keep her away from cold air—for example, do not keep her near an open window or door.

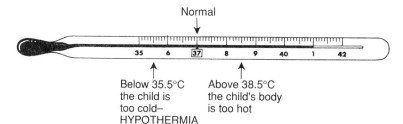

Normal

Below 35.5°C
the child is
too cold–
HYPOTHERMIA

Above 38.5°C
the child's body
is too hot

Fig. 17–5 A thermometer showing
dangerous body temperatures.

- Warm the room if necessary.
- Measure the child's temperature regularly (every 6 hours) (if possible with a thermometer which records low temperatures).
- If the methods described above are impossible or not effective, it may be necessary to put bottles of warm water in the bed beside the child. Wrap them in cloth, and be careful that they do not touch and burn her.

Fever

The temperature of the surroundings affects malnourished children more than normal. They can also become *too hot* on a hot day or if the room is too warm, especially if they have severe skin lesions. 'Fever' may be due to simple overheating and not to infections.

If a child becomes too hot (body temperature above 38.5 °C):

- Make sure that she is treated for infection.
- Make sure that she is not overheated—if necessary, cool the room and reduce her clothing a little (but be careful not to let her become cold).

Hypoglycaemia

Low body temperature may be the only sign of hypoglycaemia. Weakness, stiffness, twitching, or convulsive movements are other signs.

If you suspect hypoglycaemia:

- Do a *Dextrostix* test to show whether the child's blood glucose is below 40 mg per cent.
- If the blood sugar is below 40 mg per cent, or if she is unconscious or convulsing, give 50 per cent dextrose solution (1 ml/kg body weight) if possible intravenously.

To prevent hypoglycaemia:

- Treat infections.
- Feed the child frequently during the day and the night.

17.9 THE PHASES OF RECOVERY

Early recovery

When a child is severely undernourished, the gut wall becomes thin and is not able to digest and absorb food normally. The tissues of her body are not able to work and to use nutrients in the normal way.

As she begins to take food and, as infections and other problems are treated, her gut wall begins to recover. As nutrients begin to reach her tissues, her cells also recover and start to work normally again. This process of *early recovery* takes time—usually 5–10 days, depending on how quickly the infections and other problems are controlled.

During this phase, you must feed the child in small amounts, frequently. If you give too much food too quickly, the nutrients may overload her gut and other tissues. Overloading can cause heart failure and other serious problems, and the child may die.

Catch-up growth

As a child's cells recover, they become able to use more nutrients to rebuild lost tissues. Her appetite increases, and the process of *'catch-up' growth* begins.

During this phase, you can give her plenty of food. You should give food with concentrated energy and nutrients.

17.10 APPROPRIATE FEEDS

The child should continue to breastfeed frequently, whenever she is willing. If breastfeeding has stopped, the mother may be willing to start again (see Section 10.15), especially if the child is still very young.

Other feeds are usually made from milk, sugar, and oil, until the child has recovered enough to start taking a more normal diet. Milk feeds should be given by cup, or cup and spoon (except when tube feeding is necessary), and never from feeding bottles.

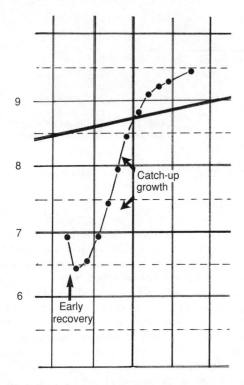

Fig. 17–6 Part of a growth chart showing the phases of recovery from severe malnutrition. This child had kwashiorkor, and lost weight during the phase of early recovery, as she lost oedema fluid. This shape in the growth line is sometimes called the '*tick sign*'.

Cleanness and safety of milk feeds

Bacteria can multiply very easily in milk feeds. Malnourished children are at great risk from infection. So it is essential that you prepare feeds very cleanly. Clean all the utensils very thoroughly in soap and hot water. Boil them if possible. Use boiled water to make up the feeds. Wash your hands well, and follow all the other rules of food hygiene in Box 7.1.

Feeds for early recovery

For early recovery the child needs:

- About 100 kcal *energy* per kg body weight per day.
- About 0.6 to 1.0 g *protein* per kg body weight per day. This small amount is enough, because the cells are working slowly.
- Additional *potassium* and *vitamins* (see Section

17.12). The cells will only begin to work properly when the micronutrient deficiencies are corrected.

- It is also helpful to give extra *magnesium* and *zinc*.

The feed must be easy to eat and to digest, and not too concentrated. You must control the volume. *Dilute milk feeds* with vitamin and mineral supplements are usually the most suitable.

How to make dilute milk feeds for early recovery

Dried skim milk (DSM)/sugar/oil mixture This mixture contains 80 kcal and 0.5 g protein per 100 ml:

DSM   15 g ⎫ made to
sugar 100 g ⎬ 1000 ml
oil   40 g ⎭ with water.

Full cream milk/sugar/oil mixtures These mixtures are suitable if DSM is not available. They contain 80 kcal and 0.5–0.7 g protein per 100 ml:

200 ml fresh full cream milk + 100 g
    sugar + 30 g oil
or 100 ml evaporated milk + 100 g
    sugar + 30 g oil
or 30 g whole milk powder + 100 g
    sugar + 30 g oil

   made up to 1000 ml with water.

Mix the sugar and the oil, and then add the milk and water.

Full cream milk/sugar mixtures These mixtures can be used if DSM and oil are not available. They contain about 75 kcal and 1.7 g protein per 100 ml, so there is more protein than is ideal.

500 ml fresh milk + 100 g sugar
or 250 ml evaporated milk + 100 g sugar
or 65 g whole milk powder + 100 g sugar

   made up to 1000 ml with water.

How much of a dilute milk feed to give (see Box 17.2)

- Give the child a total of 120 ml of feed/kg body weight/day.
- Divide the total volume into a number of small feeds.
- If the child has vomiting or diarrhoea reduce the volume and increase the frequency of feeds.

Transitional feeds

Some children do not tolerate an immediate change from dilute milk feeds to concentrated, high-energy

> **Box 17.2.** Quantities of dilute milk feeds for early recovery
>
> Give 120 ml/kg body weight per day.
> 120 ml DSM or full cream milk/sugar/oil mixtures give 100 kcal and 0.6 g protein.
> 120 ml full cream milk/sugar mixtures give 90 kcal and 2.0 g protein.
>
> Quantities to give per feed
>
> | Frequency | No. of feeds in 24 hours | Volume per feed (ml/kg body weight) |
> |---|---|---|
> | 2 hourly | 12 | 10 |
> | 3 hourly | 8 | 15 |
> | 4 hourly | 6 | 20 |
>
> **Example.** A child who weighs 8 kg needs a total of 960 ml mixture/day.
> - If given 2 hourly, the child needs 80 ml mixture per feed.
> - If given 3 hourly, the child needs 120 ml mixture per feed.
> - If given 4 hourly, the child needs 160 ml mixture per feed.

feeds. It is necessary to give *transitional feeds* for a few days.

How to make transitional feeds

1. Mix equal quantities of dilute milk feed and high-energy feed. (This saves having to make three different recipes for different children every day.)
2. Or mix *either*:
   (a) 1 litre of fresh full cream milk with 50 g sugar;
   or
   (b) 500 ml evaporated milk with 50 g sugar plus 500 ml water;
   or
   (c) 150 g whole milk powder plus 50 g sugar made up to 1 litre with water.

How much transitional feed to give

Give the child 120 ml/kg/day.

Feeds for catch-up growth

For catch-up growth, the child needs:

- a high-energy intake (150–200 kcal/kg body weight/day);
- sufficient protein (4–5 g/kg body weight/day);
- micronutrients, especially potassium, iron, zinc, and vitamins (see Section 17.12).

The feeds must be easy to eat and digest. They also need to be concentrated, to enable the child to get all that she needs in a reasonable volume. It is best to use locally available foods that are culturally acceptable.

To achieve high-energy intakes:

- Feed the child frequently, at least six times a day.
- Add oil, margarine, butter, sugar, honey.
- Use fat-rich foods such as groundnuts, avocado, undiluted buffalo milk, sheep's milk.

To achieve high-protein intakes:

- Use milk; or locally available staples mixed with legumes, meat, or fish.

What the mixture should contain

The mixture should contain 100–135 kcal and about 3.3 g protein per 100 ml. Box 17.3 gives some recipes.

How much feed to give for catch-up growth

Start with 150 ml/kg/day, and then increase the amount, (see Section 17.11).

17.11 FEEDING THE CHILD

Early recovery—dilute milk feeds

- If the child is *not dehydrated*, start dilute milk feeds immediately.

Box 17.3.   High-energy feeds

These mixtures contain about 135 kcal and 3.0–3.3 g protein/100 ml.

DSM feed

90 g dried skimmed milk ⎫ made up to
65 g sugar ⎬ 1000 ml
85 g oil ⎭ with water.

1. Mix milk powder and sugar then mix in oil.

2. Add warm (not hot) water, previously boiled, to 1 litre.

3. Mix thoroughly using a rotary egg beater or electric blender if possible.

4. Clean the beater or blender *very thoroughly* afterwards.

Fresh milk feed

900 ml warm cow's or goat's milk (previously boiled)

70 g sugar

55 g oil

Add water to make the volume up to 1000 ml if necessary. This mixture needs to be blended with an electric blender, or the oil may separate. If separation is a problem, use the cereal mixture below.

Milk/cereal feed

900 ml cow's milk

50 g sugar

50 g cereal flour

40 g oil

1. Mix the sugar, flour, and some milk to a smooth paste.

2. Add the rest of the milk, and heat over a low flame, stirring all the time. Boil for 2–3 minutes to cook the flour.

3. Remove from heat, and stir in the oil.

Add boiled water to make quantity up to 1000 ml if necessary.

Groundnut/cereal porridge

100 g cereal
100 g groundnut paste
100 g sugar

Make a thick porridge with the cereal, add the groundnuts and sugar. Use to make 1000 ml porridge.

Legume/cereal porridge

200 g cereal flour
100 g bean flour
 40 g oil
Use to make 1000 ml thick porridge.

Corn soy milk (CSM) feed

200 g CSM
 40 g sugar
 50 g oil

1. Mix CSM with cold water, add sugar and oil, stir into hot water, and boil stirring frequently for 5–10 minutes.

2. Add water to 1000 ml.

Note. The ingredients for these feeds need to be weighed on accurate scales, which can weigh to within 5 g. If your ward does not have an accurate weighing scale, find one in a laboratory, or a bigger hospital or pharmacy, and work out the number of measures, such as cups and spoons, which give the required weight of each ingredient (see Table A4.4, Appendix 4). If this is impossible, use Table A4.4 to convert weights to volume measures, but this is not very accurate. Then write out the recipe for the feed in volume measures, giving the appropriate numbers of cups, spoons, etc.

• If the child *requires rehydration*, start dilute milk feeds after 4–6 hours of ORS (or after not longer than 8–12 hours of ORS).

For very sick children, who are not able to drink, it may be necessary to give feeds by nasogastric tube.

• Use a fine tube.
• Use the tube for the shortest possible time.
• Use tube feeding only for dilute feeds during early recovery—not for high-energy feeds during catch-up growth. (This is to avoid the danger of overfeeding.)

Days 1–2

Give dilute milk feeds:

• Give 120 ml/kg body weight per 24 hours.
• Divide into 12 two-hourly feeds.

Example
A child of 7 kg needs 7 × 120 ml = 840 ml/24 hours. Give (840/12) ml = 70 ml at each feed. So give 70 ml two-hourly day and night.

Day 3

Continue to give the dilute milk feeds.

• Give 120 ml/kg body weight per 24 hours.
• If the child is feeding satisfactorily, divide into eight three-hourly feeds.

Example
Give a 7 kg child (840/8) ml = 105 ml at each feed. So give 105 ml three-hourly day and night.

Days 4–5

• If the child accepts dilute milk feeds well, start transitional milk feeds. Give 120 ml/kg body weight per 24 hours.
• If she does not, continue dilute milk feeds.

Continue to give eight three-hourly feeds per 24 hours.

Catch-up growth—high-energy feeds

From day 6

When the child takes transitional feeds well:

• Start a high-energy feed. Give 150 ml/kg body weight per 24 hours. Divide into six four-hourly feeds.

Example
A child of 7 kg needs 7 × 150 ml = 1050 ml/24 hours. Give (1050/6 ml) = 175 ml at each feed. So give 175 ml four-hourly day and night.

• Increase the volume progressively day-by-day (e.g. 170, 190, 210 ml/kg body weight per day) until the child leaves some of each feed—in other words she is having as much as she wants. Some children take 250 kcal/kg/day or more during this phase.

If the child has *mild diarrhoea* (4–5 stools per day), introduce and continue the high-energy feeds as above, provided she is not dehydrated, and is passing normal amounts of urine.

If the child develops *severe diarrhoea or vomiting*, or if she refuses feeds:

• Return to more dilute, smaller, more frequent feeds (as for Day 3).
• Examine her for signs of infection (such as ear, throat, or other respiratory infection).

Third week onwards

Continue with high-energy feeds, but it may be appropriate to give increasing amounts of family foods. You can make high-energy, high-protein foods from family foods if you add oil, legumes, etc. (see Section 17.10 and Chapter 11). Add other family foods, such as pumpkin, pawpaw, mango, and dark green leafy vegetables to provide important micronutrients, such as vitamins A and C and folate. If possible, add meat or fish to provide micronutrients such as iron and zinc.

The child need not stay in hospital during the whole catch-up phase. The family can take the child to a *Nutrition Rehabilitation Unit* (NRU), either as an in-patient or as a daily out-patient. It may be possible for them to take the child to a normal health centre every day.

The arrangement depends on the facilities available, and how far away the family live. It also depends on the child's condition. It is usually safe for the child to go home if:

• She is eating well and gaining weight.
• Infections are controlled.
• The family has the resources and information needed to continue to give her high-energy feeds.
• There is someone at home who can care for her full time and bring her to the NRU or health centre every day.

Return to good family diet

When the child has a normal weight-for-height (see Section 17.14, and Appendix 5 Tables A5.4 and A5.5) she does not need special high-energy foods. She can

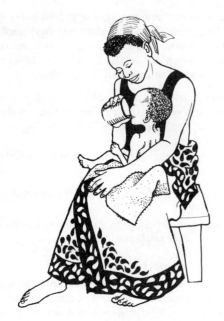

Fig. 17–7 Feed malnourished children often.

now have good mixed meals and snacks (see Chapter 11). Breastfeeding also should continue until she is at least 2 years old.

17.12 MICRONUTRIENTS

In the early recovery phase children need vitamins and minerals (especially vitamin A, folate, potassium, zinc).

- to help tissues heal;
- to destroy free radicals;
- to restore appetite.

During catch-up growth, a child's requirements for micronutrients increase, because of the rapid growth of new tissues. As growth increases, a child may suddenly show signs of severe deficiency—for example of vitamin A.

So give vitamin and mineral supplements during both early recovery and catch-up growth. Give iron, however, only during the catch-up phase.

If suitable preparations of micronutrients are not available, micronutrients must come from food.

Vitamin A

Give *all* children one dose of vitamin A by mouth, either as a capsule, or as oil, at the start of treatment:

- children aged 12 months or more: 200 000 IU vitamin A;
- children aged less than 12 months: 100 000 IU vitamin A.

Give children with signs of vitamin A deficiency or measles:

- A second dose the following day, and a third dose after 4 weeks (see Box 19.4). Give a further dose after 6 months.

Treat any sign of a corneal lesion immediately (see Section 19.8).

Folate

Anaemia is often due to folate deficiency. Give 5 mg (1 tablet) folate daily until the child is eating home food and is no longer anaemic.

Multivitamins

If a multivitamin preparation is available, give that in the recommended dose. However, these preparations may not contain enough folate or vitamin A.

Iron

Malnourished children are often deficient in iron. However, iron increases free radicals, and can make infections worse.

So do NOT give iron during early recovery.

During catch-up growth, give ferrous sulphate (in a dose of 2–4 mg iron/kg/day) and continue for 3 months.

Potassium

All children with severe malnutrition are deficient in potassium and need potassium supplements.

Prepare a solution with 7.5 g potassium chloride in 100 ml boiled water. Give the child 2–4 ml of the solution per kg body weight per day for 2 weeks, added to milk feeds. Start to give the solution as soon as she has passed a normal amount of urine.*

---

* If available, give the following also:

- magnesium (12 mg/kg/day) as chloride (48 mg/kg/day) or acetate (71 mg/kg/day). To 1 litre of water add 48 g magnesium chloride or 71 g magnesium acetate and give 1 ml/kg/day in divided doses with meals.
- zinc (2 mg/kg/day) as zinc acetate (5 mg/kg/day). (Zinc acetate is preferable to zinc sulphate, 5 mg/kg/day.)
- copper (0.2 mg/kg/day) as acetate (0.6 mg/kg/day), chloride (0.4 mg/kg/day), or sulphate (0.7 mg/kg/day).

17.13 CHOICE OF DIETARY TREATMENT

There are two main choices for dietary treatment of severely malnourished children after the early recovery phase. Which you choose depends on where you work and what foods are available. You can:

1. Give high-energy milk feeds until the child reaches her normal weight-for-height, and then start on family foods. With this diet, most children regain their lost weight in about 4–6 weeks.

2. Start earlier on family foods, but enrich them so that the child gets enough energy and nutrients for catch-up growth (see Box 17.3). With this diet, the family can learn about better feeding. How fast the child grows depends on whether the family foods can be enriched adequately.

Using family foods may enable a child to be treated at an earlier stage at home, or as an out-patient, or in a nutrition rehabilitation centre. This is helpful if the family or hospital can only manage in-patient treatment for the early recovery phase.

17.14 MONITORING RECOVERY

With adequate treatment, even severely malnourished children usually recover enough to go home in 8–10 weeks.

To treat a child successfully, it is necessary to monitor her progress. You need to measure and record:

1. On admission:
   - weight;
   - length or height (if you are measuring the child's weight-for-height);
   - arm circumference (this helps with follow up—see Section 17.18).

2. Every day:
   - the amount, frequency, and type of food the child eats. This will tell you if she has a good appetite, and if she is getting enough nutrients and fluids (see Fig. 17–9).

3. Daily or at least three times a week,
   - weight:
     - to notice when oedema has gone and 'catch-up' growth begins;
     - to prescribe treatment according to the most recent weight (antibiotics, other medication, feeds, supplements);
     - to decide when to discharge the child.

Plot the weight on a chart for daily weights. Figure 17–8 shows an example. However, if you do not have printed charts, you can make your own out of any squared paper. You can draw a chart and photocopy it, or draw one on a stencil for duplication, or you can adapt temperature charts.

Weight changes during recovery

Overall, whatever her weight on admission, a child should gain about 2–3 kg in 8–10 weeks.

Early recovery (5–10 days)

When a child is still taking milk feeds, weight gain is usually slow. A child with oedema should *lose* weight at first, as she loses the oedema fluid (see Figs 17–6 and 17–8). But her appetite, mental state, and general condition should improve.

'Catch-up' growth

When she is taking high-energy feeds, weight gain is much faster. A child can gain as much as 10–20 g a day for each kilo of body weight during this phase of treatment, if she takes enough energy and nutrients. She may gain about 50–100 g each day, or 350–700 g a week for about 1 month. Marasmic children in particular should gain weight very rapidly if they are given enough energy and nutrients.

Return to normal rate of growth

When the child has regained lost weight, and returned to a normal weight-for-height, her weight gain slows down. She should now be eating family foods, and should continue to grow, but at a normal rate.

Deciding if the child has gained enough weight

- If you are able to measure the child's weight-for-height, then she should achieve a weight-for-height within the normal range, that is, above the 3rd centile, (see Appendix 5 Tables A5.4 and A5.5) or, better, above 90 per cent of reference (see Section 14.17).

- If you can only measure weight, look for the rapid 'catch-up' increase in weight, followed by normal growth. Her growth line should *move towards* the normal range. However, if she is already stunted, her growth line may not rise above the 3rd centile weight-for-age curve. She may remain underweight, even though she is receiving adequate treatment, and has a normal weight-for-height.

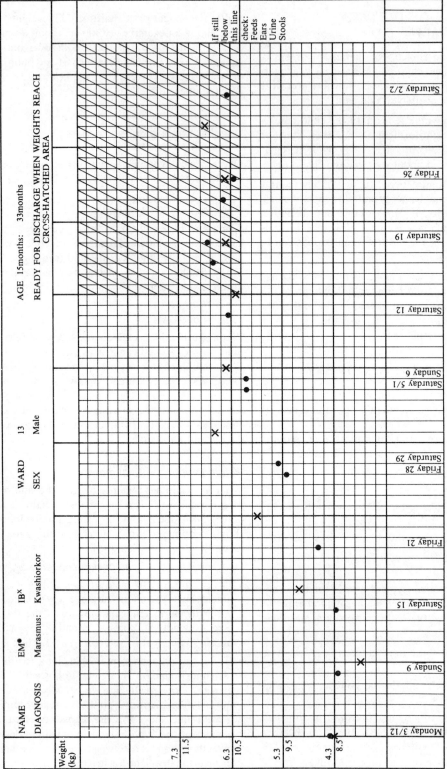

Fig. 17–8 Example of a weight chart used to monitor recovery of malnourished children in hospital. The weights of two children are shown, one with marasmus (shown by the dots) and one with kwashiorkor (shown by the crosses). There is a scale of weights on the left. There is a separate scale for each child, starting with the child's weight on admission. This makes it possible to use the same type of chart for children of different weights and ages. For example, the child with kwashiorkor weighed 8.5 kg on admission; the child with marasmus weighed 4.3 kg on admission. Both admission weights are plotted on the same line.

Food intake chart

John			Weight on admission	5.5 kg
Day	Time	Food	Amount	Remarks
Day 1	10.0 am	Milk feed	55 mL	—
"	12.0 n	Milk feed	55 mL	—
"	2.0 pm	Milk feed	55 mL	Passed urine
"	4.0 pm	Milk feed	55 mL	—
"	6.0 pm	Milk feed	55 mL	small vomit
"	8.0 pm	Milk feed	55 mL	—
"	10.0 pm	Milk feed	55 mL	loose stool
"	12 mn	Milk feed	55 mL	Passed urine
Day 2	2.0 am	Milk feed	55 mL	small vomit
"	4.0 am	Milk feed	55 mL	—
"	6.0 am	Milk feed	55 mL	loose stool
"	8.0 am	Milk feed	55 mL	Passed urine
"	10.0 am	Milk feed	55 mL	+22 mL KCl
"	12 noon	Milk feed	55 mL	Passed urine
"	2.0 pm	Milk feed	55 mL	—

Fig. 17–9 Part of a chart showing a record of a child's intake of milk feed.

Failure to respond to treatment

If a child fails to gain weight satisfactorily:

- Check that her weight has been measured and recorded properly.
- Make sure that the feed is being made up correctly.
- Make sure that she is being offered enough feed during both day and night.
- Make sure that she is taking enough of the feed.
- Make sure that she is getting vitamin and mineral supplements.

If the child has a poor appetite, or fails to gain weight on an adequate diet:

- Make sure that recommended treatment has been given.
- Look for an infection, such as TB, ear infection, or urinary infection, parasitic infection, or malaria, which was not found before.
- Look for another problem, such as a heart problem or AIDS.

A child who is unable to take enough feed may somtimes need to be tube fed. Give the same volumes of feed, at the same times, but by nasogastric tube.

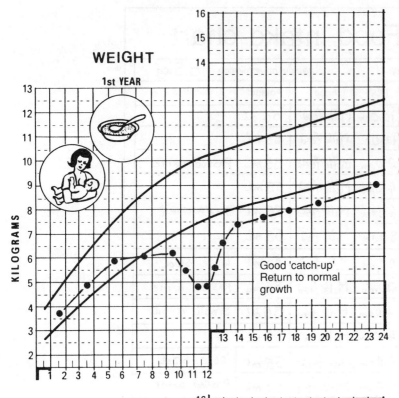

Fig. 17–10 Growth line of a child recovering from severe malnutrition. Good 'catch-up' and return to normal growth, although growth line continues below the 3rd centile curve.

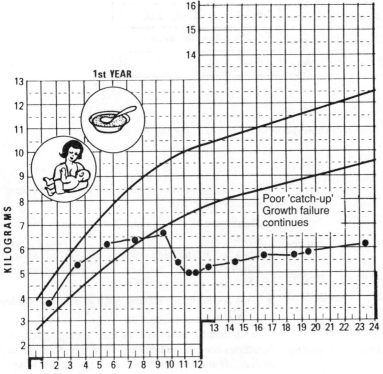

Fig. 17–11 Growth line of a child after severe malnutrition. Poor 'catch-up', and growth continues poor. This child has not recovered, and continues to be at risk.

17.15 SOCIAL AND EMOTIONAL CARE

Comfort and affection for the child

The child needs affection from family members and health workers. The child's mother or another close relative should stay with the child to help take care of her. The mother holds, comforts, and talks to the child, and keeps her warm, clean, and dry. The mother helps to feed the child; and learns how to look after her and feed her when she goes home.

Mental stimulation

When the child begins to recover, she needs mental stimulation with games, toys, and stories appropriate to her age and home background.

Health workers should help families to find ways to play with and talk to children to stimulate them. Try to arrange for some play activity at some time every day, for example, in the afternoon, when the ward is less busy. If there are any older children in the hospital, they may like to help to play with the younger children, or to make toys out of local or waste materials for them.

Support and sympathy for the family

- Be friendly towards the mother or other relative who cares for the child, and make her feel welcome.
- Be polite and respectful to the family, even though they may be poor and in a difficult situation.
- Show the mother how to care for the child, and make her feel an essential person in the child's recovery.
  - When she does something well (for example, she gets the child to take some food), praise and encourage her.
  - If she is having difficulties (for example, if the child is not willing to eat much), encourage her to go on trying.
- Spend time talking with her, asking about the family's situation. Take an interest and listen to what she says. You need to learn why the family thinks the child became ill and to understand their situation.
- Show sympathy to the mother and family. Families of undernourished children are often poor and they often have other problems also. For example, the child's parents may be separated. A mother or father or grandparent may be alone, caring for several children and also trying to earn money to feed them.

Show that you understand the family's problems, and that you are concerned and want to help.
- Be careful not to make the family feel guilty, or that you blame them for the child's illness. If families feel that health workers blame them, they may be afraid to bring their children for help. They may be unwilling to talk about their problems or to co-operate with the treatment.

Help with social problems

Families of malnourished children often have social problems. Sometimes there is nothing that you can do about these problems, but if you listen and sympathize that can help.

Sometimes you may be able to arrange for the family to get some practical help, for example, from social services, or from a voluntary agency or religious organization, or from a feeding programme. Sometimes community leaders or a village health committee might be able to help a family to get some sort of social support.

Before you talk to the family about feeding the child, try to find out if there is someone who could help with their problems. Try to learn who in your area can give any help, so that you know what might be available.

17.16 HELPING MOTHERS TO LEARN IN HOSPITAL

Undernutrition is often due to poverty. But it can help if the family learns how to feed the child better with the food that they have. So an important part of the care of malnourished children is education of the family. Families need to understand how to feed the malnourished child when she goes home, and how to feed and care for other children, especially younger children, to prevent malnutrition.

Plan how you will help mothers in hospital to learn any new skills that they may need, and how you can make the learning interesting. Think about how to reach the rest of the family, to encourage them to support the mother when she is at home.

Caring for the child

One way for a mother (or other relative) to learn, is to care for the child herself and to watch the child recover. Show mothers everything you do for their child, and explain why it is necessary. Let them do as much as

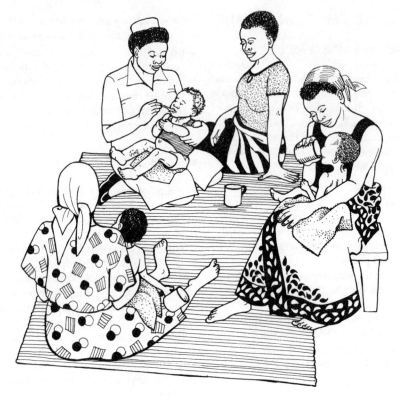

Fig. 17–12 Encourage and help mothers to care for their children in hospital.

possible themselves. Show them how to do it, and supervise them while they learn.

All mothers should be able to give children feeds from spoons and cups. They may be able to help with:

- the preparation of feeds;
- measuring feeds;
- giving tube feeds;
- weighing children;
- filling in weight charts;
- keeping the child clean and warm;
- stimulating and playing with the child.

Learning from each other

Mothers in hospital learn from each other. Encourage mothers who have been in the ward for some days to show others how to feed children or how to measure feeds. They may help each other to understand how feeding helps a child to recover.

You need to make sure that what mothers tell each other is accurate. But you may learn some practical tips about feeding children from their experience.

Other useful ways for mothers to learn

When their children are beginning to recover, you may find these ways of helping their mothers to learn useful:

- group discussions and role play;
- preparing songs and dances;
- demonstrations.

These are all described in more detail in Chapter 28.

Group discussions

You can arrange for mothers to have discussions in small groups of four to eight, using a *starter*, such as a *role play*. You can also have very informal discussions, for example, when a few mothers are sitting together in the ward. You can ask one of them how her child is getting on, and ask her to talk to the other mothers about the child's treatment. Encourage mothers to discuss what they have noticed and how they feel. This can lead to a discussion about feeding children to prevent undernutrition.

Songs and dances

Help mothers to make up songs and dances about

nutrition problems and how to overcome them. They can then sing the songs to other mothers in the ward, or to other family members, or they can just sing them together. It is important to get songs with a useful message.

Demonstrations

Food and cooking demonstrations may be helpful for mothers when their children start to eat family food. Let mothers who have been in the ward longest and whose children are recovering demonstrate to mothers who have not been in the ward so long.

17.17 TALKING TO OTHER MEMBERS OF THE FAMILY

When a mother goes home she will need the support of other members of the family to care for her child. When you talk to the mother, try to learn whose support is most important. The child's father? The grandmother? An aunt?

Try to talk to someone else in the family, and make sure that they know what you discussed with the mother in hospital. Then they can support her if other family members are not helpful. Talk to the family when they come to visit. Or ask the mother to ask other members of the family to come and see you.

Another possibility is to take the mother home and talk to the family there. You can also talk to neighbours about how they might be able to help.

17.18 FOLLOW UP—CONTINUING CARE AT HOME

When a child leaves the ward, arrange for her and her family to be followed up, and for care to continue. Follow up may be by a community health worker, or at a health centre near where the family live. The child may return to the ward for one or more visits.

Make sure that the child is fully immunized. Encourage the family to make use of family planning and other services.

1. Keep a record of the child's name, number, and other essential details on a follow-up register in the ward or clinic, so that you know if she has been followed or not.

2. Make sure that the family has a growth chart for the child, and make sure that the family understand the purpose of the growth chart.

3. Fill in as much information as possible including:
   - the child's weights before the illness, if known;
   - her lowest weight during the illness;
   - the weight on discharge;
   - any infections and their treatment;
   - the child's immunization status;
   - what you discussed with the mother for the child's management at home.

4. Make sure that there is enough information on the card to enable another health or nutrition worker to understand the family's situation, without asking all the same questions again.

5. Give the family a date to come back, and write it on the growth chart or record card. The first few visits probably need to be every week. When the child is progressing well, visits can be less often, for example every month.

6. Explain to the mother that she can come back before the appointment if the child is not well. Try to make her feel that you would welcome her if she came back, and not blame her if the child becomes ill again.

7. If possible, visit the family at home, or ask a colleague who works in the community to visit. Even one or two home visits are helpful. It helps you to understand the family and their situation, and why the child became undernourished. This makes it easier to help them care for her. If you take the family home when they are discharged, make sure that their address and directions about how to get there are written in the follow-up register, so that you know how to get there again.

8. If a child fails to come to the clinic or hospital for follow up, you should record this in the follow-up register. Try to visit this family to find out what has happened.

17.19 WHAT TO DO ON A FOLLOW-UP VISIT

Often you will follow a family up in a health centre or hospital. Sometimes you will visit them at home. How to visit a family at home is described in Section 27.2.

If you do a home visit, you will learn more about the family. You will have to carry scales to weigh the child, or an arm circumference tape. (It helps therefore if the child's arm circumference was also measured in hospital.)

Many of the steps are similar wherever you do the follow up:

1. Greet the mother and ask her how she and the child are getting on. Ask her how she feels she is doing.

2. Listen to what she has to say;
   - about the child (is she better? active? playing? eating well?);
   - about other problems.

3. Ask the mother if she is managing to do what you discussed with her before; ask what problems she has doing those things.

4. Notice the child's behaviour and general appearance.

5. Weigh the child, and plot the weight on her growth chart. You can then see if she is gaining weight and growing again.

6. If the child is gaining weight well then, whatever the mother is feeding her, it must be enough.
   - Praise the mother, and encourage her to continue.
   - Let her tell you what she is doing—it may help you to help another family.

7. If the child is not gaining weight well, try to find out why. Help the family to do something about it before the child becomes seriously ill again.
   - Examine the child for signs of infection. If she has an infection, arrange treatment.
   - Discuss again with the family how they are feeding her. Try to find out if they are having any difficulties, and help them to find a way to overcome the difficulties.
   - Try to find out if the child is being abused or neglected. If so, arrange for a welfare worker to visit.

8. Discuss again some of the ideas that the mother has learnt, and reinforce them.

9. Give any other kind of health care that may be appropriate, such as:
   - immunization for the child;
   - treatment for worms;
   - antenatal care for the mother;
   - family planning for the parents.

10. If the child is losing weight, and is not able to eat enough, consider readmitting her to hospital.

THINGS TO DO

Role play

Ask trainees to role play talking to a family of a malnourished child.

1. Role play admitting the child to hospital, and asking the questions which give the information that you need to start treatment.

2. Role play talking to the family after a few days, to learn more about the child and the family.

3. Role play discussing with the parents how to feed the child.

Demonstrations

4. Demonstrate how to keep a child at the right temperature.

5. Demonstrate how to prepare feeds for severely malnourished children (for early recovery and catch-up growth). Ask trainees to work out how much to give to children of different weights and how frequently to feed them.

Practical exercises

6. Ask trainees to plan (and, if possible, cook) suitable high-energy feeds for undernourished children from locally available foods.
   For example, you can make 1000 ml of food which gives 1350 kcal and at least 30 g protein with:
   (a) 150 g maize flour and 150 g pounded ground-nuts; *or*
   (b) 150 g cassava flour, 100 g soybean paste, and 50 g oil; *or*
   (c) 100 g rice, 100 g beans, 2 (80 g) eggs, and 70 g margarine.

7. Ask trainees to think of toys using local or waste materials that they could make for children in hospital. They could collect the necessary materials, and demonstrate the toys to each other.

8. Ask trainees to write a song for in-patients, explaining how to feed children when they go home.

Field visit

9. Take trainees to a hospital which cares for severely malnourished children. Ask them to:
   a. Talk to staff who care for the children, and ask how they treat them.

b. Ask about the difficulties of caring for these children.

c. Watch staff preparing feeds. Discuss the recipe, and the reasons for it. Notice how good their hygiene is.

d. Ask some mothers about their child's illnesses, how the child is being treated, and if she is getting better.

e. Ask them if the child is hungry or unwilling to eat, and how they manage to feed the child.

f. Ask to see how they monitor children's recovery and weight gain.

g. Discuss with the mothers why they think that their children became ill.

h. If there is an opportunity, practise feeding an anorexic child.

Discuss the observations in class.

10. Arrange for one or two trainees to escort a child home from hospital, or from a health centre, or to go on a 'follow-up visit'. (This is easiest if the family do not live too far away.)

Ask them to visit the family as far as possible in the way described in Sections 17.19 and 27.2. They can report their visit to the class, and discuss what they found and how they would plan to help the family.

11. Discuss who in your area or community may be able to give help to families with social problems. Trainees could visit possible sources of help, and ask what they might do for undernourished families.

USEFUL PUBLICATION

WHO (1981). *Treatment and management of severe protein–energy malnutrition*. WHO, Geneva.

18　Undernutrition in women

18.1 THE STORIES OF TWO WOMEN

The story of Mari

Figure 18–1 shows a picture of Mari, who is 27 years old. She has two children, a boy of 6 years and a girl of 3 years. Soon she will have her third baby.

The family have a small farm. Mari works on the farm in the morning and then she works around her house in the afternoon. Sometimes she goes to meetings of the women's organization, and she is learning dressmaking. Sometimes she visits friends. Mari went to the antenatal clinic today. She weighed 70 kg. At the beginning of this pregnancy she weighed 60 kg. She eats three meals a day—porridge and milk in the morning, maize and vegetables at midday, and maize with beans or sometimes meat in the evening. She eats about 2400 kcal a day. She breastfeeds all her babies for 2 years.

The story of Lila

Figure 18–2 shows a picture of Lila. She, too, is 27 years old, and breastfeeds her babies. This is her fifth pregnancy. Her first born is a boy, who is now 7 years old. The next baby, born 20 months later, was very small and died soon after birth. Then came a girl who is nearly 4 years old. She was LBW too, but she did not die. Then Lila had a boy who is now 21 months old. He is underweight and often sick.

Lila works hard on a farm 3 miles from her home for a small wage. She finds the work very tiring, especially when she is pregnant. When she gets back to her house, she is too tired to do anything but cook the family's meal.

Lila is very thin—much thinner than when she married. Then she weighed about 60 kg. But after the last baby was born, she weighed only 45 kg. Now, at the end of pregnancy, she weighs only 49 kg. She has tea for breakfast. At midday, she may eat a left-over snack if there is something, but often she eats nothing. In the evening, the family eats maize or cassava and some green vegetables. They cannot afford meat or even beans. Lila usually eats about 1800 Cal a day. She has eaten less for the last 2 months, because she is frightened of having a difficult delivery.

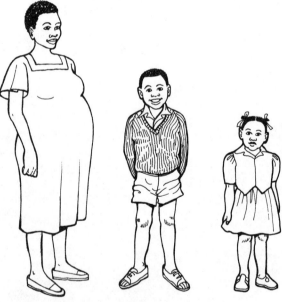

Fig. 18–1 Mari and her children.

Compare the stories of Mari and Lila. Mari has enough to eat, but Lila does not. The story of Lila shows some of the problems of undernutrition in women.

- Lila is very tired, and she finds it difficult to work.
- Lila has no energy to do extra things like going to the women's organization meetings.
- Apart from her first baby, all her babies have been small or undernourished, and one died.
- She has gained very little weight during this pregnancy—and she is getting thinner with each baby.

Many women have the same problems that Lila has. Even many women who are not pregnant are undernourished.

18.2 HOW WOMEN BECOME UNDERNOURISHED

They may have been undernourished in childhood

Many undernourished women have been under-

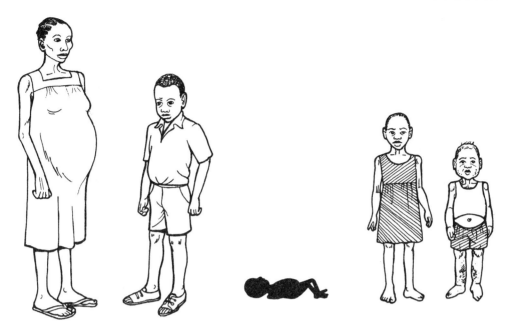

Fig. 18–2 Lila and her children.

nourished all their lives. Girls who were LBW babies, or who were undernourished in the first 3 years of life may be stunted, and grow up into short women.

They may not eat enough food to cover their energy needs

If the family is poor, all family members may lack food. The most serious problem may be lack of energy. In some communities, it is the custom for men to have the largest share. A woman may not get a fair share of the food.

They may have a heavy physical workload

Women may spend many hours in physical labour every day. They may spend more hours working each day than men. So they need a lot of energy. If they use more energy working than they get in their food, they lose weight and become undernourished.

Women farmers have to work harder at certain times, for example, when planting and harvesting. These may also be times when there is less food available, and women may lose weight. If men are away and not available to help, women may have very heavy workloads.

Women become more tired when they are pregnant, and they reduce their physical activity if they can. But many women have to continue with the same workload during both pregnancy and breastfeeding. We do not

yet know exactly what effect this has, but, if women are not eating enough, hard physical work must make them more undernourished.

Lila does not eat enough Calories. Lila works hard and she is pregnant, so she needs about 2500 kcal per day (see Section 2.11 and Appendix 2). However, she is getting less than 1800 kcal per day. This lack of energy makes her feel tired. She finds it difficult to work hard, and she is not able to do anything extra.

They may not eat enough different sorts of food

If a woman does not eat enough different foods, she may lack certain important nutrients, such as vitamins and minerals. For example, women may lack the iron or folate that they need to prevent *anaemia* (see Chapter 20). Anaemia is the commonest kind of undernutrition in women. Lila's tiredness may be partly due to anaemia.

They may not get extra food when they are pregnant

Pregnant women need extra energy and nutrients (see Table 18.1, and Sections 2.11 and 3.5). Women who do not get the extra food that they need may become undernourished during pregnancy.

Women who are poor may be undernourished with poor stores of nutrients before they become pregnant. They may be unable to increase their food intake, and pregnancy makes them *more* undernourished.

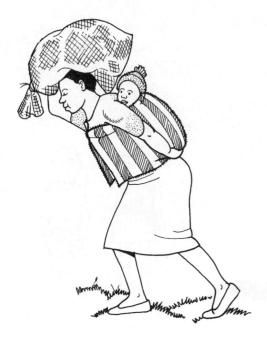

Fig. 18–3 Many women have a heavy workload.

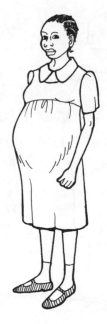

Fig. 18–4 Some girls have babies when they are very young.

They may not get extra food while they are lactating

Lactating women need extra energy and nutrients to make breast milk (see Table 18.1). A woman who does not get enough food when she is breastfeeding uses more of her own stores to make breast milk.

They may have babies when they are very young

For the first few years after the menarche (start of periods) a girl is still growing. If she becomes pregnant it may interfere with her own growth. She and the baby compete for the same food.

18.3 WEIGHT GAIN DURING PREGNANCY

Well nourished women gain on average about 10 kg during pregnancy. The 10 kg is made up *approximately* like this:

- The baby weighs about 3.0 kg.
- Increase in the size of the mother's uterus and breasts, plus increased blood and fluid in her body, plus the placenta make another 4.0 kg.
- The fat store which the mother builds up weighs about 3.0 kg. The fat is used after the baby is born to make breast milk.

During the first 6 months of pregnancy most of the extra food is needed to build up the mother's tissues and fat store. Only a small amount is needed for the growing fetus.

During the last 3 months of pregnancy more of the extra food is needed for the growing baby, and to build up the baby's stores of fat, iron, and vitamin A.

Table 18.1. Change in daily nutrient needs during pregnancy and lactation (see Appendix 2)

	Pregnancy	Lactation
Energy (kcal)		
Well nourished, moderate activity	+100	
Well nourished, heavy activity	+200	+500
Undernourished, moderate/heavy activity	+285	
Protein (g)	+7	+20
Iron (mg)	+ at least 28	−22*
Vitamin A (RE)	+100	+350
Folate (µg)	+230	+100
Vitamin C (mg)	+20	+20

* While not menstruating.

18.4 HOW UNDERNUTRITION AFFECTS PREGNANCY AND CHILDBIRTH

Effects on the woman

Women who are very short (less than 151 cm high) because of stunting in childhood are more likely to have difficult births. Women who had vitamin D deficiency while they were growing may have deformed pelvic bones which make childbirth difficult.

If a woman does not eat enough, she cannot build up stores of fat and other nutrients. She uses her own muscles and other tissues to provide the energy, protein, fat, vitamin A, iron, and other nutrients for the baby's growth. Instead of gaining 10 kg during pregnancy, she may gain only 6 kg or less, like Lila. Some undernourished women may not gain any weight at all during pregnancy. Some weigh less after the baby is born than before they were pregnant. After each pregnancy, they weigh less and look thinner.

Effects on the baby

Women who are stunted or undernourished before or during pregnancy have smaller babies. Their babies are more likely to be low birth weight (see Section 16.6), especially if the mother gains less than 6 kg during pregnancy. In some communities, it is customary to eat less during the last 3 months of pregnancy to prevent the baby from becoming too large and making the birth more difficult.

A girl who becomes pregnant within 2 years of her menarche is twice as likely to have a low birth weight baby as an older girl.

If a woman is deficient in iodine at around the time of conception, her baby is more likely to have a congenital abnormality (see Chapter 21).

Effects of giving a pregnant woman extra nutrients

When undernourished women are given extra food during pregnancy:

- They gain more weight.
- The birth weights of their babies increase.

The gain is greatest with very thin undernourished women. If women are well nourished, extra food may not increase the weights of their babies.

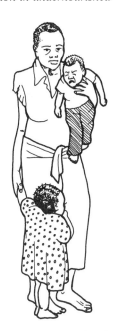

Fig. 18–5 Undernourished women often have undernourished children.

Eating well should not make the baby too large to deliver, if the mother herself is not too small. Very short mothers are at risk of difficulty with childbirth whatever the size of the baby.

Giving iron and folate prevents anaemia and can also increase the baby's birth weight (see Chapter 20). Giving high doses of iodine prevents iodine deficiency disorders (see Section 21.8). Pregnant women should never be given high doses of vitamin A (see Section 19.9).

18.5 LACTATION IN UNDERNOURISHED WOMEN

Effects on the mother

An undernourished woman may not have built up stores of fat and other nutrients before the baby was born. She may not be able to eat extra food when she breastfeeds. The energy and nutrients to make breast milk must come from her own body tissues. So breastfeeding can make an undernourished woman more undernourished. Her weight may fall below the weight that she was before she was pregnant.

It may take up to 6 months after stopping breastfeeding for a woman to build up her nutrient stores again.

The amount of breast milk

A *moderately undernourished* mother can produce enough breast milk for her baby, if the baby continues to suckle often. *Severely malnourished* women may produce 20–30 per cent less breast milk than well nourished women. But many continue to produce 500 ml or more a day if the baby suckles enough. Possibly, to keep up the supply, a baby needs to suckle more often if his mother is undernourished than if she is well nourished.

The nutrients in breast milk

Undernourished women produce a good-quality breast milk using nutrients from their own tissues, and from whatever food they are able to eat.

In severely malnourished women:

- The amount of fat in the breast milk may decrease, so there may be a little less energy (about 10 per cent less).
- The amount of protein remains high because it is made from the mother's own tissues. There may be a slight decrease in some of the anti-infective factors.
- Probably the amount of iron remains adequate, even if the mother is anaemic.
- A woman who has low levels of iodine in her body, may not provide enough iodine in her breast milk.
- The nutrients that are most likely to decrease are the vitamins, because they can only come from the mother's diet. Vitamin A is particularly important. A woman who is undernourished may have no stores of vitamin A in her own body and she gets very little in her food so she cannot secrete enough in her breast milk.

Effects on the baby

Babies of severely malnourished mothers are more likely to outgrow the supply of breast milk before 6 months of age. These babies' growth may slow down after 3–4 months of age, instead of after 6 months of age. Some babies may become deficient in vitamin A.

However, even when there are slightly smaller amounts of some nutrients, *breast milk is always better than any artificial food.*

Effects of food supplements on lactation

Sometimes breastfeeding women are given food supplements to increase their milk supply. But it is not yet certain that it is possible to increase a woman's breast milk this way. Supplements may increase the woman's own energy (which is, of course, good), but they may not increase her breast milk output.

It is more helpful for a woman to eat more food before and during pregnancy, so that she builds up better stores of nutrients from which to make breast milk. If a woman eats extra before the baby is born, she will have a healthier baby. She is also more likely to have enough breast milk to feed the baby exclusively for 6 months.

If food supplements are given during breastfeeding, they should certainly be given to the mother, and not to the baby. Where food supplies are limited, supplements may only be given for the first 6 months. However, if possible, they should continue for at least a year, or throughout lactation. This would help the mother to build up her nutrient stores.

18.6 WOMEN WHO HAVE TOO MANY BIRTHS TOO CLOSE TOGETHER

When babies are born close together:

- The mother's body does not have time to rebuild its store of nutrients between pregnancies.
- The mother is likely to have a large number of children.
- It is more difficult for the mother to care for the children.
- Each baby is breastfed for a shorter time.

Mothers may be pregnant or lactating all the time. If they do not eat enough, like Lila, they may lose weight and become thinner with each baby.

Babies born within 3 years of the previous baby are more likely to die than children born after more than 3 years.

18.7 THE CYCLE OF UNDERNUTRITION IN WOMEN

Girls who are undernourished may be stunted and may continue to be undernourished when they are women. They may have low stores of nutrients in their bodies before pregnancy, and they may be unable to eat well to build up stores during pregnancy. Their children are at risk of low birth weight, of lack of breast milk, and of undernutrition in childhood. Their daughters may be stunted, and may become undernourished women.

This is a *cycle of undernutrition* that occurs when girls and women are not well fed. It is important to feed girls and women well to help them break out of this cycle.

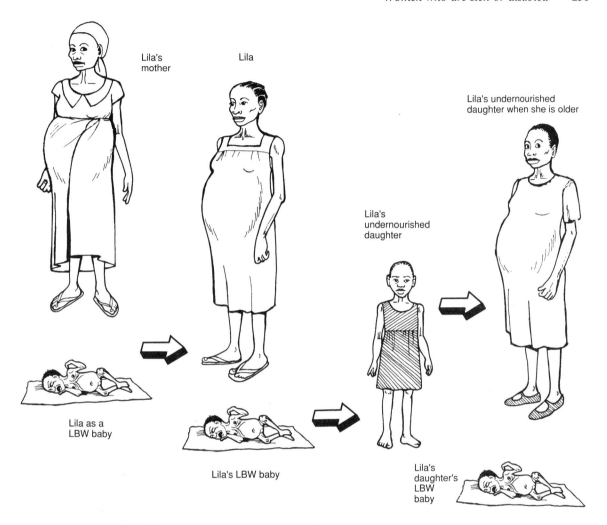

Fig. 18–6 Lila, her mother, her daughter, and her daughter's baby.

Lila's mother was undernourished, and Lila was born small. She grew up into an undernourished woman, and her daughter was LBW, and undernourished as a child. Lila's daughter is likely to grow into an undernourished woman, and to have LBW babies.

How can we stop undernourished women having undernourished babies who grow into undernourished women?

18.8 WOMEN WHO ARE SICK OR DISABLED

Infections and other illnesses

Illness and infection make it more difficult for people to work hard. They may grow less food, or earn less money to buy food. So they are poorer, and their families may be more undernourished. Worm infections are common in some areas and interfere with nutrition and ability to work (see Section 16.12).

Undernutrition makes many illnesses worse—especially infections, due to either worms or microorganisms. So this is another example of the infection/undernutrition spiral which we showed in Fig. 16–5. This spiral can interfere with the development of communities.

What you can do

Help women with worm and other infections to get treatment.

Physical and mental disability

Women who are physically or mentally disabled, or who have chronic illnesses, may have difficulty getting enough food for themselves and their families. They may have difficulty budgeting, storing, preparing, and cooking food. They may have difficulty breastfeeding or caring for their children. If they are mentally ill or have a disease like AIDS their relatives and friends may avoid them.

How you can help chronically sick and disabled women

These women and their families need special help. You may be able to get help for them from:

- their community, community groups, and community leaders;
- religious groups;
- community health workers and other workers;
- social workers;
- voluntary agencies.

18.9 HOW TO PREVENT UNDERNUTRITION IN WOMEN

Growing more food

Home economic workers and agricultural extension workers may be able to help families to produce more food, so that women can get a larger share.

Increasing income

Community development workers may be able to help women to develop income-generating projects. If women can earn money, they can feed both themselves and their families better. When women are better nourished, they have more energy and can earn more.

Reducing workloads

Appropriate technology projects can develop ways to reduce women's workloads, and hence their energy needs. For example:

- Wells which provide water nearer to homes reduce the work women have to do to fetch water.
- Improved cooking stoves may reduce the amount of fuel needed, so they can reduce the work of fetching fuel (or the cost of buying it; see Section 24.4).
- Village-based mills can reduce the work that women have to do to make flour.
- Child care centres can help to look after children so

that women do not have to carry them to their fields. Child care centres can also give women a chance to work to earn money.

Teaching schoolchildren

The school curriculum should include these topics:

- the special food needs of girls and women before and during childbearing;
- the importance of not having babies too close together, or when the mother is too young.

Education in the community

Community workers might discuss these topics with appropriate groups in the community.

- Women need to eat enough food, and enough different kinds of food *before pregnancy*, *during pregnancy*, and *during breastfeeding* for their own health, and for the health of their babies.
- A strong healthy wife is an advantage to a man—to work hard, to develop her skills, and to bear healthy children. A man can help his wife continue to be strong and healthy, if he helps her to have enough food to eat, and not too much work.
- If children are born too close together, the woman and the baby may both be weak.

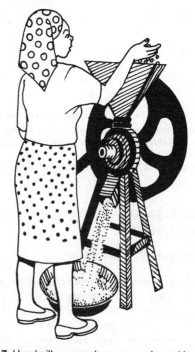

Fig. 18–7 Handmills can reduce women's workloads.

18.10 HOW COMMUNITY HEALTH WORKERS (CHWs) MIGHT HELP

CHWs might help local groups to work out how women in the community could eat better. For example, perhaps women could:

- eat an extra snack every day; *or*
- eat more of certain important foods, such as fresh fruit, green vegetables, and beans; and meat, liver, or fish if they are available.

CHWs might learn about local traditions which are helpful for women's nutrition, and encourage them to continue. For example:

- eating special nutritious foods during pregnancy— such as finger millet or soured porridge;
- killing a goat to provide meat for a newly delivered woman, and drying the meat in strips, so that the woman can eat more of it later on;
- letting the woman rest more during pregnancy, or helping her with heavy work;
- letting her rest after delivery, and feeding her special foods to help her to regain her strength and to produce breast milk.

CHWs who visit families at home might:

- help women to find ways to get more food and to eat better (including helping them to get help from agricultural and community development workers);
- discuss with the men in the family about how they can help women to eat more and work less;
- find out who can help and support women, so that they can rest more during the last 3 months of pregnancy, and the first 1–2 months after delivery.

18.11 HOW OTHER HEALTH WORKERS CAN HELP

When you give family planning care

- Emphasize the importance of spacing births for the nutrition of the *mothers*, as well as for the babies. It is best if a family leaves a space of at least 3 years between babies and if there is a space of 6 months after the mother stops breastfeeding before she starts a new pregnancy.
- Help mothers who have just had a baby to find a suitable method of family planning for their needs, which does not interfere with breastfeeding.

- Explain how breastfeeding can protect against a new pregnancy for 6 months if the mother is breastfeeding exclusively and her periods have not returned (see Section 10.4).

When you give antenatal care

- Discuss with each woman what she eats, and how she can eat more if necessary. It is especially important for her to increase her intake of foods rich in iron, vitamin C, folate, and vitamin A.
- Help to prevent anaemia (see Chapter 20). Make sure that you always have enough iron and folate tablets for all the women who need them.
- Explain that eating well should not make the baby too large to deliver. Advise very short women (less than 151 cm) to eat well, to come for antenatal care regularly, and to deliver in hospital if possible. They may have difficulties whatever the size of the baby.
- If there is a supplementary feeding programme which gives food to pregnant and lactating mothers, make sure that any woman who needs help receives it (see Chapter 29).
- If possible, weigh women at each antenatal visit, and chart the weight. Measure the height of the uterus to check the growth of the baby. (In some places there are charts for this.)

When you give postnatal care

- Discuss with the mother how she can eat a good diet after delivery to help to regain her strength and to build up her nutrient stores again.
- If a woman is likely to be vitamin A deficient, give one high-dose vitamin A capsule **not later than 8 weeks after delivery**. (Do **not** give high-dose vitamin A capsules to any woman who is or who might be pregnant. They may harm the baby; see Section 19.9).
- Support and help her with breastfeeding (see Chapter 10).
- Discuss family planning.

When you weigh and immunize children or treat them for illnesses

- Think about the mother's nutrition as well as the child's nutrition. If necessary discuss how she can eat better.
- Continue to give mothers support for breastfeeding, and help with family planning.
- Try to prevent undernutrition in all children—boys and girls. Take particular care to check the growth of

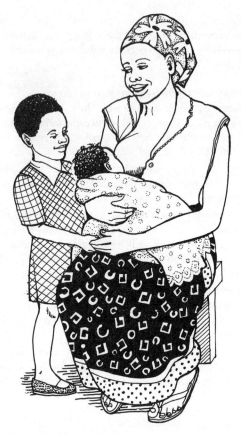

Fig. 18–8 Emphasize the importance of spacing births.

girls and make sure that they receive equally good care to break the 'cycle of undernutrition' in girls and women.

THINGS TO DO

Field visit

1. Take trainees to visit an antenatal clinic, to talk to some mothers and to look at their antenatal records.

   a. With each mother, they should try to find out how much weight she has gained during her pregnancy.

Does she know her pre-pregnant weight? Is there any record of it? Has she records from any previous pregnancies?

   b. Ask trainees to discuss with each mother what she is eating now that she is pregnant, and if she is eating differently from before. Has she received any advice from anyone about what to eat? What is the advice? Is she able to follow it? Why?

From this exercise trainees learn about women's weight gain during pregnancy. Also, they may learn how difficult it is to advise a pregnant woman about what to eat, and how difficult it is for her to follow any advice.

Role play

2. Ask trainees to role play a health worker discussing with a group of men the feeding and care of wives and daughters. Afterwards, discuss the role play.

   Make sure that you cover:

   a. nutrient needs of pregnancy and lactation;
   b. women's workloads;
   c. feeding of young and adolescent girls;
   d. birth spacing;
   e. reasons why women are more at risk of undernutrition than men.

Discussion topic

3. Ask trainees to make a list of local customs which affect the nutrition of girls and childbearing women.

   a. Discuss which customs are helpful, which are harmless, and which are harmful.
   b. Discuss how they could encourage helpful customs and discourage harmful ones.

USEFUL PUBLICATIONS

ACC/SCN (1990). *Women and nutrition*, Nutrition Policy Discussion Paper, no. 6. ACC/SCN, Geneva.
Children in the Tropics (1990). Childbearing and women's health. *Children in the Tropics*, **Vols 187–8**.
WFHPA (1984). *Improving maternal health in developing countries*. UNICEF, New York.

19 Vitamin A and other vitamin deficiencies

19.1 VITAMIN A DEFICIENCY (VAD)

Vitamin A deficiency (VAD) is one of the most important nutritional diseases among young children because:

- It damages the eyes and can cause blindness.
- It may increase the risk of infection and death.

How vitamin A deficiency occurs

VAD occurs when:

- A child or older person does not eat enough to cover her needs.
- The store of vitamin A in her liver is finished (see Section 4.2).

VAD is most common among young children because:

- They grow quickly so their needs are greater.
- They have many infections.

Infections can cause VAD because:

- A sick child does not want to eat much, so she eats too little vitamin A.
- A child with diarrhoea or other gut infections, including worms, absorbs less vitamin A than normal.
- Many infections, especially measles and diarrhoea, increase vitamin A needs.

Most children with vitamin A deficiency also lack energy, protein, and other nutrients—they may have protein–energy malnutrition (PEM). Undernourished children often eat little fat or oil, which makes VAD deficiency more likely. Fat and oil help the absorption of vitamin A so, when the diet is low in fat, less vitamin A is absorbed. Vitamin A is one of the nutrients that destroys free radicals (see Section 17.2).

Signs of VAD often occur when a child is *recovering* from infection, or during treatment for PEM. This is because a child grows rapidly at these times, and vitamin A needs increase. Severe eye damage is uncommon in school-age children or older people, but they may have night blindness (see Box 19.1). They may

have low stores of vitamin A, which is especially important among pregnant or breastfeeding women. The baby may be born with low stores of vitamin A and may not get enough from breast milk.

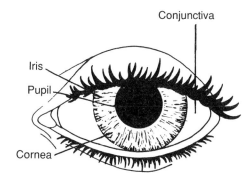

Fig. 19–1 Diagram of the eye.

The effects of vitamin A deficiency

Vitamin A deficiency affects the eyes and the lining of the gut and the respiratory system. Vitamin A deficiency causes xerophthalmia and leads to increased risk of infection.

Xerophthalmia

This is a range of disorders that affect the eye and that can lead to blindness (see Box 19.1). Probably about a half million children around the world develop serious xerophthalmia each year due to vitamin A deficiency. This is the main cause of blindness among young children. More than half of the children die. Many more children have mild vitamin A deficiency, but we do not yet know how many in most areas.

Increased risk of infection

Children who lack vitamin A are more likely to get gut, respiratory, and other infections and to die from them than children with enough vitamin A. Even mild vitamin A deficiency, with no signs of xerophthalmia, may increase the risk of infection and death. This is because:

255

Box 19.1.   Xerophthalmia

The signs of xerophthalmia occur in approximately the following order.

Night blindness (Fig. 19–2)
The child cannot see in the dim light of evening (dusk). Families describe how the child falls over things or knocks them over when she moves around. She cannot see to eat. Often there is a local name for night blindness—such as 'chicken blindness'. It is an important sign because families recognize it and because it can easily be cured. To find out if a child has night blindness, ask the relatives. Night blindness is cured in 1–2 days by vitamin A.

Bitot's spots (Fig. 19–3)
These are foamy, soapy whitish patches on the white part of the eye. Bitot's spots may not disappear completely after treatment especially in older children and adults. But they do not affect the sight.

Conjunctival xerosis (Fig. 19–3)
Xerosis means dryness. The conjunctiva (the covering of the white part of the eye) looks dry and slightly rough or wrinkled, instead of wet, smooth, and shiny. It is difficult to recognize conjunctival xerosis without special training. Bitot's spots which usually occur at the same time, are easier to see. Conjunctival xerosis is cured in 1–2 weeks by vitamin A.

Active corneal lesions (Fig. 19–3)
The cornea is the clear part of the eye that you see through, in front of the brown iris. If the cornea is damaged, the person cannot see properly and may be blind.

Corneal xerosis
The surface of the cornea is cloudy and dry. Some people call these 'fish scales over the eye'. Early corneal xerosis can be cured in 1–2 weeks. However, it can become more serious very quickly, in hours or days. More serious lesions are incurable. So a child with corneal xerosis needs treatment urgently with large doses of vitamin A.

Corneal ulcers
If xerosis is not treated early enough, ulcers (holes) may form on the surface of the cornea. Vitamin A can cure the ulcers, but usually a scar remains which may affect the eyesight.

Keratomalacia
If xerosis or ulcers are not treated, the whole cornea becomes cloudy and soft. The cornea may burst, and part of the inside of the eye may come out. Often one eye is worse than the other. Giving vitamin A immediately stops keratomalacia becoming worse and may save some sight, especially in the better eye.

Corneal scars
The cornea is white, and the person can see little through it. There are several causes of corneal scarring, and it can be difficult to know which is responsible. If the family can tell you that the scars appeared after the child had measles, or another infection, or undernutrition, then they are probably due to vitamin A deficiency.

- *Resistance* to infection is decreased. The cells which line the gut and respiratory tract secrete less mucus. Bacteria can stick to the cells and cause infection more easily.

- *Immunity* against infection is decreased. The white blood cells cannot fight infections so well.

19.2 PEOPLE WHO ARE AT SPECIAL RISK OF VAD

People who live in 'at risk places'
Vitamin A deficiency is commonest in certain areas, and at certain times.

- *'At risk places'* are dry areas, where it may be difficult to get vitamin A rich vegetables and fruit, such as mangoes and green leaves, for all or part of the year.

- *'At risk times'* are dry seasons or droughts, when little vitamin A rich food is available for a long period.

Everyone who lives in these areas is at risk of VAD, particularly children, mothers, and old people. You may see signs of VAD mainly at the end of the dry season when people's liver stores of vitamin A are finished.

Some babies, especially if their mothers lack vitamin A
Babies who are not breastfed or who stop breastfeeding

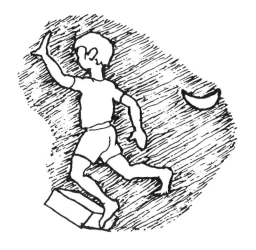

Fig. 19–2 A child with night blindness.

early and who are given dilute bottle feeds or other foods which contain little vitamin A may develop VAD.

Babies whose mothers lack vitamin A may be born with low stores, and they may not get enough from breast milk. LBW babies are also born with a low store of vitamin A. If their mothers also have low stores, there may not be enough in breast milk.

Children who are undernourished or sick

These children are at increased risk of VAD:

- children under the age of 5 years who are undernourished, especially those with severe PEM;
- children who have measles or diarrhoea, especially diarrhoea which continues for more than 14 days, that is, persistent diarrhoea.

Possibly children with other infections such as pneumonia are also at increased risk.

Other groups at risk

Old people, school-age children, and pregnant adolescent girls; prisoners; refugees and displaced people

living in camps may also be at risk if they have vitamin A poor diets.

19.3 WHAT YOU CAN DO ABOUT VAD

You can:

- know how important VAD is in the community;
- watch over children at special risk;
- recognize the warning signs of xerophthalmia;
- treat or refer children with, or at high risk of, xerophthalmia;
- help to prevent vitamin A deficiency.

19.4 KNOWING HOW IMPORTANT VAD IS IN THE COMMUNITY

VAD is an important problem in some areas and not in others. To find out how important VAD is in your area, ask the following questions:

- *Has anyone done a survey?* Examine a number of children aged 0–5 years old for signs of xerophthalmia. Box 19.2 shows how to decide if VAD is an important problem.

  You can see that, even when the problem is serious, only a very small number of children have eye signs. You need to examine a large number of children to find out if such a small proportion are affected. This is not often practical. However, if someone has already done a survey in or near your area, you should know about it.

- *Do many families report night blindness?* This is an easy sign to use to find out about VAD, because families recognize it themselves. However, it is not a reliable sign to use by itself.

- *What do health workers report, and what do health records show?* Health workers in the area may already know from experience if many children have

---

Box 19.2. Criteria for deciding if vitamin A deficiency is a public health problem
(WHO/UNICEF/USAID/HKI/IVACG 1982)

Vitamin A deficiency is a serious community health problem if, among children aged 0–5 years, at least:

- 1% have night blindness; *or*
- 2% have Bitot's spots; *or*
- 0.01% have corneal dryness or ulcers or keratomalacia; *or*
- 0.05% have corneal scars.

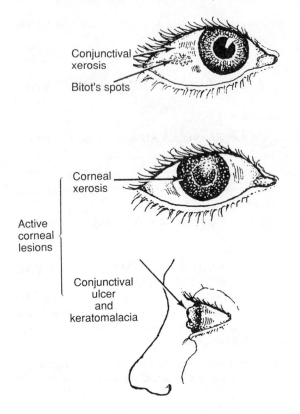

Fig. 19-3 Eye lesions in xerophthalmia.

xerophthalmia. They may know that many children have night blindness or Bitot's spots. They may know that many children with PEM or measles develop xerophthalmia.

Ask health workers who may be able to help, and ask to see any available records, for example in the local hospital or district or provincial health office.

- *Are vitamin A rich foods available to families?* Is it an 'at risk place' or an 'at risk time'? There may be no vitamin A rich foods available. The vitamin A rich foods which are available may be too expensive for poorer families to buy, or farming families may sell vitamin A rich foods, such as eggs and milk.

  If families cannot get vitamin A rich foods, children are likely to have vitamin A deficiency.

- *Do children eat vitamin A rich foods?* Foods may be available, but families may not give them to small children. Children may not like foods such as dark green leaves or families may not like to give young children whole small fish.

If you cannot examine eyes, but you suspect that there

may be a problem, ask your supervisor or local health committee to try to find out more.

19.5 WATCHING OVER CHILDREN AT SPECIAL RISK

If you know which children are most likely to have VAD, you can watch over them and help the families who need it most. Most 'at risk' children live in 'at risk places'. But you may find children who are at risk in any community. For example:

- *children of families who cannot afford to buy enough vitamin A rich foods.* In towns, fruits and vegetables can be very expensive, especially at certain times of year;

- *children who are not given vitamin A rich foods* even if they are available, or children who refuse to eat them;

- *children with protein–energy malnutrition*;

- *children with infections*, particularly measles and persistent diarrhoea;

- *babies (especially LBW babies) born to mothers who lack vitamin A*, such as poor mothers who live in 'at risk places';

- *babies who are not breastfed*, and who eat little vitamin A rich food.

19.6 RECOGNIZING THE WARNING SIGNS OF XEROPHTHALMIA

Xerophthalmia is a serious condition which can lead to blindness very quickly. Also, children with xerophthalmia may become very ill with infections, because lack of vitamin A causes low resistance. Therefore all nutrition workers must be able to recognize the early warning signs of xerophthalmia. Then they can get urgent treatment for the child. The warning signs which are easiest to recognize are:

- *night blindness*—the family reports that the child cannot see in dim light;

- *Bitot's spots*—whitish soapy patches on the outer white parts of the eye;

- *active corneal lesions*—cloudiness or sores on the clear, front part of the eye.

19.7 TREATING OR REFERRING CHILDREN WITH OR AT HIGH RISK OF XEROPHTHALMIA

A child needs treatment with vitamin A if he or she:

- has any signs of xerophthalmia;
- has or has just had measles.

Treat children with any signs of active corneal lesions IMMEDIATELY or send for treatment urgently.

Even 1 hour's delay can make the difference between the child having sight or being blind.

If you have a high-dose vitamin A preparation available

- Give the three treatment doses described in Box 19.4.
- If there are active corneal lesions:
  - Cover the eye with an eye shield, to prevent the child pressing or rubbing the eye, and making it worse.
  - Apply tetracycline eye ointment three times a day. Do *not* use eye ointment which contains steroids.

- If there are corneal ulcers apply atropine ointment or drops to prevent prolapse of the iris.
- Treat the child for infections and malnutrition (see Chapter 17).
- Explain to parents how they can prevent vitamin A deficiency in the future.

If high-dose vitamin A preparations are not available

- Feed the child large helpings of liver, carrots, mangoes, or red palm oil, *or* give any vitamin preparation which contains vitamin A, *or* give fish liver oil—*if these are readily available, and if they can be given without causing delay.*
- If the child has active corneal lesions, cover the eye with an eye shield.
- Refer *immediately* to a health centre or hospital where high-dose vitamin A preparations are available.
- Explain to the parents how they can prevent vitamin A deficiency in future.

Box 19.3. Preparations of vitamin A

Vitamin A in oil is absorbed quickly when given by mouth. Most vitamin A preparations also contain vitamin E which improves absorption.

Capsules of vitamin A in oil ('high-dosage capsules') are usually best. Each capsule usually contains 200 000 IU in oil.

For a dose of 200 000 IU:

- The person can swallow the whole capsule,
- Or you can cut off the tip and squeeze the oil on to the tongue (see Figs 19–5 and 19–6).

To give a smaller dose:

You need to count the total number of drops in your type of capsule to be sure of the exact number which will give the dose.

For example, many capsules give 12 drops if you cut the tip off 1 mm from the end. If you have these capsules:

- If the child needs 100 000 IU, squeeze 6 drops on to her tongue.
- If a baby needs 50 000 IU, squeeze 3 drops on to her tongue.

Oily solution of vitamin A. This solution comes in a bottle, to measure and give with a dropper or multidose dispenser. Usually 1 ml contains 100 000 IU *but the concentration varies*, so you have to work out how much to give.

Unopened, and stored carefully in the dark, the solution lasts for 2 years. After the bottle has been opened, it loses its strength after about 6–8 weeks.

Ampoules of watery vitamin A contain 100 000 IU in 2 ml. If the child cannot take the oily solution by mouth, for example because of persistent vomiting, you may have to give vitamin A by injection. Injections must always be the watery solution. (This method is not recommended, however, because of risk of infection. Give oral therapy if possible.)

Sugar-coated tablets, each containing 10 000 IU vitamin A.

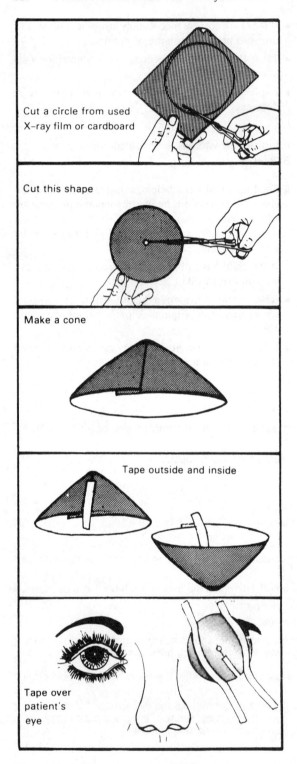

Cut a circle from used X-ray film or cardboard

Cut this shape

Make a cone

Tape outside and inside

Tape over patient's eye

Fig. 19–4 How to make an eye shield.

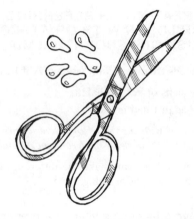

Fig. 19–5 High-dose vitamin A capsules.

19.8 HELPING TO PREVENT VAD

There are a number of ways in which different kinds of nutrition worker can help communities to prevent vitamin A deficiency.

Help families to give children enough vitamin A rich foods

This is the best long-term *sustainable* way to prevent vitamin A deficiency.

- Discuss with families the special needs of young children and pregnant and breastfeeding mothers for vitamin A rich foods. Explain the risks of not eating enough.
- Encourage childbearing women to eat plenty of vitamin A rich foods.
- Encourage mothers to give their babies colostrum which is an excellent source of vitamin A.
- Encourage mothers to breastfeed for at least 2 years. Breast milk is a very important source of vitamin A, provided the mother is eating plenty of vitamin A rich foods. A baby can get most of the vitamin A that he needs from breast milk up to the age of 2 years, if he continues to breastfeed frequently. (A baby needs 300 RE/day, and breast milk has 60 RE/100 ml, so a baby only needs 500 ml breast milk to get all the vitamin A that he needs.)
- Discuss with families which local vitamin A rich foods are best value for money (see Appendix 3) and which foods young children like.
- Encourage families to give vitamin A rich foods, such

Box 19.4. Dosage of vitamin A for treatment (from WHO/UNICEF/IVACG Task Force 1988)

	Aged under 1 year or weight less than 8 kg	Aged over 1 year and weight 8 kg or more
Immediately	100 000 IU by mouth	200 000 IU by mouth
Next day	100 000 IU by mouth	200 000 IU by mouth
4 weeks later (or on discharge from hospital; or if xerophthalmia becomes worse)*	100 000 IU by mouth	200 000 IU by mouth

* Xerophthalmia is most likely to become worse in children with severe PEM—watch these children carefully.

If you have to give vitamin A by injection, the dose is half the dose by mouth:

- 50 000 IU for those under 1 year;
- 100 000 IU for those over 1 year.

Note. 100 000 IU = 30 000 RE.

as green leaves, liver, red palm oil, mangoes, or pawpaws to young children. Meals should contain a little oil to help absorption of vitamin A.

- Show families how to prepare vitamin A rich foods in ways that children like. For example:
  - mashing green leaves with oil rich food (e.g. groundnuts) and staples;
  - mashing carrots with sweet potato;
  - using red palm oil in children's meals.
- Show families how to grow vitamin A rich foods such as dark green leaves.
- Show people how to dry vegetables and fruits in a way that preserves vitamin A (see Section 6.3). Then they can have a supply for most of the year.

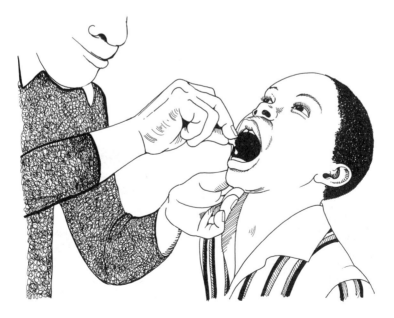

Fig. 19–6 Giving a high dose of vitamin A.

Encourage people to use foods fortified with vitamin A

Fortification can be a good way to prevent vitamin A deficiency among people who buy most of their food and who do not grow it. Fortification may become more important as more people live in towns. Some examples of foods fortified with vitamin A are:

- margarine;
- some weaning foods, such as 'Lishe' in Tanzania;
- some dried skimmed milk (DSM), corn soy milk, and some oils used in feeding programmes.

Give high-dose vitamin A capsules

This is an effective short-term way to prevent VAD (Table 19.1). However, it depends on having vitamin A preparations, which may need to be imported, and on good distribution.

The aim is to give large doses of vitamin A to people who are 'at risk', to fill up their liver stores. The main groups at risk are:

- young children;
- newly delivered mothers (for their own health, and so that their breast milk contains enough vitamin A).

Encourage people to come for their doses and explain that it is safe. It is important at the same time to encourage families to grow and eat vitamin A rich food, and not to depend on capsules for ever.

Table 19.1. Doses of vitamin A to prevent deficiency (WHO/UNICEF/WACG Task Force 1988)

Women 0–8 weeks after childbirth (not later)	200 000 IU
Infants 6–12 months and older children who weigh less than 8 kg†	100 000 IU
Children over 1 year and under 6 years old	200 000 IU

* Record that you have given the dose:
- in your own records;
- on the child's growth chart;
- on the mother's health card.

† If a non-breastfed baby aged 3–6 months is at risk of VAD give 50 000 IU.

Whom to give vitamin A capsules to

This depends on your local situation and country programme. You may include these groups:

- Children at increased risk, such as those with severe PEM (see Section 19.1), with measles, severe acute or persistent diarrhoea, or with pneumonia.
- In places and at times of special risk, such as the dry season:
  - All children from 6 months to 6 years of age every 3–6 months. (Exactly how often depends on how severe the problem is and what resources are available in the community.)
  - All mothers not later than 8 weeks after childbirth.

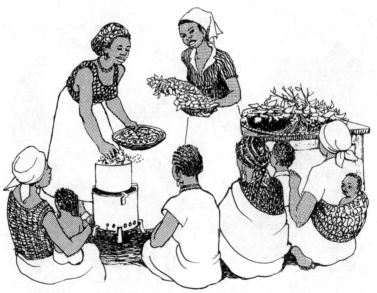

Fig. 19–7 Encourage parents to give vitamin A rich foods to young children.

Do *not* give:

- High doses of vitamin A to pregnant women, or to any woman who could soon become pregnant, because it may cause abnormalities in the baby. This means that you should *not* give high doses of vitamin A to a mother more than 8 weeks after childbirth.
- More than the recommended dose. Side-effects are rare if you give the correct dose. An overdose may cause headache, nausea, vomiting, and diarrhoea, which usually stops in a day.
- More than one dose every 3 months, except when you are treating a child for xerophthalmia, or the child is at increased risk (e.g. has measles or is severely malnourished).

How childbearing women can take vitamin A

Pregnant and breastfeeding women can safely:

- eat vitamin A rich foods;
- take regular vitamin supplements which contain vitamin A, provided the dose does not contain more than 10 000 IU (3000 RE) vitamin A per day;
- have a high dose of vitamin A in the first 8 weeks after childbirth, because women rarely become pregnant at this time;
- take one sugar-coated tablet of 10 000 IU daily for 14 days.

Encourage families to take their children for immunization

Many children develop xerophthalmia after measles. Vitamin A is sometimes given to children when they are immunized, in particular with their measles vaccine, at 9 months of age.

19.9 VAD AMONG REFUGEES AND DISPLACED PEOPLE IN CAMPS

Refugees and displaced people are at risk of VAD if their rations do not provide much vitamin A; *and* they cannot buy or barter vitamin A rich foods outside the camp.

To prevent vitamin A deficiency in camps:

- Give high-dose capsules to people with signs of xerophthalmia.
- Give high-dose capsules to young children and newly delivered women.
- Give rations which provide vitamin A, for example,

yellow maize if acceptable, or oils or cereal products fortified with vitamin A.
- Give enough rations so that people can exchange some for fresh vegetables and fruits from outside the camp.
- Encourage people to grow green leaves when this is possible.

19.10 MONITORING AND EVALUATING VAD PREVENTION PROGRAMMES

What you do depends on your particular job and your type of programme, but you may need to:

- monitor the production or purchase and use of vitamin A rich foods;
- monitor supplies of high-dose preparations;
- monitor the number of people in the community who have received a high dose and follow up non-attenders;
- collect data for evaluating the programme, such as the number of children with night blindness or the number of child deaths;
- tell the public about the progress of the programme;
- report any problems to the programme supervisors.

19.11 THIAMINE DEFICIENCY— BERIBERI

Thiamine deficiency causes *beriberi*. It occurs occasionally where people eat mainly refined ('polished') rice or a starchy root such as cassava and very little other food. Beriberi is commonest in women of childbearing age and their infants, and sometimes in active young men.

Symptoms of beriberi include:
- loss of appetite;
- severe weakness, especially of the legs;
- sometimes paralysis of the arms and legs;
- sometimes cardiac failure with acute oedema of the body.

Ways to prevent beriberi include:
- giving parboiled rice or unpolished (less highly refined) rice;
- giving foods rich in thiamine (wholegrain cereals and legumes);
- giving fortified foods, such as blended cereals;
- giving thiamine supplements.

19.12 NIACIN DEFICIENCY— PELLAGRA

Pellagra occurs occasionally in people who eat a very poor diet which consists mostly of maize, for example, refugees and prisoners. Women, old people, and young children are particularly at risk. Men may get enough niacin if they drink beer.

Symptoms of pellagra. The parts of the skin that are exposed to the sun develop a dark, peeling rash. Some people have severe diarrhoea or mental changes.

Ways to prevent pellagra include:
- giving foods which are rich in niacin, such as groundnuts;
- fortifying maize or sorghum or other foods with niacin;
- giving a different cereal;
- giving niacin supplements.

19.13 VITAMIN C DEFICIENCY

People who do not eat enough vitamin C may not absorb enough iron and may develop iron deficiency anaemia (see Chapter 20). Severe vitamin C deficiency also results in a disease called *scurvy*. Scurvy occurs occasionally among people who do not have fresh foods or other sources of vitamin C for 2–3 months.

People who may not eat enough vitamin C include:
- Refugees who cannot get fresh fruit and vegetables.
- People who live in dry areas where no fresh fruit and vegetables are available. This is especially likely to happen during a drought.
- Urban people who cannot afford fresh fruit and vegetables.
- Old people and unmarried men who live alone and do not eat many fresh foods.

The groups who most often have scurvy are adolescent boys and pregnant and lactating women.

Symptoms of scurvy. Scurvy causes internal bleeding which can result in:
- swollen bleeding gums, which may lead to loss of teeth;
- swollen painful joints, particularly of the knee, hip, and elbow.

Scurvy can cause death.

To prevent scurvy, ensure that people have a source of fresh fruit and vegetables. If necessary, give vitamin C supplements to people who are at risk.

19.14 VITAMIN D DEFICIENCY

Vitamin D deficiency is called **rickets** if the bones are still growing, and **osteomalacia** if they have finished growing. Vitamin D deficiency is not common in Africa. However, it is becoming commoner as more people live in crowded cities.

People who are at risk of vitamin D deficiency are:

- *Low birth weight babies.* LBW babies are born with low stores of vitamin D. If their mother also lacks vitamin D, they get little from breast milk. Mothers may keep them covered and out of the sun because they are worried about them.
- Babies of mothers who lack vitamin D. There may be little vitamin D in breast milk from a mother who lacks vitamin D.
- Children who live in crowded shanty towns and play mainly inside.
- Children whose mothers go out to work and leave them inside the house all day.
- Adolescent girls who do not go outside often and who become pregnant—because their vitamin D needs are particularly high.
- Women who cover themselves in public and who live in houses or apartments with no private garden or courtyard.
- Old or disabled people who stay indoors all day and who eat a poor diet.

Rickets

Rickets occurs in young children and teenage girls. The bones become soft and may bend.

Signs in babies:
- The bones of the skull may be soft.
- The fontanelle (soft spot) takes a long time to close.
- There may be swelling of the bones in wrists and ankles.
- The chest may be deformed, and there may be swellings at the ends of the ribs.
- The baby may have repeated respiratory infections.

Signs in children:
- The skull may look enlarged.
- The muscles are weak, and the child may learn to walk late.
- The legs may bend outwards so the child walks like a duck.

- Sometimes the legs are bent inwards, and the child has 'knock knees'.

Adolescent girls may complain of pain in the back and legs. Severe rickets in girls can cause pelvic deformities which can result in difficulties during childbirth.

Osteomalacia

Osteomalacia occurs in women who lack vitamin D. The body cannot absorb enough calcium from food, and uses calcium from the bones. The bones become soft and can break easily.

Symptoms include:

- severe pain in the bones;
- muscle weakness;
- deformity of the pelvis, causing difficulties in childbirth;
- broken bones, especially in people who are old or disabled.

A woman's breast milk may lack vitamin D, increasing the risk of rickets in her baby.

How to prevent and treat vitamin D deficiency

Eating foods which are rich in vitamin D can help, but these foods are usually expensive. There is no need to buy special 'tonics' or cod liver oil. Sunshine is free and better.

To prevent vitamin D deficiency, go outside in daylight for at least 10 minutes every day (or most days) with the face and arms uncovered (see Section 4.8).

To treat a child with rickets, let the child stay in the sun for 30 minutes each day for about a month. If the parents are worried that strong sunshine may harm the child, reassure them that the sun in the early morning or evening is not harmful.

THINGS TO DO

Demonstration

1. Let trainees study pictures which show signs of xerophthalmia and learn to recognize the warning signs. Try to see real cases in a hospital or health centre.

2. Show trainees pictures of people with other vitamin deficiencies which may occur where they will work (e.g. pellagra in a refugee camp). Ask them to identify the signs and which vitamin deficiency causes them.

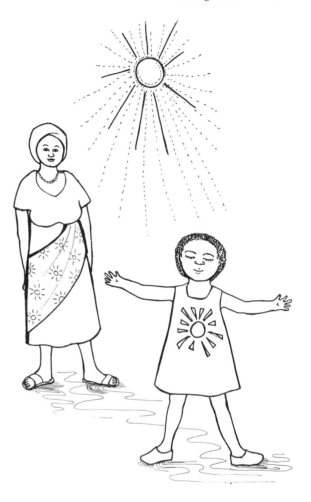

Fig. 19–8 Sunshine prevents vitamin D deficiency.

Projects

3. Ask a few trainees to do a simple survey of night blindness among young children in a community.

   a. Ask a number of families with children aged 1–5 years if the children have night blindness.

   b. As they talk to families, they should learn the names that communities have for the symptom.

   Discuss the findings in class.

4. Ask trainees to find out the cheapest source of vitamin A in a community. Ask mothers which of these foods children like.

   a. Trainees can use Table 9.1 to calculate the cost of 100 RE in different local foods.

   b. They can use the food composition Tables (Appendix 1) and tables of Vitamin A needs (Table 4.1 and

Appendix 2) to calculate how much of each of the cheap local vitamin A rich foods a child needs to eat to cover her daily vitamin A needs.

Discuss the answers.

Discussion and role play

5. Discuss with trainees whether there could be groups of people in their community who are at risk of vitamin D deficiency. If there are, role play a nutrition worker advising a mother to take herself and her young children into the sun each day. Discuss afterwards.

6. Ask trainees to list the sorts of people in their communities who could be at risk of vitamin C deficiency. Discuss why they are at risk.

USEFUL PUBLICATIONS

HKI (no date). *Know the signs and symptoms of xerophthalmia*. HKI, New York.

Sommer, A. (ed.) (1982). *Field guide to detection and control of xerophthalmia*. WHO, Geneva.

Vitamin A Technical Assistance Program (VITAP)/HKI (1990). Vitamin A reference manual. Available from HKI, New York.

WHO/UNICEF/IVACG Task Force (1988). *Vitamin A supplements: a guide to their use in the treatment and prevention of vitamin A deficiency and xerophthalmia*. WHO, Geneva.

20 Nutritional anaemia

20.1 WHAT ANAEMIA IS

Anaemia means that the blood does not contain enough *haemoglobin*—the substance that makes blood red. People sometimes call anaemia 'weak blood' or 'thin blood' or 'pale blood'. When there is not enough haemoglobin, it is more difficult to get oxygen to the cells.

The commonest cause of anaemia is *iron deficiency*, or lack of the nutrient *iron*. Iron is needed to make haemoglobin (see Section 4.10). Iron deficiency anaemia (IDA) is a *nutritional anaemia*. Nutritional anaemia means that the body cannot make enough haemoglobin and healthy red blood cells because it lacks the necessary nutrients.

There are other less common causes of anaemia, for example, sickle cell disease. Infections can also make people anaemic, especially malaria and hookworm. However, we do not discuss these other diseases in detail.

20.2 WHY NUTRITIONAL ANAEMIA IS IMPORTANT

Anaemia is the most widespread nutrition disorder in the world

Anaemia is found in all countries, rich and poor, and it affects women and children particularly. In many parts of the world about 50 per cent of all women and children are anaemic.

Anaemia affects how people function

Anaemia reduces people's ability to work, increases their tiredness, and slows learning in children.

Reduced ability to work
Anaemic men and women cannot do as much work as healthy men and women. They may be just as strong, but they have more difficulty continuing to work for a long time. Reduced ability to work is very serious. A person in a paid job may not be able to earn as much money—especially if they are paid 'piece rates'. A person doing unpaid work—for example on their own farm, or caring for their family, may not be able to do so much.

It may be more difficult to do anything extra—such as going to a women's group meeting, or a literacy class; or playing with children. So anaemia may be one reason why a family is poor or receives less care.

Increased tiredness
Anaemia can make a person feel tired, apathetic, and 'not well'. People who feel tired all the time may lose interest in trying to make things better. This also contributes to poverty and lack of care in the family.

Slower learning
Children who are anaemic have less energy for playing and learning. Throughout childhood, they may learn and develop more slowly than healthy children.

Anaemia increases the risks of childbearing

Increased risk of death for the mother
An anaemic woman is more likely to bleed severely or to become very ill and die during delivery.

Increased risk of sickness and death for the baby
The baby of an anaemic mother is more likely to be low birth weight, and to become sick or die during early childhood.

20.3 SIGNS AND SYMPTOMS OF ANAEMIA

Paleness of the tongue and inside the lips
Haemoglobin in the blood gives the red colour to the tongue and inside the lips. When there is too little haemoglobin, the tongue and lips look paler than normal. This is the main sign of anaemia to look for. However, it is usually only possible to see paleness if the anaemia is moderate or severe.

Tiredness
An anaemic person does not feel well. She may feel tired and apathetic. She may feel dizzy, or have headaches. She may lose her appetite, or feel nausea. A person who is iron deficient with low iron stores, may feel tired before her tongue and lips look pale.

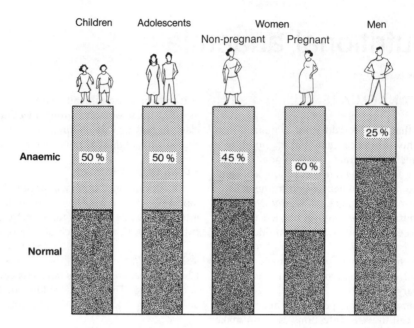

Fig. 20-1 Proportion of people in developing countries who are anaemic (De Maeyer 1989).

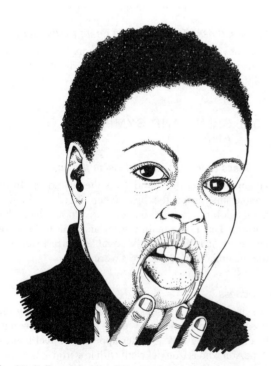

Fig. 20-2 Examining the lips and tongue for anaemia.

Breathlessness

An anaemic person may feel breathless or she may feel her heart beating faster. Her legs may swell. These are all signs that the heart has to work harder to pump the blood around the body to get enough oxygen to the cells.

Variability of symptoms

The symptoms of anaemia (except persistent paleness) can be caused in other ways, for example:

- by lack of food;
- by infections or by other illnesses such as a weak heart;
- by mental illness, such as depression;
- by simple tiredness due to hard work;
- by lack of 'fitness', for example, when a person who is not regularly active does hard physical work.

On the other hand, people who are anaemic may not complain of symptoms:

- A person who is anaemic may not be aware of being weak or tired until the anaemia is very severe.
- People who are anaemic but who have to work may force themselves to overcome tiredness.
- Children may show no obvious signs. They are only found to be anaemic when they have another illness, and the health worker notices that the child's tongue and lips are pale.

20.4 FINDING OUT IF SOMEONE IS ANAEMIC

So the *symptoms* of anaemia are very variable, and they can be caused by other conditions. The only *sign* you can look for is paleness, which is not very reliable.

So to know whether a person is anaemic or not, you need to *measure the amount of haemoglobin in their blood.*

Measuring haemoglobin

Haemoglobin is measured in *grams per 100 ml of blood.* It is not possible to say exactly what the 'normal' haemoglobin is, because it varies from person to person. We can say however, that haemoglobin below a certain level means anaemia (Table 20.1 and Fig. 20–3).

Table 20.1. Haemoglobin levels in anaemia (from ACC/SCN 1991a)

	Haemoglobin level (g/100 ml)
Haemoglobin below these levels means anaemia	
Children 6 months to 5 years	11
Children 6 years to 14 years	12
Men	13
Women (not pregnant)	12
Women (pregnant)	11
Mild, moderate, and severe anaemia	
Mild	Below the values given above, but more than 10
Moderate	7–10
Severe	Below 7

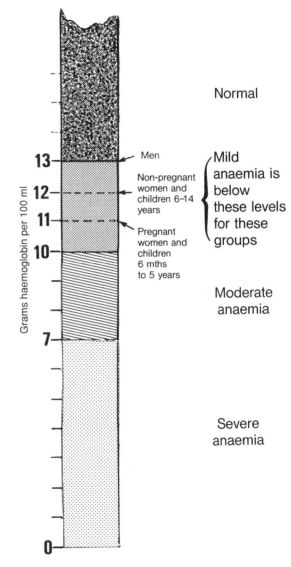

Fig. 20–3 Levels of haemoglobin in mild, moderate, and severe anaemia.

The haemoglobin does not usually go much above about 16 g/100 ml even in men. You can usually see the paleness of a person's tongue and the inside of their lips if their haemoglobin is below about 10 g/100 ml. It is not usually possible to see paleness if the anaemia is mild.

20.5 HOW NUTRITIONAL ANAEMIA DEVELOPS

Red blood cells last for only about 4 months, so the body has to replace them continually.

The nutrients needed to replace red blood cells include:

- *iron*—to make haemoglobin;
- *folate*—for the development of the red blood cells;
- *protein*—to build the red cells and haemoglobin.

When a person gets plenty of these nutrients in their food, or when they have enough in their body stores, they can make new red cells as fast as the old cells wear out.

But a person may not get enough nutrients in their

food, or their body stores may be low, or the need for new red cells may increase. Then the body may not be able to make new red blood cells fast enough, and the person becomes anaemic.

Iron deficiency

Iron deficiency can occur when:

- The person does not get enough iron from their food.
- The need for iron increases, for example, during growth or pregnancy.
- Blood (and therefore iron) is lost from the body:
  - during menstruation and childbirth;
  - in parasitic infections such as hookworm, schistosomiasis, and whipworm (*Trichuris*).

Iron stores

The body can *store* some iron in the tissues. This store provides iron at times when there is little iron in the food, or when the need for iron increases. The body also *saves* iron. When red cells die, most of the iron is kept and used again. However, when red cells are lost from the body, their iron is lost with them.

When a person needs more iron than she gets from food, she is *iron deficient*. Her body uses stored iron. If iron deficiency continues, the store is used up, and she develops *iron deficiency anaemia (IDA)*. To get more iron, she needs to eat plenty of iron-rich food (see Section 4.10).

When a person's iron stores are low, more iron is absorbed from food (see Fig. 4–11). Increased absorption of iron helps, but it is usually not enough to prevent a fall in haemoglobin. Because it may be difficult to get enough iron from food alone, people (especially childbearing women) may need to take iron supplements.

If people lose more iron than they take in:

- The total amount of iron in their bodies decreases

    ↓

- They become iron-deficient.

    ↓

- Their stores of iron are used up.

    ↓

- They can no longer make enough haemoglobin.

    ↓

- They develop anaemia.

Folate deficiency

Folate deficiency is a less common cause of anaemia than iron deficiency. Folate deficiency occurs when:

- There is not enough folate in food.
- The need for folate increases, for example, during growth, but particularly during pregnancy.
- Red blood cells are destroyed inside the body faster than usual, for example, in malaria, sickle cell anaemia, and thalassaemia. The body has to replace the red cells faster than usual, so more folate is required.

Unlike iron, folate cannot be reused. The body stores very little folate, so we must eat enough nearly every day.

When red cells are destroyed inside the body, as in malaria, sickle cell anaemia, and thalassaemia, iron deficiency is not usually a problem. In these conditions, the iron can be saved and used again.

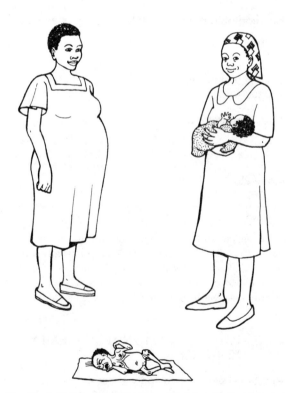

Fig. 20–4 Childbearing women and babies who are low birth weight or not breastfed are at risk of nutritional anaemia.

20.6 GROUPS WHO ARE 'AT RISK' OF NUTRITIONAL ANAEMIA

Some groups of people are more likely to be iron or folate deficient than others. They are 'at risk' of anaemia. High-risk groups are:

- women, especially during pregnancy or soon after delivery;
- babies who are low birth weight or not breastfed;
- young children—especially if they are malnourished;
- adolescents, who are growing fast, especially girls;
- older men and women, especially if they are poor.

Women

Women are at risk of nutritional anaemia because:

- They lose blood with menstruation. Anaemia is especially likely if menstruation is heavy.
- During pregnancy, they must provide the growing fetus with a store of iron. Iron is transferred to the baby even if the mother's stores are low. The baby gets a good store of iron, even if the mother becomes anaemic.

  Closely spaced pregnancies are especially likely to cause anaemia. Iron is transferred to the new growing fetus before the mother has had time to replace the iron stores used up during her previous pregnancy.

- During pregnancy, their bodies make red blood cells faster than normal.

Young children

The first 6 months of life

A baby is born with an iron store from his mother. The iron in breast milk is very well absorbed. Even if the mother is iron-deficient, her milk contains the usual amount of iron. Normally, these two sources of iron are enough for at least the first 6 months of life.

- *Low birth weight (LBW) babies.* Babies who are small at birth have smaller iron stores than bigger babies. Babies who are born too early have not had time to build up their stores of iron before birth. Low birth weight babies may become iron-deficient after about 2–3 months of age.

- *Babies who are not breastfed.* Iron from artificial feeds is not as well absorbed as iron from breast milk. Babies fed on formula which is iron-fortified get

more iron, but it may not be enough to prevent problems. Babies fed on animal milk alone are likely to become anaemic by about 4 months of age.

From 6 months to 3 years of age

By 6 months of age, a baby is growing fast, and his iron needs are increasing (see Table 4.2). He has used up the store of iron that he was born with, and has outgrown the supply from breast milk. He must start to get iron from other foods.

Many children become iron-deficient between 6 months and 3 years. Weaning foods often consist mainly of food from which it is difficult to absorb enough iron. Infections which are common at this age interfere with the absorption, storage, and use of iron, as well as reducing food intake.

- *Malnourished children.* Most malnourished children lack iron and are anaemic. When a child who is severely malnourished starts to recover, iron deficiency may become more severe. This is because, as the child's tissues starts to grow again, iron needs increase.

Older children

Older children also need plenty of iron, because they are growing. However, iron needs per kilogram body weight decrease with age, and older children are at less risk of anaemia than younger ones. Even so, many older children are mildly anaemic, but they only become severely anaemic if they have some other problem, such as hookworm or schistosomiasis.

- *Children with sickle cell anaemia or thalassaemia.* These children are making new red blood cells faster than normal. They do not usually become iron-deficient, but they often become deficient in folate.

Adolescents

Just before puberty, children grow very fast for about a year, and their iron needs increase. Boys and girls both need extra iron, but girls are more likely to become deficient because they are also starting to menstruate.

It is important for girls to build up their stores of iron before they start childbearing.

Men

Men who eat a good mixture of food usually get enough

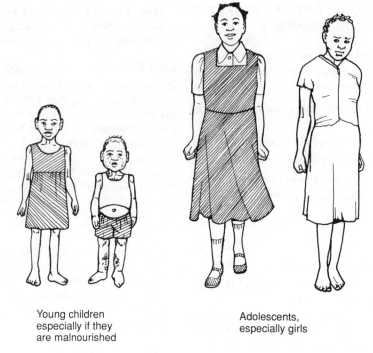

Young children
especially if they
are malnourished

Adolescents,
especially girls

Fig. 20–5 Other groups who are at risk of anaemia.

iron and folate. Men who eat a poor diet or who have hookworm or schistosomiasis may get anaemic. They do not develop severe anaemia nearly as often as child-bearing women and children, because their iron needs are less.

Older men and women

Elderly men and women may eat less than younger people. If they have poor teeth, they may eat more soft food, such as cereals, from which it is difficult to absorb iron. They may have difficulty eating some of the foods from which iron is well-absorbed, such as meat, or they may be too poor to buy it. They may not bother to eat green vegetables, which can supply folate or fresh fruit which provides vitamin C.

20.7 WHAT YOU CAN DO ABOUT NUTRITIONAL ANAEMIA

- Learn to recognize anaemia.
- Find out if anaemia is a problem in your area.
- Help to prevent nutritional anaemia.
- Help people who are anaemic to get treatment.

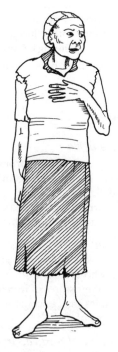

Fig. 20–6 Older men and women are at risk of anaemia, especially if they are poor.

Learning to recognize anaemia

Suspect anaemia in a person who:

- has signs or symptoms as in Section 20.3;
- is in a high-risk group (see Section 20.6).

If you suspect that a person might be anaemic, examine her tongue, and inside her lower lip, and try to decide of she is paler than a healthy person. It is easy to recognize severe anaemia. When you have looked at a lot of people's tongues, you should be able to recognize moderate anaemia also. It is difficult to recognize mild anaemia.

Finding out about nutritional anaemia in your area

- Find out the results of any surveys done in your area, or in the country, or even in the region.
- Find out how many cases of anaemia are reported from hospitals and health centres, especially from MCH and maternity services, and among malnourished children.
- Find out what percentage of babies in the area are low birth weight.
- Find out if the diseases that contribute to iron deficiency are common in the area—hookworm, schistosomiasis, and whipworm.

Helping to prevent nutritional anaemia

- 'Watch over' people who are particularly at risk. Help them to improve their diets, or to get and take iron and folate supplements.
- Encourage people to build and use latrines, or to join in water and sanitation schemes to prevent diseases such as hookworm and schistosomiasis.

Increasing people's intake of iron and folate

Discuss with families how they can help women and children who are most at risk of nutritional anaemia to get more iron and folate. You can suggest that family members who are 'at risk':

- eat more of the family's usual food, especially iron-rich foods (see Appendix 3).
- eat more foods which increase iron absorption (see Section 4.10):
  - fresh foods which contain vitamin C, such as citrus fruits and tomatoes;

- foods which contain haem iron—such as meat, offal, and fish; even a small amount of meat or fish helps a lot; liver and kidney are also good sources of folate;
  - sour fermented porridge.
- eat more green vegetables. Green vegetables contain folate. Green vegetables contain vitamin C, but some also contain antinutrients which interfere with iron absorption (see Section 4.10). Advise people not to overcook vegetables, because it destroys both vitamins.
- avoid foods which decrease iron absorption. For example, do not drink tea or coffee with meals.

Other important ways in which you can help to prevent iron deficiency are:

- Encourage pregnant and recently delivered women to get and take *iron and folate tablets*. This may be the most effective thing to do. One of the main difficulties may be for health workers to get enough tablets for all the women who need them.
- Find out what women usually eat around the time of delivery. Do these foods help to increase a woman's intake or absorption of iron? If they do, encourage women to eat them.
- Encourage mothers to breastfeed. Breastfeeding from soon after delivery helps to reduce the mother's blood loss, as well as providing iron for the baby.
- Encourage families to space pregnancies at least 2 years apart. One reason is to give a woman's body time to build up her iron stores again.
- Make sure that low birth weight babies are given iron supplements from the age of 2 months, as well as breastfeeding.
- If appropriate, discuss foods which are fortified with iron.

Iron-fortified foods

Some foods have extra iron and folate added during processing. Commercial weaning foods and some brands of infant formula are examples. The iron is usually well absorbed, though it is not clear how effectively these foods prevent anaemia. Mothers who have heard about iron may wonder if they should give these fortified foods to their children.

However, fortified foods are often more expensive than unprocessed foods. Also, there are many other reasons why it is better for a mother *not* to feed her baby artificially, on either formula or cow's milk. If a mother has money to buy these foods, she could spend it more usefully on some liver, meat, or fish.

Helping people who are anaemic to get treatment

If you find or suspect that a person is anaemic, you may want to send them to a more experienced health worker:

- to measure the haemoglobin and decide how severe the anaemia is;
- to arrange for other laboratory tests of the person's blood to find out if they have malaria, sickle cell disease, thalassaemia, or folate deficiency;
- to arrange for examination of their faeces to find out if they have hookworm, schistosomiasis, or other parasites (see Section 16.12);
- to check for blood loss from other causes—for example, heavy menstrual bleeding;
- to get the necessary treatment.

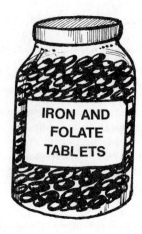

Fig. 20–7 Iron and folate tablets to prevent and treat nutritional anaemia.

Box 20.1.   Doses of iron and folate for prevention and treatment of nutritional anaemia (ACC/SCN 1991a)

Note. 1 iron and folate tablet contains 200 mg ferrous sulphate (= 60 mg iron) plus 250 µg folate.

	Daily dose	Course
PREVENTION		
Pregnant women		
Where prevalence of anaemia low	60 mg iron + 250 µg folate (1 tablet)	} Especially 2nd half
Where prevalence of anaemia high	120 mg iron + 500 µg folate (2 tablets)	} pregnancy
Newly married girls	60 mg iron + 250 µg folate (1 tablet)	4–5 months
Preschool children	30 mg iron (liquid or tablet)	} 2–3 weeks several
Schoolage children	30–60 mg iron (1 tablet)	} times a year
TREATMENT		
Pregnant women		
Severe anaemia	180 mg iron + 750 µg folate (1 tablet 3 times a day) + antimalarials (in endemic areas) + albendazole (if hookworm load heavy) + antimicrobial (if necessary for other infections)	} Until haemoglobin normal and no longer rising + 4 weeks
Moderate anaemia	120 mg iron + 500 µg folate (1 tablet 2 times a day)	
Infants and young children	3 mg iron per kilogram body weight (liquid or tablet)	Take care not to overdose
Adolescents and adults		
Mild anaemia	60 mg iron (1 tablet)	} Give with folate if
Moderate/severe anaemia	120 mg iron (1 tablet 2 times a day)	} available

Give iron orally unless there is severe vomiting or the patient is persistently not taking tablets.

20.8 TAKING IRON AND FOLATE TABLETS

It is sometimes difficult to get people to take iron or iron and folate tablets for the 4–5 months that is usually necessary to treat anaemia. The reasons are:

- The supply of tablets may not be enough for all the people who need them.
- People do not understand the need to take the tablets for a long time.
- Some people find that iron tablets cause side-effects, such as stomach pains, nausea, constipation, or diarrhoea, and that they make the faeces black. This is most likely with larger doses of 2–3 tablets a day.

What you can do to help

- Try to make sure that there are enough tablets available for community workers and others who give them to people.
- Take time to explain to communities and individuals why pregnant women and sometimes other people need iron and folate and why they need to take them for several months.
- To prevent side-effects, suggest a smaller dose to start with (e.g. 1 tablet daily) and increase to the full dose after 1–2 weeks. It also helps to take the tablet with a meal.

THINGS TO DO

Class exercise

1. Ask trainees to use Table 4.2 to find out how much iron a pregnant woman needs to eat each day if she eats plenty of haem iron. Liver is one of the richest sources of haem iron.

   a. Use the Food Composition Tables in Appendix 1 to find out how much haem iron liver contains.

   b. Ask trainees to calculate how much liver a pregnant woman needs to eat if all her iron comes from liver.

   c. Could most women eat this much liver?

   Use this example to discuss the difficulty pregnant women have eating enough iron.

Project

2. Ask trainees to make a list of locally available iron-rich foods and to find out their cost. Use formulae at the end of Table 9.1 to find out the cost of 10 mg iron from each food. Discuss if haem iron is more expensive than non-haem iron.

Field visits

3. Take trainees to visit a clinic or hospital, so that they can talk to some pregnant or recently delivered women about what they usually eat. They should try to find out whether the women ate any food containing haem iron:

   - in the last week;
   - in the last month;
   - at any time during pregnancy.

   The trainees should ask to examine the women's tongues and lips for anaemia. If the women have had their haemoglobin measured, trainees can compare the results with their own assessment.

4. When trainees see children being weighed, or children in a health centre or ward, encourage them to think about the children's haemoglobins as well as their weight.

   Trainees can look at the children's tongues, and inside their lower lips, to see if they are anaemic. They can compare the children's tongues with their mother's tongues, or with a colleague's tongue.

5. Ask health staff if there are any older children or other patients whom they know to be anaemic. Ask if trainees could see the patient, and ask what the haemoglobin is. Trainees should explain what they want to do, and ask the patient to show their tongue.

   These patients may have anaemia due to other diseases and not nutritional anaemia. However, examining them may help trainees to learn to recognize a person with a low haemoglobin.

Group work with stories

6. Put trainees into small groups. Ask groups to read these stories, and to make lists of all the things in them that could be due to anaemia.

   List 1. The *symptoms* that the people themselves notice.

   List 2. What their friends and family may notice.

   List 3. The *signs* that a health or nutrition worker should look for to check for anaemia.

   Write down possible causes of the anaemia in each case. Discuss conclusions in class.

   The story of Asha

   Asha has four children; the youngest is 7 years old. The family have a very small farm, and they grow rice. They usually have enough rice to eat, and they eat it with whatever vegetables they can get—sometimes a few beans, sometimes green vegetables growing round the house, which Asha stews for a long time. Sometimes

Asha has some coconut to cook the vegetables with. Often the family have to eat the rice by itself or with a little sauce.

For the last year or so Asha has been feeling more and more tired. She has found it very difficult to work, even though she does not have a baby now. She has become breathless more easily than before, and her periods have been heavy. She decided to go to the health centre.

The health worker listened to Asha's story. She examined Asha, and looked at her tongue and the inside of her lower lip. 'Your tongue is very pale, and I think that your blod is thin. I would like to arrange for you to have a blood test. Tell me what you usually eat.'

Two schools

The nurse lived about a mile from the health centre. On her way to work, she passed two schools. In one of the schools, most of the children were from a village that had been there for as long as anyone could remember. Most of the children in the other school were from families in a new agricultural scheme. The nurse noticed every day that the children from the agricultural scheme made much more noise than the children in the old village school. She decided to visit the schools to find out why.

The nurse talked to the teachers, who seemed to think that the 'noisy' children were quicker at learning than the 'quiet' children. She examined the children, and asked them to put out their tongues. She noticed that many of the 'quiet' children had pale tongues, but that most of the 'noisy' children's tongues were redder in colour.

The nurse took faeces samples from the children, and she found that many of the 'quiet' children had hookworm, but only a few of the 'noisy' children had hookworm. Then she enquired about where the children defecated. She learned that the children from the old village defecated in the bush, as their families had always done. The new village had pit latrines, and most of the children were using them.

She asked some of the children what they ate at lunch time. The children in the new school said that the teacher had taught them all to bring a midday meal to school, with a staple, some legumes, and some fresh fruit. The children in the old school often had no midday meal at all. Those who had some money bought sweets or biscuits.

Baby Fatimah

Fatimah's mother had a job as a secretary. Her boss wanted her to come back to work as soon as possible after her baby was born, so she decided to bottle feed Fatimah. She bought powdered full cream milk, and she budgeted carefully, so that she had enough to make feeds of the correct strength all through the month. Baby Fatimah gained weight well, and her mother decided not to start solids for a time. When Fatimah was 6 months old, she had a nasty cough and cold, which would not get better, and one evening her mother took her to the doctor. The doctor examined Fatimah, and looked in her mouth. 'Baby's tongue looks very pale, I think she may be anaemic. I would like to test her blood.'

USEFUL PUBLICATIONS

ACC/SCN (1991). *Controlling iron deficiency*, Nutrition Policy Discussion Paper, no. 9. ACC/SCN, Geneva.

Children in the Tropics (1990). Iron and folate deficiency anaemias. *Children in the Tropics*, **Vol. 186**.

DeMaeyer, E. in collaboration with Dallman, P., Gurney, J. M., Hallberg, L., Sood, S. K., and SeiKantia, S. G. (1989). *Preventing and controlling iron deficiency anaemia through primary health care*. WHO, Geneva.

21 Iodine deficiency disorders

Nutritionists estimate that about 1 billion people or 12 per cent of the world's population are at risk of iodine deficiency, and that 20–30 per cent of the people at risk show signs of deficiency. Most of them live in isolated places far from the sea.

21.1 CAUSES OF IODINE DEFICIENCY

Lack of iodine in food

The most important cause of iodine deficiency is lack of iodine in food which *continues for a long time*.

The thyroid gland at the front of the neck stores iodine (see Section 4.11). This store enables the gland to continue producing thyroid hormones for a number of months, even when there is little iodine in the person's food. But after some time, if the amount of iodine in the diet does not increase, signs of deficiency appear.

Goitrogens

Goitrogens are substances in food which reduce the amount of iodine that the thyroid takes up from the blood. If a person lacks iodine, goitrogens make the deficiency worse. One important goitrogen is the toxin in bitter cassava roots or leaves which have not been properly processed (see Section 7.8). Other goitrogens occur in some kinds of millet and in contaminated water.

21.2 IODINE DEFICIENCY DISORDERS (IDDs)

This is a group of disorders that iodine-deficient people may develop. Which type of disorder a person has and how severe it is depends on the following factors.

How much iodine is available to the thyroid gland
This depends on:

- how much iodine is stored in the body;
- how much iodine the food contains;
- whether or not the food also contains goitrogens.

For the unborn baby, how much iodine is available depends on how much is in the mother's blood; and for the breastfeeding baby, on how much there is in breast milk. Both depend on the mother's diet.

How much the person needs
Needs are higher:

- during growth of infants, children, and adolescents;
- during pregnancy and lactation.

How IDDs develop

- If there is not enough iodine in food, the level of iodine in the blood falls, and the stores of iodine in the thyroid gland are used up.
- The thyroid gland enlarges to collect more iodine from the blood. The enlarged gland is called a *goitre*.
- If the enlarged thyroid gland produces enough thyroid hormone, the person's body works normally. The goitre is the only abnormality.
- If the gland fails to produce enough thyroid hormone, the person becomes *hypothyroid*.

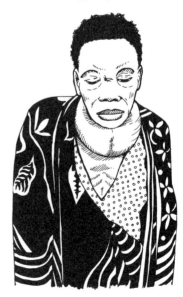

Fig. 21–1 A goitre is an enlarged thyroid gland.

277

21.3 GOITRE

Goitres vary in size from those that you can only feel to those that you can easily see.

Goitres often start in childhood and gradually enlarge, particularly during puberty. In women they may continue to enlarge, but in men they usually stop enlarging and may get smaller. A goitre often gets bigger during pregnancy and lactation because the body needs more thyroid hormone at that time. It may continue to increase in size with each new pregnancy.

Giving iodine can reduce the size of some goitres, especially in young people with smaller goitres. In adults who have had a large goitre for a long time, iodine may not reduce the size of the goitre very much. Iodine is also not very effective if the goitre is *nodular*, that is lumpy.

Large goitres are ugly and uncomfortable. Sometimes the swelling presses on the trachea and causes difficulty breathing. It may press on the oesophagus and cause difficulty swallowing. It may press on blood vessels and interfere with the flow of blood. Surgery may be the only useful treatment when this happens.

21.4 HYPOTHYROIDISM

A *person* who is hypothyroid:

- feels cold easily;
- moves slowly and lacks energy;
- thinks slowly and appears unconcerned ('apathy');
- may be sleepy;
- has a dry skin;
- may be constipated.

A *child* who is hypothyroid also:

- grows slowly, and may be very short;
- may not do well in school.

These problems all improve if you give the person iodine.

Women who are hypothyroid during pregnancy may also have:

- miscarriages or stillbirths;
- low birth weight babies;
- babies with congenital deformities.

Babies born to hypothyroid mothers may have *cretinism*. You can prevent these effects if you give iodine to women before pregnancy.

21.5 CRETINISM

There are two types of cretinism—*neurological* and *hypothyroid*. Some people show signs of both types. Which type is commonest varies from area to area.

Box 21.1.   How to examine and classify goitres

Examination
- Stand or sit facing the person (see Fig. 21–2).
- Place your two thumbs on either side of the person's trachea, several centimetres below the larynx ('voice box').
- Roll your thumbs gently over the thyroid (which lies next to the trachea). This is called 'palpation'.
- If each lobe of the thyroid is smaller than the end joint of the person's thumb, there is no goitre.
- If one or both lobes is larger than the end joint of the person's thumb, then there is a goitre.
- Ask the person to bend their head back and look upwards. Try to see the goitre.
- Ask the person to look straight forward, and try to see the goitre again.
- Notice if you can see the goitre from a distance of about 10 metres, or only from close up.

Classification
Grade   0: No goitre. Lobes smaller than end joint of thumb.
Grade 1A: Thyroid lobes larger than ends of thumbs.
Grade 1B: Thyroid gland visible with head bent back.
Grade   2: Thyroid gland visible with head in normal position.
Grade   3: Thyroid gland visible from about 10 metres.

In a community survey:

Grades 2 and 3 are called *visible goitre*.
Grades 1A, 1B, with grades 2 and 3 are called *total goitre*.

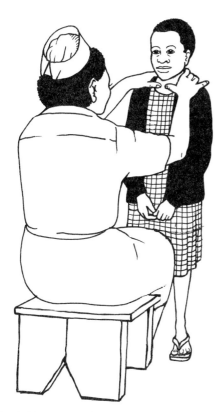

Fig. 21–2 How to examine the thyroid gland.

Neurological cretinism

The baby has damage to the brain and nervous system. The effects vary from those that are mild and difficult to find to severe mental and physical handicap. The effects may include:

- deafness and *mutism* (the child cannot speak);
- squint (the eyes are not held straight);
- weakness and stiffness especially of the legs;
- severe mental handicap.

Neurological cretinism is likely if the mother is iodine-deficient in the early part of pregnancy, when the baby's brain and nervous system are developing.

Neurological cretinism cannot be treated. Giving iodine does not help. The child remains handicapped throughout life, and may die young. You can, however, prevent neurological cretinism if you give iodine to mothers before conception. This is one of the main reasons why it is important to prevent iodine deficiency.

Hypothyroid cretinism

The baby has signs which are similar to those listed under 'hypothyroidism' in older people. The baby may:

- not feed well;
- fail to gain weight;
- be constipated;
- feel cold;
- seem very sleepy;
- have a thick dry skin;
- have a hoarse cry;
- develop slowly and be mentally handicapped.

Hypothyroid cretinism is likely if the mother is iodine-deficient in later pregnancy. Breastfeeding may partly protect the baby and effects of iodine deficiency may become worse after weaning.

If you give the baby iodine, the signs may improve or disappear. The earlier the baby gets iodine, the better the result. Treatment may not be effective if it is started after a child is about 1 or 2 years old. So it is important to try to find and treat hypothyroid babies as early as possible.

It is even better to give mothers iodine before or during pregnancy to prevent deficiency altogether. (Hypothyroid cretins can also be treated with thyroid hormones, but these are not available in many places.)

21.6 WHY IDDs ARE IMPORTANT

- Iodine deficiency delays social and economic development in the area because:
  - There are more handicapped people who need care from the community.
  - Cattle, goats, chickens, and other domestic animals are also iodine-deficient. They grow more slowly and reproduce less.
  - Local people are mentally slower and less energetic than healthy people. It is more difficult to *motivate* them.
- Iodine-deficient children are difficult to educate and they are less likely to get good jobs when they grow up.
- Children with cretinism often die young. Severely disabled children who survive can be a burden on their families and communities. Less disabled people, if they are physically strong, may be able to do simple manual tasks.
- A large goitre may reduce a person's chances of marriage or employment.

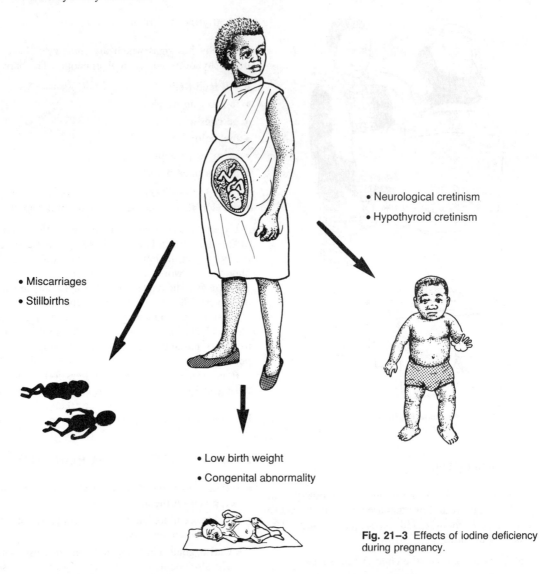

- Neurological cretinism
- Hypothyroid cretinism

- Miscarriages
- Stillbirths

- Low birth weight
- Congenital abnormality

Fig. 21–3 Effects of iodine deficiency during pregnancy.

21.7 HOW TO ASSESS THE SEVERITY OF IDDs IN AN AREA

There are two *indicators* which are useful. It is best to use both indicators if possible (Table 21.1).

1. Prevalence of goitre

Find the percentage of people or children in a community who have goitre. Goitre is the only widespread sign of iodine deficiency that is easy to recognize, and that does not need laboratory tests. Most surveys count only *total goitre*, that is the presence or absence of goitre of any size. They do not record *grades* of goitre.

2. The level of iodine in urine

The level of urinary iodine is a measure of the amount of iodine in the body. Collect samples of urine from at least 40 people. Send the samples to a laboratory which can estimate the concentration of iodine in them (see ICCIDD in press, in Appendix 6).

Organizing a survey

Usually the most convenient method is to do goitre surveys and urine collection on children aged 6–12 years old from schools in poor or remote villages.

Table 21.1.   Classification of severity of IDDs

Severity of IDDS	Prevalence of goitre	Mean urinary iodine (μg iodine/100 ml)
Using goitre and urinary iodine		
Mild	10–30%	3.5–5.0
Moderate	20–50%	2.0–3.5
Severe	30–100%	Less than 2.0
Using goitre only		
Mild	5–20% of children	
Moderate	20–30% of children	
Severe	More than 30% of children	

If you cannot do a survey, you know that there is a severe IDD problem if:

1. More than 10% of people have a *visible* goitre.
2. Many men have large goitres.

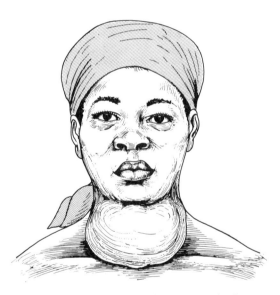

Fig. 21–4 A large goitre may reduce a person's chances of marriage or employment.

School-age children are easy to reach and they show well how much iodine deficiency there is in the area *now*. Goitre in adults may be the result of previous deficiency.

21.8 PREVENTION AND TREATMENT OF IDDs

To prevent and treat iodine deficiency disorders, it is necessary to give people iodine. Giving iodine can:

- prevent all IDDs;
- reduce the size of some goitres;
- correct some of the effects of hypothyroidism;
- make people who lack iodine *feel better* (even if the size of their goitres does not decrease much).

There are several ways to give iodine:

- adding iodine to salt;
- giving large doses of iodine by mouth or by injection;
- adding iodine to drinking water;
- giving Lugol's iodine.

Adding iodine to salt

Most people eat some salt. It is possible to add iodine to almost any kind of salt during processing. This is called *iodizing*. (The chemical kind of iodine added is usually *potassium iodate* or *potassium iodide*.) Iodizing does not alter the taste or appearance of the salt.

Iodizing salt is an effective way to control IDDs if:

- The amount of iodine in the salt is carefully monitored and controlled. This is easier where there are only a few producers of salt.
- Iodized salt reaches the people who lack iodine.
- People who lack iodine want and can afford to buy the iodized salt.

Iodizing is less effective when there are many small producers, because it is difficult to monitor and control the addition of iodine to the salt.

Iodizing salt may be the best long-term way to give iodine. But it takes a long time before iodized salt regularly reaches the consumers who need it. Therefore it is often necessary to give iodine in some other quicker way first.

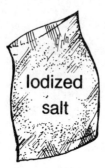

Fig. 21–5 Adding iodine to salt helps to control IDDs.

Giving large doses of iodine—iodized oil

You can give iodized oil by mouth or by injection. It usually contains 480 mg iodine in 1 ml of oil. This may be the best way to give iodine before iodized salt becomes available.

The groups that most need iodine, in order of importance, are:

- women of childbearing age (including lactating women);
- children aged 0–15 years;
- men to age 45 years.

It is not necessary to give iodine for prevention to babies under the age of 1 year if they are breastfed. They should get the iodine that they need from breast milk.

Old people need less iodine. If they have been iodine-deficient for a long time, they have a greater risk of side-effects. They are not usually given large doses.

Iodized oil by mouth

This is easier and safer than injections. The iodine is stored in the body, and should prevent iodine deficiency for 1–2 years. The dose for all ages is 1 ml of iodized oil. You may have capsules, or you can give the oil by syringe on to the tongue (but without touching the tongue).

Iodized oil by injection

One injection prevents iodine deficiency for 3–5 years. The iodine slowly enters the body from the injection site. The thyroid gland collects and concentrates it.

The dose for people aged 1–45 years is 1 ml. Give a baby under 1 year of age who is not breastfed, or who needs treatment for iodine deficiency 0.5 ml. Give an older person with a nodular goitre 0.2 ml.

For small children inject the oil into the buttocks or thighs. For older children and adults, inject into the upper arm.

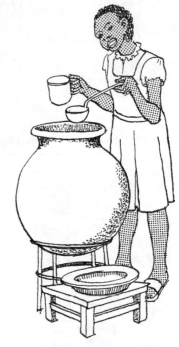

Fig. 21–6 Iodine can be added to the drinking water of a school.

Adding iodine to drinking water

In some situations this is a more practical way to give iodine. Sometimes iodine can be added to public piped water supplies. Sometimes iodine is added directly to a container of drinking water—for example, in a school. The iodine solution can be prepared locally, and distributed in dropper bottles to schools or households. Add a measured number of drops of solution to drinking water each day to give each person on average about 150 µg iodine per day.

Giving Lugol's iodine

Sometimes this is the easiest way to give iodine. Lugol's iodine is cheap, and is widely available in small hospitals and health centres, usually for antiseptic use. Iodine in

Lugol's solution is stored only in the thyroid gland and not elsewhere in the body, so you have to give it more often than iodized oil.

The exact dose has not been worked out, but a useful guide is:

- Give 1 drop of Lugol's iodine (which contains 6 mg iodine) every 30 days; *or*
- Dilute the Lugol's iodine and give a solution containing 1 mg iodine every 7 days—for example, put one drop in 30 ml water and give a teaspoonful.

21.9 WHAT A NUTRITION WORKER CAN DO TO HELP PREVENT IDDs

Watch for signs that IDDs are a problem in the area where you work

The most important sign to look for is goitre. Notice especially if women develop goitres during pregnancy. If you suspect that IDDs may be a problem, discuss it with your supervisors, so that you can find out more about it and can if necessary get help to control it.

Consider ways to give iodine to people 'at risk'

There may be no IDD control programme in your area, but some people have iodine deficiency. Discuss with your supervisor how to give iodine to people who are most at risk. For example:

- Is it possible to give pregnant and lactating women Lugol's iodine?
- Can you put iodine into drinking water in schools?

Help with an IDD control programme

If there is a programme in your area, you may need to:

- explain the purpose of the programme to the public;
- help with surveys;
- monitor supplies and sales of iodized salt;
- monitor supplies and distribution of iodized oil;
- report any problems to programme supervisors.

Explain to people that it is dangerous to eat unprocessed bitter cassava

Eating bitter cassava that is raw or not processed properly is a risk (see Section 7.8). This may be most likely to happen when food supplies get low, in the 'hungry season'.

THINGS TO DO

Demonstrations

1. Show trainees pictures of people with iodine deficiency disorders.
2. Demonstrate how to examine for goitre. Let trainees work in pairs and practise examining for goitre with each other.

Discussion

3. Discuss the effects of IDDs on a community. Which effects are most important? Are they likely to occur where trainees will work?

Project

4. Ask trainees to find out what sorts of salt are available in the area. Are they iodized or not?

USEFUL PUBLICATIONS

Dunn, J. and van der Haar, F. (1990). *A practical guide to the correction of iodine deficiency*. ICCIDD, Adelaide.

Hetzel, B. S. (1988). *The prevention and control of iodine deficiency disorders*. ACC/SCN Nutrition Policy Discussion Paper, no. 3. ACC/SCN, Geneva.

Hetzel, B. S. (1989). *The story of iodine deficiency*. Oxford University Press, Oxford.

22 Overnutrition and related disorders

22.1 OBESITY

People who eat more than they need to cover their nutrient needs are likely to become *overweight* or *obese*. **Overweight** means that the person is *too heavy* for their height. Their weight is above the range of weights of healthy people.

A few very active people (such as some boxers and weight lifters) are overweight because they have developed large muscles. You can usually see if a person is overweight because of muscles. Most people who are overweight are *too fat*. Being too fat is called *obesity*.

How to recognize obesity

Adults

- Examine the person. It is easy to see if someone is very obese.
- Measure height and weight. Use Table A5.7 in Appendix 5 to decide if a person is too heavy for their height. Or use Fig. 22–2. Or calculate the person's *'body mass index' (BMI)* (see Box 22.1).
- A quick way to tell if a man is obese is to find out if his waist is bigger than his chest. If it is, he is obese. You cannot use this method with women.

Children

- Examine the child. It is easy to see if a child is very obese.
- Measure weight-for-height (see Section 14.17). The child is overweight if above the 97th centile (120 per cent) of reference weight for height (see Tables A5.4–A5.6 in Appendix 5).
- If it is not possible to measure the child's height, measure weight for age or, if the child is under 5 years old, use the growth chart.

  A child whose weight is above the 97th centile curve is *overweight*. In Chapter 14 we explained that 3 out of every 100 healthy children have weights a little above the 97th centile curve. So if a child's weight is just above the 97th centile curve, he may be healthy. But if it is a long way above it, he is obese.
- If you are monitoring a child's weight on a growth chart, examine the growth line. If it is rising faster

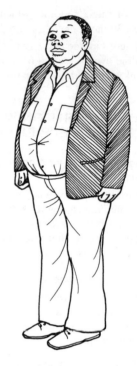

Fig. 22–1 This man is obese.

than the reference curve, and it is not because the child is 'catching-up' lost weight, the child may be becoming obese.

22.2 WHY BEING OVERWEIGHT MATTERS

People who are overweight are at greater risk of several disorders. These include:

- coronary heart disease;
- strokes;
- high blood pressure;
- adult-type diabetes;
- gall stones and other digestive disorders;
- back problems;
- arthritis of the knee and hip.

284

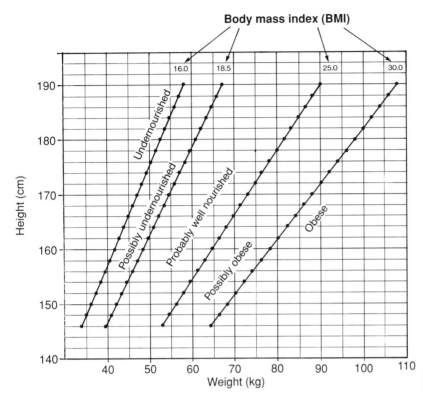

Body mass index (BMI)

Fig. 22–2 Weights-for-heights of adults.

Box 22.1. Body mass index (BMI) (Beaton *et al.* 1990)

One way to assess the nutrition of adults is to calculate their 'body mass index' or BMI.

$$BMI = \frac{Weight\ in\ kg}{(Height\ in\ metres)^2}$$

Example. Hannah weighs 55 kg. Her height is 160 cm.

$$So\ her\ BMI = \frac{50}{1.60 \times 1.60} = 21.$$

If the BMI is:

- below 16, the person is undernourished;
- 16–18.5, the person is possibly undernourished;
- 18.5–25, the person is probably well nourished;
- 25–30, the person is possibly obese;
- over 30, the person is obese.

You cannot use BMI to assess nutrition in pregnant women.

These disorders may result in earlier death or in disability, which makes it difficult to work and support or care for a family.

Obese people are also more likely to have accidents and broken bones, and to become tired quickly.

Overweight children risk becoming overweight adults. They may be unable to run or play games as well as healthy children. Other children may tease them.

22.3 WHY PEOPLE BECOME OBESE

People become obese when they eat more Calories than they burn for energy. The extra Calories are changed into storage fat. People eat many Calories when:

- They eat large amounts of food at each meal;
- They eat a lot of energy-rich foods such as:
  - *fatty foods*, especially those which contain little fibre—for example, cooking oil and fat, butter, margarine and fried foods such as chips, samosas, and sausages;
  - *sugary foods* especially those which contain little fibre—for example, sugar, honey, sweets, biscuits, cakes, jam, and ice cream and drinks such as sodas and sweet tea.
- They eat energy-rich snacks between meals;
- They drink a lot of beer.

People burn few Calories when:

- They do little physical activity. A woman who is sewing burns fewer Calories than a woman who is sweeping. A man who is doing office work burns fewer Calories than a man who is cutting wood.
- They have a low basal metabolic rate (BMR).

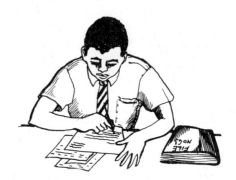

A man doing office work burns fewer calories

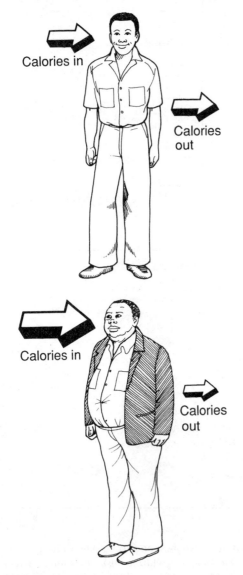

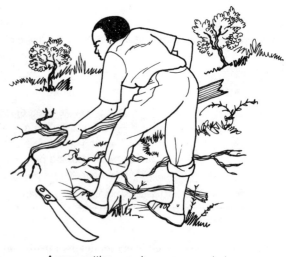

A man cutting wood uses more calories

Fig. 22–3 When 'Calories in' are more than 'Calories out' the person becomes obese.

Fig. 22–4 People use fewer Calories when they do not take much exercise.

22.4 WHY MORE PEOPLE ARE OVERWEIGHT NOW THAN IN THE PAST

More people are overnourished now than in the past, because the life style of many people has changed. For example:

- People eat foods which contain more fat and sugar than before. For example, a family may eat chips instead of maize porridge.

  100 g chips gives about 560 kcal;
  100 g maize porridge gives about 100 kcal.

  People may eat more fried food because:
  - Frying is a quick way for busy housewives to cook food.
  - Fried 'fast foods' are favourite meals for people who work in towns, and who cannot go home regularly.
- People eat fatty or sweet snacks instead of fruit or starchy foods.
- Modern meals often use highly processed foods which contain less fibre than traditional meals. Low-fibre meals may not make people feel as full as high-fibre meals. Also the nutrients from low-fibre meals are digested and absorbed more quickly, so a person may become hungry sooner and may eat more.

  Figure 22–6 shows that people eating modern diets get much more of their energy from sugar and fat, and less from starch than people eating traditional diets.
- Some people drink much more alcohol.
- People are less active. This is often the most important cause of obesity. For example, many people go to work by bus or car instead of walking. They work in offices instead of on farms. Some women have piped water and kerosene stoves so they do not have to carry water and wood. They can buy milled maize instead of pounding it themselves.

22.5 PEOPLE WHO ARE AT RISK OF OBESITY

Adults are at risk of obesity:

- *if they have enough money:*
  - to buy plenty of energy-rich foods such as butter and sugar;
  - to use cars instead of walking;
  - to employ other people to work for them.

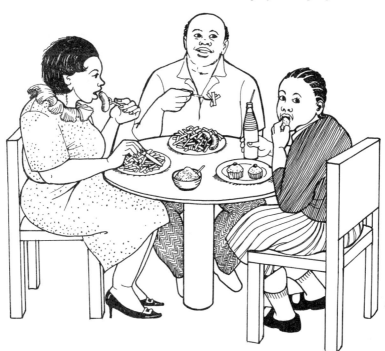

Fig. 22–5 The life style of many people has changed. Many people now eat more sweet and fatty foods.

- *if they live in towns:*
  - energy-rich foods are often easier to get in towns;
  - people in rural areas are usually more active.

- *if they do only light work*, for example, if they mostly sit down at work.

- *if they are middle-aged or old*. They may be less active, but eat the same as when they were younger, so they slowly become fatter.

- *after childbirth*. Women who are well nourished during pregnancy lay down a store of fat, to make breast milk. Women need some extra nutrients for the baby during pregnancy and lactation, but not too much. If women continue to eat extra and if they are less active after childbirth, they may not use up the store of fat. Some women gain weight and become obese. Women are especially likely to keep their fat stores or to gain weight if they do not breastfeed.

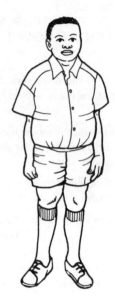

Fig. 22–7 Some children are obese.

22.6 CHILDREN WHO ARE OBESE

Children are sometimes obese because:

- *They have a disease.* This is rare.

- *They eat more Calories than they use.* The reasons are the same as with adults. They may eat too much energy-rich food, or take little exercise, or both. A child who is overweight becomes less active, because it is more difficult to run about. So he may become more obese as he becomes older.

Children at greatest risk of obesity are those:

- from richer families, who buy many sweet and fatty foods;
- who are overfed on formula.

Young children should not get used to eating too many sweet and fatty foods, or they will be at risk of developing obesity later.

22.7 OTHER CONDITIONS RELATED TO OVERNUTRITION

Coronary heart disease and stroke

Atheroma and thrombosis
Over several years, patches of fat build up in the lining

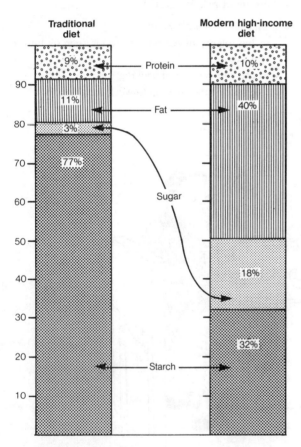

Fig. 22–6 The nutrients from which people get their Calories.

of some arteries, making them narrower. This is called *atheroma*. Sometimes a clot of blood forms where there is a patch of atheroma, and it blocks the artery completely. This is *thrombosis*. When an artery is blocked, the part of the body which it supplies receives too little food and oxygen. It cannot work properly, and may die.

If an artery in the heart is blocked, the person has *coronary heart disease* (CHD) or ischaemic heart disease (IHD). If an artery in the brain is blocked, the person has a *stroke* and may be paralysed down one side of the body.

Coronary heart disease

Usually, a patch of atheroma has been quietly building up in the blood vessels for several years. The person has severe chest pain on exercise, which passes when he rests. He may become unable to do much physical work. He may have a '*heart attack*', when part of the heart is damaged, and he may die suddenly.

This is one of the commonest diseases associated with a modern 'Westernized' diet and life style. It is one of the main causes of death and disability among middle-aged adults, especially men. These people are usually supporting a family. The whole family is affected if the wage earner dies or cannot work.

Factors which increase the risk of CHD and stroke

We do not yet know all the things which increase the risk of CHD and stroke, but the following are important:

- Smoking.
- Obesity. Obesity is just *one* risk factor. CHD and stroke also occur in people of normal weight.
- High blood pressure. Eating too much salt is one thing which increases the risk of high blood pressure in *some* adults (Section 4.15). Obesity, too much alcohol, and not enough exercise also increase the risk of high blood pressure.
- High blood cholesterol. A high level of low-density lipoprotein (LDL) cholesterol in the blood may increase the risk of CHD and stroke. The type and amount of fatty acids in food affect the blood cholesterol (see Section 2.5).
- Not enough exercise.
- Diabetes.
- Drinking too much alcohol. Small amounts may reduce risk, but large amounts increase risk.

There may be other factors too, such as stress, and undernutrition in early childhood, that increase the risk of CHD and stroke.

Diabetes

In diabetes, the level of glucose in the blood is too high, and glucose is passed in the urine. A hormone *insulin* controls the movement of glucose from the blood into the body cells. Obesity interferes with the action of insulin and is one of the causes of diabetes which starts in adults. (Children have a different kind of diabetes.)

The best way to control diabetes in adults is to reduce obesity. Fibre may help to protect against adult diabetes and may be helpful in control. Fibre in food slows down the digestion and absorption of sugars. The body can more easily control the glucose if it comes into the blood slowly.

22.8 HOW TO PREVENT OBESITY AND RELATED DISORDERS

Treating obesity is difficult. It is better to help people to stay a normal healthy weight.

Advice to prevent obesity

- Eat meals which contain plenty of fibre, and not too much fat or sugar.
- Eat snacks which are not energy-rich. Eat foods such as fruit or maize cobs, and avoid foods such as sweets, chips, crisps, and cakes.
- Do not drink too much alcohol.
- Take regular exercise. The best type of exercise is one which moves all parts of the body and makes you breathe a little faster than at rest (but not gasp for breath). For example, walking briskly or uphill, digging the garden, dancing, or playing football. But any physical activity, such as walking to work or using stairs instead of the lift, can help.

  Exercise needs to be for a minimum of about 150 minutes a week. Doctors recommend that we exercise for about 20 minutes a day, or an hour three times a week.

Foods which people think of as 'fattening'

Some people think of certain foods as 'bad' or 'fattening'. It may help to explain these points to them:

- Fatty foods are *not* 'bad' foods; it is essential to eat a certain amount of fat, especially essential fatty acids. Fatty foods cause overnutrition only if you eat too much.
- Starchy foods such as potatoes and bread are not 'fattening'.

Box 22.2.   Healthy eating to prevent obesity and related disorders

Plenty of: *Moderate amounts of:*

Cereals and roots   *Fat, fatty foods, fried food*
Legumes   *Sugar*
Vegetables   *Meat*
Fruit   *Salt*
Fish   *Tea and coffee*

Very little:
Foods rich in saturated fats
Alcohol

+ Plenty of exercise and no smoking

- Fruits and other foods which contain unrefined sugar are not 'fattening', because they contain fibre. They are not energy-rich.
- There is no need to eat refined sugar, because it gives Calories only. You can get all the energy that you need from other foods, which contain other nutrients and fibre. But it is all right to eat *some* sugar.

Advice to reduce the risk of CHD and stroke

Encourage people who may be at risk:

- to stop smoking;
- to take more exercise;
- not to become overweight;
- not to eat too much fat, especially saturated fat, such as vegetable oils;

- to eat more vegetables and fruits:
  - Fibre may reduce the absorption of fat, and lower blood cholesterol.
  - Micronutrients help to destroy free radicals, which may cause some of the damage to blood vessels.
- to eat less salt, especially if they eat more than other people—for example, if they eat a lot of salty food, or if they add a lot of salt to food;
- to have treatment to lower blood pressure if it is high.

22.9 HOW TO HELP PEOPLE LOSE WEIGHT

Obese people often ask nutrition workers how to lose weight. You need to discuss with them how they can

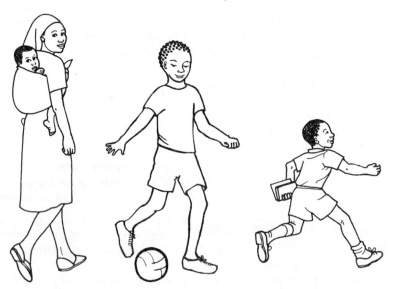

Fig. 22–8 Regular exercise helps to prevent obesity and related disorders.

change their eating and living habits so that they eat less *and* exercise more. When they have a satisfactory weight they must be willing to eat differently and exercise more for the rest of their lives. Otherwise slimming is a waste of time. It may help to suggest that people make changes in their meals gradually. Then they are more likely to continue to eat a healthier diet.

There are different ways to lose weight which suit different people. For most people the best advice is:

- *Eat smaller amounts of food at each meal.* Eat good healthy 'mixed' meals, but take less. It may help to drink a glass of water before meals to 'fill you up'. At each meal, stop eating before you feel quite full.

- *Eat less fatty foods.*
  - Boil, steam, or grill food instead of frying it. 1 cup of boiled potatoes gives about 100 Calories. 1 cup of chips gives about 600 Calories.
  - Cut the fat off fatty meat. Cut the skin off chicken (most of the fat is under the skin).
  - Spread less butter or margarine on bread. Cut the bread thicker.
  - If you must eat chips, cut potatoes thicker.
  - Do not eat crisps, samosas, or other fatty snacks.

- *Eat less sugar-rich food.*
  - Add less sugar or no sugar to tea, coffee, and porridge.
  - Use less sugar when you cook.
  - Drink fewer sodas.
  - Instead of sweet or fatty snacks, eat boiled maize cobs, non-sweet biscuits, and bread or fruit (see Section 8.6).

- *Eat more fibre and bulky foods.*
  - Eat more starchy foods such as cereals (wholegrain if possible), potatoes, cassava, bananas, plantains, and legumes.
  - Eat more fresh vegetables and fruits.

- *Drink only small amounts of beer and other alcohol.*

- *Take exercise every day.* Exercise for at least 20 minutes a day, or an hour 3 times a week, as described above.

Why most slimming diets do not work for long

There are many slimming diets advertised in newspapers and magazines. But most are difficult to follow because they contain very few Calories, so they leave you feeling very hungry. Some are expensive, and some may be dangerous because they do not supply enough minerals, vitamins, or other nutrients. People should check with a health worker before they start a commercial slimming diet.

Some people who eat very low Calorie diets adapt to the low energy intake by reducing their basal metabolic rate (BMR), and using *less* Calories. When they stop the diet, their bodies continue to use less energy, so there are more spare Calories to change into fat. Many people gain weight again very quickly again after dieting.

On some diets, people 'burn' muscles, instead of storage fat for energy. They may lose a lot of water and minerals, so they lose weight quite quickly. As soon as they eat normal foods, they gain weight again, so they become discouraged.

It is much better that obese people lose weight slowly and regularly, by taking more exercise and eating healthy mixed meals.

Some people find that it is helpful to join a health club when they start to change the way that they eat and live. Try to find one which advises good mixed meals and plenty of exercise.

22.10 TOOTH DECAY AND GUM DISEASE

Many people have tooth decay or gum disease, which often starts in childhood. These problems are becoming more common because people eat more sugar and less fibre.

Tooth decay (or *dental caries*) means holes slowly forming in the teeth. Teeth with holes may be painful, and may prevent a person from eating properly. The bone around the tooth may become infected resulting in an abscess. If a tooth is severely damaged, or an abscess forms, the tooth may have to be pulled out.

Gum disease (or *periodontal disease*) is damage to the tissues that hold and support the teeth. The person may notice bleeding gums, an unpleasant taste in the mouth, and bad smelling breath. However, gum disease is not usually painful, so a person may not be aware of the damage. However, the teeth may become loose and fall out.

People who lose many teeth cannot eat properly— often they can only eat soft food. So tooth decay and gum disease may be a cause of poor nutrition especially among old people.

22.11 THE CAUSE OF TOOTH DECAY AND GUM DISEASE

Many bacteria live in our mouths. When we eat, some of the food sticks to our teeth. The bacteria multiply in this food, forming a layer of yellow-white *plaque*. The bacteria also form waste substances such as acids which damage the teeth and gums.

You may be able to feel plaque on your teeth with your tongue—it feels furry, or you can scrape some off with your fingernail. You may feel it in your mouth when you wake up in the morning. Most plaque forms between the teeth and the gums where food sticks most easily.

If you do not clean away the plaque every day, it becomes hard, called *tartar* or *calculus*. Only a dentist can remove calculus. Plaque grows on the calculus and is more difficult to brush off than plaque on teeth.

Bacteria multiply fastest in sweet foods and drinks which stick to the teeth. For example:

- sweets;
- lollies;
- cakes;
- biscuits;
- sugar;
- ice cream;
- sodas and other sugary drinks;
- honey;
- jam.

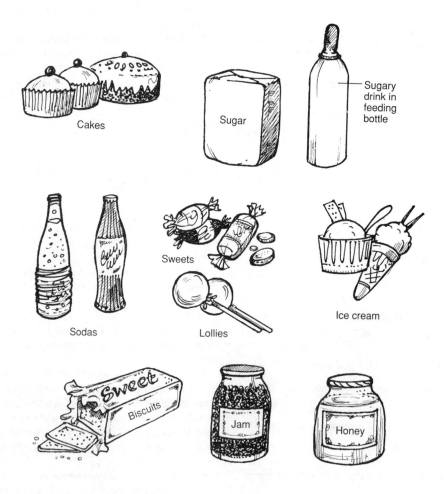

Fig. 22–9 Sweet foods which are bad for teeth.

Each time we eat sweet sticky foods, the bacteria multiply fast and form waste substances for about 2 hours. If we eat sticky foods many times each day, the bacteria make waste substances all day. All day the teeth are covered in acid which damages them.

Sweet foods which are not sticky are not bad for the teeth. Fruits and some vegetables and sugar cane contain sugar, but it is not sticky. Most of the sugar is still inside the plant cells, which have fibre in their walls. You have to chew to get the sugar out. As you chew, the fibre acts like a brush. This helps to remove plaque, and prevents sugar from sticking to the teeth. Recently dentists have found that *tannin*, a substance in tea and some chewing sticks, prevents plaque forming.

22.12 HOW TO PREVENT TOOTH DECAY AND GUM DISEASE

Clean teeth properly at least once a day
Proper cleaning of teeth removes plaque and prevents calculus forming. It is better to clean teeth properly

once a day, than to clean them quickly three times a day. Use a brush or chewing stick, and clean between the teeth and around the back teeth. Some people pull a piece of strong, thin string (*floss*) between the teeth to break up the plaque. Then brushing sweeps the plaque away. Washing the mouth with water after meals also helps to remove bits of food.

Clean a baby's teeth with a cloth or soft brush as soon as they appear. Let the baby help you.

Eat less sticky sweet food
- Eat smaller amounts of sweet sticky foods and drinks.
- Eat sweet sticky food and drink less often during the day.
- Do not give a baby a bottle or feeder which contains sweet drinks—for example, 'dinky feeders'. Breast-feeding is best for teeth too.

A good rule to give people is: *Do not eat sweet food or drink sweet drinks between meals.*

Eat foods which contain fibre
- Eat fruits and vegetables and other fibre-rich foods instead of refined foods—especially those which contain refined sugar.
- When you eat sweet sticky foods or sweet drinks, eat foods which contain fibre at the same time. The fibre foods help to prevent the sweet foods sticking to the teeth.

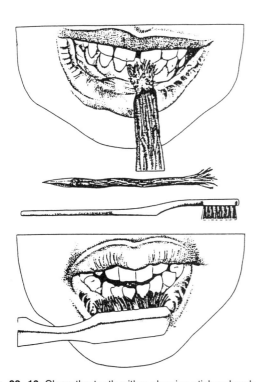

Fig. 22–10 Clean the teeth with a chewing stick or brush every day. Clean all the surfaces of the teeth. Try to get the bristles between the teeth and move the chewing stick up and down.

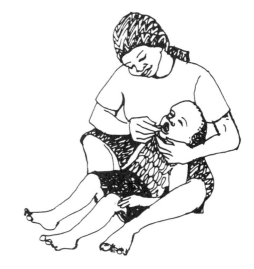

Fig. 22–11 Parents should help a young child to clean her teeth thoroughly until the child can do it herself.

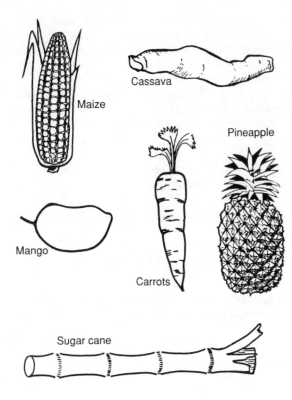

Maize

Cassava

Pineapple

Mango

Carrots

Sugar cane

Fig. 22–12 Eat fibre-rich foods instead of sweet, sticky foods.

22.13 BUILDING HEALTHY TEETH AND GUMS

Children need good mixed meals to build strong healthy teeth and gums.

The mineral *fluoride* makes the *enamel* (the hard surface of the tooth) stronger, which helps to prevent decay. But too much fluoride may cause *fluorosis* (see Section 4.13). Dentists may 'paint' fluoride on to the outside of children's teeth. This can help to repair small holes in the teeth. Fluoride which the child eats does not help to repair damaged teeth.

Toothpaste with fluoride may be useful where the level of fluoride in the water is low, but is unnecessary in areas where fluoride levels are high, and may add to the problem of fluorosis.

We are not really sure how much fluoride children need, or whether it is better to eat fluoride, or 'paint' it on the surface of the teeth, or to use toothpaste which contains fluoride.

THINGS TO DO

Class exercise

1. Ask trainees to work out the BMI for the following people, and to decide whether or not they are obese.

	Weight (kg)	Height (cm)	Answer BMI	
Mary	55	165	20	Not obese
Fanny	70	150	31	Obese
Solomon	75	160	29	Possibly obese

Some trainees like to work out their own BMIs.

2. Ask trainees to use Table A5.6 in Annex 5 to decide which of these children is overweight:

	Weight (kg)	Height (cm)	Answer
John	38	130	Overweight
Grace	25	124	Not overweight
Beth	42	134	Overweight

Discussion

3. Ask trainees to write down what they ate yesterday and how they think they should improve their meals. Discuss their ideas in class.

4. Ask trainees to demonstrate eating and living habits which may help to cause obesity. For example:

   ● adding lots of sugar to tea;
   ● not taking exercise;
   ● eating many energy-rich snacks;
   ● frying food;
   ● drinking too much beer.

   Then discuss how to help people to change these habits.

5. Ask trainees to write down any sweet, sticky foods that they ate yesterday, and to remember if they ate a fibre-rich food at the same time. Ask them to discuss whether they think that they should change their diet to help to prevent tooth and gum disease.

Practical exercises

6. Arrange for trainees to measure the weights and heights of some adults.

a. They can use Table A5.7 to see if anyone is overweight.

b. If they cannot weigh people, give trainees some weights and heights already taken and ask them to decide who is overweight.

7. Without telling trainees, weigh the sugar put out at a teabreak. Weigh the sugar again afterwards.

a. Work out the average amount of sugar used per trainee.

b. From this calculate the average Calories from sugar eaten per trainee.

Discuss the results.

8. Collect some sweet foods, including sweets, sugar, jam, sodas, sweet fruits, sugar cane, etc. Or collect pictures of these foods, or their packets. Ask trainees to divide them into 'sticky' foods which are bad for teeth, and 'fibre-rich' foods which are not bad for teeth.

9. Ask trainees to bring a toothbrush or chewing stick to class, and to demonstrate thorough cleaning of teeth. Discuss how to make sure that:

- the brush goes between the teeth (for example, brushing up and down);
- plaque is removed from between the gums and the teeth (for example, brushing sideways at the bottom of the tooth).

Discuss how easy it is not to clean the back teeth thoroughly.

Project

10. Watch children at a shop or kiosk where they can buy ice cream or sweets in a rich part of your town. Count how many of them look too fat. Compare their size to the size of children in a poorer part of town.

USEFUL PUBLICATIONS

Dickson, M. (1983). *Where there is no dentist*. Hesperian Foundation, Palo Alto, California.

WHO (1991). *Diet, nutrition and the prevention of chronic diseases*. Technical Report Series, no. 797. WHO, Geneva.

23 The food paths

23.1 WHAT IS A 'FOOD PATH'?

The foods that people eat come from different places.

- Maize, beans, and vegetables come from farms or gardens.
- Milk and meat come from cattle, goats, and other animals.
- Fish comes from the sea, rivers, or lakes.

You can think of foods travelling along 'paths' from the places where they are produced to the people who eat them. These paths are the *food paths*. At the beginning of a path, the food is built up from nutrients. At the end of the path, the body breaks the food down into nutrients again and then uses them for energy and body building. The path in between is sometimes short and simple, and sometimes long and complicated.

Figure 23–1 shows a food path for maize, and Fig. 23–2 shows how the food path continues with the preparation, eating, and using of the food. Maize is produced, dried, and stored. Later it is milled, cooked, and eaten by the farmer's family.

Figure 23–3 shows a food path for fish. Notice that the path divides, because some fish are eaten fresh, and others are dried before people eat them.

These food paths are short and simple, because the same families produce and eat the food. Usually, some of the food is eaten by the families who produce it, and some is sold and eaten by other families. Often the food is processed and transported long distances before it is sold. When food is sold, it makes the food path longer and more complicated. Figure 23–4 shows the food path for maize which is bought by traders and then sold.

A farming family produces the maize and then decides how much to sell and how much to keep. Traders buy the maize, and transport, store, and mill it. If the harvest is good, the country may export some maize. If the harvest is poor, it may import some. Traders sell the milled maize to shops who sell it to people to eat.

In order to buy food, families must have enough money. The money path is often as important as the food path. Figure 23–5 shows the money path and where it joins the food path. Figure 23–6 shows the different food paths put together.

The paths of many foods are becoming longer, because food has to be transported long distances and packaged and processed for growing urban populations. Imported foods are handled by many people and have very long food paths indeed. The food path of breast milk is the shortest of all.

Governments try to make sure that enough food travels along the food paths so everyone has enough to eat throughout the year. This is called *food security* (see Chapter 25).

23.2 THINGS THAT ALTER THE AMOUNTS OF FOOD TRAVELLING ALONG FOOD PATHS

If everyone is to have enough to eat, many different sorts of food must move along food paths.

- Enough food must be produced.
- Enough food must be stored.
- Enough food must get to the places where it is needed.
- Families must have enough money to buy foods which they cannot produce.
- Each person in the family must eat enough food.

Some factors help people to have enough food, for example, good weather, credit for farmers, and good stores.

Some factors prevent people from having enough food, for example, drought, poor roads, and low wages. These are *blocks on the food path*. Blocks are like trees falling across the path, which make it difficult for food to move along. People get less food. Sometimes they get *no* food, and there is famine.

Even if enough food is available, some people may not get enough because they are sick. They may have a poor appetite, or the infection may increase their nutrient needs, or decrease the amount of nutrients that they absorb.

So there may be blocks at the end of the food path even after the food is inside the person's body. It is difficult to do anything about some of the blocks. For example, you cannot change the weather, and it is difficult for nutrition workers to change food prices or wage rates. But there are some things which you *can* do

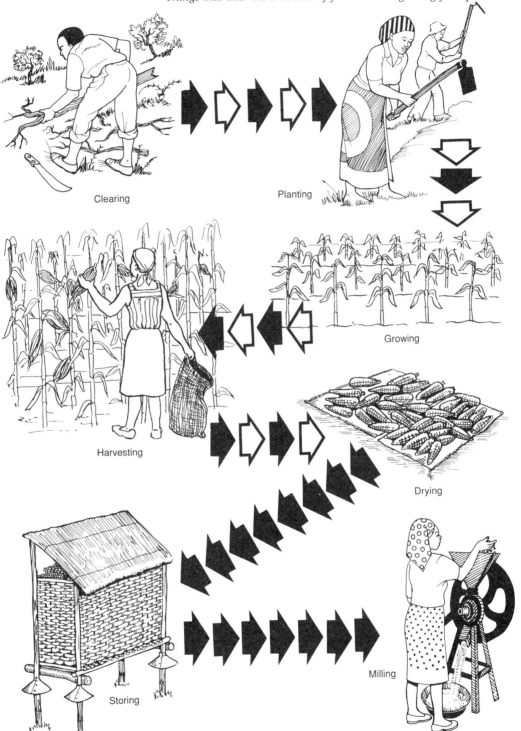

Fig. 23–1 A food path for maize. Black arrows show the path for food alone; white arrows show the path for money, and where food is bought and sold (see also Figs 23–2 to 23–5). Black and white arrows show where the paths combine (see Fig. 23–6).

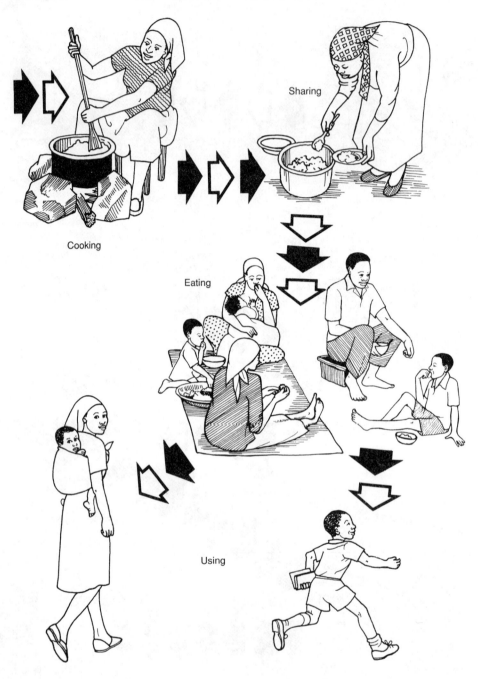

Sharing

Cooking

Eating

Using

Fig. 23–2 How the food path continues.

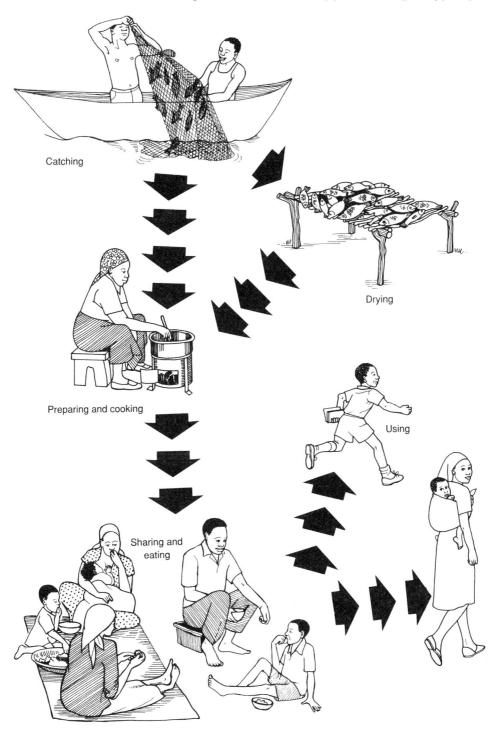

Catching

Drying

Preparing and cooking

Using

Sharing and
eating

Fig. 23–3 A food path for fish.

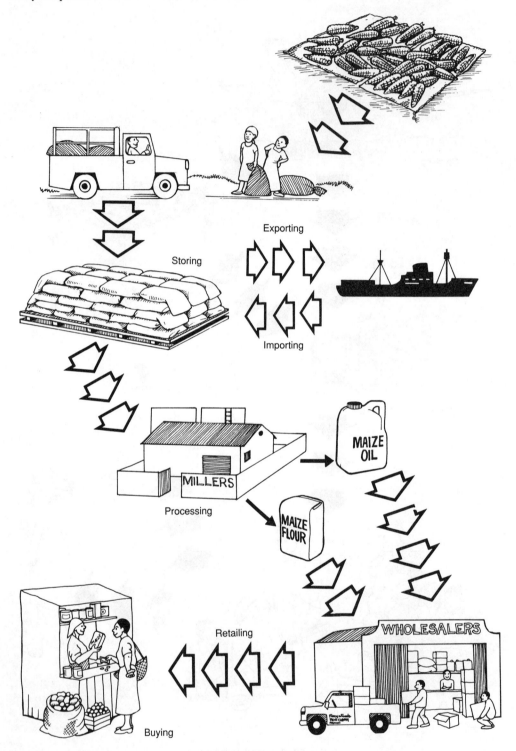

Fig. 23–4 The food path for maize which is bought by traders and then sold.

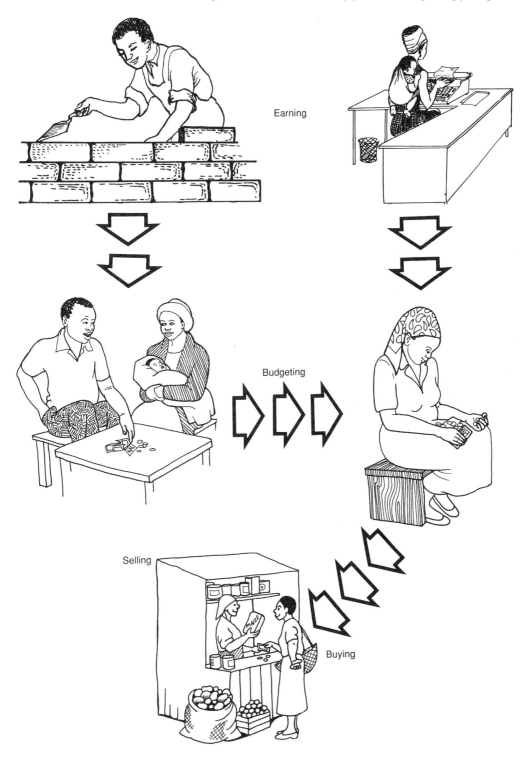

Earning

Budgeting

Selling

Buying

Fig. 23–5 The money path.

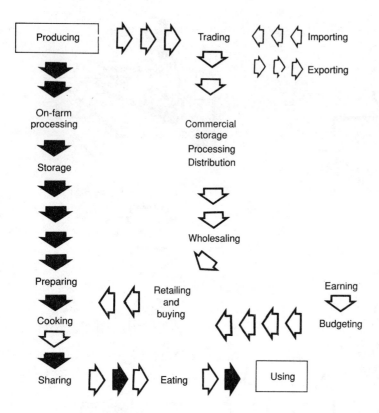

Fig. 23–6 The different food paths put together.

to help families to eat enough food. The following chapters suggest things which you can do at each stage of the food path.

Look at Box 23.1. Where on the food path do you work? Even if you are not one of the people listed, your work probably affects one or more stages of the food path in some way.

23.3 DIFFERENT STAGES OF THE FOOD PATH

In the following sections we discuss each stage of the food path and give examples of the common blocks on it and how you can help to remove them. But each country and community is different. You need to decide

---

Box 23.1. Different nutrition workers involved at different stages of the food path

Stage of food path	Nutrition workers
Production Storage	Agricultural worker
On-farm processing	Home economist Nutritionist
Trading	
Buying Preparing	Home economist Nutritionist
Sharing and eating	Home economist Nutritionist
Using	Health worker

which blocks are important where you work and what other blocks there are. This helps you to decide what you and other workers can do to help local people to remove important blocks. The main stages of the food path which can be blocked are:

- production;
- storage;
- distribution and marketing;
- buying food;
- preparation;
- sharing and eating;
- using food in the body.

23.4 BLOCKS TO FOOD PRODUCTION BY FAMILY FARMERS

Shortage of land

Shortage of land may result from:

- Rapid increase in population (see Sections 24.6–24.8).
- Unequal distribution of land. Some families have large farms, some have small farms, and some have no land at all.
- Environmental damage to land, particularly erosion (see Section 24.2).
- A lot of land used for commercial cash crops. In some places rich farmers or large companies use large areas of land for cash crops (which are often exported) so there is less for family farmers.
- Civil disturbances and wars which make people leave their farms.

Land is not fertile

Land may not be fertile because:

- It is too dry, swampy, salty, or mountainous. Farmers use land like this when there is not enough fertile land.
- It is environmentally damaged because of erosion, deforestation, overgrazing, or overcultivation, or burning bush fires (see Section 24.2).

Shortage of water

Shortage of water reduces yields from crops and animals. It is an important block to the amount of food produced in home gardens (see Sections 24.9–24.14). Water may be short because:

- Rainfall is low. One reason may be because of deforestation in or outside the country.

- There is no irrigation system.
- People do not store water during the rainy season to use later ('water harvesting').
- Water supplies are a long way from gardens.

Crop and livestock diseases and pests

Plant and animal diseases and pests cause large losses of food. Some of the most important are locusts, cassava mealy bug, spider mites, maize streak virus, weevils, and army worm among crops, and rinderpest and trypanosomiasis among livestock.

The causes are:

- the natural occurrence of the disease or pest;
- inadequate control methods.

Shortage of labour

A shortage of labour reduces food production on some farms, especially on farms managed by women, and at planting and harvesting times. The reasons for labour shortages are:

- Incomes from small farms are so low that many rural men and young people work in towns, estates, or mines or for large farmers to try to earn more money.
- Agricultural wages are too low to attract workers from towns.
- Women farmers have many tasks in addition to food production (see Sections 23.15–23.17).
- Many children nowadays go to school, so they have less time to work on the family farm.
- In some families the young adults are ill or have died (for example, from AIDS or civil war).

Shortage of inputs

Farmers need many *inputs* to produce food. For example, seed, fertilizer and other chemicals, and tools. They may need small-scale irrigation systems or water for animals. They may need oxen to plough fields or donkeys or bicycles to carry goods to market. Fishermen need boats, fuel, and nets. Many family farmers and other food producers cannot afford these things because:

- Rural incomes are low.
- Many farmers, especially women farmers, pastoralists, and fishermen, etc. cannot get low interest credit or loans, because they have no *collateral* (property which can be taken if they fail to repay the loan).
- There are not enough co-operatives to help food producers to get the inputs that they need for a reasonable price.

Lack of incentives

Farmers, fishermen, etc. are discouraged from producing food for sale if:

- They are paid low prices for their produce. Farmers may not be sure when they plant how much traders will pay for the crop.
- They are paid late.
- It is difficult to get inputs.
- Their tenure of their land is insecure (for example, short-term tenants, squatters, and share-croppers).

The reasons why some farmers are paid low prices are both political and economic. Governments may want to provide cheap food for growing urban populations. Low incomes make it difficult for producers to improve farming and fishing methods.

Disasters

Natural disasters, such as floods, fires, or storms, may destroy crops growing in the field and stored food. They may also destroy the means to produce more food (such as seed, oxen, boats, and tools). Man-made disasters, such as civil war, may do the same. Farmers produce less food if they think that they will not be able to harvest it. Sometimes they have to leave their farms and live in camps.

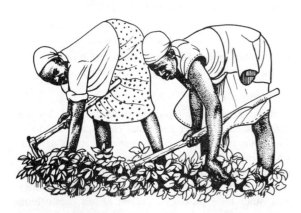

Fig. 23–7 Many women have little help on their farms.

23.5 INCREASING FOOD PRODUCTION

What you can do depends on your job, and which part of the food path your work affects. Here are some of the things that you may be able to do.

Help with resources and training

- Identify farmers (especially women farmers), fishermen, etc. who do not produce enough food, so that the authorities can target resources or training to them.
- Identify the sort of resources (e.g. credit, irrigation, tools) and training that can help them.
- Help to provide the training that they need.
- Advise family farmers, pastoralists, fishermen, etc. of services which are available (such as information, veterinary care, pest control, low-cost chemicals).
- Help family farmers and food producers to get low interest loans and credit.
- Give special support to women farmers (see Sections 23.15 and 23.16).
- Try to persuade commercial farmers to provide their labourers with land for growing food.

Encourage sustainable food production

- Encourage food production methods that use land, water, labour, and other resources efficiently and that protect the soil, trees, and environment (see Chapter 24).
- Encourage families to produce a variety of foods, including traditional foods (see Box 24.2) and foods that mature at different seasons, so that the family has enough to eat throughout the year, especially during the hungry season before the main harvest.
- Encourage sustainable fishing methods, including fish farming.
- Encourage home, community, and school gardens.
- Support schemes for small-scale irrigation for family farmers.

Help to improve incentives for food producers

Nutrition workers cannot do much but it may be important to support and lobby for policies and plans which:

- make inputs such as seed, agricultural chemicals, and credit available to farmers at fair prices in the appropriate season;
- ensure that farmers, fishermen, etc. are paid fair prices for the food they produce (and that not too much profit goes to traders), and that farmers are paid promptly;

- make it easier for small-scale food producers, especially women, to get low-cost loans and credit;
- give family farmers legal title to land;
- increase the area of land available to family farmers (e.g. through irrigation schemes);
- increase agricultural wages and rural job opportunities.

23.6 ON-FARM FOOD STORAGE AND PRESERVATION

Blocks to storing and preserving food on farms

Producers sell food

Farmers may sell much or all of the food that they produce because:

- They need money urgently, for example, for taxes, school expenses, repaying a loan, a marriage.
- They do not have good stores, and they know that they will lose much of the food if they keep it.

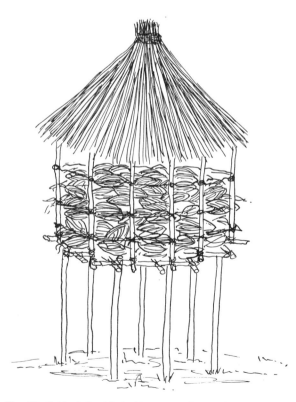

Fig. 23–8 Much food is lost because of poor stores.

Farmers may not get much money for their crops because food prices are usually low after the harvest when many farmers sell at the same time; prices are higher later in the year when many families want to buy food.

Fishermen sell most of their catch because they need the money and have no way to store or preserve fish for their families.

Pests or moulds destroy the food

Much food may be lost or spoilt during storage by moulds, such as the one which produces aflatoxin, and by insects, rats, and mice, because:

- The stores and the methods of storage are poor.
- Foods are not dried enough before storage.

Post-harvest losses of fresh and dried fish are high due to poor facilities for processing and distribution.

Lack of equipment or knowledge of food preservation

Families may not preserve and store foods such as vegetables and animal foods because they do not know how to or do not have the necessary equipment.

Improving food storage and preservation

Ways to help people improve food storage and preservation include:

- Showing families how to handle harvested food and improve food stores and storage methods. It is especially important to make sure that people dry cereals, roots, and legumes properly and that they use any chemicals safely.
- Developing, improving or encouraging simple methods for preserving foods—such as drying vegetables or souring milk or porridge.
- Demonstrating better methods for preserving fish, and promoting better transport and storage facilities for fish.

23.7 COMMERCIAL STORAGE, DISTRIBUTION, AND MARKETING

As more people move off the land and live in towns, the number of people who buy food increases. This means that there must be an efficient system for distributing and marketing food. Nutrition workers cannot influence these stages of the food path very much. But

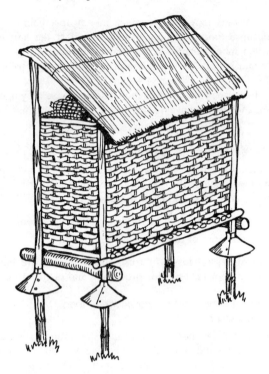

Fig. 23-9 An improved maize store.

it may be interesting to know the main blocks and how they might be moved.

Blocks to food distribution and marketing

- Markets far from food-producing areas. Food may be needed a long way from where it is produced. This increases the costs and difficulties of marketing food, particularly fresh foods such as fish, meat, milk, and vegetables. Refrigerated trucks are often not available or they increase costs too much.
- Poor roads.
- Shortage of lorries and spare parts.
- Shortage or high cost of fuel.
- Inefficient marketing systems.
- Poor stores.

Things which improve food distribution and marketing

- Improving transport and storage systems;
- Improving the management and efficiency of marketing systems;
- Improving large-scale food processing;
- Having fair, and sometimes controlled, prices for both traders and customers.

23.8 BLOCKS TO BUYING FOOD

Most families, even farming families, buy some food. Here are the main blocks to buying enough food.

Lack of money

Lack of money to buy food is the main reason for hunger and undernutrition in many places. Some reasons why people have little money for food are:

- They are unemployed or underemployed.
- Wages are low.
- A family cannot sell the things it produces (such as food, baskets, charcoal) or its skills (such as driving or carpentry, domestic work or herding animals) because other people do not want or cannot afford to pay for them.
- There are a large number of *dependent* people—that is, young children, old people, disabled people—in the family compared to the number of earners and producers. In many families grandparents or older children look after younger children, because their parents have died.
- A family must spend money on other things (e.g. school expenses, taxes, rent, someone in hospital).

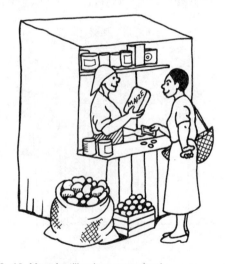

Fig. 23-10 Most families buy some food.

The block 'lack of money for food' occurs when family incomes are low *compared to* the price of foods, especially staple foods. So another cause of this block is high food prices. Prices may be high because:

- The cost of producing food is high.
- Transport costs from farm to market are high.
- Costs of imported foods are high.
- There is a shortage of food so traders can raise prices. When food is in short supply, or likely to be in short supply, people often hoard food which increases prices still more.

Not budgeting enough money for food

Sometimes families spend much of their income on other things and do not have enough left over for food, because:

- *They give priority to other things.* This often happens when men decide how the family's income is spent. A man may not buy enough food or give his wife enough money to buy food. He may not know the importance of good mixed meals. If a man does not buy and prepare food himself, he may not understand how much it costs to buy all that a family needs. He may spend so much on beer or entertainment that there is not enough left over for food.

- *Women earn very little money.* Women usually give food a higher priority than men. Often, women can decide how to spend the money that they earn. But many women earn low wages and so cannot budget enough for food.

Buying 'poor value' foods

Some families spend a lot on poor value drinks and foods such as sodas, sweets, 'health foods', and tonics. These foods contain mainly sugar. They give poor value for money and mean that there is less money for good value foods. Reasons why families buy poor value foods are:

- Children demand them.
- People do not know which foods are nutritious and which are not.
- Advertising encourages people to buy these foods, or to think that they give them extra energy or strength.
- Healthy foods may be difficult to get, or less convenient to drink or to carry. For example, fruit and fresh milk are often more difficult to get than sodas.

- Healthy foods sometimes seem expensive. (For example, groundnuts and fruit may be more expensive per kilogram than sweets—but they give many more nutrients.)

Some families, especially those who have just moved to towns, may not know which foods give best value for money. They may use the little money that they have on foods which contain few nutrients. For example, they may buy cabbage instead of carrots or spinach. Or bottled fruit 'juice' instead of fresh fruit.

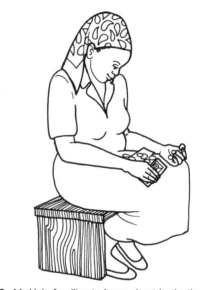

Fig. 23–11 Help families to learn about budgeting.

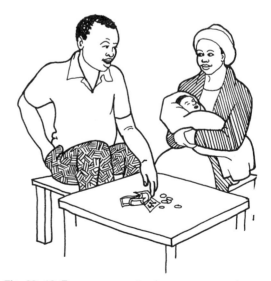

Fig. 23–12 Encourage men to give women enough money for food.

23.9 HELPING PEOPLE TO BUY ENOUGH FOOD

We need to look for ways to help the poorer families in a community to have more money. Some ways in which you may be able to help these families are to:

- Help community groups, particularly women's groups, to start or improve income-generating activities—for example, making bread or clothes, processing foods, or raising poultry, goats, or rabbits.
- Encourage family farmers to grow cash crops which give a good return for labour and other inputs without reducing too much the amount of food they produce for home use (Box 23.2).
- Encourage local planners and business people to start or expand businesses or industries to increase jobs (for example, small-scale food processing).
- Encourage planners of development projects to target resources and opportunities (e.g. for work) to poorer families in the area.
- Support local plans and policies which:
  - provide better wages and more jobs for men and women;
  - control or subsidize food prices;
  - help poor people in times of trouble through cash-for-work or food-for-work or other feeding programmes (see Chapter 29).

You may also be able to help families to spend their money better if you can:

- 'watch over' poorer families especially when they have less money than usual and try to help them (see Chapters 26 and 27);
- help families to learn about budgeting and about buying good value foods—both raw foods and cooked meals (see Chapter 9);
- encourage men to learn about family food needs and to give women enough money to buy good foods;
- encourage families to have fewer children so that there is enough money for food for everyone (see Sections 24.6–24.8).

23.10 FOOD PREPARATION

Blocks on this stage of the food path may be less important than blocks on the food production or money parts of the path. Not being able to get enough food is usually a more important reason for undernutrition.

However, it is often easier to improve food preparation and sharing than to move blocks on other stages of the food path. You can help families to make the best use of the food that they have.

Sometimes there are families who have plenty of food, but their children do not eat enough. Nutrition

---

Box 23.2. Cash crops and nutrition

It is important that farmers produce the right balance of crops for sale and for family use. The family must have enough to eat but it must also have enough money for other essential things. The type of cash crop must be suitable for small farmers. It should not need too much land or other inputs such as expensive fertilizer. Cash crops often provide work for landless rural families.

Families who grow cash crops may not have enough food if:

- Very little land is left for family food crops.
- The family receives payment for the cash crop only once or twice a year. It is difficult to budget this money over several months, especially where there are no banks. So families run out of money before the next harvest and cannot buy enough food. Sometimes they are forced to borrow money at high interest rates and so become deeper and deeper in debt.
- All the money earned from cash crops belongs to men. If a family is not used to buying most of their food, the man may not budget enough of the money for food.
- Traders or marketing boards reduce the price paid, or the cash crop fails. Then families have less money to buy food. Farmers cannot change quickly from growing cash to food crops.
- Women work on the cash crops and so have less time to:
  - grow family food and raise animals;
  - process and prepare food;
  - feed and care for children;
  - earn money which they control themselves.

workers can help these families too. Blocks to food preparation may result in:

- *Infrequent meals.* This is an important cause of young children becoming undernourished, and of older children and adults being hungry and unable to work and study well (see Chapter 11).
- *Contaminated, unsafe meals.* These increase the risk of infection, which can make undernutrition worse.

Blocks to food preparation

Shortage of fuel

Shortage of fuel means that families may cook only once a day. Cooked food may be kept for other meals. Bacteria may multiply in the food and cause diarrhoea. Families may not have enough fuel because:

- There is little firewood near the home. In many places most of the trees and bushes have been cut down. Many women and children spend much time and energy collecting firewood and other fuels such as dung or straw.
- Fuel is very expensive to buy—for example, charcoal, kerosene, and in some areas firewood.

Shortage of time and labour

Women may be too busy to prepare food often. This happens most often during the planting and harvesting seasons or among women who work outside the home for long hours. The block may also occur in families where the mother is absent, ill, or sick.

Shortage of equipment

In many homes there is little equipment for food preparation and cooking. It is much easier to prepare good clean meals when you have a stove that you can easily control, and a table, and enough pans and utensils.

Lack of information

It is difficult for some people to know how to prepare good clean mixed meals. The people who need most help are:

- people who have just moved to a town and must use unfamiliar foods;
- single men or youths cooking for themselves;
- old people living alone;
- people in refugee camps who receive unfamiliar foods.

Shortage of water

Water is important for:

- washing roots, fruits, vegetables, etc.;
- soaking beans, cereals, etc. before pounding, souring, or cooking;
- washing hands;
- boiling food, making tea;
- washing utensils.

Many families walk long distances to collect water or must pay a lot to buy water. The amount of water that a family has affects the way they prepare food, and how clean and safe meals are.

Helping families to prepare food better

Ways to help families to prepare enough clean food include:

- helping families to use less fuel (Box 24.1, p. 320) and to protect and plant trees for firewood;
- supporting activities (such as child care centres) and labour-saving technologies that reduce women's workloads (see Sections 23.15–23.17);
- helping families learn how to prepare meals in a clean, safe way (see Chapter 7);
- supporting schemes for improving domestic water supplies; helping the community look after and keep clean their wells, boreholes, etc.

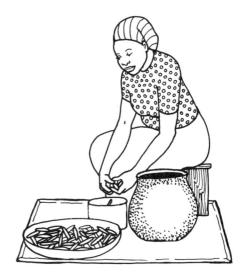

Fig. 23–13 Help families to prepare food in a clean safe way.

23.11 BLOCKS TO EATING ENOUGH

Not getting an adequate share of food

Families may share meals according to social customs and not nutritional needs. When there is only just enough food, some people (usually women and children) may not get enough.

The family may believe that it is important to give the wage-earner the best food. Men may demand special treatment. In an unstable marriage or partnership, the woman may want to please the man who supports her and her children.

It is sometimes difficult for a busy mother to give young children enough attention at meal times—especially if they are born close together, so that there is more than one who needs help with eating.

Children may all eat from the same plate of food. Older children learn to eat fast and finish the food quickly. Younger children who eat more slowly may not get enough.

Artificial feeding

Anything which makes a mother feed her baby artificially is a block on the short breastfeeding food path (see Chapter 10). For example:

- hospital practices which interfere with new mothers starting to breastfeed;
- incorrect advice and lack of support of breastfeeding mothers from health workers;
- mothers not knowing how to continue breastfeeding when they work away from home;
- stopping breastfeeding because of a new pregnancy;
- promotion of formula milks by the manufacturers.

Some methods of weaning (see Chapter 11)

Young children do not get enough nutrients if:

- they start weaning foods after about 6 months of age;
- they have too few meals or snacks each day;
- the weaning food is very 'bulky';
- they do not have enough different sorts of food.

The causes of this block may be:

- shortage of money to buy nutrient-rich weaning foods such as groundnuts, fish, and oil;
- the mother not having enough time to feed the child

as often as necessary, and not having anyone (such as a grandmother) to help;

- traditional beliefs about child feeding—'Babies have always been fed this way!';
- lack of information on children's needs, and on appropriate foods to give babies;
- the mother is absent, ill, or mentally disabled.

Poor appetite

Poor appetite is one of the most important blocks to eating enough food, especially among young children. The causes of a poor appetite are:

- gut, respiratory, and other infections;
- undernutrition, especially kwashiorkor;
- misery or jealousy;
- teething, or a sore mouth or teeth.

Lack of teeth

This block affects mainly old people who have lost their teeth and so can only eat soft foods.

23.12 WAYS TO HELP PEOPLE TO EAT ENOUGH

- Help people—especially men—to learn about the special needs of mothers and young children in order to encourage fairer distribution of food (see Chapters 8 and 12).
- Help mothers to breastfeed exclusively for 6 months and to continue breastfeeding for 2 years or more (see Chapter 10).
- Discourage bottle feeding. If a baby cannot breastfeed, teach the family to feed the baby with a cup.
- Help parents to get the family planning advice that they need, so that they can space their children and give each enough attention. Discuss with them the advantages of matching family size to family resources (see Section 24.8).
- Discuss with parents how to improve weaning:
  - Start giving babies weaning food at 6 months.
  - Make nutrient-rich weaning foods.
  - Feed small children five times a day.
- Encourage parents to give a small child her own plate of food, to help her to eat it, and to make sure that she eats enough.

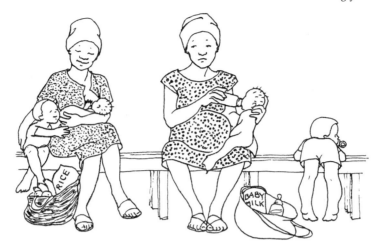

Fig. 23–14 Bottle feeding is a block on the breast milk food path.

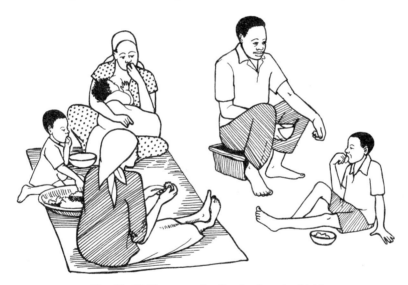

Fig. 23–15 Encourage families to share food fairly.

- Try to prevent infections among young children.
  - Encourage families to take children for immunizations.
  - Encourage them to prepare food cleanly and safely and to protect water supplies to prevent diarrhoea.
  - Discuss how to prevent AIDS, which can be passed to children.
- When children are ill, treat them early. Make sure that they continue to eat during the illness, and eat extra during recovery.
- Help people to learn about the special food needs of old people.

23.13 USING FOOD IN THE BODY

At the end of the food path, food enters the body and breaks down into nutrients again.

Blocks to the body using nutrients

Infections

Infections and worms decrease absorption of nutrients, increase nutrient needs, and increase loss of nutrients (see Sections 16.3 and 16.12). Infections are commoner and more serious when:

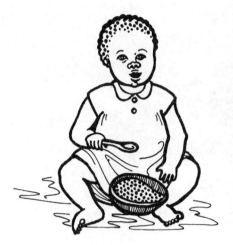

Fig. 23–16 Encourage families to give a child her own plate of food.

- People are undernourished.
- Housing is poor.
- Living conditions are crowded.
- Water and sanitation are inadequate.
- Children are not immunized.
- Health services are inadequate and infections are not treated early enough.

Antinutrients

Substances in some foods interfere with the digestion, absorption, and use of nutrients. For example:

- Phytate in cereals reduces the absorption of iron and zinc.
- Goitrogens in cassava interfere with the use of iodine by the thyroid gland.

Helping people to use nutrients

Help people to prevent and control infections:

- Help communities to get better water supplies and sanitation and efficient food inspection systems.
- Discuss with parents how they can prevent infection if they:
  - prepare clean safe meals;
  - keep the house and its surroundings as clean as possible;
  - keep the children clean;
  - bring children for immunization.

- Explain why it is important to give food and drink to adults and children when they are ill. Help them to do this.
- Explain when it is important to take sick children for treatment promptly.

23.14 BASIC CAUSES OF BLOCKS ON THE FOOD PATHS

You can see that most blocks on the food paths can be moved if people have more resources:

- more money;
- more land;
- more time;
- more fuel;
- more information and skills;
- better services (e.g. health and agriculture);
- more facilities (e.g. wells);
- better housing and living conditions.

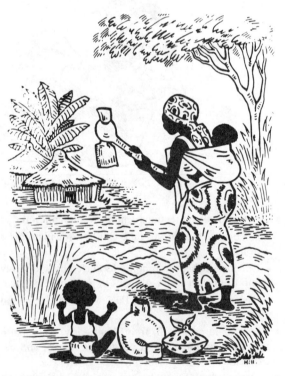

Fig. 23–17 In Africa, women produce about 80 per cent of the family food.

The basic cause of poor nutrition is *lack of resources.* If you think about your community, your country and the world, you see that a major problem is *unequal distribution of resources.* If all the land, money, and food were shared more equally, it would be easier for everyone to have enough to eat.

The amount and distribution of resources within a community or country depend on many things, such as the land and its fertility, climate and weather, water supplies, industries, the population size, its density, and growth rate—also economic conditions in and out-side the area, how much trade there is and the prices of imports and exports, investment and aid from outside the community or country, as well as government policies and organization, and whether the country is peaceful and stable.

One of the important but difficult things that you, a nutrition worker, can do to improve nutrition is to encourage the more equal distribution of resources within your country or community. Perhaps you can:

- support and vote for a politician or councillor who wants to give poorer families more land or higher wages or better health services;
- help poorer families to develop the confidence and skills they need to ask for more resources (see Chapter 28);
- encourage the education of girls and women;
- make sure that development programmes help the poorest families in an area.

Land, forests, and water are some of the most im-portant resources in a community or country. We have already seen the terrible famines which result from erosion, deforestation, and drought. So another way to improve nutrition is to protect these precious resources from environmental damage. Help people to use them in a sustainable way, so that they preserve them for their children and grandchildren.

In many places the population is increasing too fast for local resources to support. Overpopulation is one cause of environmental damage. So another important task for nutrition workers is to help people to plan their families to match land, income, etc., so that they do not use up resources.

23.15 WOMEN AND THE FOOD PATH

In most families women and men have separate but supporting responsibilities. Often women are re-sponsible for providing food for the family, as well as

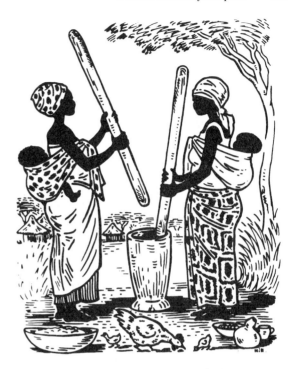

Fig. 23–18 Women process and prepare food.

making a happy home and caring for children. For example:

- In Africa, women produce about 80 per cent of the family food. They grow almost all the traditional foods such as roots, legumes, and vegetables.
- Women help to care for animals, especially small animals and poultry.
- Women and children gather wild foods such as green leaves and fruits.
- Women process food (e.g. threshing and pounding cereals, souring milk, cleaning and drying fish).
- Many women earn money to buy some or all of the family food.
- Women collect firewood and water to prepare food.
- Women prepare meals and clean up afterwards.
- Women feed young children (including breastfeeding them).
- Women feed and care for old or sick relatives.

So it is women, more than men, who move food along most stages of the food paths. If women receive more support and training, more food will move along the food paths and families will get more to eat.

23.16 WHY WOMEN NEED SUPPORT AND TRAINING

- In many places, women do not have the same rights to land as men. Land reform programmes usually give the title of land to men. Some land reform laws have actually taken away women's traditional rights to communal land.

- It is difficult for women to get loans or credit or to join co-operatives, because they do not have 'collateral' (i.e. they do not own cattle, land, etc.).

- Few women are politicians or on national or local councils and committees. So they do not help to make decisions which affect their lives and work and different stages of the food path. The reasons include social customs and women's lack of time, and sometimes their lack of confidence and education.

- Agricultural programmes have developed better farming methods and inputs such as improved seeds and tools mainly for cash crops which are usually produced by men. Only a small part of foreign aid for agricultural development has helped women.

- Most agricultural extension workers are men. They work mainly with men farmers and usually still give most attention to cash crops.

- Most agricultural training courses are designed for male farmers. For example, timetables often conflict with women's other duties.

- Most women are less educated than men, and so find it difficult to get training and information.

- Many women have very heavy workloads.

The women who have the heaviest workloads are:

- *Poor rural women.*

- *Women who are heads of families*, who receive no support from husbands or other relatives. Nowadays many women are heads of families and the number is increasing. A woman may be a temporary head if her husband is working away from home. Or she may be the permanent head if she is not married or is divorced, or if her husband is dead or sick. If the husband or another relative does not send money, these women must work very hard to support their families.

    Families in which women are the permanent heads of household are often the poorest and most undernourished in the community.

- *Older women who look after many grandchildren*, if their children or their partners are dead or work away from home. This is becoming more common in areas where AIDS is a problem.

- *Women who have many closely spaced children.* A woman who is often pregnant has less time and energy to provide good meals. She may be anaemic during and after her pregnancy. Caring for a new baby and all the other children takes much time. Many women of childbearing age are pregnant or breastfeeding 80 per cent of the time.

The heavy workload of women is the cause of blocks at several places on the food path. It is difficult for women to find enough time and energy to do all that is needed to feed the family sufficiently. Women who have much other work have less time and energy to:

- cultivate and produce food;
- earn money for buying food;
- collect enough fuel to cook frequent meals;
- encourage young children to eat;
- prepare special food for sick children and encourage them to eat and drink;
- join women's organizations, literacy classes, etc., where they can learn better ways to produce, process, store, or prepare food;
- attend young child or antenatal clinics.

At certain times, such as during planting and harvesting, women's workloads are even heavier. Women may be undernourished and lose weight, especially if they are pregnant or breastfeeding. They have even less time to care for young children, and to feed or breastfeed them often, so young children are often undernourished at these times too.

23.17 HOW TO HELP WOMEN

Examine development schemes planned for your area

Find out what effect they are likely to have on food supplies of poorer families, and on women's workloads and incomes. If a scheme is likely to have a *bad* effect, tell the planners. Often small changes can prevent bad effects. For example, making sure that women have control of some of the new income from the scheme, or providing child care facilities.

Help to empower women

- Encourage women to become members of village or district councils and other groups which decide how to use local funds.

- Help women to learn about and improve their legal rights. Teach schoolchildren the legal rights of women and men.
- Help women to get inputs and credits for food production.
- Discuss the roles, needs, and rights of women with men too. Changes in the status and roles of women are unlikely to come unless men support them.
- Help women to start co-operatives and saving schemes.
- Ask agricultural extension officers to work more with women farmers to improve the crops that women produce.

Reduce women's workloads

- Help women to get labour-saving tools and equipment, such as handmills.
- Help them to build or buy stoves that use less fuel and that are suitable for local conditions (Box 24.1, Fig. 24–3).
- Support activities to bring water supplies nearer people's homes.
- Try to persuade employers to give paid maternity leave.
- Help women to find ways to get bicycles or donkeys to carry loads.
- Help to organize child care centres where working mothers can leave their children safely.

Help women to get education and training

- Encourage parents to send girls to school, to allow them to attend regularly, and to complete primary school—and to go to secondary school if possible.
- In schools teach students about women's special problems and needs and why good nutrition is particularly important for girls.
- Help to organize training:
  - to manage women's groups, funds, saving schemes, and co-operatives for example;
  - to improve the production, marketing, processing, and preparation of food.
- Help at literacy classes and adult education for women.
- Explain to men how education and training for women also helps to improve the family food supply, meals, and nutrition.

Improve community health care for women

- Promote child spacing and family planning. Help to prevent adolescent pregnancies (see Section 24.8).

- Encourage women to attend antenatal classes and other health care services for women. Make sure that these services can help women with anaemia and other nutritional disorders.
- Help women to learn about nutrition by discussions at health centres, community growth monitoring sessions, women's group meetings, and adult education classes.

Help families of needy women

Know about, watch over, and, when necessary, help poor families where the mother is:

- head of the family without support from relatives;
- old;
- disabled or sick;
- very young;
- frequently pregnant;
- has many young children.

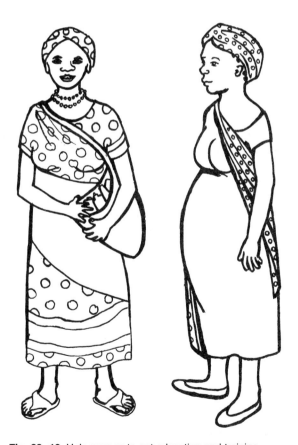

Fig. 23–19 Help women to get education and training.

Box 23.3.   Customs and practices which affect food paths

How old and new customs and practices affect the food paths
Old customs which help enough good food to reach people
- Traditional methods of agriculture and fishing which preserve the soil, fish stocks, etc.
- Giving special foods such as chicken or sour fermented porridge to women who are pregnant or recently delivered.
- Giving newly delivered women a rest from work for some time.
- Breastfeeding for 2 years or more; and breastfeeding at night.
- Eating fresh or whole foods instead of highly processed foods (for example, eating dark green leaves instead of cabbage, fresh fruit instead of bottled drinks).
- Having 2 or more years between babies.

Old customs which may block food paths
- Having large families.
- Men controlling the family food budget.
- Bulky weaning foods.
- Men being given the biggest share of the family food.
- Not sending girls to school.

New practices which help food to move along food paths
- New sustainable methods of agriculture which increase yields.
- Modern methods of large-scale food storage, processing, and marketing.
- The use of grain mills which reduce women's work.
- More girls going to school. Women with more education are likely to feed and care for their families well and have fewer children.
- More families using electricity, piped water, and other modern technology which makes food preparation easier and cleaner.
- More families listening to the radio and reading newspapers and magazines, from which they get useful new information about food production, budgeting, and preparation, and about feeding children and prevention of infections.
- More families using effective methods of contraception to space children and reduce family size.
- Women having more control over the money that they earn.
- More children attending clinics for immunization, growth monitoring, and early treatment of infection.

New practices which may block food paths
- Bottle feeding.
- Women going out to work and leaving babies with young, inexperienced carers.
- Fewer extended families and many women, including adolescent girls, raising families on their own.
- People preferring foreign foods, such as wheat (for bread), that may not be easy to produce locally.
- Practices which lead to babies being born too close together, i.e.
  - starting sex soon after giving birth;
  - breastfeeding only partially or not at all before the baby is 6 months old.
- Eating poor value 'convenience foods' instead of fresh whole foods.

What you can do
- Discuss with people local customs and practices which influence the way in which food moves along the food path. Help them to identify the customs and practices which help everyone to have enough food, and those which may block food paths.
- Help people to plan ways to change 'blocking' customs and practices.
- Encourage customs and practices which help food to move. For example:
  - Encourage breastfeeding and discourage bottle feeding.
  - Encourage families to share food by nutritional needs.
  - Encourage men to give women more control over the family budget.
  - Encourage girls to stay at school as long as possible.

THINGS TO DO

Class exercise

1. Ask trainees to choose a local food and to draw a food path for it. Ask them to mark places where the path may be blocked.

Group discussion

2. Ask groups to make a list of common blocks to food production.
   a. Discuss how each block might be removed.
   b. Discuss the importance of women in food production, especially in relation to these blocks.

3. Ask trainees to talk about families they know who do not have enough money for food.

   a. Why do these families not have enough money?
   b. What can nutrition workers do to help?

4. Ask trainees to discuss how infection blocks food paths and to make a list. In class, combine the lists from the different groups, and discuss how to remove these blocks.

USEFUL PUBLICATIONS

ACC/SCN (1990a). *Women and nutrition*, Nutrition Policy Discussion Paper, no. 6. ACC/SCN, Geneva.

ACC/SCN (1990b). Policies to improve nutrition—what was done in the 80s. *SCN News*, no. 6.

UNICEF (1990). *Strategy for improved nutrition of children and women in developing countries.* UNICEF, New York.

Gillespie, S. and Mason J. (1991). *Nutrition—relevant actions* Nutrition Policy Discussion Paper, no. 10. ACC/SCN, Geneva.

24 Nutrition and the environment

24.1 NUTRITION, THE ENVIRONMENT, AND THE SOIL

Food production is closely linked to the environment. One of the worst tragedies of this century is the damage that people all over the world are doing to the environment. Damaging the environment affects food production because:

- Soil fertility decreases.
- Rainfall decreases.

In some places the Sahara Desert is advancing 10 km each year. In other places too land that was once cultivated and fertile is now useless. Crops fail to grow, or have a very poor yield. About 37 000 square kilometres are lost to deserts in Africa each year. The problem is similar in other parts of the world.

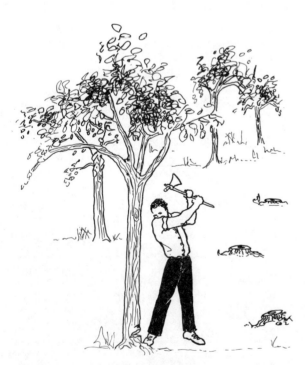

Fig. 24–1 People are cutting down more trees than they plant.

24.2 HOW THE ENVIRONMENT IS BEING DAMAGED

Some of the ways in which people are damaging the environment are:

- cutting down more trees and bushes than they plant;
- overgrazing grassland;
- overcultivating the soil.

Cutting down too many trees and bushes

Many trees are cut down to clear land for agriculture and for firewood and timber. People are cutting down trees much faster than they are planting them. This is called *deforestation*. Trees and bushes protect the soil.

- Trees prevent heavy rainfall from carrying soil away and flooding rivers. The water sinks into the ground, soaks into the roots, and rises slowly up the trees and out through the leaves into the sky, to collect as more rain. So trees recycle the rain.
- Fallen leaves and the animals and plants that live in forests keep the soil fertile and able to hold water.

When trees and forests are lost, rainfall decreases, and the soil becomes less fertile. When soil is not protected, it can be washed away by heavy rain, or blown away by wind. This is called *erosion*.

Sometimes people burn trees, bushes, old grass, and crops to clear land for planting, or to promote growth of new grass for grazing. Burning in a small area sometimes has short-term benefits. But it destroys young trees and bushes and their seeds and harms the fertility of the soil. This can cause erosion.

Overgrazing grasslands

As the number of people has increased, so has the number of cattle, goats, sheep, and other domestic animals in Africa. But there is less land available for grazing because so much has been taken for crops, plantations, game reserves, and towns.

So in many places there are more animals and less land. When there are too many animals, they eat almost all the grass and bushes. The soil is uncovered and can be eroded by wind and rain.

Overcultivating the soil

Soil contains many micro-organisms and nutrients, so it is a living system. When plants that grow on the soil are eaten or burnt, nutrients are removed. The soil needs to be nourished and restored with animal manure, compost, or other plant and animal waste, or chemical fertilizer.

If nutrients are removed faster than they are replaced, the soil loses its fertility and the land gives lower yields. The soil is more easily eroded. It may become dry and blow away. Or, when it rains, water runs off the soil or washes it away instead of soaking into it. Soil cannot be replaced—and may take many centuries to restore.

In many places nutrients are removed from soil faster than they are replaced because:

- Farmers use the same land to grow crops every year. They cannot leave fields fallow (resting) because they do not have enough land.
- Farmers cannot afford fertilizers.
- Farmers use animal dung and waste from crops for fuel so they cannot use it to fertilize soil.

Helping people to protect the environment

- Help to preserve trees (see Section 24.4).
- Discuss with farmers and communities the dangers of overgrazing, overcultivation, and deforestation.
- Help farmers to prevent erosion and preserve soil fertility by farming practices such as those discussed in Section 24.14:
  - planting trees and bushes to make windbreaks;
  - building water breaks;
  - *terracing* sloping land (Fig. 24–2) and *alley cropping*;
  - feeding soils with animal manure, green manure, and compost;
  - *mulching* and *intercropping*.
- Encourage the use of natural pest control and natural fertilizers (also see Section 24.14).
- Teach schoolchildren about protecting the soil, trees, and their environment.
- Join and encourage others to join organizations which try to protect the environment.

24.3 NUTRITION AND TREES

Trees and bushes are linked to nutrition because:

- They keep the soil fertile, prevent erosion, and recycle rain water.
- They provide food—for example:
  - fruits such as plantains, mangoes, and oranges;
  - oil seeds, such as coconuts and palm nuts;
  - green leaves, such as acacia leaves;
  - herbs and sap (sometimes used to make drinks).

Some people eat the animals, insects, or birds which live in the forests; the mushrooms which grow beneath the trees; or the honey from bees which have hives in the trees. Sea foods, such as prawns and fish, live in the mangroves on the edge of the sea.

- Trees and bushes provide fuel for cooking and for processing foods such as smoked fish. Most rural families use wood or charcoal for cooking because it is the cheapest fuel.
- Trees and bushes provide food for animals such as goats and camels.

24.4 HOW TO HELP PRESERVE TREES AND FORESTS

- Help families and communities to plant and care for trees, particularly trees for food and fodder, and quick-growing trees for fuel and trees which protect or nourish the soil.
  - Encourage people to plant trees in their gardens or farms, and on unused land, along roads and rivers.
  - Ask the local forestry officer about the best kinds of trees to plant and how to care for them.

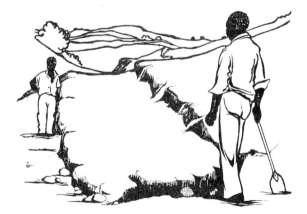

Fig. 24–2 Terracing sloping land helps to prevent erosion.

Box 24.1. Fuel-efficient stoves

Figure 24–3 shows examples of stoves that use much less wood than a 'three-stone fire' (Fig. 8–1) or traditional charcoal stove and gives less smoke.

A stove must be designed so that it:

- suits the fuel used in the area;
- suits the way in which women like to cook;
- provides heat and light if necessary;
- is cheap;
- is easy to maintain and lasts for several years.

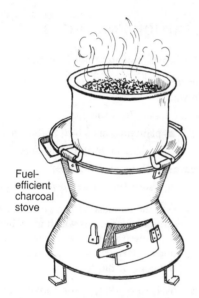

Fuel-efficient charcoal stove

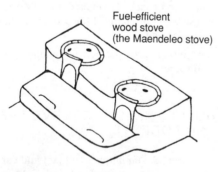

Fuel-efficient wood stove (the Maendeleo stove)

This stove uses 30 –50% less wood than cooking on three stones. The stove insert, made out of fired clay is bought. The rest of the stove is built by women using local material, mainly sticky soil and stones

Fig. 24–3 Examples of fuel-efficient stoves.

- Encourage people to use wood for fuel efficiently:

  - To use fuel-efficient stoves (Box 24.1; Fig. 24–3). Ask home economists, community development workers, or leaders of women's groups about stoves which have been made and successfully tested in your area.

  - To dry firewood thoroughly and store it in a dry place if possible. Dry wood gives more heat than fresh wet wood.

  - To prepare food in a way which reduces cooking time (e.g. soak legumes before cooking; cut food small).

  - To put lids on cooking pans.

24.5 NUTRITION, FAMILY SIZE, AND POPULATION GROWTH

In many countries the population is increasing at more than 3 per cent a year, which means that it doubles in size every 20 years (see Figs. 24–5 and 24–6). The population increases faster than the amount of food that is produced, and faster than governments can build new schools and health centres or develop new jobs.

Many of the people in growing populations are young and in need of good food, health care, and education. About 20 per cent of the population is under 5 years of age, and 50 per cent are under 16 years.

Where people live is changing too. The percentage of people living in urban areas in Africa was about 14 per cent in 1965, and nearly 30 per cent at the end of the 1980s. By the year 2000, about 50 per cent of people will live in towns.

1. Soak beans before cooking

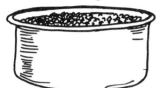

2. Cut food into smaller pieces

3. Put a lid on the pan

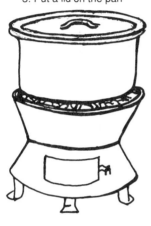

Fig. 24–4 Ways to reduce the cooking time of foods.

The reasons for the increasing population are:

- *Each woman has, on average, more babies.* Women have more babies mainly because they have pregnancies closer together than in the past. This is because they:
  - start having babies at a younger age;
  - breastfeed exclusively for a shorter time;
  - start sex sooner after a baby is born;
  - may become fertile again sooner if they are better nourished;
  - cannot get family planning easily.
- *Fewer children die than in the past.* This is because it is now possible to prevent or treat many illnesses. However, we do not yet know how much difference AIDS will make to population growth.

24.6 HOW FAMILY SIZE AFFECTS THE FOOD PATH

It is difficult for parents with many young children to care for them properly and to give enough attention to each.

If a family is large, with many closely spaced children

- Each baby cannot breastfeed for so long.
- Each child may get less food and care. Children who are born closer together are less healthy than children who are well spaced. They may be undernourished, and may get less stimulation to help them develop normally.
- The mother does not have enough time between pregnancies to rebuild her nutrient stores and become strong again. She may become more and more undernourished, and anaemic, and have small weak babies.
- The mother is likely to be overworked (Chapter 18).
- The family's land or income is less likely to provide enough food and other necessities for everyone. There may not be enough money to send everyone to school.

If a family is small, with a few well spaced children

- Parents can feed and care for each child better. There is more food for everyone and more money for other necessities.
- Children are healthier, and have a better chance to develop normally.
- Children are more likely to be well educated, get good jobs, and be able to support their parents in old age.

24.7 HOW AN INCREASING POPULATION BLOCKS THE FOOD PATH

Shortage of land to grow food

A larger population means that there are more families, with more children. But the amount of land remains the same. So each family has less land. When parents die, the land is divided between the children. If there are many children, the farms get smaller. Some children may not get a share.

As the number of people on fertile land increases, some families move to the dry marginal lands where farming is more risky and yields are lower. Some families end up with no land at all.

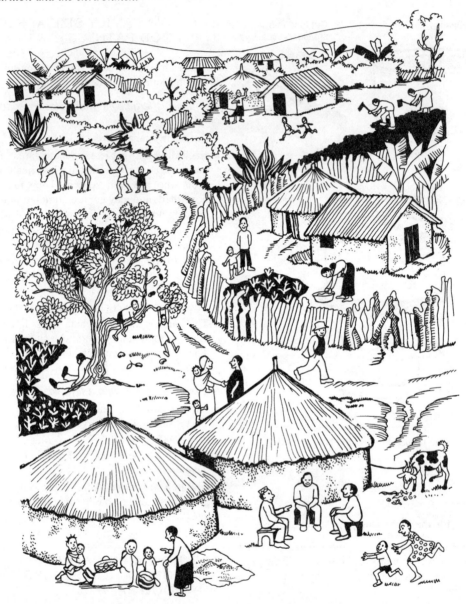

Fig. 24–5 How many people are there in this village? By the time these children have grown up, the population of the village will have more than doubled.

Low family income

Because there is not enough land, some people have no land. They have to look for work with other people who have larger farms or plantations. Because prices paid for food are low, agricultural wages are very low. Agricultural labourers and their families are usually very poor.

Many people move to towns to look for work. But the rapid increase in the number of people in towns, especially young people, means that there are not enough jobs for everyone. This means that many people do not have money to buy enough food.

Lack of government funds

The increasing population means that governments must spend money to build and staff more health

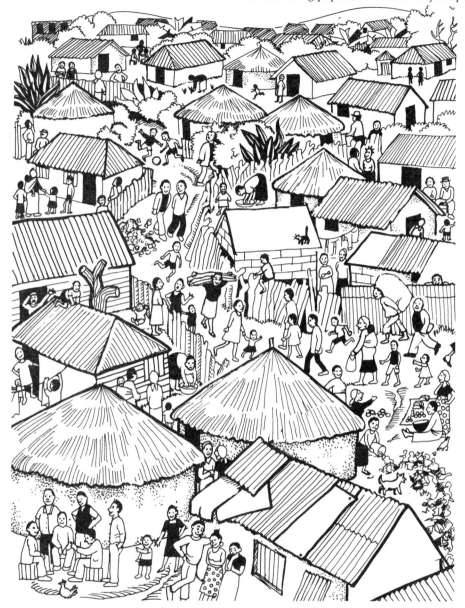

Fig. 24–6 The same village (Fig. 24–5) 30 years later. How many people are here now?

centres, schools, and other services. So there is less money to develop new industries and new jobs, for agriculture and food research, for training and extension services.

Poor living conditions

There are not enough houses for everyone, and not enough clean water. So people in towns live in large slums, with poor housing and poor sanitation and water supplies. Children are often ill with diarrhoea and other infections.

Families in towns may be separated from their extended families. Young women may not have anyone to help them to feed and care for children.

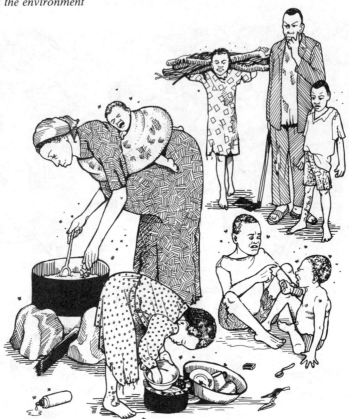

Fig. 24–7 A family with too many closely spaced children.

24.8 DISCUSSING FAMILY SIZE, POPULATION, AND NUTRITION

Your aim should be to help people to *match their family size to their family resources.* If families have only the children that they can feed and care for properly, the result should be smaller families and slower population growth. To help people make wise decisions about family size and child spacing, you need to:

- Encourage people, especially women, to believe that it is possible to decide when to have children and how many to have.

- Understand why some families have many closely spaced children. For example, wanting children for support in old age; wanting many children for pleasure and prestige; wanting a child of a particular sex; women giving in to men's desires and demands; family planning services not being easily available.

- Discuss with men, women, and schoolchildren the problems of a population that increases faster than

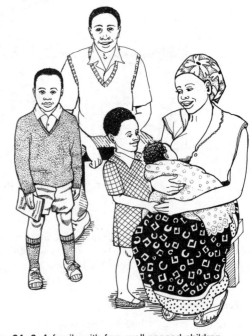

Fig. 24–8 A family with few, well spaced children.

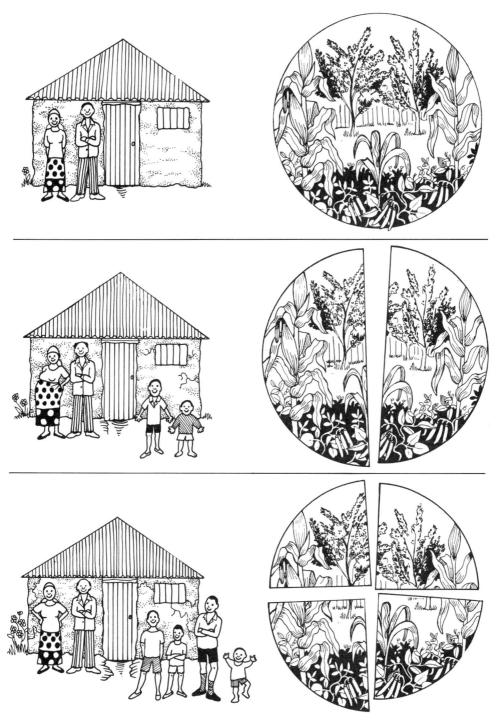

Fig. 24–9 The bigger the family, the more the land must be divided.

the food supply, jobs, and schools. Encourage them to think about the problem in relation to their own community and environment.

- Discuss the advantages of having a few healthy well-educated children, compared with having many undernourished poorly educated children. Include older people in discussions—they may influence their children's and grandchildren's attitudes to family size.
- Encourage couples and groups (such as women's groups) to discuss how many children they want and how many they can afford.
- Encourage men to respect women's opinions about family matters.
- Help women to have the confidence to discuss these things. Encourage the education of girls and women. Women with a good education or their own income often have more independence and confidence to plan their families. They usually want smaller families, and often start childbearing later.
- Discuss the problems of early sexual activity and pregnancy with adolescent girls and boys and their families, teachers, and employers. It may not be acceptable to provide adolescents with contraceptives, but they need to understand their own feelings and the pressures and risks that they face, and they need help to develop the confidence to say 'no'.

Help with family planning services

You should be able to tell people where they can get family planning services. You should encourage people to use the service and know how to refer them.

Family planning should help mothers to have at least 2–3 years between pregnancies. To fully restore her strength and nutrient stores, a mother should wait 6 months after stopping breastfeeding before she becomes pregnant again.

Health workers who advise about family planning should:

- Explain how exclusive breastfeeding for 6 months and frequent breastfeeding (8–10 times a day) can delay the return of the mother's fertility (see Section 10.4). Breastfeeding can protect a mother against a new pregnancy for at least 6 months, if her periods have not returned,
- Explain that, when her periods return or when her baby is 6 months old, she should use another method of family planning to be certain of avoiding another pregnancy.

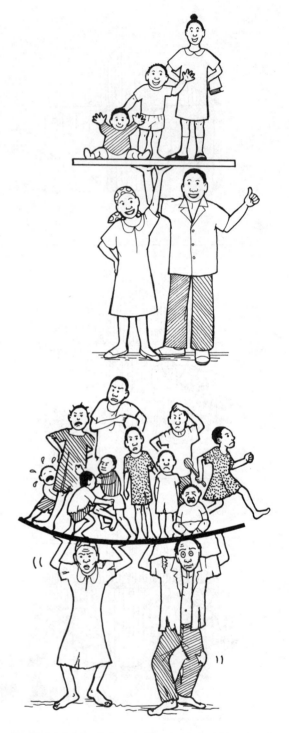

Fig. 24–10 Which family can care for their children best? Encourage parents to match their family size to their family resources.

- Advise a method which does not interfere with breastfeeding. The safest are: progesterone-only pills, depo-provera, and IUDs.
- Give information and counselling to adolescent girls and boys, and contraceptives to young mothers.

24.9 HOME GARDENS

Home gardens (kitchen gardens) are an important source of food for families in both rural and urban areas. Some gardens include crops and small animals such as chicken, goats, and rabbits, and sometimes fishponds. In some places there are school gardens and community gardens. This section is about home gardens, but it can help you to start and improve school and community gardens too.

In rural areas many people work gardens in the traditional way, growing trees and different plants mixed together. This is an efficient way to use land and labour. Trees protect smaller plants from too much sun and rain, and they help to conserve the soil, animals provide manure, and the plants provide food.

A garden costs little money, because the family does the work, using simple tools. It is not necessary to use commercial chemical fertilizers or pesticides, and there is no cost for transporting the food.

Therefore helping to start or to improve a garden may be one way in which you can give practical help to a poor and undernourished family. Home gardens can provide:

- food for the family;
- food for the animals;
- herbal medicines;
- wood and other material for fuel;
- wood for timber;
- materials for thatching, fencing, baskets, and mats;
- cash crops, extra food, and sometimes timber for sale;
- a way for children to learn to grow food.

24.10 THE TYPES OF FOOD THAT GARDENS PROVIDE

When you discuss starting or improving a garden with a family, you need to think of:

- the types of food which the family is able to grow on the land available;
- which foods can provide the nutrients that the family needs.

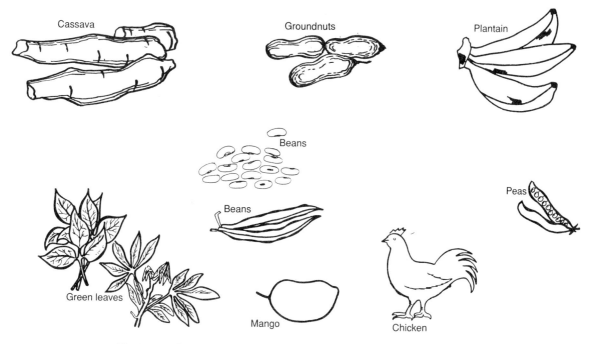

Fig. 24–11 Some traditional foods which can increase household food security.

Box 24.2.   Traditional foods

We use the words *traditional foods* to mean foods which farmers in a country have produced or gathered for several generations. We also include some newer foods such as round (Irish) potatoes which have similar advantages.

Examples of traditional foods are: cassava, yams, sweet and round potatoes, millets, sorghum, plantains, many legumes, vegetables, and fruits, small animals, insects, and poultry. Often these foods are produced by women. Some, such as insects, wild birds, and mice, are caught by children.

Until recently, governments and international agencies have not given as much attention or resources to the production and processing of traditional foods as they have given to major cereals (maize, rice, wheat) and export crops (such as coffee, sugar cane, and tobacco). One reason is that many traditional foods do not store well and so the amounts traded are quite small. Most are eaten by the families who grow them.

Traditional foods are important because
- They increase the *family food security* (see Chapter 25). Many traditional foods are available throughout the year. So families can use them before the maize or rice harvest or if these crops fail. Having cassava, yams, or plantains is like having a permanent store of food.
- They can often grow on poor soils and need little fertilizer. Some need little water or are resistant to pests and diseases. Some, for example, round potatoes, sweet potatoes, and cassava, produce more Calories per hectare than some cereals.
- Families can produce them on small areas of land such as home gardens (see Section 24.9)—for example, cooking bananas, vegetables, and fruits and small animals and poultry.
- They often require labour at different times to cereal crops, so they spread the workload.
- They are an important source of income for women. Women produce, process, and sell many traditional foods, such as legumes, vegetables, and eggs, or they make these foods into snacks (for example, fried bean cakes) or beer for sale.
- They are valuable sources of important nutrients. African vegetables (such as cowpea leaves) and fruits (such as pawpaw) are rich in many micronutrients.
  - Round potatoes contain good quality protein compared to other roots.
  - Small animals and poultry are good sources of complete protein and haem iron.
  - Nuts and oil seeds, such as simsim, are rich in essential fatty acids and energy.
- Many traditional foods, such as fruits and nuts, make good snacks.

Many wild traditional foods can still be collected. They provide important nutrients especially in the hungry season. For example, wild green leaves, including leaves from trees; wild fruits, such as baobab and figs, and wild insects, birds, animals, and honey.

Nowadays governments realize that traditional foods are an important part of a nation's plans to prevent food shortages (that is, to increase food security; see Chapter 25). Governments are investigating methods of production and processing which increase yields and reduce labour.

How to help to increase the amounts of traditional foods eaten and sold
- Look around local gardens and farms and find out which vegetables, fruits, and other traditional foods grow well. Tell other families about them.
- Ask agricultural officers and research workers about suitable traditional foods and how to produce and process them.
- Help people, particularly women, to start co-operatives or food processing or marketing schemes to process and sell more traditional foods.
- Encourage families to grow suitable crops which increase their food supplies throughout the year. These may be crops which:
  - are available all the year—e.g. cassava;
  - are drought-resistant—e.g. pigeon peas;
  - mature quickly—e.g. 'early maturing' or 'fast-growing' cow peas.

  Give special help to poor families who need these crops most if the cereal harvest is poor.
- Find out about wild foods in your area. Tell people which contain important nutrients, especially micronutrients which are low in local diets (for example, folate, vitamin A).

Gardens do not usually provide the main part of the family's energy, but they may supplement it, and they can provide important nutrients and special foods which may be expensive or not easily available otherwise. Gardens may provide:

- *Staple foods* (for example, cassava, yams, taro, sweet potato, plantain) which help to:
  - feed the family during the hungry season before the main cereal harvest;
  - protect families against failure of the main cereal harvest;
  - increase the food supply for poor urban families, who have to buy most of their food.

- *Legumes* (for example beans, cow peas, groundnuts) that are useful for sauce or relish and that are an important source of protein, energy, minerals, and B vitamins.

- *Chickens and goats* and other animals, e.g. rabbits, which provide meat, eggs, and milk.

- *Vegetables and fruit* (especially green vegetables) which may be the family's main source of vitamin A, vitamin C, and folate or which provide flavour for food, such as onions or peppers. Fresh vegetables and fruit and other foods that provide vitamins are often expensive or difficult to buy.

- *Honey*, which can provide concentrated energy and sweetness and which may not be available in other ways.

24.11 GARDENS IN TOWNS

Urban families often start gardens to increase their food supply. Usually they grow food mainly for the family's meals. If the garden is small, they may grow a few vegetables.

People in towns start a garden only when they feel sure that:

- the garden will provide enough food to be worth the cost in money and time;
- the authorities will not destroy the garden or prevent the family from using the land;
- thieves will not steal from the garden.

Explain to authorities how gardens help poorer families and increase food supplies. You may be able to persuade them to allow people to have gardens.

24.12 PROBLEMS TO CONSIDER WHEN PLANNING GARDENS

When you discuss starting gardens with families, you need to consider:

Land
Land may be a problem in both rural and urban areas.

In rural areas the increasing population means that many families do not have enough land. They may have to use steep land, dry marginal land, or land with poor soil.

In towns there may be very little land available, and people may not be able to get a legal right to the land that there is.

- If there is a plot near the house, the family may be able to grow some vegetables.
- Sometimes only a plot far from the house is available. Families then have to walk further to work in the garden. They may prefer to grow crops such as maize, beans, and pumpkins, which do not need much watering and looking after, rather than green vegetables, which need more work. Food is more likely to be stolen from gardens which are far away from the house.

Box 24.3. Gardens and vitamins

There are three vitamins which many women and children lack.

Vitamin	Source
Vitamin A	Liver, fish, red palm oil, orange fruits and vegetables, green leafy vegetables
Folate	Liver, kidney, fish, legumes, fresh vegetables
Vitamin C	Fresh vegetables and fruits, fresh plantain, cassava, yams, potatoes, milk

Cross out the foods which are difficult or expensive for most families to buy. Underline the foods which grow in gardens in your area. You may find that gardens are the main source of these three vitamins.

- If there is no garden, families can sometimes grow vegetables in boxes or cans outside the house.

Water

Lack of water is the main problem in many places. Carrying water to a garden takes a lot of time and energy. In towns gardening may only be possible:

- in the rainy season; *or*
- if the garden is near water; *or*
- if water is not expensive to buy.

Labour

Gardens and animals need much attention, especially at the beginning. It is often necessary for men to clear the ground to start a new garden. Women who have much other work or who are employed may not have enough time for a garden. Or they may only have time for a small garden. Children may be too busy at school to help much. Women know the size of plot that they can manage through the year.

Fencing

A garden needs a fence to prevent cattle, goats, chickens, and wild animals entering and damaging it and to discourage thieves. A live hedge of a sharp thorny plant or a legume takes time to grow. Sometimes it is easier to fence the animals in.

Pests

Sometimes vegetable and other crops suffer from pests and diseases. Ask advice from the agricultural worker about methods of control which are suitable for gardens and safe and cheap. Usually natural methods are best. Chemicals are expensive and they may be dangerous if not used properly. Improving the fertility of the soil may help plants to resist pests and may reduce the need for chemicals.

24.13 TRADITIONAL GARDENS

Many traditional gardens are very efficient, and you can learn from them. There is often a mixture of plants of different heights, forming *layers* (see Fig. 24–12).

1. The top layer contains tall trees, which protect the other layers and hold moisture. Their fallen leaves add nutrients to the soil.
2. The next layer contains fruit trees such as banana or pawpaw.
3. The next layer contains bushes such as coffee, maize, peppers, sugar cane, and cassava leaves.
4. At ground level there are plants such as beans and pumpkins.
5. Below the ground are root vegetables such as potato and taro.

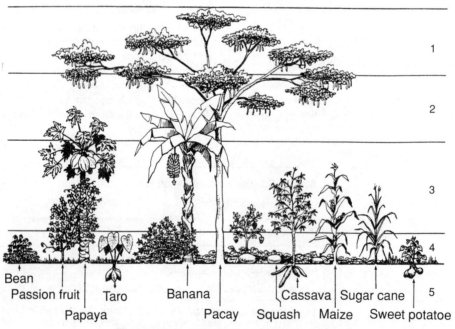

Fig. 24–12 An example of a good home garden.

Box 24.4. A successful kind of home garden

A Chagga garden on Kilimanjaro can give the family food and many of the other things that it needs. This type of garden makes efficient use of the land, it keeps the soil fertile and protects it from erosion, and it costs very little.

- A typical Chagga garden is about ½ to 1 hectare.
- The trees and shrubs protect the shorter plants from heavy rain and from too much sun.
- The family keeps a few cows, goats, and chickens and sometimes a pig.
- Manure from the animals and compost from household waste fertilizes the soil.
- There is food for the family and the animals all the year round including: bananas, legumes, vegetables, sweet potato and taro; eggs, meat, and milk; honey.

The garden also produces:

- coffee and some food for sale;
- wood for fuel and building;
- thatch for roofs;
- plants for fencing, medicine, and killing insects; sharp, thorny plants round the edge of the garden make a fence to keep animals out.

The men in the family sell the coffee, chickens, and eggs. The women sell any bananas, vegetables, and milk that the family do not need.

(Adapted from Fernandes *et al.* 1985)

24.14 IMPROVING GARDENS

If there is no garden, or if the soil is poor, or if it does not produce many nutritious foods, you may be able to help.

When you visit a family, look at their plot, and discuss how they use it. To grow more food, and to improve the quality of crops, a family may need to find ways to prevent soil erosion and to improve soil fertility. To have enough of all nutrients, a family may need to produce different types of foods.

If you are an agricultural extension worker, you know what improvements families can make. Remember that poor families cannot afford chemicals, and results are often better with natural and traditional methods.

If you are another kind of worker you should discuss with an agricultural worker what you can advise, or ask an agricultural worker to talk to community groups or visit individual families.

These are some of the things that you may want to suggest, or to help the family to get advice about.

Preventing erosion

Ways to prevent soil being washed away include:

- *terracing*—that is, building flat *terraces* or steps in gardens which are on sloping land (see Fig. 24–2);

- building water breaks, that is, small dams, banks, or ridges, to spread out fast flowing water during the rains;

- *alley cropping*, that is, growing crops between rows of trees or hedges;

- planting grass to cover open ground;

- planting trees or hedges as wind breaks;

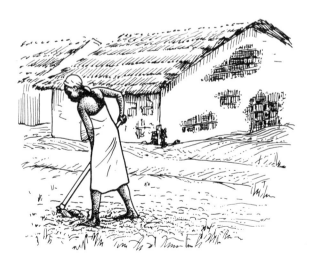

Fig. 24–13 When you visit a family, look at their plot and discuss how they use it. You may be able to help.

● not allowing cattle or goats to overgraze land, avoiding having too many animals, and allowing the grass to grow between periods of grazing.

Maintaining fertility

To keep soil fertile, it is necessary to replace lost nutrients and allow soil time to recover. Ways to do this include:

● Letting soil 'rest' for a time. Growing crops continuously can make soil lose its fertility. But where people do not have enough land, it is difficult to let it rest.

● *Crop rotation*, that is, growing different crops in different years. Different crops use up different nutrients, and some put nutrients into the soil.

● *Mixed cropping or intercropping*, that is, growing a mixture of plants together, for example, maize and beans. Beans add to the soil some of the nutrients such as nitrogen which maize takes out.

● Making *compost* from plant waste to add to the soil. This is an important way to return nutrients to soil. There are many ways to make compost. Figure 24–14 shows one way.

● *Mulching* which means spreading plant material like cut grass or banana leaves on the soil around the plants. This keeps soil dark, cool, and moist and discourages weeds from growing. It reduces soil damage from heavy rainfall. The leaves rot down into the soil.

There are a number of other methods of maintaining and improving soil fertility. Find out what agricultural workers are promoting.

Growing new types of plant

After a garden has grown for some time, it is often not necessary to use seeds. To grow more vegetables, gardeners divide the roots of a plant, or plant a potato, or take 'cuttings'.

If a gardener needs seeds to start a garden or add new types of vegetable, it is important to:

● get fresh, good quality seeds; if seeds are stored or kept for a long time, few of them grow;

● choose a suitable *variety* of seed.

THINGS TO DO

Discussion

1. Show pictures of land with environmental damage. Discuss ways in which nutrition workers can help communities to protect their environment and to use sustainable methods of food production.

A compost heap

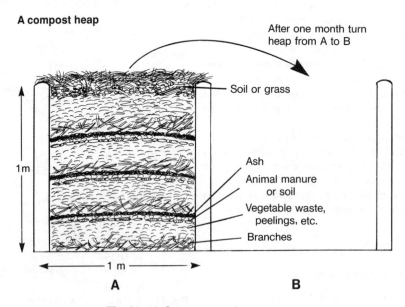

Fig. 24–14 One way to make compost.

Demonstration

2. Demonstrate a locally used fuel-efficient stove. Ask trainees to suggest other ways to save fuel.

Field visits

3. Take trainees to visit a place where there is environmental damage (e.g. soil erosion, deforestation, overgrazing).

   a. Discuss reasons for the damage and how nutrition workers might be able to help communities to do something about it.

   b. Discuss what else could help to restore the environment.

4. Take trainees to visit some gardens in your area.

   a. Look at the arrangement of the garden—with intercropping, layering, terracing, etc.

   b. Make a list of the foods produced.

   c. Find out how and when the family uses each food.

   d. Find out what problems they have with the garden (e.g. shortage of water).

Project

5. Ask trainees to find out where families who want to start or improve their gardens can get help, for example, from successful garden owners, agricultural workers, or from a horticultural institute.

6. If trainees are on a course of a year or more and you have some land:

   a. give each a small garden;

   b. or have a communal garden.

   This helps trainees to learn how to grow different foods. In a communal garden, you might keep some livestock.

USEFUL PUBLICATIONS

FAO (1988). *Traditional food plants*, Food and Nutrition Paper, no. 42. FAO, Rome.

FAO (1988c). *Field programme management. Food and nutrition: population and nutrition—a training pack*, FAO Rome.

FAO (1989a). *Edible plants of Uganda*, Food and Nutrition Paper, no. 42/1. (Author, P. Goode.) FAO, Rome.

FAO (1989b). *Forestry and food security*, Forestry Paper, no. 90. FAO, Rome.

25 Food security

25.1 'FOOD SECURITY' AND 'FOOD AND NUTRITION SURVEILLANCE'

Betty works at a rural health centre. When young children come for growth monitoring, she and her staff record whether or not the children are underweight. Betty reports the percentage of underweight children in her monthly returns.

Silas is an agricultural extension worker in the same area. His tasks include measuring rainfall each month, predicting the yields of the main crops, and recording the price of staple foods in the market.

Betty and Silas collect these data for *'food and nutrition surveillance'* which is part of their country's *'food security'* system.

25.2 FOOD SECURITY

'Food security' means that everyone is able to get enough food throughout the year to satisfy their nutritional needs. It means that enough food of different sorts must travel along the food paths. It means that all families must have enough land, money, or other resources to get the foods that they need.

A secure supply of food is necessary for good nutrition, but it does not, by itself, mean that everyone is well nourished. This is because other things such as infections, appetite, the energy concentration of weaning foods, and people's workloads also affect nutrition.

'National food security' means that a country has enough food for everyone. But this does not mean that *every family* has enough food, because the food may not be evenly distributed. *'Family'* or *'household food security'* means that every family always has enough to eat.

Governments promote national and household food security in different ways. These may include:

- promoting sustainable methods of food production;
- improving food distribution and marketing;
- deciding how much food to import and export;
- having stores of staple foods (called a *strategic food reserve*) that they use to stabilize supplies and prices, and in times of food shortages;

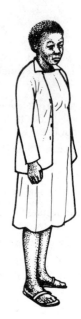

Fig. 25–1 Betty works at a rural health centre.

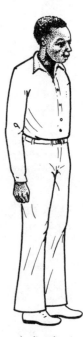

Fig. 25–2 Silas is an agricultural extension officer.

- controlling and/or subsidizing the price of staple foods and other essentials so that poor families can afford enough food;
- trying to increase incomes of the poorest families:
  - fixing minimum wages;
  - encouraging employment opportunities;
  - encouraging suitable cash crops for small farmers (e.g. coffee).

Families try to have enough food all year by:

- deciding how to get the most money and food from the family's resources such as land, skills, labour, time (for example, men working in town for wages while women grow food at home);
- growing crops which mature at different times;
- selling livestock when grain stores are low and the family needs money to buy more;
- buying cheaper foods when money is short (e.g. buying cassava instead of rice);
- budgeting wages or money from cash crops so that there is always enough for food—or having credit with local foodstores.

25.3 FOOD AND NUTRITION SURVEILLANCE (FNS)

In the sections on removing the blocks on the food paths we have listed ways to help families to be 'food secure'. An important part of food security is *food and nutrition surveillance (FNS)*. FNS means:

- monitoring the supply of food at different points along the food paths, to see and remove blocks quickly;
- monitoring the nutrition of at risk groups, such as young children, to find out where and when there are nutrition problems, and whom they affect. And then doing something to deal with the problems.

The aim of FNS is to improve food security and prevent undernutrition. The data collected in FNS are used in several ways:

- *To warn that people may be short of food.* This may occur when food supplies are low (e.g. if the rains fail), or when people do not have enough money to buy food (e.g. if unemployment is high).

- *To provide planners and administrators with information.* FNS can show where there are blocks on the food paths, and whether particular programmes and policies are likely to remove them.

- *To monitor the effects of 'structural adjustment' on food supplies and nutrition.* 'Structural adjustment' is the action that governments take to deal with debt and other economic problems. Sometimes structural adjustment includes reducing food subsidies or health services. This may mean that poorer families cannot buy enough food. It may increase undernutrition among children and other groups at risk.

25.4 COLLECTING AND REPORTING DATA FOR FNS

An FNS needs to receive regular information so that it can monitor changes over time. It needs information on:

- food supplies at different places along the food paths;
- families' ability to get food (their access to food);
- nutrition of 'at risk' groups.

The *indicators* may be:

- data which people collect routinely (for example, rainfall, crop forecasts, weight-for-age of young children);
- data which people collect periodically and specially for the FNS (for example, surveys of stored foods, how households spend their money, height-for-age or arm circumference of young children).

Box 25.1. What an FNS system consists of

1. Collecting and reporting data:
   - on food supplies;
   - on families' access to food;
   - on nutritional status.
2. Analysing and interpreting data; finding reasons for poor food security.
3. Action to prevent or correct poor food security.

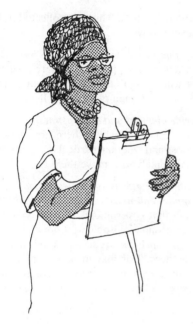

Fig. 25–3 Collecting data for an FNS.

The amount and type of data collected depends on:

- the reason for collecting the data;
- the resources for analysing the data (it is often quicker and easier to collect information than to analyse it);
- the resources for doing something about the situation.

For example, if there are few resources to do anything about a food shortage, then it is only necessary to collect a few simple indicators to show where the worst areas are.

Examples of indicators for FNS

Food supplies

- Crop forecasts (from records of areas planted, and effects of pests or diseases, and rainfall).
- Numbers of livestock, availability of feed, effect of disease.
- Fish catches and losses during processing and transporting.
- Harvested yields of staple crops and other foods, and estimates of post-harvest losses.
- Amounts of stored staple crops.
- Changes in population (a rapid increase, such as

many refugees coming into the area, may lead to land and food shortages; migration to towns, mines, etc. may lead to labour shortages on farms.)

Access to food

- Prices in the shops of staple foods eaten by low-income groups.
- Wages of low-income workers.
- Rates of unemployment and underemployment.
- Forecasted or actual yields of cash crops grown by small farmers and their farm prices.

Indicators that warn of food shortages:

- *If prices increase compared to the minimum or average wage*, some people cannot buy as much. For example, if the price of maize increases, but the minimum wage stays the same, the number of families who cannot buy enough is likely to increase.

- *If there is an increase in the number of people selling things* (such as jewellery, household goods, animals, or land), people are probably having difficulty buying food. If a family has to sell equipment and resources that they use to produce or market food or earn money (for example, oxen, bicycle, sewing machine, land) they are at risk of having less food or money in the future.

- *If there is an increase in the number of animals (especially small animals) for sale and a decrease in their price.* If many people sell animals it may mean that there is a shortage of animal feed because of drought or poor harvests. Or it may mean that the family needs money to buy food because of an increase in the price of staple or because of a poor harvest.

Box 25.2 shows how a rise in the price of a staple food and a fall in the price of animals can warn of serious food shortages. This situation is most obvious in rural areas, because in towns prices are often controlled, or food is imported.

Nutrition of young children

This is an indicator of the effects of poor food security. You can compare the proportion of children who are undernourished in different places, and in the same place at different times. This tells planners and administrators when and where there are food security problems. If malnutrition increases, it suggests severe food shortages in an area. It indicates a need to investigate the situation. (Malnutrition in an individual child can be due to infection, bulky weaning foods, etc., as well as shortage of food in the family. But if the

---

Box 25.2. Example of poor rainfall leading to food shortage

Rains fail

↓

Harvest of maize is poor

↓

Less maize stored on farm
Less maize sold

↓

Farmers have less cash
Less food on market
Traders hoard maize

↓

Price of maize rises

↓

Pastoralists sell animals to get enough money to buy maize
Price of small animals decreases
People sell possessions to get money to buy maize
People borrow money to buy maize

↓

Less maize bought and less eaten

↓

Hunger and undernutrition increases
People unable to work as hard as usual

Poor harvests also mean that there is less agricultural work. Farmers have less money to spend, so there is less money in the community, and more unemployment. So for many families, incomes go down, while food prices go up.

---

number of malnourished children in a community increases, it is more likely to be due to lack of food in the area.)

Indicators of undernutrition used for the FNS are:

- Weight-for-age. This is used most often, because the information is routinely collected from growth charts. Collect data from community growth monitoring as well as health centres.
- Weight-for-height and height-for-age collected in surveys.
- Birth weights—often routinely collected.

Measuring children does not *warn* about food shortages—because malnutrition shows that there *already are* shortages. But these indicators show which areas or groups need help most, so that resources can be *targeted* to them.

25.5 ANALYSING DATA

Data must be analysed and interpreted to find out what they mean and to decide what to do. Data that may warn about food shortages need to be analysed quickly so that, if necessary, authorities can do something in time to prevent them. Analysis is done at different administrative levels (for example, community, district, or central) depending on where there are resources for action.

If FNS data show a food security problem, the next step is to find out where the blocks are on the food paths—and how to remove them. For example:

- Poor yields of beans may be due to bad weather, lack of fertilizer, or crop disease.
- An increase in the cost of maize may be the result of a poor harvest, a problem with distribution (such as an increase in the price of petrol), removal of a price subsidy, or civil unrest in the area leading to hoarding.

25.6 ACTIONS TO IMPROVE FOOD SECURITY

It is only useful to collect and analyse data if it is possible to improve the situation or to make better policies and plans. Some of the ways governments promote food security are listed at the beginning of this section.

If FNS data warn of food shortages, action must be taken quickly. The type of action depends on where the block is on the food path. If the block is early on the path, there is a better chance of removing it before food shortages occur. For example, if an insect pest threatens a staple crop, it may be possible to control it before it does much damage. But, if floods interfere with food distribution and raise food prices, it is likely that many poor families will suffer before much can be done.

Prevention or control of food shortages

Actions which authorities can take include:

- moving food from the strategic food reserve on to the market; or using it for feeding programmes;
- importing more food, or moving food from another part of the country to an area with problems;
- starting a feeding programme for vulnerable groups (see Section 29.2);
- starting a Cash-for-Work programme or a Food-for-Work programme for needy families (see Section 29.5);
- providing loans so that needy families can buy food (which they pay back later in cash, food, or labour);
- increasing subsidies to producers or consumers on basic foods and other essentials (e.g. fuel);
- providing seeds for planting if supplies have been eaten or lost;
- increasing health care of at-risk groups.

25.7 NUTRITION WORKERS AND FNS SYSTEMS

Nutrition workers often help to collect data for FNS as Betty and Silas do. Sometimes you may help to interpret and use the data.

An important time to watch over a community is when something new or unusual is happening. For example, when there is a drought or a flood, or when pests attack the staple food, or food subsidies are re-

duced, or there is civil unrest. Or when a development programme starts, or a new crop (e.g. soybeans or tobacco) is introduced. Sometimes development programmes do not help poorer families or women. Sometimes it means that they have less land to grow family food or less time for child care.

You may be able to help set up a local FNS system to collect and analyse data and to take action at community or district level. Many food problems are local, and can be dealt with by local action. Box 25.3 gives an example of the type of data which you could collect and use locally.

Using local data

You can help the community to plot data like that in Box 25.3 on simple graphs each month to show how it changes over time. Here are examples of what you might find.

Example 1

The rainfall graph shows that there was much less rain than usual during the maize growing season. This warns community leaders that the harvest will be poor. So:

- They ask the marketing board to bring some extra maize into the area.
- They encourage farmers to plant a 'drought-resistant' crop (such as pigeon peas) that they can sell for cash so that they have money to buy maize.

Example 2

The health centre returns show that the percentage of underweight children has increased a lot. The local council asks a senior health worker to find out why and to suggest a plan of action.

- The health worker finds that two local factories have closed and many men are unemployed so their families do not have cash for food.
- She suggests that they start a feeding programme for short-term relief.
- She suggests that the council starts a training programme for unemployed workers so that they can start small local industries.

Example 3

The local agricultural officer has recorded the supplies and prices of beans for several years. He knows that supplies are low and prices are high just before the harvest.

- He suggests that the authorities buy a reserve store of beans earlier in the season. Then they can put it on the market later and keep the price down.

Box 25.3.   Local food and nutrition surveillance

Example of chart to collect monthly data from one place e.g. village, location (adapted from Brown 1990)

Place	*Month*	*Year*
Rainfall (collected in simple guage)	Days rain:	mm rain ....
Maize harvest forecast	Better than normal/normal/worse than normal	
Market prices	Maize – kg Beans – kg Goat meat – kg Cooking fat – 250-g tin Beer – bottle Kerosene – bottle	
Birth weights	Number of births:	No. <2500 g (LBW) .... % <2500 g ....
Weight for age of young children	Number of children:	No. underweight .... % underweight ....

25.8 SIMPLE NUTRITION SURVEYS

A survey of the weights, heights, or arm circumferences of young children is a quick easy way to get a general idea of the nutrition of a community. It can tell you how many families have undernourished children and which types of families or areas have nutrition problems. It can indicate whether you need to investigate the situation more closely.

A simple nutrition survey may be useful:

- for nutrition surveillance;
- for planning community activities and for monitoring and evaluating them;
- for planning development programmes so that they help undernourished families, and for monitoring their effects on nutrition.

A simple survey of body measurements may be part of a bigger survey which also examines micronutrient deficiencies (e.g. vitamin A deficiency, anaemia) and which collects data on the cause of undernutrition.

Planning a survey

The important things are:

- Plan the survey with the community and its leaders.
- Decide which young children to examine—all the children or a sample. Try to measure at least 100 children and make sure that they include all the types of children in the community rich and poor, sick and healthy, living in different areas.
- Decide which measurements and other data (such as age, location, family occupation or income group) you need and can analyse.
- Decide when to do the survey—nutrition may vary with the season.

A survey using growth charts

Weigh children aged 6 months to 3 or 5 years and find out their ages to the nearest month (see Section 14.10). Mark the weight of each child on one growth chart. Then you

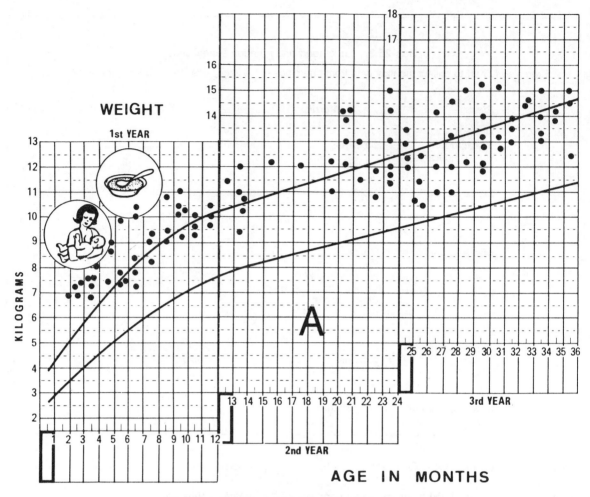

Fig. 25–4 Weights of children from Area A in Zambia.

can see how many children are underweight (below the 3rd centile) and how many have healthy weights for their age. If only a few children (about three in every 100) have weights below the 3rd centile, then the community is probably well nourished.

If many children have weights below the 3rd centile then most of these children are likely to be malnourished and the community has a nutrition problem. A simple survey like this also shows the ages when most children are malnourished.

A survey in two areas of Zambia

Figures 25–4 and 25–5 show the weight charts used in a survey of two areas of Zambia. Figure 25–4 shows the result of a survey of 103 children in area A. You can see

that all of the weight dots are above the 3rd centile curve. So probably most of the children in Area A are growing well.

Figure 25–5 shows the result of a survey of 107 children in Area B. You can see that 32 of the children have weights below the 3rd centile. So about one-third of the children may not be growing well.

The children in Areas A and B were different children living in different places at the same time. There were many differences between the families and the conditions of the two places. The survey showed that the conditions affected the children's growth.

You can also do surveys of children in the same place at different times. The number of children who are not growing well may vary from year to year. For example,

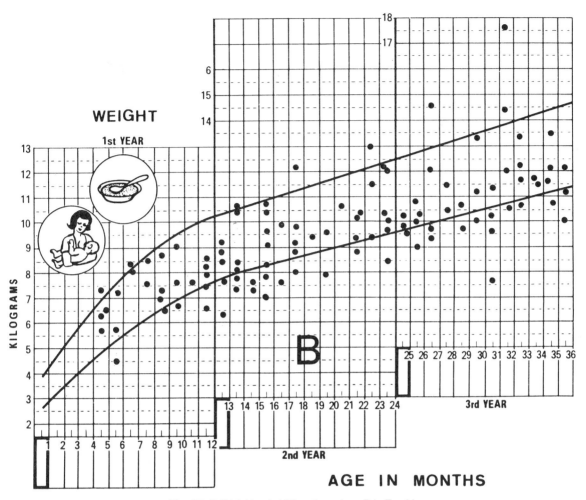

Fig. 25–5 Weights of children from Area B in Zambia.

if the number of underweight children increases, you would want to try to find out why, so that you could plan what might be done to help those families.

A survey using arm circumference

The advantage of an arm circumference survey is that you do not need to know the children's ages accurately and it is easy to carry a tape from house to house.

Measure the arm circumference of children aged 1–5 years (see Section 14.18). Record the results on an arm circumference chart or on a sheet of paper and count how many are:

- above 13.5 cm or in the green Shakir band—these children are probably well nourished;

- between 12.5 and 13.5 cm or in the yellow Shakir band—these children are moderately undernourished;

- below 12.5 cm or in the red Shakir band—these children are severely undernourished.

If only a few children have an arm circumference below 13.5 cm then the community is probably well nourished. If many children have an arm circumference below 13.5 cm, the community probably has a nutrition problem.

A survey using arm circumference in Zambia

Figures 25–6 and 25–7 show the results of a survey of children's arm circumference in Zambia. These children are from the same areas as in the survey of weights in Figs 25–4 and 25–5. But notice that in this survey we have left out the children below 1 year old, because arm circumference is not such a useful measure at this age.

Figure 25–6 shows that in Area A there were 65 children, but none of them had an arm circumference below 13.5 cm. Figure 25–7 shows that in Area B there were 82 children: 19 of them had an arm circumference below 13.5 cm; of which 5 had an arm circumference below 12.5 cm. So about 22 per cent of the children are wasted, showing that they are moderately or severely undernourished.

The results are very similar to the results of the survey of children's weights. In this survey, we knew the children's ages. But if we did not know their ages, we could simply count how many children had arm circumferences above and below 13.5 cm. The results would be exactly the same—without the need to plot them on a chart (Table 25.1).

Table 25.1.   Tally of arm circumferences of children aged 12–35 months in two areas of Zambia

	Area A		Area B	
	Number	%	Number	%
Total	65		82	
MUAC more than 13.5 cm	65	100	63	78
MUAC 12.6 to 13.5 cm	0	0	14	16
MUAC 12.5 cm or less	0	0	5	6

A survey using a thinness chart

You can fix a thinness chart to a wall or use a mobile chart (see Section 14.17).

Weigh children aged around 2–5 years (it is difficult to use the chart with younger children). Stand them against their weight on the thinness chart and note the colour of their height. Record the number of children in the green (lower) 'well nourished'; yellow (middle) 'moderately malnourished'; or red (upper) 'severely malnourished' bands.

If not more than about three in 100 children reach the yellow band and none reach the red band, the community is probably well nourished. If many children are in the yellow or red bands, the community has a nutrition problem.

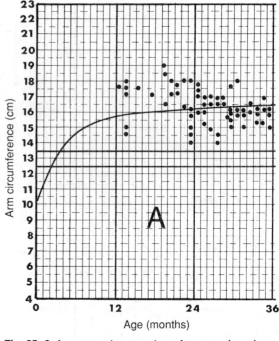

Fig. 25–6 A survey using arm circumference—Area A.

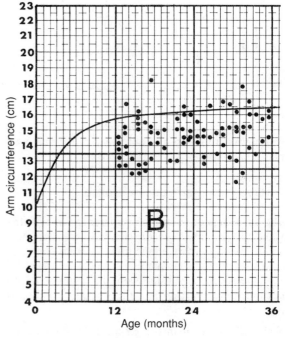

Fig. 25–7 A survey using arm circumference—Area B.

THINGS TO DO

Discussion

1. Put trainees in groups. Ask them to decide which are the best local indicators to give an early warning of food shortages.

Learning from other workers

2. Find out if agricultural or other workers are collecting information for food and nutritional surveillance. If so, ask one of them to come and tell trainees what they collect and how they use it.

3. Let trainees ask an agricultural worker whether the next harvest is likely to be good, and which indicators he uses to estimate yields.

Projects

4. Ask a health centre for the records of the percentage of underweight children for the previous year.

   a. Ask trainees to study these records to see if there are any changes during the period.

   b. If so, discuss reasons why these changes may have occurred.

c. Ask the health centre staff what they observed, and what they did about it.

5. Let the trainees do a simple survey of 100 children in an area nearby.

   a. Weigh the children or measure their arm circumferences. You can either plot the weights on a chart, or do a simple tally of MUAC.

   b. Measure all the children under the age of 3 or 5, or all the children between 1 and 5 years old in a small area, or measure children in every fifth or tenth house in an area until you have measured 100 children.

   c. Be careful that you see all the children in the houses that you choose or the survey will not be accurate. You may have to come back to find any children who were out the first time.

USEFUL PUBLICATIONS

Beaton, G., Kelly, A., Kevany, J., Martorell, R., and Mason, J. (1990). *Appropriate uses of anthropometric indices in children*, ACC/SCN Nutrition Policy Discussion Paper, no. 7. ACC/SCN, Geneva.

FAO (1990). *Conducting small-scale nutrition surveys: a field manual*, Nutrition in Agriculture, no. 5. FAO, Rome.

26 Working with communities

The job of many nutrition workers is to work with people and local officials to improve nutrition in an area. The nutrition of poorer families is especially important. Previous chapters of this book give the technical information that you need. This chapter and Chapter 27 discuss how to use the technical knowledge when you work in a community.

This chapter covers the following topics:

- learning about your community;
- learning about malnourished and 'at risk' families;
- working with groups in the community.

Chapter 27 discusses:

- working with malnourished and 'at risk' families.

26.1 LEARNING ABOUT YOUR COMMUNITY

The word 'community' in this book means all the people who live in one area and whose lives affect each other—such as a village, a plantation, or a housing block.

In any community there are people who are rich and people who are poor, people who are powerful and people who are weak, people with many years of schooling and people with only a few years. There are people with many skills and people with many needs.

You need to understand the problems and priorities of different groups, the nutrition problems of undernourished and 'at risk' families, and the causes of these problems. You need to know what *resources* the community has for dealing with problems.

As you get to know people, you learn:

- the problems that affect the *whole community* (such as lack of enough fertile soil, or shortage of clean water);
- the problems that affect *individual families*, such as a mentally ill mother.

You also learn what is *normal* for the community at different times of year, and what *most* people do. When you know what is normal, it is easier to know when things change. For example, you will notice when there is less rain than usual, or when the price of maize

increases. When you know how families usually live, you notice families who are unusual and who need extra help.

As you learn about the community, you start to become part of the community. For example, you are invited to weddings, or called when someone has a problem. But remember that it takes time for people to learn to like and trust you.

26.2 HOW TO LEARN ABOUT A COMMUNITY

- *Learn customs and language.* If you are new to a community, you should learn the social customs so that you can greet and show respect to everyone, and so that people find you polite and friendly. You may need to learn the local language or dialect.

- *Study reports* of surveys of the area, or any other documents on the area that may be available—such as local development plans. Try to see the reports from the health and agricultural departments, or the minutes of meetings of groups involved with nutrition work.

  Most nutrition workers are too busy to do surveys themselves. But you should know what other people have found out.

- *Listen* to people talking in markets, bars, buses, or other public places. What do they talk about? Encourage people to talk to you—most people like to talk about themselves and their town or village to a friendly listener.

- *Watch* how different sorts of people live, what they buy, how they spend their time. Notice how these things change at different times of the year.

Listening and *watching* are skills that many of us need to learn.

- *Ask about the community.* Decide what you need to know, and then plan how to ask questions so that you get reliable answers.

  First, find a friend who knows the community very well—perhaps a health worker or a teacher who has lived in the community for a long time. A friend like

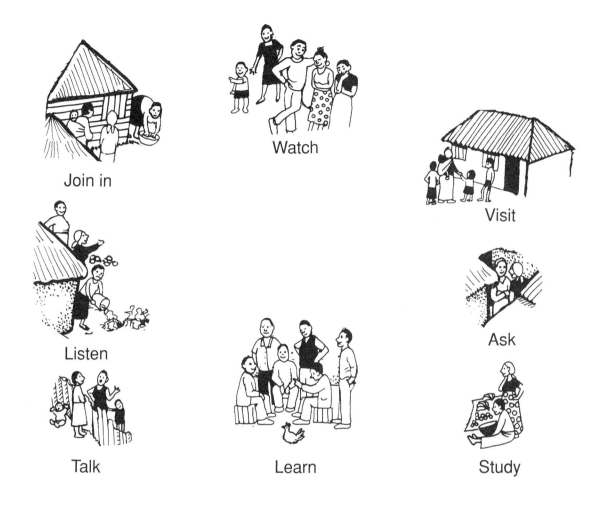

Fig. 26-1 Learning about the community you work with.

this can tell you many things which it may be hard to find out in other ways. For example, what people think about their leaders, local customs, important local friendships and quarrels.

Ask political, administrative, and religious leaders for information. Ask them how to learn about families in the community. If necessary, ask permission to talk to families and other community workers.

- *Talk with people*—chat with them. Talking with people helps you to understand them, and may also

make more people interested in nutrition. When you talk with people, explain what your job is and that you want to understand and help. Show that you do not want to force the community to do things, but you have knowledge and skills, and the community has knowledge and skills, and, if these are all shared, they could be useful. Show that you want to work with the community.

- Talk with the community's opinion leaders.
- Talk with other workers in the community,

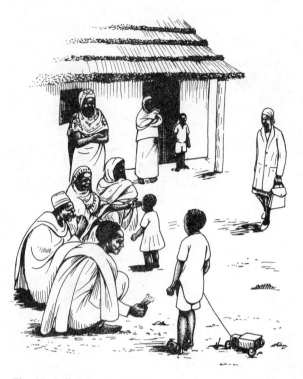

Fig. 26–2 If you are new to a community, you need to learn about their customs.

especially those who work with poor families or with self-help groups. Spend a day working with them if you can.

- Talk about yourself so people know you as a friend as well as a nutrition worker. Ask for local advice for yourself, for example, which is the best place to get fresh eggs?

- *Visit families and places.*
  - Visit different kinds of families in the community to learn about their lives and problems. Make sure that you visit both well nourished and undernourished families so that you understand the differences between them.

    Talk to the leaders and visit and talk with families who are not 'at risk' so that you know what is usual. This will help you to understand the problems that poorer families have. Then you can be tactful and gentle when you talk with 'at risk' families.
  - Visit families where a health or other worker tells you that there are malnourished children.

    Try to learn why they have problems, and the kind of help that they need.

Try to visit families at different times of the day, and at different times of the year. Also visit when special things are happening—for example, when someone is sick, or when the mother is expecting a new baby, and when the baby is born.

- Visit a health centre and a children's ward to see the sorts of nutrition problems that women, children, and others have, and which types of families are affected. Talk with them about their situation.

- Visit shops and stalls in the area where poorer people live. Ask the shopkeepers what these families buy, and if they often need credit. Do shopkeepers think that some families do not have enough food? When does this happen most?

- *Join in* local activities such as celebrations, dances, public meetings. Help sometimes with weeding, harvesting, minding children, or other work. In this way people learn to know, like, and trust you. They know that you are not proud, and that you enjoy working with the community. If you do not live in the community, try to stay overnight sometimes. Often you learn more talking to people in the evening than during the day.

The answers to questions may be different at different times of year and as time passes. So keep on listening, watching, and being aware of what happens all the time that you are working in an area.

26.3 WHAT YOU NEED TO LEARN ABOUT A COMMUNITY

General information

You need to build up a general picture of the community, and to know where to go for official information and support:

- How many people live in the area?
- Who are the political and religious leaders?
- Who are the government and other officials?
- Which firms, organizations, large farmers, and businessmen employ many people in the area?

You need to learn which of these services are in the area, and where they are:

- markets and shops;
- banks, post offices, etc.;

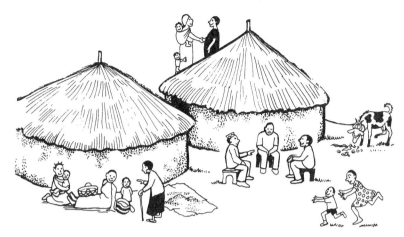

Fig. 26–3 Talk with people wherever you meet them.

- services which give loans and credit, both official and unofficial, such as money lenders;
- buses or other public transport. (How much does it cost to get to the nearest market or health centre?)

You need to learn the general problems in the area:

- environmental problems (such as erosion, variable rainfall, or lack of firewood);
- problems of civil unrest;
- problems of unemployment and low wages;
- problems of overcrowding and poor transport.

Political and administrative structure

Learn what you can about:

- how plans and decisions which affect the community are made. Who makes them (such as councillors and administrative officers, development committees)? Are 'ordinary people' involved?
- which of the political leaders and government officials are just, helpful, honest, and hardworking?
- which leaders and officials care about the poorest people in the community?

Opinion leaders

Learn who are the opinion leaders in the community. These are people who influence others, although they may not be official leaders—for example, a community health worker or a wise farmer, whom people admire and copy. These people may know more about families in the community than the official leaders.

Relationships between different groups and families

Learn about different groups in the community, and how they get on and work together—for example, the religious groups, the government officers, the people of different tribes.

- Which groups are friendly, and help each other; and which disagree and oppose each other?
- Are there quarrels and friendships which affect improvements to the community? For example, are some leaders blocking land reform?
- What is the status and educational level of women?

About education

- Do most children go to primary school? How long do most stay? Do girls stay as long as boys?
- What is the educational level of most: young women, young men, older women, older men?
- What proportion of adults can read?

About earning money

Learn about the economic level of different families, what types of families may not have enough money for food, and when money problems are most likely to occur.

- What are the common occupations of families in the community? What kinds of jobs and wages do men have? What kinds of jobs and wages do women have? What kind of jobs and wages do children have?

- Is there more work available at certain times of year?
- In most families do both men and women earn money?
- Do many families produce things (e.g. crops, fish, eggs, processed foods, crafts, beer) for sale?
- Do many women earn an income? Can they spend their money as they want?

About credit and saving schemes

- Can families borrow money or get credit? From whom?
- Are there any savings schemes?
- Are there times of the month or year when some families often need credit or to borrow money?

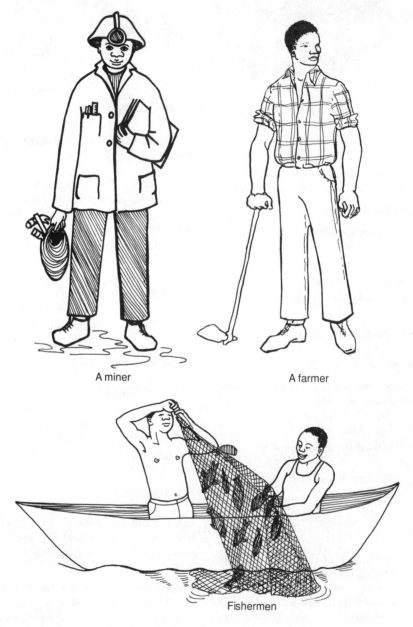

A miner   A farmer

Fishermen

Fig. 26–4 What kinds of jobs do men have?

- Are many families in debt to money lenders or other people who charge high interest rates?

About producing, and storing foods

Learn what you can about the beginning of the food paths and the blocks which may occur there. Then you can recognize families who may have problems with food supplies and nutrition.

- Which foods are produced in the area?
- Do family farmers own, rent, or sharecrop their land, or other resources, such as equipment?
- How many families grow their own staple food?
- Do they grow enough for the whole year?
- How much of the food produced does the farmer or fisherman sell?
- How much does the farmer's or fisherman's family eat themselves?
- Is the family able to keep enough for their own needs?
- How many families have home gardens?
- What are the problems of producing food in the area?
- Are there times of the year or month when some families may be short of food? What are the reasons for this? What do people eat then?
- Which part of the work for food production is done by women, which is done by men, and which is done by children?
- How are food crops stored? Is much lost during storage?

About buying, processing, and preparing food

- Who buys foods? Who decides which foods to buy?
- How much do staple foods cost? Do prices change with the season?
- Which foods are processed or preserved in the home or community? Who does this work? Does it take much time? Is there a grain mill in the area?
- How do people prepare food? Is it done in a clean way?
- How often each day do most families cook? eat meals or snacks?
- How do families cook food? What fuel do most families use?
- Do people buy meals and snacks from food sellers? What sorts of people sell these foods? What sorts of people buy them? How much do they cost? Are the foods safe and clean? Are they nutritious? Good value for money?

About sharing and eating food

Learn how families share food and how they feed young children and other 'at risk' groups. This helps you to decide what changes you need to discuss with families.

- How is food shared between the family? Do women and children get a fair share? Are there times when some members of the family have extra or less food?
- Who has most influence on decisions which affect children and the way in which they are fed?

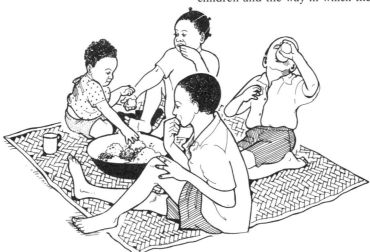

Fig. 26–5 How do families share food, and how do they feed young children?

- How many mothers breastfeed their babies exclusively for 6 months? How many give supplements before 6 months of age? How many mothers bottle feed their babies?

- At what age do young children start to have weaning foods? Who decides when and how to feed young children?

- Which foods do families think are good weaning foods? What do they actually use? How often do they give them? Do they give the food by cup? spoon? hand? bottle? Who gives it to the baby?

- How do families prepare weaning foods? Do they usually cook them with the family food or separately? How do they keep the food and how long for?

- Do young children eat from the same plate as older children, or do they have their own plate of food?

- How do families feed children and older people when they are sick or recovering?

- Do many people eat foods away from home—for example, do they carry food with them to work or school, eat school meals, use canteens, or eat in hotels or eating houses?

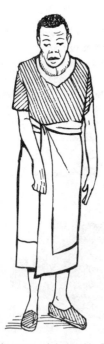

Fig. 26–6 Learn about people's health. Do many women have a goitre?

About health in the community

Learn about people's general health and nutrition, and at what time of year most poor health occurs.

- What illnesses are common? Are there any which are especially common among certain groups, or in certain areas or at certain times of the year (such as malaria)? Is HIV infection common?

- Are there many underweight and malnourished children? In what types of families?

- Are many women anaemic? Thin? Do many women have a goitre? Are there many low birth weight babies? Pregnant adolescents?

- What is the average family size? Do many women have pregnancies less than two years apart? Is the population increasing rapidly? Are family planning services available? Do parents know about them and use them?

What interests and worries people

Learn what interests people, and what worries them. This helps you to plan nutrition activities that are supported by the community, and to know which people will help you most.

- What are people worried about (for example, late rains? AIDS? rapid population growth?)

- What are people angry about (for example, an increase in the price of maize)?

- What are people happy about (for example, a new well in the village) or hopeful about (the government has promised that there will be regular rubbish collections)?

- Are there often burglaries or attacks on people? Is there fighting in the area? Does this affect the amount of food which people store or grow? Does it affect employment in the area?

About resources in the community

Learn about resources which might help with nutrition problems and undernourished families. For example:

- Agriculture, livestock, fisheries, forestry, and home economics and nutrition extension services. These may give information and help on food production, marketing, storage, processing, and preparation.

- Health centres and community health workers who provide health monitoring and care, and education for health, hygiene, and nutrition.

- Women's groups which help members to learn new information and skills for food production, processing, sale and buying, and on food cleanness, cooking, and feeding. They may have income earning or saving schemes and adult education classes.

- Voluntary agencies and religious and civic groups which support child care and early learning centres, health care, nutrition education, and income earning or saving schemes, or which give help to very poor families. Sometimes these groups want to help, but it is difficult for them to find the families most in need.

- Feeding programmes which provide temporary supplies of free or low-cost food. These may be linked to nutrition education, growth monitoring, and health care. They may provide meals in primary schools or support rural development through 'Food-for-work' programmes. Sometimes there are emergency feeding programmes in times of disaster or for refugees.

- Child care centres which care for young children so that mothers can work. They may give meals to the children, education to parents, and health care.

- Schools which teach children about food production, nutrition, home economics, and health and hygiene. They may monitor health or give school meals or snacks.

- Youth groups, such as Young Farmer's Clubs, where young people learn about producing and preparing food, feeding the family, and health care.

- Social and welfare services which provide special help for needy families, single parents, or orphans.

About 'safety nets'

Learn about 'safety nets' which provide support for families who need help. For example, relatives or neighbours may help in times of trouble; shopkeepers may give credit; trade unions and religious organizations may help members; sometimes community councils help families with undernourished children or sick parents.

About organizations you could work with

To plan nutrition activities you need to learn:

- What programmes and projects which affect nutrition already exist in the area? For example, rural development schemes, pre-school feeding programmes, urban gardening schemes, food processing co-operatives, saving schemes. Are they successful? Do they reach families who need help most?

  Do they really improve the nutrition of these families? What do the people in these programmes think about them?

- Which organizations deal with food and nutrition activities (such as community councils, voluntary organizations, schools)?

- Which community groups can you work with and which are particularly concerned with needy families? For example, women's groups and religious or civic groups.

- What official community structures are there which you could work with? For example, village health committees, community development committees.

- Are there any funds or support for nutrition work in the community (e.g. from voluntary organizations, religious or civic groups, rich business people, landowners, politicians)?

- Are there other people in the community with special skills, who might help with nutrition activities and education (such as artists, child care workers,

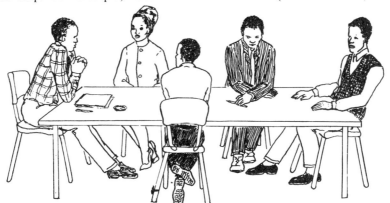

Fig. 26–7 What official community structures are there with which you could work, such as village health or community development committees?

teachers, etc.)? Are there people with time to help (such as the wives of businessmen)?

About other workers who are your colleagues

It is important to know other workers in the community who are interested in helping undernourished families. These are your colleagues, and you should look for ways to work with them—for example, health workers including community health workers, traditional birth attendants, and healers; agricultural, fisheries, and forestry workers; home economists and social welfare and community development workers; and staff of voluntary agencies and religious groups.

Your colleagues may be pleased when you ask for their advice and when you offer to help them when you can. For example, in one place in Kenya, the nutrition worker at a health centre works with the staff of a voluntary agency to help women's groups. They advise the women on good food for their families, give them seeds, and help with a cockerel exchange programme.

In some places, the agricultural worker attends the health centre and finds out which families have agricultural problems so that he can help them.

26.4 LEARNING ABOUT MALNOURISHED AND 'AT RISK' FAMILIES

When you have learnt about the community in general, you need to find out about the families who need help most. These are the malnourished families, or the families who are 'at risk' of undernutrition. By 'at risk' we mean families who could easily become undernourished, but who may not be undernourished now. You may need to work with the following groups.

Families who cannot get enough food

Families may have difficulty getting enough food, because they lack money, land, or labour, or because the food path is blocked in some other way. Some or all members of the family may not get enough nutrients to cover their needs.

Some families never have enough food. Some families have enough food at some times and not at others. Some families may have just enough food most of the time, but they may not have enough if there is an extra need, such as a sudden extra expense.

These families need help to get more food. They may need help to get a job, or more pay, or to produce things that they can sell. They may need help to produce more food or store it better, or to budget their money better, or to use food more efficiently.

You may be able to help with some of their problems. Your colleagues may be able to help with other problems. Some things you may not be able to help with.

Families with other difficulties

Some families can get enough food, but one or more of the members is malnourished or 'at risk' of becoming malnourished because of some other difficulty.

Children may be malnourished or 'at risk' because:

- A baby is bottle fed.
- A child is often sick.
- They are not fed often enough.
- The family food is too bulky for small children.

Sometimes children are not fed well or often enough because:

- The mother is too busy (for example, working and caring for a family, with many young children, with no support from a husband or from relatives, with a busy job outside the home).
- The mother is sick or disabled or mentally ill.
- There are problems between husband and wife.
- The mother is absent.
- The mother is very young—adolescent mothers are likely to have undernourished children and to be undernourished themselves.

Sometimes pregnant or breastfeeding women, or sick or old people are undernourished because the family does not know their special food needs. These families need immediate advice and help from a nutrition worker.

Families who get enough food

Families who can get enough food are usually well nourished and healthy. These families do not usually need help. However, childbearing women may be at risk of anaemia, so pregnant women should attend antenatal clinics. Young children need immunizations and regular weight checks. You may need to talk to mothers about the dangers of bottle feeding, and about how to prevent and treat common infections.

Sometimes you may need to advise these families about the problems of obesity (see Chapter 22).

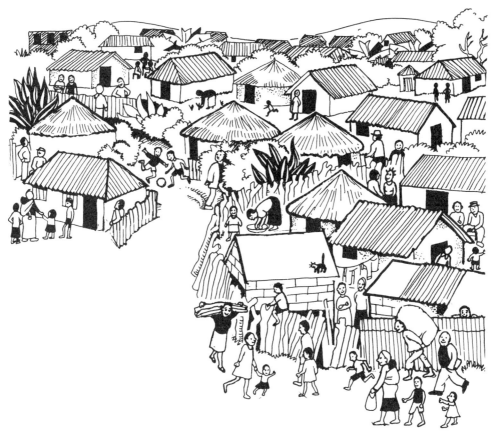

Fig. 26–8 It can be difficult to find families who are 'at risk' of malnutrition.

26.5 FINDING FAMILIES WHO ARE MALNOURISHED OR 'AT RISK'

To help families who are malnourished or 'at risk' of undernutrition you must *find* them. It can be difficult to find these families. You may not see all those who are at risk in the community. Often these families cannot afford the time or money to get to a health centre or child care centre. They have not the time or confidence to join a women's or youth organization. Their homes may be hidden along small paths or back streets far from the road or centre of the community, so you are less likely to see them. Often when a nutrition worker finds a family like this, she is surprised and says: 'I never knew that a family lived there!'

You are not likely to have time to 'watch over' *all* the families in a community *all* the time. So you need to know:

- which *types* of families may be malnourished;

- *where* most of them live;
- *when* families are most at risk.

These are things that you learn about as you work in the community.

Types of families who may be malnourished and where they live

Poor families

Poor families are always 'at risk' of undernutrition because:

- They do not produce enough food to feed themselves, for example, farmers with little land.
- They do not produce enough cash crops or goods to earn money for all their food.
- Their wages are too low or too irregular to buy enough food.

Poor families often live in certain areas such as plantations or estates, slums or shanty towns. Often they are squatters or agricultural labourers. .

Weak families

Families may be 'at risk' of undernutrition if, for example:

- They lack one or both parents because of death, sickness, or separation.
- They have many members who are not productive because they are too young, too old, sick, or disabled.
- The mother is very young and is not ready to care for children.

Socially isolated families

Families who have recently moved (into town, or into a new rural area such as a resettlement scheme) are 'at risk' of undernutrition because:

- They may be cut off from their relatives and friends who can help them.
- They may not know which foods are good value or where to get help in times of trouble.
- They may also be poor if they are unemployed or have very low wages, and they may live in poor houses.

Families in isolated places are at risk of undernutrition because:

- They may live on infertile, marginal land.
- They are far from health and other services (including *you*).
- They are far from markets, supportive relatives, or neighbours.

Families in refugee and displaced people's camps are another important 'at risk' group.

When families are most at risk

There are certain times when families are most at risk of hunger and undernutrition. Nutrition workers need to know these times so that they can watch over 'at risk' families more closely then.

At certain seasons

Families may be more 'at risk' of undernutrition when:

- Stores of food are low, for example in the pre-harvest season.

- They need extra energy for heavy agricultural work—such as during planting or harvesting. Planting often occurs during the rainy season when infections are common.
- Women are more busy than usual with agricultural work, so they have less time to feed or breastfeed babies.

Before payday

Families may not have enough food in the days before payday, especially if workers are paid monthly or irregularly.

When there is a disaster

Food production and employment may decrease when there is drought, flooding, an epidemic of an animal or plant disease (such as cassava mealy bug), war, or civil unrest.

When there are extra expenses and financial losses

Large expenses and losses may put the family into debt, and they may not have enough money for food. For example:

- An accident or sickness, especially of the family wage-earner. There may be expenses associated with hospital admission or a funeral. There may be loss of labour or income or long-term disability which prevents a person working.
- Loss of possessions, especially those used by a family to produce food or earn money. For example, theft of cattle or a donkey, destruction of a fishing boat, loss of a house by fire or flooding.

If you know when families are likely to be at risk, you can plan to help them most at these times.

26.6 FINDING INDIVIDUAL MALNOURISHED OR 'AT RISK' FAMILIES

When you know the *types* of families who are at risk of malnutrition, it is easier to find the *individual* families who are at risk. When you know *where* most of these families live—for example in an urban slum, or on a coffee or sisal estate, or on marginal farming land—you can visit that area more often.

You may notice the family yourself

When you are in the area, you notice that something is wrong. For example:

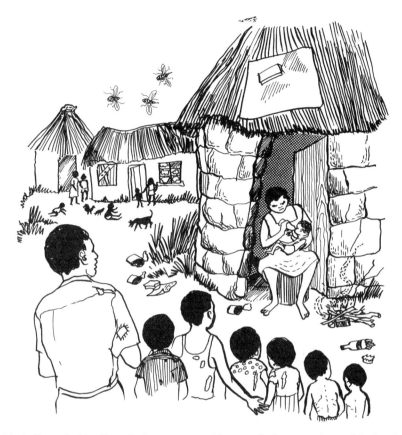

Fig. 26–9 Try to find families who have many problems and who are undernourished or 'at risk'.

- You see a woman who is very thin.
- You pass a home where there is no food cooking at mealtimes; or where children are alone and crying.
- If you are a teacher, you notice a child who often misses school, or who is tired and dirty.
- If you work in a health centre, you may see a family with a sick or undernourished child or mother, or you may see a growth chart which shows that a child is not growing well.

Other people tell you about a family who is 'at risk'

- Friends, neighbours, employers, or shopkeepers sometimes tell you about a family who is in trouble.
- Workers from voluntary agencies, or religious groups who work with needy people tell you about families with nutrition problems.
- Other workers in the community tell you of families with nutrition problems. For example, a school teacher can report about children who are under-nourished, or tired, or who do not attend school regularly.

26.7 'WATCHING OVER' AND HELPING FAMILIES AT RISK

You can 'watch over' and visit families who are at risk of undernutrition; or you can ask a community health worker (CHW) or other community worker to watch over the family. You may be able to do something to help, especially at times of special risk. For example:

- Help people get low interest loans or credit for special expenses.
- Help to start a child care centre for children of single mothers, or for children whose mothers work on an estate, especially during the planting and harvesting season.
- Encourage estate workers' families to start home

gardens; you or a colleague may be able to help the families get the land and start the gardens.

• Encourage women to join women's groups where they can learn an income earning skill.

• Start discussion groups with parents or with women's groups about topics such as feeding sick children, feeding pregnant mothers, budgeting money, family spacing.

• Help to start a feeding programme in a poor urban area, or in an area with a sudden food shortage, or during the hungry season.

26.8 CO-OPERATING WITH OTHER WORKERS

You need to co-operate with other workers and community leaders in the area, both to find the families who need help and to help them. Tell your colleagues what you are interested in, and help each other when you can.

A schoolteacher will be pleased if a health worker can visit and try to help the families of children whom she is worried about. The health worker can also visit the school to check the health of the children.

Different workers may tell each other when an area has a particular nutrition problem. For example, the agricultural worker tells the health worker that the cassava has been eaten by insects in the field across the river. The health worker tells the agricultural worker that many malnourished children come from families squatting on unused agricultural land.

If other people tell you about families in trouble, make sure that you *try* to help the family. This makes it easier for you to ask them for help again.

26.9 WORKING WITH GROUPS IN THE COMMUNITY

Why you need to work with groups

To help a community to move blocks on their food path, and increase their food security you need to work with a *group*. It is easier for a *group* to decide to change things than it is for an *individual* person or family. People are suspicious of a person with new ideas, who starts to do things differently by herself.

A group of people can decide together to try something new—for example, making a different weaning food, or a new kind of food store. Groups can share experiences, and work out for themselves what is prac-

tical for them. Women can support each other even if relatives or other people disapprove. People who are not sure about a new idea, can get the confidence to try it out. For example, a mother is more likely to give her child enriched porridge if she knows that her neighbour is doing the same.

In a small community, such as a small village, the best group to work with might be the whole community. In a larger community, it is easier to work with a smaller group within the community.

Different groups and some ways to work with them

A community consists of many different groups. Some of these are 'permanent' groups, such as a village health committee, or a religious group. Other groups may form just for a time to deal with a particular problem such as a new water supply. Below we discuss some of the people and groups, and some of the ways in which you can work with them.

Policy makers, decision makers, and administrators
These include politicians, district officers, and councillors. You may:

• advise and inform them about the nutrition situation and how it might be improved;

• visit government officials to seek help for and to represent undernourished and 'at risk' families;

• work for a fairer distribution of resources to all families in the community, or for special help for undernourished families;

• work with the planners of a development scheme to make sure that 'at risk' families get their share of the benefits of the scheme.

• act as a link between your own organization and the community.

Official groups such as the Community Development or Health Committee
You may:

• speak at meetings and give nutrition information and advice;

• train community health workers so that they can teach families, for example, how to feed sick children or grow drought-resistant foods such as millet or pigeon peas;

• train traditional birth attendants (TBAs) about the special nutrition needs of mothers and babies, and encourage them to support breastfeeding.

Organized groups such as classes of schoolchildren or staff who prepare meals at hospitals or canteens

You may:

- teach staff who prepare meals about:
  - the quantities of food needed;
  - hygiene;
  - cooking methods.
- teach schoolchildren about healthy mixed meals and poor-value snacks, about how to care for their teeth, and about how to feed babies.

Consumer and voluntary groups

You might be a member of a group which tries to help families with nutrition problems. You might get information for a civic club, for example, on the price of a handmill which they plan to donate.

Self-help groups such as young farmers' or women's groups

You may:

- arrange for a health worker to give a talk about weighing children;
- help to start a breastfeeding mother's support group;
- help a group to start a garden for vegetables; or a scheme to produce and sell eggs;

- arrange for leaders of a new group to attend a course on management and bookkeeping;
- help a group to write a request for funds to a voluntary agency.

26.10 PROBLEM-SOLVING WITH COMMUNITY GROUPS

An important way to help people remove blocks on their food path, is to help them to solve problems themselves. This means helping people to develop the attitudes and confidence that they need to:

- *Recognize that they have a nutrition problem.*
- *Identify the causes of their nutrition problems.* They need to understand how much these problems are due to *lack of resources* (such as land or fertilizer) and how much they are due to *lack of information* (such as not knowing the best kind of weaning food).
- *Decide what to do about these problems.* They discuss possible solutions, and exchange opinions and ideas, to find practical things that they can do themselves. They think about the resources they need, and what they have.
- *Prevent nutrition problems occurring again in the future.*

Box 26.1 explains these steps through the example of Grace, a home economics worker.

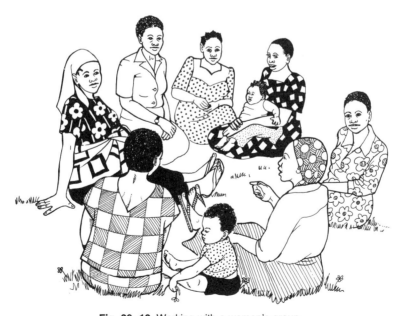

Fig. 26–10 Working with a women's group.

Box 26.1.   Example of how to help a community group to solve a nutrition problem

These are the steps that it may be useful to follow.

1. Work with the group to recognize and identify a problem

Example. Grace, the local Home Economics Worker, often attended meetings of a women's group on a tea plantation. Grace noticed that several of the young children were very thin and quiet. Some had growth charts. These showed that the children were not gaining weight at a healthy rate. She asked the members of the women's group if they were worried about the health of their children. They said that they were worried, and they thought that most were small for their age. But they did not think there was anything they could do about it. If Grace would help them, they would like to make the children more healthy.

2. Help the group to identify the causes of the problem

The group holds discussions to identify the blocks on the food path.

Example. The group discussed with Grace *why* the children were thin. They decided that one of the blocks on the children's food path was that they were not fed enough during the day. The women labourers worked all day away from home, and left the young children in the care of other children who did not know how to feed them properly.

3. Work with the group to think of ways to remove blocks on the food path and to decide which ways are most effective and feasible

Example. After discussing other possibilities, the women decided to start a child care centre on the plantation. This would help all the mothers on the plantation, so that better-off families would be interested in supporting the child care centre, as well as 'at risk' families.

4. Help the group to list the resources they will need to remove the block

For example: information, skills, tools, labour, buildings, money, food, time, etc. Find out which of these resources are already available, and which must be found—for example, requested from government officials, employers, voluntary agencies, civic groups, etc.

Example. The group listed the resources they needed:

- shelter for children and store for equipment;
- child minders to look after the children;
- training in child care for these minders;
- foods, fuel, and equipment for a midday meal for children and child minders;
- toys for the children.

After visiting families on the plantation, they found that the following resources were available:

- Grandmothers and pregnant mothers were willing to look after children once a week in return for a meal;
- Fathers were willing to build the shelter and store. Better-off labourers agreed to provide some timber. Poorer ones agreed to provide the labour.
- Most mothers agreed to contribute food and fuel and to provide cooking equipment. The poorer ones would fetch water and do the cleaning.

Grace helped the group to find the other resources that it needed:

- *Land for the shelter and store.* The husband of one of the group, who was a foreman, asked the plantation manager for land. Grace helped him to explain why the child care centre was needed. The manager provided the land.
- *Roofing material.* The local Rotary Club gave this.
- *Training for child minders.* A teacher at a nearby kindergarten, who was a friend of Grace, offered to train the minders one evening a week for 6 weeks.
- *Toys.* The same teacher showed the women's group and some of the older children how to make toys from local materials. Some of the kindergarten children drew pictures to decorate the new centre.

5. Work with the group to make a detailed plan for removing the block on the food path

Suggest that the group invite some 'at risk' families to help them so that they are involved in planning the scheme. This plan should include details of:

- who is to do what and when they will do it;
- who will supervise, monitor, and evaluate the scheme.

Example. The women's group invited some of the poorest families to the meetings at which they planned the child care centre. They made out a time-table for constructing and equipping it. Grace helped the group to plan the meals and she advised on food cleanness.

A woman who could not work on the plantation because she was disabled with polio offered to supervise the women who looked after the children, the food supplies, and cleanness in return for meals. She would report each month to the group.

As the plans progressed, the poorer women realized that the women's group used their suggestions and that they were important members of the group. They took a bigger part in meetings.

6. Help the group to start and to manage the scheme

As the group becomes more experienced, you gradually do less. But you are there at times of trouble, and when the group is discouraged.

Example. The child care centre started. There were some problems with the grandmothers coming late for work. There was one outbreak of diarrhoea. Grace helped the group to solve these problems. Soon she was able to visit the centre only once a month.

7. The group decides how successful the scheme is and what improvements are needed

Example. After 6 months, Grace helped the women's group to examine the growth charts of the children who attended the child care centre. Almost all the children were growing at a healthy rate. But some of the poorer children who did not attend had flat growth lines. The women decided to explain the value of the centre again to those children's parents.

8. The group shares the successes and failures of the scheme with other similar community groups

Example. Grace told mothers on another plantation about the child care centre. They invited the disabled supervisor to come and tell them how to start one themselves.

26.11 HOW TO HELP GROUPS TO DISCUSS A PROBLEM*

Group discussions can help communities to solve problems. They can help people to change their attitudes and to decide that they want to do something differently. You do not give advice or tell the group what to do. You help people to think about and discuss their situation and agree about what they might do. The *process* of identifying problems, their causes, and possible solutions helps people to develop new skills and more confidence.

You can use this method when you work with women's and other community groups, or when you train community workers. For example, you may help a women's group to identify bottle feeding as a community problem, to identify lack of support for young mothers as an important cause of bottle feeding, and to decide to form a breastfeeding support group.

A good number for a group is 5–6 people. A nutrition worker may be an ordinary member of the group, a special resource person, or the *facilitator* of the group.

What a group does

- They share experiences, ideas, and information.
- You listen and find out what they know already, and what they need and want to know.
- You share useful information with the group or help them to get it.
- You encourage them to discuss their nutrition situation, if they have any problems, or what they feel needs to improve.

---

* Section 26.11 was written with the help of staff from AMREF, Nairobi.

- You encourage them to suggest ways in which they can solve problems or improve the community's nutrition. If necessary, you suggest some ideas. The group discusses and decides which is best for them. It is very important to discuss *several alternatives* and not just one.

Preparing for group work

Find out all that you can about local nutrition problems and their causes

Ask several different sorts of people in the community and your colleagues which problems seem to be most important. Then learn all that you can about the problems, their causes, and possible solutions. Then you have the technical information if the group needs it.

Help the group to choose one problem which is important to them

Reasons for choosing a particular problem might include:

- It affects and worries many people.
- It causes bad effects such as poor growth or absenteeism from work.
- It is possible to solve it with common action.

Examples

1) A colleague who works with young mothers, finds that many of them worry about not having enough breast milk and they give babies watery dilute porridge from 1–2 months of age.

2) A group of young men complains about their pay. They have problems budgeting, because the food they like is very expensive.

Decide on a 'starter' for the discussion

A '*starter*' is something which '*poses*' or *presents* a problem, and which 'starts' people thinking.

A starter can be a short drama, a story, a song, a real object, or a picture (see Box 26.2)). A 'starter' must not be too detailed or complicated. It must pose only one problem. The group needs to think about one specific thing at a time.

- A 'starter' does *not* give *information*, like a poster, a chart, or a radio programme.
- A 'starter' does *not* give a *solution* to the problem. It is important for the group to work out their own solution.

A solution that comes from outside may not be possible for the group to carry out. Or the solution may be possible, but if people do not see a need, they may lose interest.

Holding a problem-posing group discussion

- The group meets and watches or listens to the drama, story, or other starter.
- If you are the 'facilitator', you ask questions around the group.
- Go slowly so that everyone has time to think and to give their opinions and ideas. Listen with respect. Do not give any answers yourself. Never say that something is 'wrong'.
- Encourage shy and quiet people to share their ideas and experiences, and to help make decisions.

Questions to ask the group

1. *Who were the people in the story? What did they do?* This is to make sure that everyone heard or saw the same things. For example, a young mother, a hungry child, an angry man.

2. *What happened in the story? What was the problem?* Make sure that everyone gives an opinion. When someone mentions the problem that you want to discuss 'hold on to' that answer and ask other people if they agree. Eventually the group should agree about what the problem is. For example, the mother in the story thinks that she does not have enough breast milk.

3. *Does this happen in our community?* Let everyone tell their experiences. Many people find it easier to discuss a personal problem if they talk about it in relation to someone else.

If the group agrees that the problem exists in their community ask:

4. *Why does this problem happen?* Ask everyone to give their opinions. Then discuss each idea and guide the discussion towards agreement. For

example, the mother has no one to advise her about breastfeeding.

5. *What are we, here and now, going to do about the problem?* Allow plenty of time for discussion. You may need to guide the group, and make some suggestions. But be careful not to dominate the group. Local people will have much better ideas than you about what *they* can do about a problem.

Deciding what to do

Eventually the group should agree about what they will do. Then they can decide what each person will do, and when.

For example, they may decide to encourage all new mothers to breastfeed exclusively for 6 months. The women can take it in turns to visit and support each new mother, and they will support and help each other when they have a new baby. A group may decide to arrange a community meeting to discuss how men can help overworked women, and why this is important.

A group may take several months and a number of meetings to decide what to do about a problem. Do not hurry them. Go at their speed. Try to guide the group into actions that are easy and practical and that produce some results quickly. This encourages the group and helps them to gain confidence to tackle more difficult problems.

26.12 THINGS TO REMEMBER WHEN YOU WORK WITH COMMUNITY GROUPS

- People can solve problems by themselves and improve their lives if they work together. They develop confidence in their ability to do so through the *process* of identifying and analysing their needs and problems, and making decisions.

- Do not expect a group to go too fast, especially when it is new. The process takes a long time. It may take a year to prepare a plan to solve a problem.

- Do not let a group be too ambitious. It is better to start with a small scheme which is likely to succeed. This gives people the confidence and motivation to continue to work together. You may need to suggest ideas which are possible, and to point out the difficulties of ideas which are too ambitious or which are not likely to solve the problem.

- Do not let one person dominate the group because

Box 26.2. 'Starters' for problem-posing discussions

Drama—an example

The problem
Your work in the community and your discussions with local people and other workers tell you that many mothers are anaemic. They complain of feeling tired and breathless even when they have done little work, especially when they are pregnant. Health workers tell you that many pregnant women have pale tongues and lips. They give iron and folate tablets but the women complain that they get stomach ache and probably don't take them.

The story
With the help of 2–3 friends or colleagues, you decide to tell a story about a pregnant woman who felt too tired to hoe or cook often. At the antenatal clinic, the nurse examines her and says that she has pale blood. She gives tablets and tells the woman to take two tablets each day. The woman takes them for a few days, but she gets stomach ache and as she doesn't feel any better, she stops taking the tablets.

The players
Ask some people to perform. Let them decide which parts they want to take. Tell them an outline of what they should say and do. There is no need to prepare a script. Help them to rehearse once or twice, to make sure that the story keeps to the point, and show what was planned. It should not last for more than about 5 minutes.

After the play is finished
Applaud, thank, and congratulate the players. Then start the discussion.

Pictures
Some kinds of problem are easier to pose with a picture, or a series of pictures, if you have good ones. For example:

- a picture of a poor, undernourished, pregnant, tired mother, with many uncared for undernourished children, and a weary, poor, father (see Fig. 24–7).
- a picture of a child with marasmus, or an unhappy pregnant schoolgirl, or a bad grain store with rats eating the food.

But pictures can be more difficult to use than plays or stories. Pictures made outside a community are often not right for that community. It may not show a community problem as local people can understand it. It is not easy to draw, and there may not be anyone nearby who can draw well enough to help you make your own pictures.

Be careful to use a picture which everyone can recognize. Test any picture that you want to use to make sure that local people understand it.

Other starters
Stories or songs about the community problem. For example, if bottle feeding with thin porridge is a problem, you could prepare a story or song about a family whose baby becomes thin and sick, after having some bottle feeds of thin porridge.
Real objects, for example, a feeding bottle or a growth chart showing a falling growth line; a poor value snack; a kilo of maize with a price on it.

Remember starters only show the problem, and sometimes suggest causes. They never suggest solutions or tell people what to do, in the way that posters do.

---

this makes the others lose interest. Be careful that *you* do not dominate the group.

- Do not let powerful individuals in the community take over the group. If powerful people become interested, try to keep them working for the good of the group and the poorest in the community. Watch carefully that they do not use the group to make themselves richer or more powerful.
- Watch over the activities of the group to make sure that the benefits of any schemes do reach 'at risk' and undernourished families.
- Encourage the group when it has difficulties or when

there are arguments so that it does not give up too easily. The most needy people are often the most apathetic and need the most encouragement.

THINGS TO DO

Class exercise

1. Ask each trainee to prepare a 'starter' picture on a common nutrition problem. Pin them up and discuss each one.

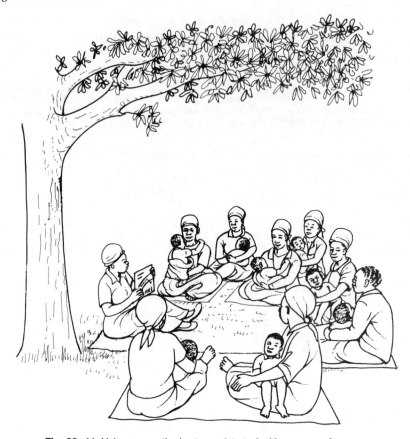

Fig. 26–11 Using a growth chart as a 'starter' with a group of women.

Group discussion

2. Ask each trainee to prepare a list of information that she wants to find out about her community when she works there. Discuss the best way to collect this information.

3. Ask trainees to describe their experiences of starting work in a community. Discuss these. Would they start differently now?

Role play

4. Ask trainees to role play a group from the community. One of them can be a nutrition worker facilitating a problem-posing group discussion.

   a. The group should prepare a 'starter' and role play asking the questions and holding a discussion.

   b. The person who plays the 'nutrition worker' must be careful not to dominate or answer questions. She must make sure that all the other people have a chance to say what they think.

   Afterwards, discuss the role play.

Project

5. Let trainees choose some pictures from this book that they think might make good 'starters'.

   a. Ask them to take the pictures, or copies of them, to somewhere where there are local people, such as a health centre, and test the pictures.

   b. They should ask people what they think the picture shows, and note the replies. If a picture is good, 8 out of 10 or more people should recognize it.

   Discuss trainees' findings in class afterwards.

USEFUL PUBLICATIONS

Shaffer, R. (1984). *Beyond the dispensary.* AMREF, Nairobi.

Werner, D. and Bower, B. (1982). *Helping health workers learn.* Hesperian Foundation, Palo Alto, California.

27 Working with families

27.1 WORKING WITH UNDERNOURISHED AND 'AT RISK' FAMILIES

Chapter 26 described how to find 'at risk' families. It is a good idea to keep a list or *register* of these families in a notebook. A register is useful whether you work in a health centre or in the community. It helps you to remember to see 'at risk' families regularly and to 'watch over' them. Or to make sure that another community worker sees them.

A follow-up register

When you hear about an 'at risk' family, write down the name, address, and any details that you have about them in the register. Leave one or two pages of the register blank for that family, to use when you see them again. Each time that you see the family make a note on 'their' page. Record the date and write brief details of their problems, what you and the family agreed to do, and when you said that you would see them again.

Why a follow-up register is useful
- It tells you whom you have and have not seen.
- It helps you to plan your work because:
  - it reminds you when to visit families;
  - it tells you which families live near each other so that you can try to visit them on the same day.
- It helps you to decide which families need your help most—for example, those families with urgent and serious nutrition problems whom you need to see more often.
- It helps you if you work at a health centre, because you can give extra attention to the children of undernourished or 'at risk' families.

Where to see 'at risk' families

You may see the children or parents of 'at risk' families:
- where you work (such as at a health centre, or in your office, or sometimes your home);

- at other places that they visit (such as at child care centres or at meetings of women's groups);
- at their homes.

The family's home is the best place to see and work with a family because:

- You meet several members of the family together, including other children.
- You see the conditions in which they live (their house, their food supplies, their farm or garden.)
- You have a better idea of what the family *can* do when you discuss with them ways to solve their problems.
- You can show them how to do things (such as prepare food for sick children) using their own utensils and foods.
- You can meet the neighbours and sometimes the landlord or employer. They may be willing to help an undernourished family, if the problem is explained to them.
- You learn about the problems of 'at risk' families and how they cope with them. This helps you when you meet with and try to help other families.

Home visiting teaches nutrition workers a lot, but it takes a lot of time and there may be transport problems. It may help you to plan your work if you can leave a definite amount of time for home visiting each week.

27.2 VISITING A FAMILY AT HOME

Working with families in their homes requires interviewing and counselling skills and a friendly, sympathetic approach. Every community is different so, if you are new to an area, try to discuss these ideas with experienced community workers.

Before you see the family

- Find out all you can about the family from their health records or from other workers who know them.

363

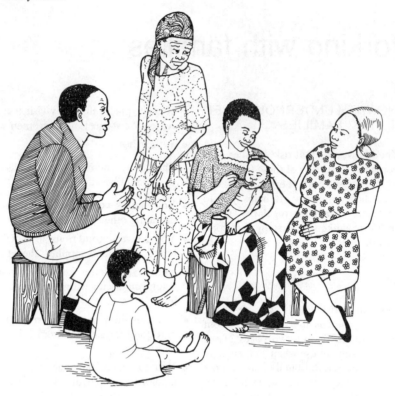

Fig. 27–1 The best way to understand a family is to visit them at home.

- Make a list of the important things that you want to learn and discuss with the family.
- If possible, ask the family for permission to visit them and get directions for finding their home.

People who work away from home

- Try to visit at a convenient time in the evening or at the weekend. This is usually better than seeing people at their workplace.
- If you must visit people at work, try to get their permission first. Then ask their employer or supervisor if you may speak with them. You may need to tell the employer why you want to see the employee. Be careful not to give him confidential information about the family. Often the employer knows when a worker has problems, and he may be sympathetic and helpful.

Learning from neighbours

Sometimes you learn things on your way to the house from the people who help you to find it. Listen carefully to what they say.

- If you do not find the family at home, talk to the neighbours. Someone may know when the family is usually at home. Someone may know about the family's problems.
- Be careful not to ask or to give confidential information or to criticize the family. Just let the neighbours talk and ask them sympathetic questions about the family

You may learn:

- if the family have some problems, such as difficulties between husband and wife, or mental illness, or alcoholism, which may be part of the reason for the child's illness;
- if the mother is away from the child often.

- Try to find out if the neighbours help the 'at risk' family. Does someone feed the children if the mother is out? Does someone dig the fields of a woman who farms alone?
- If neighbours do not help the family, or if they are unwilling to talk, try to discover the reason. Maybe the family is not liked, or they are from a different area of the country, or they behave in a strange way.

- If a neighbour mentions a problem of their own (perhaps their child has diarrhoea or their coffee bushes are dying) listen and help if you can. This helps to build up the community's trust in you.

Families who refuse to see you

Families who are 'at risk' or undernourished quite often avoid workers who try to help them. They may not trust you. They may fear that you will blame them or try to force them to do things that they cannot do or do not want to do. They may be ashamed of a malnourished child or they may feel too busy to bother—especially a woman who is both supporting and caring for a family.

Visit and try to help other families nearby to show that you can be trusted. These other families may persuade the 'at risk' family to see you; or they may help the family themselves. After some time, the 'at risk' family may be willing to see you.

When you see the family

Introduce yourself

- Greet and show respect to everyone during your visit.
- Make the family feel comfortable. Accept food, hold a baby, or help with small jobs to show that you are friendly and not proud.
- Introduce yourself, explain who you are and what your job is, and say something about why you have come to see them in a tactful and humble way. Be careful not to make them feel threatened or embarrassed by your visit.
- Ask the head of the family if you may ask some questions and discuss the family's problems.
- Ask (now or later) if you may see the house, kitchen, foodstore, garden, farm, and animals if they have them.
- Ask where they would like to talk to you. Would they prefer to go inside the house where neighbours cannot watch and listen?
- Promise the family that you will keep private information confidential (such as their income or crop yields, or health details). Be sure to keep your promise.
- Ask the family to tell you about their situation and problems in their own way.

Listen to what they say

- Listen to what they have to say. Respond sympathetically, and ask a few questions to encourage them

to tell you more and to make sure that you understand correctly what they say. Try not to ask too many questions or to 'interview' the family at this stage.

- Listen to what they say about other problems, which they may think are more important than nutrition. Sympathizing and taking an interest will help you to get to know and understand the family. Sometimes other problems are the *cause* of nutrition problems.

Help with simple problems

- If there is something that you can easily do, offer to help. For example:
  - Show them how to make up and give ORS to a child with diarrhoea (see Section 13.4).
  - Help with feeding a child who is sick (see Chapter 13).
  - Advise about treatment of a child with worms or skin sores (see Section 16.12).
  - Explain how to treat a crop pest such as mealy bugs, or how to make a grain store rat-proof (Fig. 23–9).
  - Tell them where they can get advice about credit or saving schemes.
  - Offer to talk to a teacher about a child's problems at school.
  - Show the mother how to express her breast milk to leave for the baby when she has to go to work (see Sections 10.4 and 10.17).

Helping a family in any way, even in a small way:
  - helps them to trust you;
  - helps them to see your visit as useful to them;
  - makes it easier to work with them on food and nutrition problems.

- If you offer to do something *after* your visit, write down what you said you would do, and arrange for the family to see you about it on a particular day. But be careful not to offer to do more than you are *sure* you have time to do.

- There may be a much worse problem that you can do nothing about—such as the father's unemployment or crop failure. You probably cannot find loans for farmers. Unless you are a health worker, you cannot treat most diseases.

So be sure about what you *can* and *cannot* do. If you cannot help with a problem, you must tell the family firmly. Do not raise false hopes. However, it is important

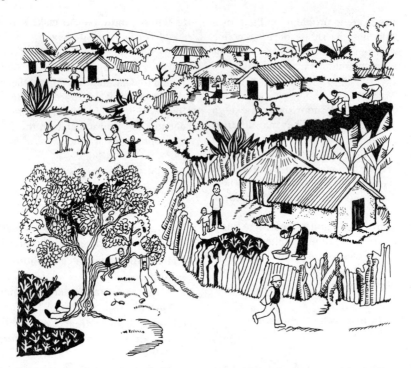

Fig. 27–2 You can learn a lot by looking around you. Notice the house and the environment.

to listen and sympathize, and you may be able to suggest someone else whom the family could go to for help.

Look around you

While you are talking with the family, you can learn a lot by looking around you.

- Notice the house, and the environment:
  - Does the family have a plot or garden to grow food?
  - Is there a toilet? Do they use it?
  - Is there a rubbish pit?
  - Is there a source of safe drinking water? How far away? How is water stored?
  - What cooking and eating utensils can you see? Is there a dish rack?
  - Can you see any food in the house? What kind of food? Is there a foodstore?
  - Is there a cooking stove or fire, and is anyone cooking or preparing any food?

You may notice things that you cannot easily ask about, but which help you to understand the family and its problems.

- Notice whether the house and environment look clean or dirty.
  - Are the children clean or dirty (this is a good indicator of home hygiene)?
  - Do the house and the family's possessions look clean?
  - What is the condition of any food?
  - Is cooked food left uncovered?
  - Are there signs of insects, pests, or dirt on food?
  - Is there a feeding bottle, tin of formula, or dummy anywhere?
  - If there is a feeding bottle: Does it look clean? Is it propped up for the baby to feed itself? Lying in the dirt? Smelling sour?
- Notice the relationship between different family members. Do there seem to be any problems? How do the parents behave with the children?
- Notice the relationship between the family that you visit and the neighbours.
- Notice the behaviour of young children, who may be at risk of undernutrition.
  - If they are active and playing, they are probably healthy.

• If they just sit miserably and quietly, they may not be healthy (although they may be shy with visitors).

Talk to other members of the family

Give other members of the family a chance to tell you about themselves. Notice:

• any other children, and whether they look well or poorly nourished;

• older people who may be able to help the mother, or who may need care themselves;

• young adults—are they employed or unable to find work?

• adolescent girls—are they at school, working, helping in the house? Are they pregnant or at risk of early pregnancy?

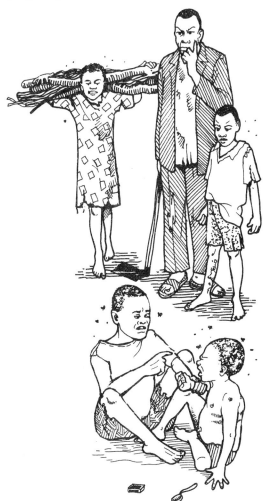

Fig. 27–3 Are the children clean or dirty?

Finding out about the nutrition and health of the family

Now you are ready to talk with the family about their food supplies and how they eat. You may need to ask more detailed questions than earlier in the visit. These are the important things that you need to find out:

• How many people are in the family, and how old are they?

• What foods does the family eat?

• What is the family's meal pattern? (How often do they eat?)

• Does the family lack any particular type of food, such as vegetables or energy-rich food?

• Do all the people in the family think that they get enough food? Who does not get enough, and why is this so?

• Which foods do they give to young children, how often, and how much?

• How do they feed babies? How often does the mother breastfeed? Does she have any difficulties breastfeeding?

• Can the family get enough food? Does it produce enough food, or have enough money to buy food?

• Are there times when the family has less food than usual?

• What do they do when there are food shortages?

• What (if anything) prevents the family getting enough food?

You also need to ask about the health of all the family members.

• Ask to see any health records that the family keep at home—especially children's growth charts. Use the information on the records—try not to ask all the same questions again, though you may need to check things which are not clear.

• You may need to examine some of them for signs of undernutrition or illness.

• If you carry scales, weigh the younger children; if not, measure their arm circumferences.

There is a check-list of questions at the end of the chapter to help you to make sure that you have the information that you need.

Diagnosing the family's nutrition problems

When you have the information on food supplies, feed-

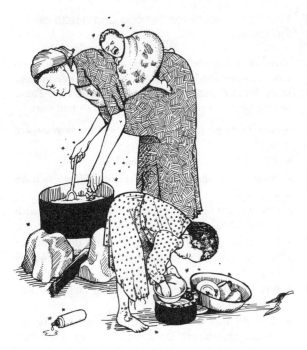

Fig. 27–4 Is there a feeding bottle anywhere?

ing, and health, you are ready to answer these questions:

- What are the nutrition-related problems of this family?
- What are the reasons for these problems? What are the blocks on their food paths?
  - Is it shortage of money, land, time, fuel?
  - Is it lack of information or skills?

Example The family has eaten little food in the past week because they are in debt and have no money until next pay day.

Example A child is very underweight, probably because he has had diarrhoea frequently. Parents do not give food when he is sick. The very dirty kitchen may be a reason for the frequent diarrhoea.

Example Father has a pale inside of mouth and complains that he cannot work hard (on a building site). He seems to be anaemic. The anaemia may be because the family eats almost no fresh vegetables or fruit and little meat or fish. But you wonder if he has hookworm.

These are what *you* think the problems and their causes are. Now ask the family what *they* think. Listen carefully to what they say.

Do not TELL the family what you think their problems are or how to solve them, because:

- You may not know all the facts, or you may be interpreting them wrongly.
- The family may not agree with you; they are then unlikely to do what you tell them.
- The family may *say* that they agree with you because they are too polite to disagree, and they want to please you.

Instead, discuss TOGETHER the problems and their causes and then offer to help the family to solve the problem.

27.3 HELPING THE FAMILY TO SOLVE THEIR NUTRITION PROBLEMS

You and the family have agreed what nutrition-related problems they have. You have some idea why they have a problem. Now discuss with the family what they want to do to solve their problems and how you can help them.

The important thing is to help people to help themselves. Help them gain confidence to solve their own problems. This is one of the most important tasks of anyone working with poor or 'at risk' families.

Discuss with the family the answers to the following questions.

Can they do better with what they have?

Discuss how they could use the food and money and other resources that they have more efficiently. The poorer the family the fewer the alternatives, but there is often something that a family can do. Sometimes they have just not thought about how they could use the things that they have in a better way.

What help or advice do they need to do this? How can you help? For example, you might be able to advise on child feeding, or food cleanness, or on growing vitamin A rich foods in the garden.

Be careful that anything that you advise is *possible* for the family and *acceptable*. Also, you need to think of the health and well-being of the whole family—not just of young children.

Example

A health worker advised a mother of a malnourished child to feed the child five times a day. When the health worker visited the family, the mother admitted that she was feeding the child only twice a day. The health worker was angry and complained to her supervisor about the mother. The supervisor went to the home and gently talked with the mother. She soon found out that the mother had a large family and spent a lot of time pounding millet every day, as well as working in the fields. She was too busy and tired to prepare five meals a day for the undernourished child. The supervisor suggested that the best way to help this mother was to ask the District Officer to get a grain mill for the village. This would save the mother an hour's work each day. The health worker worked out with the mother that she had enough millet so that she could sell the extra to pay for the cost of milling.

Example

A nutrition worker advised a mother to give her 1-year-old child fish whenever the family ate it. But the child never received any fish because:

- The grandmother did not think that fish was suitable for a young child.
- The mother thought that it was more important to give fish to her husband who earned money for the family.

The nutrition worker should have spent more time asking what foods the family were willing to give the child. Then she could have suggested ways of using these foods to make good meals and snacks for the child.

There may be something that the family can do *immediately*—such as breastfeed a baby more often, gather wild vegetables, or protect cooked food from flies.

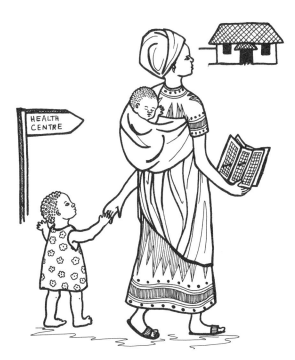

Fig. 27–5 There may be something that the family can do immediately, such as take the child to the health centre for weighing and immunizations.

There may be things which take *longer* to improve family nutrition. For example, growing more beans, terracing sloping land, or improving food stores.

Try to persuade the family to agree to do at least one thing to help themselves—for example, give the children an extra snack each day, attend the health centre, plant some vegetables.

Sometimes it helps to make a *contract* with the family. For example:

- The father promises to give more money for food, or the mother promises to attend the family planning clinic.
- You promise to visit the family once a month until the baby is growing well: to weigh the baby and to show the mother some new weaning food recipes.

What resources are there in the community to help this family?

Discuss together what the family needs to solve their problems.

- Do they need *'one-time' help* to get over a particular problem—for example, an unexpected expense such as an accident or a fire?
- Do they need *'long-term' help*—for example, because the mother is disabled or single?

It is often easier to get 'one-time' help, to get a family back to normal again, than it is to get long-term help.

From your knowledge of the community, you should know what resources are available, and how the family can get help from them (see Section 26.3). For example:

- You may be able to help the family to get a low interest loan to pay back later.
- You may be able to ask neighbours to 'watch over' the family, to report to you if they are in trouble, and to help the family if they can.
- In some places it is possible to arrange for other people to help the family at times of trouble, so that there is a network of support—for example, the community council, a women's group, a school teacher, members of the family's religious group, an employer, or fellow worker.

The community cannot help the family—what can you do?

If there are no resources in the community to help an undernourished family, what can you do?

- The best that you may be able to do is to 'watch over' them to make sure that their situation does not get worse.

- You may be able to help the children get treatment quickly if they are ill, so that they do not become more malnourished. You may be able to help the parents to get family planning advice.
- Can you visit frequently? There may be certain times of the year when the family is most 'at risk'. Can you visit more at these times? Or ask a community health worker (CHW) to visit more often?
- Can you get help for the family from *outside* the community? For example, from the government or other agency, from a voluntary organization or religious group.

Try to find at least one thing that you can do to help the family at each visit. Just knowing that someone cares about them may be enough to encourage a poor family to help themselves.

27.4 RECORDING AND FOLLOWING UP THE FAMILY

Write notes about your visit in your follow-up register, so that you remember what you discussed and agreed to do. Box 27.2 shows an example of a record of a home visit. You should write down:

- people's names so that you remember them properly;
- what you found when you examined different family members;
- important information that you collected about the family, including the family's problems and needs;
- what you think are the causes of their problems;
- how you agreed to help them and what the family agreed to do.

Do not write while you are talking because this interferes with real communication with the family. You can write your notes at the end of the visit, or as soon as you leave.

If you make your notes at the end of the visit:

- Explain to the family what you are doing.
- Tell the family that you will not use the information to make trouble for them. Sometimes it is better not to write down income or crop yields as the family may worry that the tax authorities will see it.
- Show what you have written to family members who can read.
- Leave some information with the family. If they have growth charts for the children, write something on the chart—including the child's weight or arm circumference if you measured that. Or you may be able to give the family a growth chart, or a record card.

When you leave the family

When you leave, thank the family for working with you. Confirm what you have agreed to do for them, and what they agreed to do for themselves. Make sure that they know what you *cannot* do—for example, give them free food, or a loan.

If you plan to visit the family again, ask when it is convenient. Write down the date for yourself, and write it down for the family. Do your best to keep the appointment. Tell the family where to come to see you if they have a new problem. Leave the family with a feeling that you are a friend who will help them as much as you can.

How often to visit

This depends on your workload and transport, on how far away the family live, and on how much they need your help.

When you first meet an undernourished family, try to visit or see them about once a month. See them more often if you can or if they have special difficulties. Try to see 'at risk' families about every 2–3 months. Visit more often at times of special difficulties, for example, during the hungry season, or if you hear that the wage-earner is in hospital.

When things are better for the family, visit or see them at least every 6 months. Continue to see them until they are no longer 'at risk'—for example, the children are older; the father is employed again. Try to see rural families throughout at least a whole year, so that you see them through all the seasons.

If you cannot visit the family again, try to find out what happens to them. Ask them to come to see you at a health centre, see the children at school, ask how they are when you see a member of the family in the market, or check with neighbours when you see them. Try to give the family some support until they do not need you. Make sure that they know how they can find you if they get into more difficulties and want your help.

Sometimes you cannot see a family yourself each time, but you work with a CHW who can. Try to visit the family together at least once. Ask the CHW to report to you about the family each time you see her.

27.5 HELPING PEOPLE IN PLACES OTHER THAN THEIR HOMES

Many of the suggestions for working with people in their homes may also be useful when you see and work with people in other places—such as at a health centre, a school, or at the meeting of a women's group, or at the work place.

Some extra points that may be helpful are:

- Try to speak to the person in a quiet place so that you can talk privately.
- Try to do *something* to help the family immediately. For example, show them how to make up ORS; give the address of the social welfare officer; agree to explain to the teacher why the children miss school often.

- If you need to refer the family to another worker, write a letter explaining the situation. Later, try to find out what happens and if the family needs more help.

If you refer someone to a health centre or hospital, write a letter for the health worker there. If the person is in hospital, try to visit her and talk to health staff. This may be another way to get to know and work with other workers in your community. Ask the person whom you referred to come to see you after she has been to the health centre or hospital.

Box 27.1. Advising and counselling families

When you work with individuals or families, you discuss their special situation and what they can do. This is a useful way to help a family which has particular difficulties, or which is undernourished, or 'at risk'.

Sometimes you need to *advise* the family; and sometimes you need to *counsel* them. There is a difference between advising and counselling.

Advising means telling a family what to do when you are sure that you know—for example, if a child is ill and needs treatment, and you are a health worker, or if the crops have pests and you are an agricultural worker.

- You decide the best treatment (or where to go for help).
- You explain what they should do.
- You want the family to have confidence in you.

Counselling means working it out together. For example, if a child is not getting enough food and not growing well. There are a number of possible causes and solutions to the problem. You cannot be sure which is best, or what the family can do.

- You help the family to decide what to do.
- You give them new skills so that they can feed the child better.
- You want them to have confidence in themselves.

Sometimes we want to help so much that we give advice too quickly, before we really understand the situation. But help is more likely to be successful if we take time to learn what the family feels is the problem, and what they feel able to do. So:

- Listen to what the family says about their situation, and try to really understand. To show that you are listening, pay attention, nod, say 'Aha', 'I see', 'Oh dear!', and ask a few questions to encourage them to say more ('How did you feel about that? What happened then?').

  Families may not tell you everything the first time, so be ready to listen again, and to go on listening.

- Learn to ask 'open-ended questions'. These are questions that the person has to answer with information, and not with 'yes' or 'no'.

  Example. Ask: 'What meals did Tsitsi eat yesterday?'
  And not: 'Did Tsitsi eat three meals yesterday?'
  Ask: 'How are you getting food these days?'
  And not: 'Do you have any food left?'

- Be sympathetic, and show that you understand how they feel. If you listen sympathetically to a person's problems it can really help them—even if you cannot do much else. For example, it may help an abandoned mother, a pregnant adolescent, or a lonely old person to be less depressed. They may develop more confidence and strength to earn money, or to look after themselves or their child. A poor mother may be more likely to come to a health centre if she knows that someone will welcome her and be sympathetic.

- Suggest some possible ways to solve the problem. Help the family to decide which of these solutions they might try, or any other solutions that they think of. Be careful not to tell people what they should do.

  Example. Say: 'Would you be able to add a little oil to Tsitsi's porridge, to enrich it?' or 'Some mothers find that babies like porridge with a little margarine added. Have you thought of trying that?' Do not say: 'You should add some oil to Tsitsi's porridge!'
  Say: 'Do you think you could wash Tsitsi's hands before she eats her food?' and not 'You must wash Tsitsi's hands!'
  Say: 'Have you ever tried to grow groundnuts? Do you think they would do well in this soil? Would you like to talk to the agricultural worker about it?' and not 'You should try to grow a better crop like groundnuts!'

Box 27.2. A record of home visit

Family Murithi in Mulobela Village

1st visit: 8/10/92

Family details
Mother: Wangeci Murithi
Father: Died December 1990
Children:
  Eriod born 1980 (12 y)
  Charity   b. 1982 (10 y)
  Cecelia b. 1984 (8 y)
  Mwangi b. 1986 (6 y)
  Joseph b. 1989 (3 y)
  Eva   b. 11.5.91

House: small, clean, little furniture

Plot growing:
  Maize—will be enough for about 2–3 months; three banana trees;
  kale—eaten by caterpillars; a few potatoes.

Water: Stream at end of plot.

Income: Wangeci does casual work on nearby farms and sells bananas from her trees.

Meals: Family eats two meals a day. Maize porridge with green leaves; potatoes; tea with sugar; sometimes beans.

Food available in house:
  Maize flour (dry—stored OK).

  Box of small dry looking potatoes.

  Few green vegetables; two small tomatoes.

  Empty cooking oil bottle—looks unused for some time.

Medical examination:

  Joseph: 8.5 kg; thin, scabies—underweight
  Eva: 7.1 kg; miserable, scabies—underweight
  Wangeci: ? few scabies burrows on hands?

Reasons for undernutrition:
  Lack of money to buy enough food and fuel; *plus*
  Lack of time to cook more meals a day; *plus*
  Bulky weaning food.

Action: Letter to health centre for scabies treatment for whole family—discussed need to treat whole family and wash clothes after treatment (not enough soap?).

Advised:
  Feed Joseph and Eva two extra meals each day.
  Keep porridge in clean covered bowl (so not necessary to cook more often).
  Buy groundnuts for children sometimes (price same as beans).

Promised: Ask agricultural worker to visit. Wangeci agreed to attend health centre to have children immunized and weighed.

12/11/92. Not at home—neighbour says children look better

11/12/92.
  Joseph: 8.7 kg scabies better.
  Eva: 7.5 kg playing, scabies better.

Agricultural worker gave insecticide for kale and advised on growing beans, groundnuts, and composting. Kale growing better. Has started small compost heap.

  Went to health centre once for scabies treatment but has not been back—says will come next week.

14/1/93.

    Joseph: 9.2 kg—brighter.
    Eva: 7.3 kg—diarrhoea.

Showed how to prepare and give ORS.
    Wangeci did not attend health centre—no money for bus fare.

24/2/93. Not home

10/3/93.

    Eva: 8.1 kg—eating better;
    Joseph: 9.7 kg—cheeky;
    Charity: roundworms.

(Letter to health centre for treatment for worms and for other children too, Wangeci says can pay fare now.)

    Half-eaten bowl of maize and beans on floor.
    Eriod says eating more beans now.
    Wangeci has about 6 kg beans from the garden. Advise how to store and not sell.
    Wangeci ?Pregnant?

CHECKLIST OF QUESTIONS ON FAMILY NUTRITION

This is a list to help you to remember what it might be helpful to ask a family. You should never ask a family *all* the questions!

Choose only the questions that are necessary to help that particular family.

It is better to get good answers to a few questions, than poor answers to many questions. Collect as many answers as possible as you observe the family, their home, and the farm or garden, or from health records such as children's growth charts.

General questions

- Names and sex of family members.
- Dates of birth or ages (estimated if necessary).
- Education and literacy.
- Health problems, including mental health and disability.
- Type of house and outbuildings.
- Their general condition and cleanliness.
- Availability and quality of water; sanitation arrangement; waste disposal.
- How much time or money does the family use each day to get water?

Income and occupation

- What kind of work do different family members do? Who earns money for the family?

- Does the family have a regular income? Is it the same all year?
- Who decides how money is spent?
- How much money do you (the woman who feeds the family) have to spend each week?
- Do you have money to buy food today? Do you always have enough money for food?

About farming

- Size and type of land, if any. Soil fertility, erosion.
- How many cattle, goats, chickens, or other animals do you own?
- What crops do you grow? (Try to see.)
- How much of each crop do you usually harvest?
- How much do you sell, and when?
- How much do you keep? and how long does it last?

- Is it likely to be a good or a poor harvest this year?
- Are there any problems which prevent you from increasing your yields? For example, lack of water, lack of good seed, difficulty of buying fertilizer or insecticide, shortage of labour, lack of secure tenure of the land?
- What foods do you produce in the garden?
- During which months do you get foods from the garden?
- Do you sell some of them?

About food, fuel, and meals

- Which foods does the family buy?
- How much does the family spend on food each month, or each day?

- Who decides what food to buy? and who buys it?
- Are you short of food at certain times of the month or year?
- What foods are in the house? How long do you expect them to last?
- What foods are in the store? How long will they last?
- What will you do when the food is finished?
- How many meals does the family usually eat each day?
- How many meals did you eat yesterday?
- What foods do you eat at each meal—usually, and yesterday?
- What do you plan to eat today?
- How many times a day does the family cook—usually, and yesterday?
- Which fuel does the family use? How much time or money does the family use each day to get fuel?

As you ask about the family's meals, think of the 'mixed meal guide', Fig. 8–3, and try to decide if the family are eating a good mixture of nutrients each day.

About feeding children

- What do the young children eat in a day—usually and yesterday (how many times; how much; what kind of food)?
- Does the youngest still breastfeed? (exclusively or partially? how many times by day and at night?)
- Do any children bottle feed (how many bottles a day, containing what)?
- What is each child's appetite like?
- Do the younger children share a plate of food with older children, or do they have their own plate?
- Who helps younger children to feed?

About health

Notice if anyone is chronically sick or disabled, or if their behaviour suggests possible mental illness.

Has anyone in the family been sick recently? What was the problem?

- Ask about older children and adults;
- Ask about younger children—including questions about worms, diarrhoea, cough, fever, and any other illnesses.

If a younger child has been sick recently ask about how the child ate during and after the illness.

If you can, ask tactfully if anyone has AIDS or is HIV+.

Ask if the parents use family planning, or if they would like family planning advice.

Examination of family members 'at risk'

Young children:

- behaviour—playing, or dull and apathetic;
- obviously disabled, or delayed development (for example, unable to walk after the age of 18 months);
- obvious signs of undernutrition such as kwashiorkor or marasmus;
- obesity;
- eyes—check for Bitot's spots, xerosis, or other signs of active corneal lesions; ask if the child can see in a dim light;
- inside of lips and tongue for anaemia;
- condition of teeth and gums;
- skin for scabies and other skin infections;
- signs of infections which may need treatment, such as diarrhoea and dehydration, cough and fast breathing (respiratory infection), discharging ears (ear infection);
- weight (if you have scales and growth charts);
- arm circumference.

Older girls and women:

- general appearance, very thin, average, obese, tired;
- inside of lips and tongue for anaemia;
- neck for goitre;
- height (for obstetric risk—above or below 151 cm); learn where 151 cm is on you, and measure her next to you;
- night blindness;
- skin for scabies (especially if children have it).

Notice, or ask, about possible pregnancy, especially if:

- She is adolescent and needs extra care.
- The youngest child is less than 2 years old. (Both children and the mother are at risk after a short birth interval. The mother may stop breastfeeding early.)

THINGS TO DO

Role play

1. Ask trainees to role play doing a home visit. One trainee can be the nutrition worker; others can be the family, neighbours, etc. The nutrition worker should

try to do everything described in Chapter 27. She can 'think out loud' and describe as she goes along what she notices.

Other trainees can comment and discuss after the role play.

Field visit

2. Arrange for one or two trainees to go home with a child from hospital, or a health centre, or to go on a 'follow-up visit'. (This is easiest if the family do not live too far away.)

Ask them to read Chapter 27 before they go, and to visit the family as far as possible in the way described. They should look at the chapter again when they return, to see what they forgot to look at. They can report their visit to the class, and discuss what they found, and how they would plan to help the family.

USEFUL PUBLICATIONS

Save the Children (1982). *Bridging the gap: a participatory approach to health and nutrition education.* Save the Children, Westport, Connecticut.

Werner, D. and Bower, B. (1982). *Helping health workers learn.* Hesperian Foundation, Palo Alto, California.

28 Helping people to learn about nutrition

28.1 NUTRITION EDUCATION

Nutrition education means helping people to learn new information about nutrition, and helping them to develop the attitudes, skills and confidence that they need to improve the *amount* and *sort* of food that they eat and feed to their families.

Chapter 26 on working with the community discusses ways to work with groups and families to solve nutrition problems. Those are often the best ways to help people learn, especially for communities and families whom you know to be undernourished or 'at risk'. But they take time.

There are not enough nutrition workers with enough time to discuss the problems of every family and every community so deeply. So you need to help people to learn in other ways too.

You need to try to reach as many people as possible in the community, even if you cannot give much time to them personally. It is important to help people who are not undernourished to *prevent* nutrition problems. You may be able to reach:

- individuals or families;
- small groups;
- larger groups.

To reach more people, you need to work with and train other community workers, especially CHWs.

28.2 PROBLEMS WITH NUTRITION EDUCATION IN THE PAST

Nutrition education has not always been effective, because:

- The advice was not practical or appropriate for the audience. This is often because the messages were decided by nutritionists in government offices, instead of in association with local nutrition workers and the community.
- Educators *told* people what to do, instead of *discussing* with people what they might be able to do.

- Nutrition education was not given to men—only to women. But women by themselves often cannot remove the causes of nutrition problems.
- Nutrition educators were poorly trained. They learned about *nutrition*, but not enough about *how to help people to learn*.
- Nutrition education received little money and support.

28.3 MAKING NUTRITION EDUCATION MORE EFFECTIVE

Nutrition education *can* help to improve nutrition if we use better ways to help people learn.

Know which sorts of problems nutrition education might solve

Nutrition education is most likely to help problems with the following causes.

Lack of information

For example, people not knowing:
- the dangers of bottle feeding;
- about the problem of 'bulky' weaning foods;
- why it is important to feed sick children;
- that pregnant women have special needs;
- that it is possible to space births;
- which legumes are drought-resistant;
- why it is important to eat dark green and yellow fruits and vegetables.

People not using their resources in the most efficient way

For example, nutrition education can help people to:
- budget their wages so that they buy foods which are good value and keep enough money for the end of the month;
- plan the amounts of food and cash crops that they plant;

- use fuel in a more efficient way;
- store maize or other food more safely, so that less is lost.

People living in new or 'at risk' situations, which they have not learned to cope with

For example:
- families who have recently moved into town;
- adolescent mothers;
- grandparents who have to look after grandchildren;
- families who have to use new foods—for example, people in settlement schemes or refugee camps who are given unfamiliar food as food aid.

Link nutrition education with other programmes and services

Communities and families cannot remove many blocks on their food paths if they do not have more *resources*— for example, more land, more water, more fertilizer, more money, more fuel, or more time.

Nutrition education by itself cannot remove blocks on the food path which are due to lack of resources. Nutrition education is most successful when it is *part* of other programmes which help people to develop or get more resources.

Nutrition education can help people to:
- understand how those other programmes might help them;
- decide the sort of programme that would help them most;
- make better use of those programmes.

Examples
- In an agricultural development programme, farmers learn how to use the extra food or cash that they produce, so that their families are better nourished.
- In a feeding programme, mothers learn how to use the foods that they receive, and what to do when they stop getting food aid.
- In a programme to provide women with hand mills, mothers learn that it is important to use some of the extra time that they have to feed children more often.
- In a programme which provides a better water supply, people learn how to transport and store water hygienically. They also learn the importance of washing hands before touching food, so children get less infections.

Plan nutrition education with the community

Work with the community to identify their problems and priorities, in the way described in Chapter 26. Then help them to plan:
- *who* needs to learn, and *what* they need to know;
- *from whom* they can best learn;
- *how* they should learn;
- *where* and *when* they should learn.

Example
You have worked with the village health committee on a *growth monitoring programme* to weigh all the children in a village and to give them all growth charts. Together, you have found that many young children are underweight. You have discussed with some families how the children are fed. The committee all agree that the children in the village do not grow well, because their food is very bulky. So they plan that:

- Mothers, older girls, and grandmothers (*who*)
- should learn:
  - why porridge enriched with soybean flour gives more energy than porridge made with maize flour alone;
  - how to make enriched porridge (*what*)
- from the village health worker (*from whom*)
- through discussions and demonstrations (*how*)
- at the village school (*where*)
- on Saturday afternoons (*when*).

Make sure that nutrition workers of all sorts give consistent information

People get nutrition information from many different sources, such as parents, relatives, friends, school teachers, health workers, home economics workers, family planning workers, and from the radio, TV, and newspapers. Sometimes different sources give different information, which confuses people. For example:

- A nurse may advise a woman to give her baby weaning foods from 4 months.
- A family planning worker may advise her not to give anything for 6 months.
- Her mother-in-law may say 9 months.
- She may see an old poster which says 2–3 months.
- A friend has given her baby dilute cereal in a bottle from 1 month.

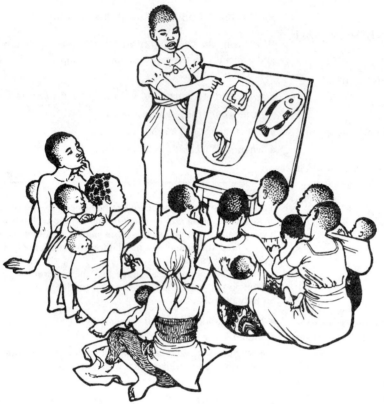

Fig. 28–1 What do you think about the way in which the mothers are learning about nutrition?

You cannot control all the information that people get. However, if you work closely with other workers in the community, you can all give *consistent*, that is, similar information. You can make sure that out-of-date posters and other materials are thrown away.

Spread information in different ways

If you spread the same information in different ways:

- It reaches more people.
- People hear the information several times. This helps them to remember and think about it.

The different ways in which you can spread information depend on what your job is and whom you want to reach. But whichever ways you use, it helps if you can *co-ordinate* them, so that people hear the information several times over the same period.

Community nutrition workers can reach these people:
- village chairmen and community groups;
- employers;
- families;
- other nutrition workers.

They may reach them through:
- visiting people at home or at work;
- talking with people in bars, markets, or buses;
- health centres and outreach health activities;
- schools and colleges and training courses;
- women's, youth, religious, and civic groups;
- trade union and co-operative meetings;
- public meetings;
- arranging displays at special functions;
- agricultural, community development, and other extension workers.

Supervisors and programme organizers can reach:
- politicians, planners, and other influential people;
- the general public, in a large part or the whole of the country.

They may reach influential people by:
- writing letters, sending them information, visiting, and talking to them;
- speaking at meetings.

Box 28.1.   Why nutrition education has not always been successful

Figure 28–1 is from the first edition of this book. We think that it shows some of the reasons why conventional nutrition education does not help people to solve their nutrition problems.

Notice these points:

1. The nutrition worker is advising the mothers to eat fish when they are pregnant
Is this sensible advice? Why may some mothers not follow it?

- Perhaps they do not understand the advice, especially if the educator uses pictures or words with which they are not familiar.
- Perhaps they do not believe the advice because:
  - It is different from what their relatives and friends tell them.
  - It is different from what they hear on the radio, or from other nutrition or health workers, or from the school teacher.
  - They do not know or trust the nutrition worker.
  - The nutrition worker does not follow the advice herself.
- Perhaps they do not have enough money to buy fish. Perhaps fish is expensive or not always available where they live.
- Perhaps they feel that it is better to spend the family income on other things such as school expenses, clothes, or entertainment. Often people do not value better food as much as nutrition workers do.
- Perhaps they do not have enough time or energy to buy and prepare fish when they are pregnant.
- Perhaps it is against cultural beliefs for pregnant women to eat fish, or other special foods.

Often nutrition advice does not fit a community's social behaviour. For example, a family shares food in a way which they believe helps to teach children not to be greedy. Or, they give the wage-earner the biggest share.

2. The nutrition worker is TELLING the mothers what to do
Is this a good way to help people to learn? Are the nutrition worker and the mothers really communicating with each other?
  The nutrition worker is standing up, while the mothers sit on the ground. Would it be better if everyone sat down together and *discussed* the picture?
  Do you think that this nutrition worker was *trained* to teach these women about improved family meals? Probably she received no training. Senior staff often do not think that training for teaching is important. They do not know that nutrition educators need special skills to teach adults.

3. All the people in the group are women
Nutrition educators often talk mostly to groups of women. They tell mothers how to feed their children better. They may make it seem as if they blame the mothers and as if it is the mothers' fault that the children are undernourished.
  But mothers cannot improve the family food supply or children's meals by themselves. Whose fault is it if a woman has little money or land for food? Or too little fuel or time to cook frequent meals? Or if she has too little education? Or if she is anaemic or often tired?
  It is good to work with groups of women, as we show in Figs 26–10 and 26–11. But it is important to include men also in nutrition education.

They may reach the general public by:

- arranging for broadcasts by radio; and in some towns and cities, TV;
- writing articles or giving interviews for newspapers and magazines;
- arranging for displays at shows and exhibitions;
- helping to develop education materials, such as posters and pamphlets, and to distribute them to community nutrition workers.

One way in which information spreads is when people *talk about it among themselves*. This is most likely to happen if people learn the information in different ways, and if the information is *consistent* and *co-ordinated* and *interesting*. For example, people are more likely to chat about 'enriched porridge' to each other if they hear about it at the health centre, then at a women's group meeting, then at a public meeting, and also from the radio and newspapers. (Many people know and talk a lot about AIDS because they have read posters

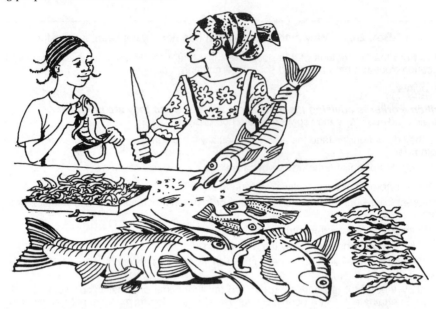

Fig. 28–2 Information spreads when people talk about it among themselves.

and newspapers, and they have heard about it from the radio, and they know families who have AIDS.)

Use 'participatory' learning methods

Choose methods in which the people who are learning play an active part, that is, they *participate*. If people just sit and listen and watch, they become bored, and they do not learn much. If they participate, learning is easier and more fun. It is also more fun for the teacher (see Sections 28.7–28.12).

Set a good example yourself

Do not suggest that people do things that you do not try to do yourself. People are more likely to listen to you if they know that your family eats good mixed meals, prepares food in a clean safe way, gives good food to sick children, spaces births, and breastfeeds babies.

Many families have less money, food, fuel, and utensils than you. Try to prepare meals sometimes with the things that poorer families have. Then you may be able to suggest more practical ways for them to improve their family meals.

28.4 FACTS FOR NUTRITION EDUCATION*

A *fact* is a statement about something which is true. A fact is a 'bit of information'. Nutrition facts are bits of

* This section was inspired by the book: *Nutrition Facts for Malawian Families* (Malaŵi Government Food and Nutrition Committee 1990)

accurate and useful information about nutrition. For example, 'All children need vitamin A to have healthy eyes.' 'Lack of iodine causes goitre.' 'Sick children need to eat often, or they lose weight.'

Nutrition workers need to know the facts or information which can help to remove blocks on food paths and improve nutrition in the areas where they work. All the nutrition workers in the area should agree about these facts. They should agree that the facts are correct; and they should agree that they are relevant to the nutrition problems in the community.

Example
- 'Using improved seed gives bigger harvests and improves family food security.'
- 'The first milk produced by mothers (colostrum) protects babies against infection.'
- 'Frequent pregnancies weaken a mother and increase the chances of her having a small weak baby.'
- 'A child who has his own plate of food gets his fair share.'
- 'Children need snacks between meals to grow well.'

Facts and messages

Facts are different from *messages*. Messages tell people *what* to do and *why*. For example:
- *Fact*. 'Dark green leaves contain more vitamin A than cabbage.'
  Message: 'Give your family dark green leaves instead

of cabbage. Dark green leaves contain more vitamin A which helps to keep eyes healthy.'

- *Fact.* 'A spoon of oil contains more energy than a spoon of porridge.'
  Message: 'Add oil to your child's porridge to give him more energy.'
- *Fact.* 'Sick children need food often or they lose weight.'
  Message: 'Give sick children soft food every 2–3 hours to prevent them losing weight.'

How to use nutrition facts in nutrition education

When all the nutrition and other community workers in an area agree about which are the important nutrition facts:

- It helps everyone to give similar consistent information to the public.
- It is easy for nutrition workers to plan the content of nutrition education activities.

Nutrition facts are the basic information that you use for example to:

- plan a talk to a community group or on the radio;
- write an article for the newspaper or a booklet for health workers, or materials for a training course.
- plan a poster, radio 'spot' (see Exercise 6 in 'Things to do'), exhibition, etc.

28.5 CHOOSING NUTRITION FACTS WHICH ARE IMPORTANT FOR YOUR AREA

The nutrition workers in an area should all know and use the same facts. You can make a list of these nutrition facts at national, district, or community level.

- Ask a group of senior nutrition, health, agricultural, and other experts to a meeting. Collect information and materials on nutrition in case they want reference material.
- Identify the most important nutrition problems and their causes.
- Together make a list of the most important nutrition facts which could help to improve nutrition. (It may help to prepare a draft list beforehand which the experts can discuss.)

- Write down the nutrition facts and, under each, write some extra information explaining why the fact is important.

Example
Frequent pregnancies weaken the mother and increase the risk of having a small weak baby.

If a mother becomes pregnant before she is fully recovered from the birth of the previous child, she may have a weak and small baby. Small weak babies are less likely to grow well, are more likely to become ill, and are more likely to die before they reach 1 year than babies who are strong and healthy when they are born.

- Make copies of the facts and extra information, and give them to all the nutrition workers and other workers who teach people in the area.
- Discuss and explain the facts together until everyone agrees.
- Write them down again, and give everyone the final list of facts.
- Send copies to anyone else who may be interested—senior health or agricultural officials, religious or community leaders.

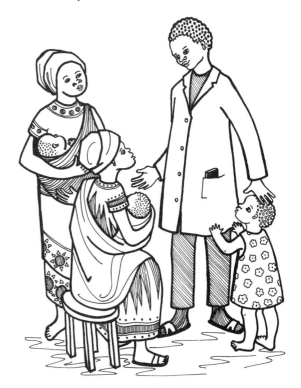

Fig. 28–3 Nutrition workers of all sorts should give consistent information to mothers.

28.6 DEVELOPING MESSAGES

Nutrition facts are for nutrition workers. Sometimes you can share a fact with families or communities and explain it. Usually you need to develop the fact into a message for it to be useful for people.

A message gives *advice*:
- It suggests something that people should do.
- It explains why they should do that.
- It tries to overcome the common reasons for *not* doing it.
- It tries to give advice in an interesting, culturally acceptable way.
- It is usually targeted to a particular group of people.

When you plan a particular nutrition activity, you need to decide which nutrition problems to try to overcome, and which nutrition fact or facts you want people to know. Then you develop the fact into a message.

Example

A problem in your area is that many young children do not grow well. One reason is that weaning foods are too bulky —they are not energy-rich, so children lack Calories for growth. The nutrition fact that families need to know is:

'Adding fat or oil to porridge gives children more energy and helps them to grow well.'

You, with the help of other nutrition workers and some local women, develop a message from the fact:

1. Make the fact into a simple message. For example, *'Add oil or fat to your child's porridge. Oil is full of energy and helps to make children grow well.'*

2. 'Pre-test' the message to find out if people can understand it and do what it suggests. For example you find that:

   - People do not have fat but they have groundnuts.
   - They believe that fatty foods give children diarrhoea.
   - They do not understand the link between 'full of energy' and 'growing well' but they do believe that fatty food gives strength and energy.
   - They do not find the message very interesting or know who it is meant for.
   - They want to know how much oil to add.

   You write and pre-test the message again until it is right. An example of the new message could be:

   'Mother—you want your baby to be strong and active? Add a spoonful of pounded groundnuts to each cup of his porridge. Groundnuts are easy to digest, and do not upset a child's stomach.'

28.7 SPREADING A MESSAGE

You also need to think of how to *spread* a message. For example, you or other nutrition workers might give a talk or demonstration at a community meeting, health centre, training centre, or school. A women's group might write a song or a drama to perform for other groups. You might make a poster or picture to display in a meeting place or health centre.

Test the song, drama, or picture again with some of the people whom you want to hear it. Make sure that they understand the message correctly.

After a talk, performance of a song or play, or display of a picture, ask people to discuss it. It is important to find out:

- who the message is reaching;
- if people understand the message;
- what they think about the message;
- if they are doing what the message suggests.

Discussing the talk, performance, or display like this is different from using a 'starter', which poses a problem (see Section 26.11). This time the performers are spreading a message, which gives information and which suggests what to do.

To find out if the message has spread, talk to people, for example, in the market or health centre some days afterwards. Ask them:

- Did they see the picture, hear the talk, etc?
- What was the message?
- What did they think about the message?
- Have they done, or are they likely to do, what the message suggested?

People who develop radio programmes or posters, leaflets, and other materials for the whole country develop their messages in a similar way. It is difficult to get messages right for a community—so it is much more difficult to get them right for a whole country. One of the 'Things to do' at the end of this chapter is to practise developing a message for a radio programme.

28.8 TALKING TO INDIVIDUALS AND FAMILIES

You may have many opportunities to talk to individual people about nutrition—for example, when you visit people at home or at work. You may be able to talk to people informally—for example, when you meet in shops or in the market. This is different from a proper home visit (Chapter 27) which takes a long time.

If you are a health worker, you can discuss nutrition when families come to you in the health centre, for example, for family planning, or to have a child immunized, or when a child is sick, or for antenatal care.

You may have only a short time, and it may seem easier just to *tell* a family what you think they should do. But remember that *telling people what to do is not likely to be effective*.

Here are some ways to help people to learn.

Explain what you are doing when you do it

Use what you do as a demonstration. For example, when you weigh a child and fill in his growth chart, ask the mother to tell you how she thinks the child is growing. For example, ask 'Do you think he has gained enough weight this month?' Explain the growth line if necessary. Mothers may be more interested and more likely to learn at the time of weighing than at some other time.

Let people take part

For example, let mothers help with weighing and with filling in their child's growth chart.

Discuss the person's situation at that time

When you see a family, discuss something about their situation at that time. Listen to what they say, and try to *suggest* one or two things that may be interesting and helpful to them *now*. Do not try to tell them too much.

For example, if you see a sick child, ask the family if they are able to get the child to eat. *Explain* why it is important to feed a child who is sick. Make some *suggestions* about how they might persuade the child to eat, and discuss what is possible for them.

If you greet a woman working in her garden, ask if her children enjoy dark green vegetables. If necessary suggest ways of adding them to children's food. If you chat with an old person who is poor, make sure that they know which foods are good value for money.

28.9 TALKING WITH SMALL GROUPS

Small groups may want you to work with them for short times—for example, a women's group may want you to be a guest for an afternoon. Or you may want to talk to a group of women in a hospital who come from different places. Or you may want to introduce nutrition into the activities of a group which has another purpose— such as adult education classes or during training of traditional birth attendants.

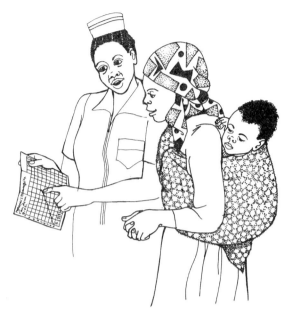

Fig. 28–4 Talk with mothers during growth monitoring.

Group discussions are a good way to work with small groups like these. They can be quite informal—for example, a group can share experiences, and talk about how their children are, and why they may be growing well or not growing well, or what vegetables they have bought this week.

You can introduce a subject and say a little about it. Or you can use a picture, or a story to stimulate discussion. Then ask members of the group to tell their own experiences of the subject. In a hospital, mothers of undernourished children can discuss why their children became ill. Discuss the problems and suggestions that the group tells about.

Ask them if they have any questions to ask you. Make sure that they have accurate information on the subject. However, it is important not to *tell* a group what to do. Ask questions, make suggestions, give information, but let the group decide.

This kind of group discussion is different from 'problem posing' discussions with communities, which take a long time (Section 26.11). You need to move a group discussion on faster. You have to give information, gently and respectfully correct misinformation, and help the group to come to a conclusion. You are not waiting for them to decide what to do as a community. But you hope that people within the group learn something useful that they can try to do.

Example

In one village a nutrition worker told mothers that small children must have their own plates for food. But many mothers did not do this because their grandmothers warned them that their children would become greedy and selfish.

In another village, a small group of mothers and grandmothers discussed, with the nutrition worker, ways to make sure that children ate enough food. Everyone, including the nutrition worker, made some suggestions which the group discussed. At the end, the group decided that the best way was to give young children their own plates. All the mothers in the group did this because they knew that the grandmothers and other mothers supported the idea.

After a few days the group met again to share experiences and any problems. They agreed that the children ate more when they had their own plates, and they decided to encourage other families to do it too. As well as improving the amount of food that the children ate, the mothers and grandmothers gained confidence to try to solve other problems.

Other ways in which groups can learn together are:

- They can study and practise interpreting growth charts together. They can bring their own children's growth charts to study.

- They can cook a new kind of recipe, such as 'enriched porridge' and try it out together, and give it to their children to eat. Different members of the group can choose, buy, or bring the food, clean and prepare, cook, and taste it. One group of mothers can give the demonstration to another group, for example in a health centre or hospital.

- They can prepare and perform songs and dances about nutrition. Most people enjoy making up songs and dances. Preparing them provides a good opportunity for nutrition discussions. You should make sure that the songs and dances give facts which are correct and relevant for the community.

  Songs help both performers and audience to learn about nutrition in a way that they understand, enjoy, and remember. Songs and poems can show what people *feel* about their food and nutrition problems.

- They can prepare dramas about nutrition to perform to other groups or at meetings. The group chooses the subject and writes their own script. This kind of drama has a written script, and it may give a 'message', so it is different from a 'starter'. The nutrition worker helps, and discusses the facts that the drama contains, to make sure that it is correct and deals with important community problems. The actors learn a lot as they prepare the drama. The actors and audience learn more if they discuss the drama afterwards.

28.10 TALKING TO LARGE GROUPS

You may have to 'give a talk' to a large group of people. This is a useful way to give a lot of people new information, to introduce and explain a nutrition fact, and to get people interested.

You may have to talk at a public meeting, for example, about starting a community growth monitoring programme or child care centre. You might be asked to talk to a class in a teacher's training college, for example, about good and poor value foods for school children or the dangers of adolescent pregnancy. Or you might have to demonstrate a better way to grow vegetables at a local agricultural show. Or you might talk to youth groups, religious groups, etc. about weaning children.

Prepare your talk carefully, so that it is appropriate for that particular audience. Make a list of the facts and ideas that you will talk about to remind you what to say. But do not read or learn a speech—just talk clearly and naturally to the audience, following your list of ideas. Try to be lively and make it fun.

Most of us can listen to a 'lecture' for about 10 minutes. Then we stop listening properly and start to get bored. To make your talk more interesting:

- Have something to show the audience.
- Get them to participate—for example, let them ask and answer questions and discuss the ideas; let them take part in demonstrations or taste food.

You may do these things before, during, or after a short talk. What you choose to do depends on both you and your audience.

Have something to demonstrate—a 'learning aid'

Demonstrations

The best kinds of learning aids in nutrition are real things such as foods and the utensils that people use. These are much better than pictures.

1. *Cooking demonstration.* For example, you may show people how to prepare enriched porridge, or 'snacks' for children, or food suitable for sick people.

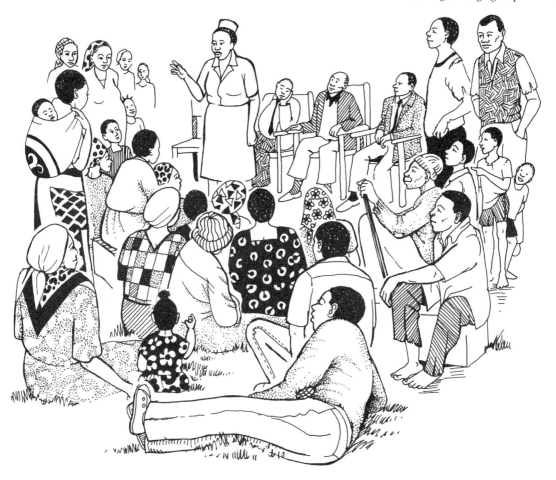

Fig. 28–5 Talking at a public meeting.

- Do as much as possible beforehand, such as cooking beans, or cleaning rice, especially if you demonstrate meals which take a long time to prepare or cook.
- Use only those utensils which local people use.
- Make sure that everyone understands each step of the demonstration.
- At the end, show how much food a child or adult needs for a meal.
- Let everyone taste the food—especially any children who may be present.

2. *Other food demonstrations*

For example:

- Ask people to choose from foods on display, three or four of which they could use to make a healthy mixed meal. Then discuss the meal that they plan.
- Compare the volume of a mug of porridge (or rice, bread, potato, etc.) with the volume of oil which contains the same amount of energy. (This might be useful in a talk about enriching porridge, *and* in a talk about how to lose weight!)
- Show a feeding bottle which has not been sterilized properly, and which smells sour.
- Use a small tin of formula milk, and count how many measuring scoops of milk it contains. Calculate how many bottles this would make, and how long the tin would last, or how much it costs per feed. (You could use an old formula tin, and fill it with flour instead of milk powder, and use it several times.)

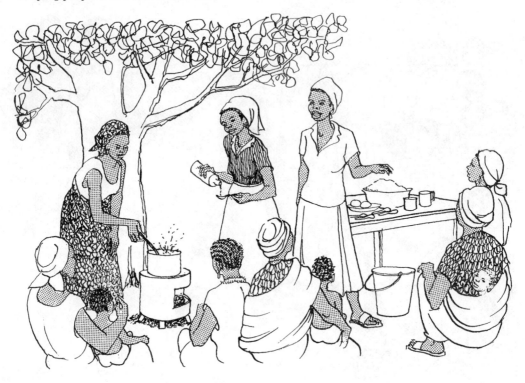

Fig. 28–6 Do food demonstrations with local women.

3. *Other demonstrations using everyday items*:

- Show a fuel-efficient stove.
- Use water and soap and show children how to wash their hands.
- Use a new chewing stick to show school children how to clean their teeth.
- Use wood, etc. to show how to make a drying rack.

Drama and stories

You could tell a story, or ask a group to perform a short play, or you can do a short 'role play' with a colleague. In some countries, people use 'puppets' for drama.

Pictures

Show the audience one or more big pictures, that everyone can see. Use pictures that show people doing things, such as cooking or eating a meal, or buying or growing food, or feeding a child. Then ask different people in the audience what the picture shows, and what they think about it. Use the discussion to introduce your ideas and information.

Slides and films

Sometimes you may be able to use slides, 'overheads', films, or videos. They can be very helpful if you have them, but you need to prepare the show carefully. Also, make sure that the equipment is available, ready, and working before you begin. Be ready to talk without them if you find that the equipment is not available, or if it breaks down.

Get the audience to participate—questions and discussions

Discussion

Always have a discussion either before, during, or after a talk, demonstration, drama, etc. Encourage the audience to give their ideas and opinions. Local people may not have as much technical knowledge as you, but they probably have much more practical experience.

Ask the audience questions

You can ask questions *generally*. For example:

- 'Do you think that soaking beans overnight is a good idea?'
- 'How can we encourage mothers to give dark green leaves to their children?'
- 'How often should we feed sick children?'

You can ask questions *individually*. For this, it helps if you know people's names. For example, 'Bibi Macha, do you find it helpful to soak beans?' Asking individually can help quieter people to take part in the discussion. When you ask general questions, nobody is embarrassed, but you may find that a few talkative people answer all the time.

When someone gives a *correct* answer:

- Say 'Yes, that sounds good', and repeat the correct answer so that everyone hears it.
- Then ask more questions such as 'Why do sick children need food frequently?' or 'Do children enjoy eating green leaves? How can mothers encourage them?'

If no one is willing to answer, you may have to make a suggestion, and ask for some opinions. For example: 'Does it help to mix the green leaves with something else? What would you suggest? Tomatoes? Onions? Soybeans?'

When someone gives an *incorrect* answer:

- You may just show that you have heard but say nothing more, and instead 'hold on to' someone else's correct answer.
- Or you may decide that it is important to gently and respectfully correct the wrong information. For example, 'Yes, it is true that bananas have yellow skins, but in fact they don't contain much vitamin A. Many people are confused by that.'
- *Never* embarrass anyone or tell them that their answer or opinion is wrong. Only inexperienced teachers do that.

Encourage the audience to ask you questions

Be ready to stop and answer questions during your 'talk'. When you answer good questions, use this opportunity to repeat and emphasize important facts. People may learn more from your answers to their questions than from your prepared talk.

Other ways to get people to participate:

- Divide the audience into 2–4 groups and ask each group to prepare two questions or problems they

---

Box 28.2. Hints on giving talks and demonstrations

Before

- Ask one or two people from the group:
  - which topic would be useful and interesting;
  - what the group probably knows about the topic;
  - how long the session should last;
  - where and when the session will be.
- Write down the purpose of your session. Complete this sentence: 'After the session the group or audience will . . . e.g. *'know why sick children need frequent meals'* or *'be able to prepare an energy-rich weaning food.'*
- Decide how to give the information or demonstrate a skill. Decide what equipment or learning aids you will use.
- Practise your 'talk' or demonstration. Make sure that it does not last too long.

During

- Arrange seating so that everyone can see and hear in comfort. Welcome everyone, and treat them with respect.
- Explain the purpose of the session, and what you will do.
- Have something to demonstrate to the audience (Section 28.10).
- Get the audience to participate (Section 28.10).
- At the end give a summary of the important things you discussed.

After

- Find out what people thought about the session. Was it useful and interesting?
- Ask people how you can improve your session in future.
- Find out if anyone tried out any of the suggestions. If so, were there any problems?

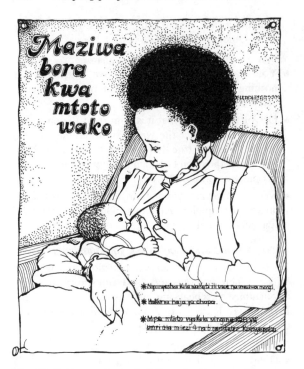

Fig. 28–7 Use posters only if they give the correct message.

want you to talk about. This makes people discuss the subject themselves and decide what they want to know about it.

- Give your audience an 'exercise' on your subject near the beginning of your talk. For example, ask them to think about or discuss with the person who sits next to them one of the following questions:
  - How long should a baby be exclusively breastfed? Why?
  - Which foods help to prevent anaemia?
  - Why it is good to have at least 2 years between births?

Afterwards people listen more carefully to your talk as they want to compare what you say with their own ideas. Afterwards you can ask a few people what they thought or discussed.

28.11 MASS MEDIA

In most countries there are nutrition programmes on the radio and television, and articles in newspapers and magazines. These can help people to learn about nutrition.

- They get information and messages to many people quickly.
- People hear about 'nutrition' and want to know more about it.
- Programmes repeat information that you give to families personally. This helps people to believe and remember it.
- *You* may learn new information.
- Some nutrition workers get groups to meet together to listen to a radio programme. After the programme the group discusses it.

However, there are some disadvantages to using mass media.

- The information may not reach the people who need it most. Many poor families do not have radios, and newspapers do not reach families who live in remote places.
- Messages may not be appropriate for every community. You may work to develop a locally appropriate message and then people hear something different on the radio. This confuses them.
- Messages through the media *tell* people about a problem and how to solve it. They give people useful information. But they do not usually persuade people to change what they do. People are more likely to change what they do if a nutrition worker whom they know and trust explains and discusses the messages.

28.12 MATERIALS TO HELP PEOPLE LEARN ABOUT NUTRITION

The best sort of learning materials are real foods and things which local people use. If you want to use materials such as posters and flipcharts, you may need to make your own, because there is a shortage of professionally produced useful materials in many places.

Good learning materials include ones which:
- *Give information which is useful to local people.* For example, how to prepare oral rehydration drinks, or how to express breast milk and feed it to a baby from a cup, or how to grow green vegetables.
- *Make people think about nutrition problems.* These materials don't tell people what to do, but they suggest questions which you can use to start discussions, or as a 'starter' for posing problems. For example, a picture of a thin pregnant girl labelled: 'How can we help this mother?'

Posters

Posters are popular. But it is important to use them only if they give the *correct* message.

In nutrition, the messages vary with local conditions. For example, messages may be different in areas where most people farm, where most people work on a coffee estate, in a poor urban area where people have to buy food, or in an area near the sea or near a lake where people can get fish. Messages may be different during a drought, and when the rains are good.

Nutrition messages are different from immunization messages, which are the same in all areas and at different seasons.

Posters are expensive and difficult to produce, and it is difficult to change the message quickly. Posters do not teach people much if you just pin them to the wall and leave them there. People soon stop looking at them. Make sure that you remove old posters, especially if they give inaccurate information. Try to find something else to cover the bare walls of your office, class-room, or health centre. Perhaps you could ask some children in a local school to make some pictures.

A good way to use posters and other pictures is to start group discussions. If they show something that is not correct, you may be able to ask the group to 'find the mistake'. But be careful not to confuse people!

Flipcharts and flashcards

Flipcharts and flashcards are popular but, like posters, they take a long time to produce, and it is difficult to get the nutrition message right. Flashcards have the advantage that you can use them in any order, and you can take some away, and add some of your own.

Booklets

Community workers sometimes find small books of pictures useful, and they are easy to carry around. The books may contain simple drawings or photographs, with a few words to explain the picture and its message. But you must be sure that the pictures show the correct important facts for the area and that people understand the pictures.

When you talk to a small group or family, show them the pictures in the book, and discuss the ideas. This can be useful to give the family information and to explain what to do, or to use as a 'starter' picture.

Locally produced materials

Try to produce pictures, posters, flashcards, and booklets with the community.

Pictures and posters and other materials which you produce yourself may be better because:

- They can show messages or pictures which are appropriate for the nutrition situation in your area. Sometimes centrally prepared materials cover topics which are not important in your area, but if you have nice materials you want to use them.

- Local people can help to prepare and test the materials. So they are more likely to understand and accept the messages.

- You can prepare new materials quickly when the nutrition situation changes.

It is very difficult to produce materials completely from the beginning. Look for ideas in professional materials and in materials produced in other communities. Often you can adapt drawings and make them suitable for your community. There may be a local artist who can help to adapt them. Some materials and drawings are produced in a way which makes them easy to copy and adapt, like many in this book. You can cut pictures out of newspapers and magazines.

Wall newspapers

Pin up nutrition pictures, newspaper cuttings, and other nutrition information on a notice board, in a school, health, or community centre. Change the things on the board often so that people keep looking at it.

You can use something in the wall newspaper to start a discussion, or as the idea for a song or a play. Then the song or play is up-to-date and more interesting.

THINGS TO DO

Class exercises

1. Ask trainees to find out if they are good at helping people to learn about nutrition. They should answer the following questions. They score +1 if they answer 'yes' and −1 if they answer 'no'. They can ask a friend to help them to answer if they like.

   - Are you a good listener?
   - Do you find out what people know before you give information?
   - Are you friendly and polite to everyone?
   - Do you give special attention to the poorer, weaker people in your community?
   - Do you encourage people to make their own decisions, even if you do not agree with them?
   - Do you feed your family in the way that you advise others?
   - Was your baby breastfed?
   - Can you explain things in a simple way?

- Do you know where to find out new nutrition information?
- Do you regularly find out new things?
- Do you consult other nutrition workers before you give nutrition information?
- Have you decided which things in this book are useful, which are not useful, and which you might adapt?
- Do you introduce only one new nutrition fact at a time?

What is your score out of 13?

Discussions

2. Show trainees a picture of a health worker teaching a group of people about feeding children. Ask them to discuss the way in which the health worker is teaching. You can show a 'good' example (Fig. 26–10) or 'bad' example (Fig. 28–1).

3. Ask groups of trainees to write down one important nutrition fact. For example,

   'Babies who start breastfeeding within an hour or two of birth, learn to suckle more easily.'

   Ask them to make a list of the sort of people who should know about the fact. For example, mothers, fathers, grandmothers, school children, teacher, health staff, and hospital supervisors.
   Then decide which is the best way to reach these different groups. For example:

   - mothers—antenatal clinics and women's groups;
   - fathers—community meetings;
   - teachers—meeting between local teachers and health staff;
   - schoolchildren—in home economics or health science lessons;
   - hospital supervisor—letter from his superior, article in medical journal.

Role play

4. Ask trainees to role play helping families learn about nutrition.

Example

A pretty young mother with a new baby lives with the baby's father who is a taxi driver and the father's mother. Ask the trainees to role play a health worker making a home visit and advising the mother to fully breastfeed the baby. Have the father, grandmother, and perhaps a neighbour in the home too. The mother is worried about losing her figure if she breastfeeds. She is worried that the father may leave her. The father's mother thinks the baby should have some bottle feeds.

Afterwards discuss the way the health worker worked with the family, and whether she could have done it better.

5. Ask some trainees to prepare talks for:

   (a) a small group, such as a women's group, or the village health committee;

   (b) a large group, such as a public meeting.

   Decide who the group is to be, what the message will be, and how you will give the talk, and choose appropriate learning aids.

   - Give the talk to other members of the class, who must role play the audience.
   - Afterwards discuss the talk. What were the good points? What could be improved?

Group work—developing a radio message

6. Ask groups of trainees to practise developing a radio message from a nutrition fact. They should work in groups and follow these steps:

   a. Choose a nutrition fact which deals with an important community problem. For example:

      'Vitamin A rich foods such as spinach, carrots, paw-paw, mango, pumpkin, and liver help young children to have healthy eyes.'

   b. Use the fact to prepare a message.

      - Decide who the message is for (e.g. mothers and fathers).
      - Decide exactly what the message should encourage people to do. This is very difficult and needs lots of discussion. (Which foods can local people get? Should they produce or buy them?)

      For example, you may choose to encourage or advise:

      - fathers to buy spinach and pumpkin seeds and dig the garden;
      - mothers to plant and care for the spinach and pumpkins and to feed them to the young children.

      Discuss why people might not want to do these things. For example:

      - Women may think that growing vegetables takes too much time.
      - Fathers may think that spinach and pumpkin are not important foods for children.
      - Mothers may think that children will not like spinach.

   c. Write the message again. You will probably have to write it several times to get it right. The message should:

      - describe exactly what people need to do;
      - explain why this is helpful;
      - overcome people's objections.

d. Pre-test the message with some people who might be the audience, for example, some mothers in a health centre or some colleagues.

- Make sure that they can understand what you mean.
- Find out if the ideas are acceptable to them.

e. Rewrite the message if necessary. Make sure that it is interesting and the right length for a short 'radio spot'.

For example:

'Fathers, young children who do not eat enough green leaves and pumpkin sometimes get serious eye diseases. Some of these children become blind. A small plot of spinach and pumpkin provides enough vegetables for all the family. Please buy spinach and pumpkin seeds this week and prepare a plot for them.

Mothers, my children enjoy a spoonful of spinach mixed with beans. They like mashed pumpkin too. I am sure that your children will like these foods too. Please spare the time to grow some spinach and pumpkins in your garden, to protect your children's eyes.'

f. Then discuss for the example:

- Which sentences explain exactly *what to do*?
- Which sentences explain *why this is important*?
- Which sentences are included to try to *overcome people's objections*?

g. If you have a tape recorder, you can record your message, and try it out with other trainees or other people. Ask if they understand it, and what they think.

USEFUL PUBLICATIONS

Malaŵi Government Food and Nutrition Committee (1990). *Nutrition facts for Malaŵian families.* Department of Economic Planning and Development, Office of President and Cabinet, Government of Malaŵi, Lilongwe.

WFHPA (1986). *Health education.* UNICEF, New York.

29 Group feeding programmes*

29.1 WHAT GROUP FEEDING PROGRAMMES DO

Group feeding programmes (GFPs) provide free or cheap food to people in need. Sometimes people get the food as payment for work. Foods for feeding programmes may come either from within the country, or from a foreign government or non-government organization (NGO), or through an international organization such as the World Food Programme (WFP). Food which organizations outside the country give is called *food aid*.

To give extra food is one way to help poor or undernourished families. But there are also problems and disadvantages with feeding programmes and food aid (see Box 29.1).

There are several types of feeding programme:

- *Feeding 'vulnerable' or 'at risk' groups.* For example, young children, and pregnant and breastfeeding mothers.

- *Institutional feeding.* For example, feeding primary and pre-primary schoolchildren, and orphans.

- *Emergency feeding.* This means feeding people during or after disasters, such as war or drought.

- *'Food for work' schemes.*

Programmes give food in different ways:

- *As 'rations' to take home.* The family or the person may eat the 'rations', or they may sell it so that they have more money to buy other food. The rations are then an *income supplement* for the family.

- *As meals at a 'feeding centre'.* People come to a feeding centre such as a school for a meal—this is 'on-site' feeding.

29.2 FEEDING 'VULNERABLE GROUPS'

Vulnerable groups are people who are 'at risk' of undernutrition. These are usually young children, and pregnant and breastfeeding mothers. Sometimes old, disabled, or homeless people also receive food.

---

* Much of the information in this Chapter is from FAO (in press) *'Food and Nutrition in Management of Group Feeding Programmes'*.

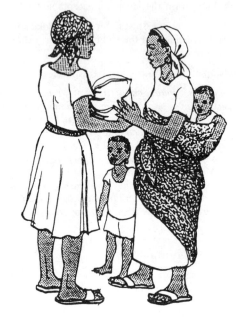

Fig. 29–1 Distributing rations to take home.

Most vulnerable group feeding programmes give rations for families to take home. Because families share food, larger rations are sometimes given to vulnerable children to make sure that they get enough.

The purpose may be to:

- increase food intake and improve nutrition while the mothers and children are most 'at risk';

- encourage women and children to attend health facilities;

- give an 'income supplement' to families in need.

How much food to give

Programme organizers decide for each programme exactly how much food to give, and for how long. International agencies have made the following suggestions.

How many Calories to give each day

Give rations containing 800 kcal per person per day to young children and to pregnant and breastfeeding

---

Box 29.1. Problems with feeding programmes and food aid

Dependency
Families may become dependent on free food. They may not want to produce more food themselves, or to make better use of what they have.

Not the best way to help families
Needy families often live in remote places. It may be difficult for them to travel to a feeding centre. There may be no one who can bring a child, especially if the mother is working. A family may spend a lot of time and effort to bring a child for food. There may be better ways for the family to use that time and effort.

Food shortage is not always the cause of undernutrition in children
If health workers have free food to give to families, they may not look for and help with other causes of undernutrition. Other causes, such as not feeding children often enough and not feeding children when they are sick, may be more important. Giving out food takes time—nutrition workers then have less time to counsel and help families.

Feeding programmes cost money
The food may be free, but transporting, storing, and distributing it cost money. This may not be the best use of available money.

There may be free food for a limited time only
It may be difficult to help families with food shortages when free food stops. Schools may not be able to continue making good meals for children. If families expect to get free food when they come to a health centre, they may not come when there is no food.

If food aid foods are used, they may not be familiar to people
Families may not like some unfamiliar foods, or they may not know how to use them—for example, some sorts of fats and oils.

Food may not reach the family members who need it most
Sometimes families share the food among other members of the family, so the needy person does not get it all. If a child has food at school, the family may give the child less food at home.

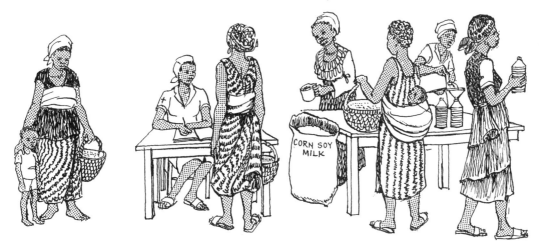

Fig. 29–2 Distributing food for young children and women. Measure the correct amount of food for take-home rations (see Section 29.10).

mothers. This provides 55 per cent of the children's energy needs, and 30 per cent of the women's needs.

How long to give rations

• *Undernourished young children.* Give rations until 2–3 months after the child's 'weight-for-height' has

reached 90 per cent of reference and the child is gaining weight at a healthy rate (see Tables A5.4– A5.6 in Appendix 5 and Section 14.17).

• *Pregnant women.* Give rations from when their pregnancy is confirmed (usually about the fourth month).

- *Breastfeeding women.* Give rations for at least the first 6 months after delivery (longer if possible; see Section 18.5). However, mothers and nutrition workers must understand that, if rations stop, it does not mean that breastfeeding stops too.

Following up children's progress

It is important to follow up children and to monitor their growth after they stop receiving rations. You need to make sure that:

- Their families are able to give them enough food.
- They continue to grow well.
- Breastfeeding continues up to 2 years or longer.

Avoiding the problems of 'free food'

Here are some ways in which nutrition workers can try to avoid the problems in Box 29.1.

Only give food when you are sure that it really is the best way to help the family

In other words, you must be sure that the cause of the undernutrition is shortage of food or of money to buy food and that there is no other way to increase family food supplies.

Give rations for a limited time

When you start to give a family free food, discuss with them the purpose of the rations. Explain how long they will receive rations. Explain clearly that they will only have this help for a limited time to help them over a difficult period.

Give the family advice and support to improve their nutrition

Give rations only as part of a programme of nutrition education, growth monitoring, and health care. Do not forget that the purpose of the programme is to improve *family food security* (see Chapter 25).

29.3 PRIMARY SCHOOL FEEDING

In school feeding programmes, children receive a snack or a meal at school to:

- *Prevent short-term hunger* (see Sections 12.1 and 30.1). Hungry children cannot concentrate or learn well. Resources which countries put into schools are wasted if the children are too hungry to learn.

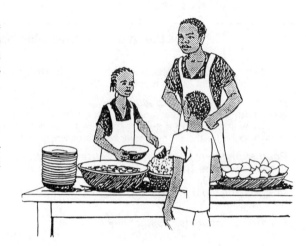

Fig. 29–3 Distributing meals at a school.

- *Improve their nutrition.* School meals improve the nutrition of undernourished children.
- *Encourage attendance at school.* If children get a meal at school, they are more likely to enrol in school, and to continue to attend regularly. They are less likely to 'drop-out' of school.

It is important to give the meal early in the school day, so that the children are more alert during lessons. It is also important for the meal to be part of other nutrition activities in school—such as health and nutrition teaching and school gardens (see Chapter 30).

Pre-primary school feeding

Children in child care and early learning centres receive a snack or a meal. This is to prevent them from feeling hungry and to improve the nutrition of undernourished children.

29.4 EMERGENCY FEEDING

Disasters such as drought and war make it difficult for people to produce or have enough money to buy food. Emergency feeding aims to:

- Provide people with at least their minimum energy and nutrient needs.
- Prevent people from leaving their homes to look for food. People who stay in their homes are more likely to survive than people who live in camps.
- Help people to provide their own food as soon as possible.

Types of emergency feeding

General feeding

All people in need receive a ration which contains at least 1900 kcal a day. At least 10 per cent of the energy is from fat. People who live for several weeks on rations which contain no fresh foods such as vegetables or fish are 'at risk' of micronutrient deficiencies. The commonest are anaemia and vitamin A deficiency. Occasionally other deficiencies such as scurvy, pellagra, and beriberi occur.

Ways to prevent these deficiencies are to:

- give rations which include foods rich in iron, folate, vitamins A and C, niacin, and thiamine;
- give foods fortified with the necessary micronutrients, for example, dried skimmed milk (DSM) or oil fortified with vitamin A;
- provide large enough rations so that people can sell or barter some for fresh, local foods;
- help people to grow fresh vegetables or to raise small animals;
- give supplements of micronutrients such as high-dose vitamin A capsules to all people at risk.

Supplementary feeding

People at special risk of undernutrition, such as young children, pregnant and breastfeeding mothers, and sick people, receive extra food. Supplementary rations usually provide an extra 350–500 kcal per person per day.

If you give take-home food for supplementary feeding, the whole family is likely to share it. To be effective, it may be necessary to:

- increase the rations up to four or five times to make sure that the 'at risk' member of the family gets enough;
- educate the family so that they increase the amount of extra food that they give to 'at risk' members;
- ask the parents to bring all the children along when they fetch the supplementary food, so that you can measure them and check that they are getting enough to eat.

If it is not possible to do these things, it may be better to give 'on-site' feeding.

Treatment feeding

Severely malnourished people receive food under medical supervision. The food may be a special preparation based on dried milk or mixed cereals (see Chapter 17).

Box 29.2.   Breast milk in feeding programmes

People often forget breast milk as a food in feeding programmes. But it is particularly important in emergencies. Nutrition workers should encourage and help mothers in these situations to breastfeed for as long as possible.

Important points to remember are:

- Even sick and malnourished mothers can produce breast milk if you give them enough food and support. It helps if you visit mothers at home to encourage them or if you ask them to come to a breastfeeding centre where mothers can support each other.
- Sometimes a woman's breast milk seems to have dried up. Encourage her to believe that she can produce breast milk again.
  - The baby must stay close to the mother and sleep with her, and must suckle often—10 or more times a day, for several minutes on each side (see Section 10.15).
  - Feed the mother to build up her nutrient stores.
  It may take 2–3 weeks for milk to flow well.
- While you wait for a mother's breast milk to return, feed the baby other milk from a cup (see Section 10.16). It may help to drip some milk on to the nipple while the baby suckles, or to put a fine tube from the cup of milk to the nipple, so that the baby sucks milk through the tube while suckling the breast (see Fig. 10–18).
- If you have to feed a baby artificially for a time, prepare the feed freshly each time—do not prepare it in advance. Watch the child carefully for signs of infection.
- Never allow the use of feeding bottles.
- Sometimes women are willing to breastfeed another baby, for example, if a baby's mother has died. This may be in addition to their own. Or, they may be willing to 'relactate' if their own baby has died or is already weaned. Encourage women to do this and, if possible, give them extra rations. Many women can produce enough milk to breastfeed two or more babies.

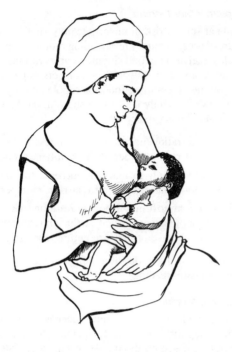

Fig. 29–4 Breastfeeding is particularly important in emergencies.

29.5 FOOD FOR WORK

People who are in need work and receive rations as part or all of their payment for the work. The work is usually on development projects which:

- protect the environment, for example, planting trees;
- increase family food security, for example, vegetable growing schemes;
- improve public services, for example, building a health centre.

Sometimes people on new settlement schemes receive rations. Each worker usually receives five individual rations or one ration per family member for each day that he works.

29.6 ACTIVITIES OF GROUP FEEDING PROGRAMMES

Important activities of GFPs are:

- involving the community;
- programme planning;
- choosing people for feeding;
- supervision;
- distributing food;
- evaluation.

Involving the community

A community is more likely to support a feeding programme if they are involved. Discuss the programme with the community, explain its purpose, and ask them to help plan, organize, supervise, and evaluate it. Ask parents to help with a school feeding programme.

29.7 PROGRAMME PLANNING

Nutrition workers may not plan a feeding programme, but they should know about the decisions that planners have to make.

Deciding objectives

The *objectives* of a programme may be to:

- improve nutrition;
- prevent short-term hunger;
- increase attendance at school;
- encourage families to come to health centres;
- give an income supplement to families or institutions.

A programme objective describes exactly what effect a programme should have.

What sort of food and how much to give

The amount and sort of ration that a programme provides depends on its objectives. Table 29.1 shows the recommended amount of energy for individual daily rations to supply for different purposes. As a general guide, about 8–12 per cent of energy should come from protein, and 20–25 per cent from fat. You may have to reduce the amount of fat in emergency feeding if fat-rich foods are scarce. The rations should also supply any micronutrients such as vitamin A and iron, if the home diet lacks them.

The best sort of food for rations is local food, if there is enough available, and if there are funds to pay for it. If local food is not available, try to give foods which are similar to local ones, so that they are familiar to people. If only unfamiliar foods are available, nutrition workers should develop recipes using local cooking methods.

Table 29.1. Suggested energy content of rations (FAO in press)

Group	Daily energy needs (kcal)	Percentage of needs to give	Calories to give daily
Vulnerable group feeding			
Children (6–60 months)	1400	55	800
Pregnant or breastfeeding	2600	30	800
Institutional feeding			
Pre-primary schoolchildren (3–6 years)	1700	55	900
Primary schoolchildren (5–12 years)	1900	55	1000 (if meal given)
		20–25	400–500 (if snack)
(5–16 years)*	2000	55	1100 (if meal given)
		20–25	400–500 (if snack)
Emergency feeding			
'Average' person† doing light work	1900	100	1900
Food for work			
'Average' active rural person†	2100	100	2100

* In many primary schools there are children aged up to 16 years.
† This is the average need per person per day if the numbers of people of different ages and sexes is the same as in a normal population.

Cereals, legumes, and oil are the foods which are used most often (Table 29.2). Some foods for feeding programmes are fortified. For example dried skimmed milk usually contains added vitamin A. Mixed ('blended') cereals such as corn soy blend, are usually fortified with several minerals and vitamins.

29.8 CHOOSING PEOPLE FOR FEEDING

Which people a programme chooses to feed also depends on the objectives of the programme.

If the aim is to improve nutrition, choose children who are already malnourished or who are at risk of becoming malnourished. Good indicators of malnutrition in children are:

- growth failure as shown on a growth chart;
- weight-for-height below 80 per cent of reference, or below 3rd centile;
- height-for-age below 90 per cent of reference, or below 3rd centile;
- arm circumference below 13.5 cm.

A child may be 'at risk' of malnutrition if he or she:

- is low birth weight;
- is a twin;
- is bottle fed;
- is the fifth or later child in the family;
- has a sister or brother who died before the age of 5 years;
- has one parent absent, disabled, sick, or with a severe social problem (such as alcoholism);
- if the parents have AIDS, especially if the child also has HIV infection;
- has an adolescent mother.

A programme may give rations to all low-income women who are pregnant or who are breastfeeding a baby under 6 or 12 months old. Or they may choose mothers who are at special risk.

Table 29.2. Examples of daily rations for different types of feeding programme (FAO in press)

Food (grams per day)	Vulnerable groups	Pre-primary school	Primary school
Maize flour (g)	175	160	180
Beans (g)	20	20	50
Oil (g)	20	20	20
Sugar (g)	–	20	–
Energy (kcal)	843	870	960
Protein (g) (% kcal)	21 (10%)	20 (9%)	28 (12%)
Fat (g) (% kcal)	25 (27%)	23 (24%)	24 (26%)

Food	Food for work	Emergencies— general rations
Cereal (g)	500	400
Legumes (g)	30	60
Oil (g)	30	20
Canned meat (g)	20	–
Blended cereal (g)	–	30
Sugar (g)	–	15
Energy (kcal)	2120	1920
Protein (g) (% kcal)	56 (11%)	55 (12%)
Fat (g) (% kcal)	43 (18%)	30 (15%)

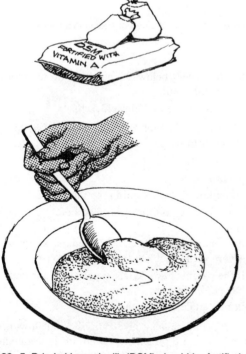

Fig. 29–5 Dried skimmed milk (DSM) should be fortified with vitamin A and mixed with cereal flour.

Mothers at special risk are those who:
- are less than 18 years old;
- had a low birth weight baby with a previous pregnancy;
- had a child who died before its fifth birthday;
- had a pre-pregnancy weight of less than 38 kg;
- had many closely spaced pregnancies;
- have a chronic health problem such as TB or HIV infection;
- have no economic or social support from the child's father or from relatives.

A programme may choose mothers and children or schools which are in 'disadvantaged' places, such as dry areas where food production is difficult, or crowded urban slums.

Sometimes undernutrition is more common in certain seasons, such as in the rainy season when there is more infection or the planting season when there is more work. People may need rations most at these times.

29.9 SUPERVISION

To make sure that food reaches the correct people in

Box 29.3. Dried skimmed milk in feeding programmes

If your feeding programme has DSM, use it with great care, because it can cause problems. For example:

- People may mix DSM with contaminated water. Germs which cause diarrhoea multiply quickly in liquid milk, especially at warm temperatures.
- People may not mix DSM with the right amount of water. They may add too much water. This makes the milk too dilute, so that it does not provide enough nutrients. They may add too little water, which makes the milk too concentrated. This can make young children very ill.
- People may give the milk to babies in feeding bottles.

For these reasons, international organizations recommend that programmes:

- Distribute legumes, meat, or fish whenever possible, and not DSM.
- Use only DSM which is fortified with vitamin A.
- Never give DSM to breastfeeding women, especially in the first 6 months after delivery. (A baby who cannot breastfeed for some extraordinary reason should have whole dried milk or infant formula by cup.)
- For take-home rations, only use DSM if it is mixed with a cereal flour, and if milk is culturally acceptable. If possible mix the flour and DSM before distributing it to feeding centres.
- For on-site feeding, mix DSM into cereal flours, porridges, or stews before or during cooking. The only situation when DSM should be used by itself is in areas where milk is part of the traditional diet, and people can use it safely—for example, soured.

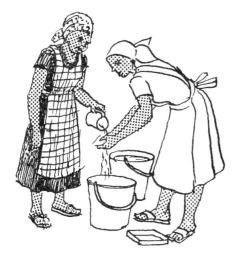

Fig. 29-6 Check that people who handle food wash their hands.

the correct quantities, efficiently and safely, it is essential to *supervise* food distribution. *Supervision* means:

- working closely with the community;
- keeping records of the food that you receive and use;
- training and supporting staff, such as kitchen workers;
- making sure that linked activities such as health care are working properly;
- monitoring attendance;
- monitoring hygiene;

- monitoring the flow of money (for wages, fuel, transport, supplies, etc.) and food.

Monitoring attendance

If someone does not come regularly for rations or meals, try to find out why. Visit them at home if possible. Perhaps the mother or a child is sick. Try to help them to get food if you can.

Monitoring hygiene

Good hygiene is very important in feeding programmes especially with 'on-site' feeding. If food is contaminated, many people become sick. Malnourished children may become dangerously ill.

Give attention to the hygiene of:

- *people* who handle food (see Sections 7.3 and 7.4); make sure that they wash their hands and have short nails and clean clothes;
- *foods* especially foods such as milk, meat, fish, and cooked meals, in which germs multiply quickly;
- *water supplies*, especially drinking water;
- *buildings* in which food is stored or cooked;
- *utensils and equipment* for preparing and cooking food, and for measuring out rations;
- *containers* for taking rations home;
- *latrines and waste disposal*.

Checking storage

Bad storage wastes food. Bags of food must not touch either the floor or the wall. The store must be clean, and must be protected from water and insects, rats, mice, birds, and thieves.

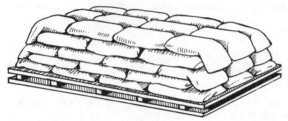

Fig. 29–7 Store food carefully to prevent wastage. Bags of stored food must not touch either the floor or the wall.

29.10 DISTRIBUTING FOOD

Measuring 'take-home' rations

Nutrition workers need to know how to measure the correct amount of each food in the ration (see Fig. 29–2).

For example, if the daily ration of maize flour for a child is 175 g, and you give rations every 2 weeks, each child should receive

$175 \times 14 = 2450\,g = 2.450\,kg$ flour every 2 weeks.

Nutrition workers usually measure rations by volume, for example, by mugs or cans. This is easier than weighing food. So you must be able to convert the weight of rations into volume measures.

For example, if you use an empty can which holds 300 g of flour, to measure the ration, each child should receive:

$$\frac{2450}{300} = \text{about 8 cans of flour every 2 weeks.}$$

Measuring food for 'on-site' feeding

Nutrition workers need to know how much food to cook for different numbers of people.

For example, if there are 300 school children, and the ration of rice for each child is 180 g per day, then the amount of rice to cook is $180 \times 300\,g = 54\,000\,g = 54\,kg$.

If you measure the rice with a large can which contains 2 kg rice, then you will need to cook $54/2 = 27$ cans of rice each day.

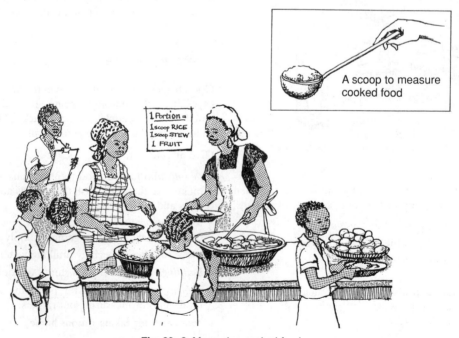

A scoop to measure cooked food

Fig. 29–8 Measuring cooked food.

29.11 EVALUATION

The purpose of evaluation is:

- to find out if the programme is running efficiently and reaching its objectives;
- to find out if there are any good or bad side-effects, and whether the objectives are still appropriate and possible;
- to use these results to alter the programme activities if necessary;
- to find out if it has had a long-term effect.

It is important to do the evaluation:

- *with the local community;*
- from time to time during a programme;
- after the programme has stopped (to look for long-term effects).

What people decide to evaluate depends on the objectives of the programme but may include:

- changes in food intake—for example, do people eat more food?
- changes in attendance at schools and health centres;
- changes in short-term hunger, concentration, and alertness among school-age children;
- changes in nutrition knowledge among families and schoolchildren.

People do not now usually attempt to measure the nutritional effects of feeding programmes (such as an increase in children's weights-for-age or weights-for-height) because it is too difficult. This is because food intake is only one of several things which affect nutrition.

THINGS TO DO

Classroom exercise

1. Try to obtain a sample of the ration that is given at a feeding programme, or find out what rations are given and prepare a sample from local foods, or examine the ration during a field visit, and do this exercise in class later.

   Ask trainees to examine the ration and to calculate:

   a. how many Calories it gives;

   b. what proportion of the Calories come from protein and fat;

   c. how much it costs using local prices for these or similar foods.

Discussion

2. Give trainees a copy of Box 29.1 and ask them to comment on it. Ask any trainees who have worked with feeding programmes to describe and discuss the advantages and problems.

3. Have a *debate* on ideas such as:
   'A feeding programme for mothers and children is not a good way to prevent PEM' or 'Foreign foods should not be used in feeding programmes'. Ask two trainees to speak for the idea and two to speak against it, and ask the others to add points to the discussion.

Practical exercises

4. Ask trainees to prepare and demonstrate recipes for children using foods from a feeding programme.

   a. Discuss the nutrient content and the time and method of preparation.

   b. Ask some children to try the foods, to find out if they like them.

5. Ask trainees to make a checklist for checking hygiene at a feeding programme.

   - You may be able to arrange to use the checklist if you visit a feeding programme.
   - If doing a formal 'check' is not acceptable, remember the list as you make informal observations on your visit.

Field visit

6. Visit a feeding programme, for example in a school, and:

   a. Ask the supervisor about the objectives of the programme, how they monitor it, and what the problems are.

   b. See how they store the food.

   c. Examine the foods and how people measure them.

   d. See how they prepare, cook, and serve the food.

   e. Notice the cleanness of the food, the equipment, and the kitchen workers.

   f. Find out what people who receive the food learn about nutrition.

   Afterwards, discuss the programme, the good things about it, and how to improve it.

7. If you visit a 'take-home' feeding programme, ask trainees to check the hygiene of food containers of people who come to collect food.

USEFUL PUBLICATIONS

de Ville de Goyet, C. (1991). *Management of nutrition emergencies in large populations.* WHO/UNHCR, Geneva.

FAO (1984). *Guidelines for training organizers of group feeding programmes: for use in Africa*, a training pack. FAO, Rome.

FAO (in press). *Food and nutrition in management of group feeding programmes*, Food and Nutrition Paper, no. 23. FAO, Rome.

Oxfam (1991). *Nutrition in emergencies—a practical guide to assessment and response.* Oxfam, Oxford.

30 Nutrition in schools

30.1 WHY NUTRITION IN SCHOOLS IS IMPORTANT

Nutrition work in schools is important because:

- If schoolchildren are healthy, well fed, and not hungry they learn better.
- If there is a feeding programme in a school, children are more likely to *enrol* and to attend regularly, and are less likely to drop out.
- Schoolchildren are tomorrow's leaders, workers, and parents.
- Schoolchildren can carry new ideas and information into a community.

Schoolchildren learn better when they are healthy and well fed

Figure 30–1 shows two girls aged 9 years, called Anna and Zela.

Anna is well fed. She has a normal weight for height.

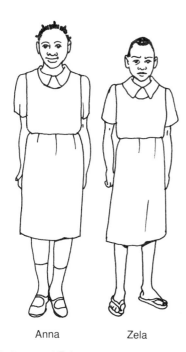

Anna   Zela

Fig. 30–1 Anna and Zela.

She eats a good breakfast, she brings a big snack to school, and she has a good mixed meal early in the evening.

Anna has missed only a few days of school. She does not feel hungry at school so she concentrates and learns well in class. She has plenty of energy for sport and play.

Zela is not well fed. She is shorter than Anna, she is also thin (with a low weight-for-height), and she is anaemic. She does not eat breakfast. She brings a small snack to school, and she eats a meal late in the evening when she is too tired to eat much.

Zela often misses school because she is sick. When she does attend, she is too hungry to concentrate and learn well in class. She does not have the energy to answer questions, or for play or sport. She is too tired to do her homework well.

So Zela gets poor grades and her teacher thinks that she is stupid. But Zela is not stupid. She is undernourished and anaemic and too tired to show how intelligent she really is.

Many things affect how well children learn. But two of the most important are:

- *The child's nutritional status.* This depends on:
  - how well the child was fed when younger;
  - the child's present diet;
  - whether the child has a heavy wormload or other diseases.

  Lack of energy and protein, iron deficiency, and iodine deficiency, can all affect children's learning. Vitamin A deficiency can affect a child's sight, which interferes with learning.
- *Short-term hunger.* Children who are hungry because they do not have enough breakfast or lunch cannot concentrate or learn well.

Schoolchildren are tomorrow's leaders, workers, and parents. They carry new ideas into a community

Most children attend primary school. Some of the important things that they can learn are:

- how good meals keep people healthy;
- how to feed their families in the future;

- how to keep food safe and clean;
- how to feed younger brothers and sisters, especially when they are sick;
- why some people become malnourished.

Children often share what they learn with their parents and other relatives. So teaching schoolchildren about nutrition helps other people in the community to learn about nutrition too.

Encourage families to send girls to school for as long as possible. Mothers with more education are able to feed and care for their children better. They have more power within the family, so they can use more resources for the children. They are more likely to have small families, and their children are more likely to be well nourished and less likely to die.

Try to help improve the nutrition of schoolgirls, so that they grow better before and during adolescence. Girls who grow well will be stronger and healthier when they become mothers. They will have larger, healthier babies. This helps to break the cycle of small mothers having low birth weight babies who grow up to become small mothers (see Section 18.7).

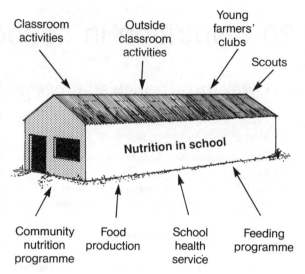

Fig. 30–3 Different nutrition activities in school.

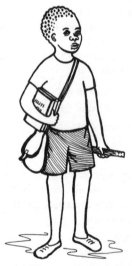

Fig. 30–2 Schoolchildren are tomorrow's leaders, workers, and parents.

30.2 NUTRITION ACTIVITIES IN SCHOOLS

Figure 30–3 shows some different nutrition activities that can take place in schools. Some activities help children to learn about nutrition. Some help to improve the children's nutrition and health.

Learning about nutrition in the classroom

The curriculum may already include nutrition, food and agriculture, hygiene, and health. You may be able to help teachers improve the way they teach these subjects. If there is not much nutrition in the curriculum, teachers can introduce something about it into other subjects, especially as examples for exercises, and in practical work, or as a topic for student projects.

Here are some examples of how some schools teach about nutrition in the class-room.

Science

- Growth and development (of children, plants, and animals).
- How germs reach food and water; what happens when you wash your hands.
- How infection and nutrition affect each other.

Home economics

Nutrition:

- the food needs of different age groups, men and women;
- feeding babies—breastfeeding and weaning;
- why breakfast and a midday meal or snack is important;
- the main nutrients in the school meals or in different midday snacks.

Foods:

- nutrients in foods and the effect of cooking and processing;
- cooking methods that preserve nutrients and give good meals;
- fuel-saving stoves and cooking methods that save fuel (see Figs. 24–3 and 24–4);
- how to prepare good mixed meals for different groups (young children, schoolchildren, mothers, old people, sick people etc.—see Chapter 8);
- how to plan a weekly menu;
- which foods are good value for money, and which are poor value for money;
- how to budget for food—for example, how to spend the local minimum daily wage, so that a family has enough food and other basic necessities.

Hygiene:

- looking at food cleanness in stores and markets;
- how to protect food in a kitchen from dirt, insects, and other pests;
- how to clean stores and kitchens;
- how to wash up;
- how to dispose of waste food, containers, and dirty water.

Mathematics

- Buying food: working out cost per kilogram of different foods.
- Measuring and weighing foods.
- How to calculate the amounts of food different numbers of students need.
- Counting bags of food in a store.
- Using store records as mathematical examples.

Languages

- Learning the names of local and foreign foods in different languages.

Geography

Finding out:
- where different foods for meals come from;
- how foods are processed, transported, and stored;
- which other countries eat the same foods.

Agriculture/gardening

- Learning about sustainable food production.
- Producing and selling food.

- Preserving and storing foods.
- Learning about seasonal variation of foods and their costs.

Reading and writing

- Writing stories and poems about food and nutrition subjects.
- Using a nutrition book to practise reading in class.

Art, music, drama

- Singing songs and act plays about the school feeding programme.
- Drawing pictures and prepare posters about food and nutrition.
- Collecting advertisements for foods, including baby foods, and discuss why they can be misleading.

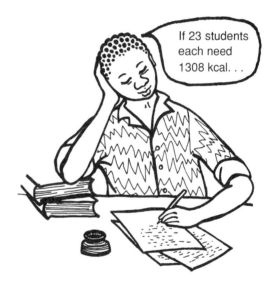

If 23 students each need 1308 kcal. . .

Fig. 30–4 Children can use nutrition examples when they learn mathematics and other subjects.

Learning about nutrition outside the classroom

Students who belong to Young Farmers' Clubs, Scouts, or other youth organizations can learn and do many practical nutrition activities. For example they can:

- learn how to produce, process, sell, and buy food;
- check the weights or arm circumferences of young children;
- teach younger children good feeding habits.

The Child-to-child Programme (see Exercise 5 in 'Things To Do') may be a useful source of ideas for these activities.

Schools can invite visitors to give talks or demonstrations about food and nutrition to students, teachers, and parents. Visitors could be experts in health, agriculture, livestock, fisheries, forestry, food storage, famine relief, etc. They could be senior government planners or officials of voluntary agencies who are visiting the area.

Schools can have nutrition exhibitions on open days or at parent–teacher meetings.

Students might take part in the nutrition activities of health services or of community groups. For example, students could help a community health worker who is caring for families with undernourished children, or they could help a women's co-operative raise funds or sell their produce.

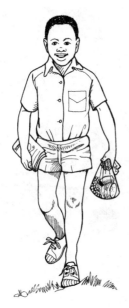

Fig. 30–5 Children sometimes carry a snack to school.

30.3 FOOD AT SCHOOL

Children get food at school in one of the following ways:

- *The children carry a snack to school* to eat during the day (see Section 12.3).
- *Food sellers* sell food to schoolchildren. Sometimes

the food is not very clean or nutritious, and it may not be good value for money.

- *The school provides a meal or snack.*
  - The meal may be free (see Chapter 29). This is usually only possible when food-aid foods are available. Parents often give small contributions of money, fresh food, labour, or firewood for the meal.
  - Parents pay some or all of the cost of the meal. Poorer families may need to pay less.

The purpose of providing a school meal may be:

- to prevent short-term hunger;
- to improve the children's nutrition. Giving good meals to children who are poorly fed can improve their growth and school performance, and it can prevent anaemia. It helps children who were undernourished when young to do as well as possible in school;
- to encourage children to *enrol* in school, to *attend* regularly, and not to 'drop out'.

A meal also provides an opportunity for practical nutrition teaching. The kitchen, store, eating place, and market are like 'laboratories' where students can learn many things about buying and preparing food, and about hygiene and nutrition.

School meals are most necessary where:

- There are many students from families who are too poor to feed them well or to give them food to carry to school. These children need a free school meal.
- Students come to school without breakfast, especially if they have to walk a long way. These children need breakfast or a snack soon after they arrive at school.
- Students stay at school all day and cannot go home for lunch or buy food. These children also need a meal in the middle of the day.

30.4 SCHOOL HEALTH PROGRAMMES

To improve students' nutrition, a good school health programme checks students' health. It tries to improve the quality and cleanness of school meals and the environmental hygiene of the school.

Checking students' health

Exactly what it is useful to look for may be different in

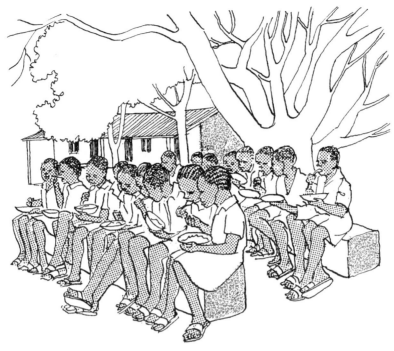

Fig. 30–6 A school meal or snack prevents short-term hunger.

different areas.* Teachers should know the signs of poor nutrition, and notice if a child shows them. Common problems are:

- *Wasting, or thinness.* Notice if any students look very thin. If a child is undernourished, try to find out why, and try to get help for the child or the family (see Chapter 27).

- *Anaemia.* Check the colour of students' tongues, to see if they are very pale (see Section 20.3). If so, treat the child or refer her for treatment.

- *Tiredness, and difficulty concentrating in lessons.* This may mean that the child has not had enough breakfast or lunch, and has short-term hunger. Check the child's diet. Discuss with the family how the child can eat more at breakfast and midday. It may also mean that the child is anaemic—check and if necessary treat for that also.

---

* Sometimes health authorities collect the weights or heights of primary school children. These are useful as an indicator of the nutritional status of the community. They are not usually useful to monitor the health of the children because:

- Changes in weights and heights in individuals are very small at this age.
- The work of processing the data is too much.

- *Iodine deficiency disorder.* Check for goitre. If many children have goitre, give iodine to everyone (see Section 21.8).

- *Vitamin A deficiency.* Ask about night blindness, especially among adolescents. If present, give advice about vitamin A rich foods.

Other ways to help students' health and nutrition

- Treating common worms (see Section 16.13).
- Referring students who pass blood in the urine or stools to a health centre for tests and treatment for *schistosomiasis*.
- Giving 'first aid' treatment for minor illnesses, such as diarrhoea, and for minor injuries such as cuts.
- Teaching children to brush their teeth thoroughly every day from an early age—starting in pre-primary school if possible.
- Advising children to avoid sweet sticky foods, and poor value snacks, and to eat good mixed meals.
- Giving advice to secondary school girls and boys on how to prevent girls becoming pregnant. Adolescent mothers and their babies are at high risk of under-nutrition.

Checking cleanness of school meals and the school environment

To help to prevent diarrhoea and other infections carried by food and water, check the cleanness of:

- the food;
- the utensils used for the food;
- the hands and clothes of kitchen workers who prepare food;
- the kitchen where food is produced;
- the water supply;
- the school toilets;
- the school compound and waste disposal system.

Ask the environmental health officer to help. He may be able to check school meals and the environment in the same way that he checks eating houses. Or he may be able to provide a checklist of points to look for—for example, whether food is kept off the ground, and if it is covered.

Checking food from food sellers

School staff should check the type, quality, and cleanness of foods that are sold near the school. Try to encourage sellers to sell nutritious foods that are good value for money, and to prepare and keep the foods cleanly. Encourage children to buy good value foods. You can discuss with community workers, parents, and teachers which foods to encourage children to buy so that they get the same advice from everyone.

30.5 SCHOOL FOOD PRODUCTION

Many schools have gardens. Some have farms, fish ponds, or livestock, or grow trees for firewood.

The purpose of a school garden may be:

- to help students learn about:
  - food production and the care of soil, trees, animals, and the environment;
  - storing, processing, and marketing of food.
- to produce food, especially fresh vegetables, and sometimes fuel for the school meal.
- to produce food to sell for school funds.
- to provide opportunities for practical work in biology, home science, and some other subjects.
- to be a demonstration garden for the community.

Things which can help to make a school garden successful are:

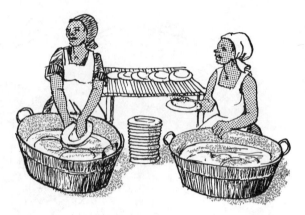

Fig. 30–7 Cleanness is important in school feeding.

- the interest of the teachers, especially the head teacher;
- the involvement of students, teachers, and parents in planning the garden each year;
- help from parents or local people to provide money, labour, seeds, etc.;
- giving groups of students their own plot and allowing them to sell or take home some of the food that they produce;
- fertile soil;
- enough water, tools, seeds, and fencing;
- labour to look after the garden during the holidays;
- a guard to prevent human and animal thieves;
- expert advice from agricultural, livestock, or fisheries extension officers, or from experienced local farmers.

THINGS TO DO

Class exercises

1. Make a diagram like Fig. 30–3 showing the nutrition activities of a local school. Discuss with trainees whether the school should try to introduce other activities and how to do this.

2. Ask each trainee to choose a school subject, such as art, geography, maths, etc. and to make notes on how to include nutrition in a lesson.

Projects

3. Ask trainee health workers to examine a class of primary school children, and to report any signs of poor nutrition.

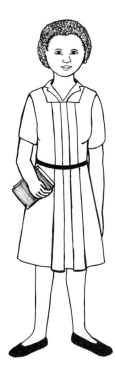

Fig. 30–8 Encourage parents to send girls to school for as long as possible.

a. Ask them to prepare a practical plan for treating these children.

b. Discuss the plan with the students and head teacher.

4. Arrange for nutrition trainees to give a 'talk' or demonstration about nutrition to school children and teachers or their parents. Trainees should assess the content of the talk and the methods used to give it with the teachers or the parents afterwards.

5. If there are Child-to-child programmes in your country get the details. Then ask trainees to examine the activities, evaluate them, and decide if they are useful or if they could be improved. If possible, arrange to visit the programme to see it in action.

Child-to-child nutrition activity sheets are: *Feeding young children: HOW DO WE KNOW IF THEY ARE GETTING ENOUGH TO EAT?* and *Feeding young children: HEALTHY FOOD.* For address see Appendix 6.

Field visit

6. Arrange for trainees to visit a school garden or farm. Observe the crops and foods produced and the methods of production. Discuss the purpose and problems of the garden with the teacher who is responsible. Afterwards discuss the garden, the good things about it, and how to improve it.

USEFUL PUBLICATIONS

Pollitt, E. (1990). *Malnutrition and infection in the classroom.* UNESCO, Paris.

Young, B. and Durston, S. (1987). *Primary health education.* Longman, Harlow, Essex.

31 Training for nutrition

There are many topics in nutrition that you may want to train people about, for example, growth monitoring, breastfeeding, and iodine deficiency.

There are many different sorts of people whom you may want to train, for example, community health workers, nurses, teachers, community leaders, and women's groups.

You may help with basic training. You may give in-service training courses or workshops about a particular topic to groups such as health or nutrition workers. You may train people 'on-the-job'—for example, kitchen workers.

But whoever you are teaching and whatever you teach them about, you need to *plan* and *evaluate* the training. We give only a short description of what to do, and a few ideas. For more information, look at the books listed at the end of the chapter.

31.1 PLANNING AND EVALUATING TRAINING

The purpose of training is to help trainees to do their work well.

When you plan *what* you teach, include only what trainees need for the tasks that they have to do in their work. Leave out things that are not useful, even if they may be interesting to know.

When you plan *how* you train, use methods which help trainees to learn well. This improves their attitude to their work and the way in which they communicate

and teach others. Both what and how you teach depend on the education and experience of the trainees, and on the particular job that they do.

Box 31.1 lists nine steps in training. But you probably will not complete the steps in this exact order. As you plan, you go backwards and forwards several times.

31.2 STEPS IN NUTRITION TRAINING

Step 1. What task are you training them to do?

Describe what task trainees must be able to do after training. For example:

- prevent and treat vitamin A deficiency in a community; *or*
- help mothers to prepare energy- and nutrient-rich porridges; *or*
- support breastfeeding; *or*
- help a community to start a growth monitoring programme.

Step 2. What do trainees need to learn in order to do the task?

Describe the knowledge, attitude, and skills that they need.

Box 31.1.   Steps in nutrition training

1. What task are you training them to do?
2. What do trainees need to learn in order to do the task—*learning objectives*?
3. How are you going to train them—*training methods and learning aids*?
4. How will you know if trainees have learned what is necessary—*assessment*?
5. What will trainees learn in each *lesson*?
6. What will the *timetable* be?
7. What *resources* do you need for training?
8. Did the trainees find the course useful?
9. Was the training effective—*evaluation*?

Knowledge

For example:

- Know the dangers of vitamin A deficiency.
- Know which local foods are rich in vitamin A, their costs, and how they are used.
- Know how a family could grow more of them.

Attitude

For example:

- Have a caring attitude towards undernourished children and their families.
- Understand and respect the reasons why it may be difficult for families to give their children more foods with vitamin A.

Skills

- *Manual* skills, for example how to:
  - examine a child and recognize signs of VAD;
  - prepare a child's meal using vitamin A rich foods.
- *Decision making* skills, for example how to:
  - decide the correct treatment for a child with VAD;
- *Communication* skills, for example how to:
  - discuss with parents how they can give a child more foods which contain vitamin A;
  - explain why a child needs vitamin A capsules.

We call the list of knowledge, attitudes, and skills that a trainee must learn *'learning objectives'*.

Step 3. How are you going to train them?

Choose *training methods* for each learning objective. Include plenty of active learning and discussion, to keep people alert and interested (see Section 31.4). Decide what *learning aids* you need.

Examples of ways trainees can learn include:

- To recognize VAD, look at photographs of children with VAD.
- To learn to examine eyes, practise examining eyes of colleagues, or children in a health centre.
- To learn to cook foods with vitamin A, help to cook appropriate foods.
- To learn how to counsel families about feeding young children, role play counselling.

Step 4. How will you know if trainees have learnt what is necessary?

Decide how you will assess their knowledge, attitudes, and skills. For example:

- Trainee can recognize Bitot's spots and corneal xerosis in a colour photograph.
- Trainee can list four local vitamin A rich foods and can demonstrate how to use them in children's meals.
- Through role play, trainee can demonstrate correct counselling techniques.
- Trainee prescribes correct treatment when given case histories of children with xerophthalmia.

Step 5. What will trainees learn in each lesson?

When you know what trainees need to learn, and how you will train them, you can decide how you will arrange the training period.

Example

Day 1, Lesson 1.

Objective. At the end of the period trainees will be able to:

- describe the dangers of VAD;
- recognize the eye signs of VAD.

Content	Method	Aids
Dangers of Vitamin A deficiency	Story/case study Show pictures of blind children Ask trainees to give examples they know	Pictures
Signs of xerophthalmia	Show and explain photos of xerophthalmia Practise looking at each other's normal eyes Trainees diagnose cases in photos	Photos of cases (or slides)

Activities to assess learning:

- Trainees demonstrate how to look at a person's eye.
- Trainees correctly recognize signs of xerophthalmia on photos or drawings.

Step 6. What will the timetable be?

Plan the course to include all the learning objectives, in a sensible order, with enough breaks and free time.

Make sure that there is a balance of classroom and practical work. It may be best to have lectures and difficult new material early in the day, and practical activities later.

Give trainees a copy of the timetable and try to keep to it (see Box 31.2).

Step 7. What resources do you need for the training?

Make a list of the resources that you need; which you already have; and which you need to get, if possible. For example:

- *Time*. 2 days teaching.
- *Funds*. Funds for meals for trainees and trainers and for foods for demonstration and for stationery.
- *Transport*. No transport needed.
- *Trainers*. Nutritionist and clinical officer or doctor.
- *Place*. School classroom.
- *Equipment*. Chalkboard, notice board, cooking utensils.
- *Supplies*. Paper and pens, scissors, tape, chalk.
- *Learning aids*. Photographs of blind children and signs of xerophthalmia; vitamin A capsules; handout sheet of vitamin A doses.

Step 8. Did the trainees find the course useful?

Decide how you will evaluate the course, and find out how you could do it better next time. For example:

- Ask trainees to fill in a questionnaire about each lesson. It is usually best to ask them to fill in the section for a lesson immediately afterwards—if they do it later, they may not remember.
- Ask trainees to discuss the lessons with each other and for a spokesperson to report the findings.
- Talk to trainees at the end of each day and ask them how they found it, what else they would like to know, what ideas they have to make it better.

Step 9. Was the training effective?

Follow up trainees, to find out if the training helps them in their work, and if they are using what they learned. If not, why not? Do they need further training? For example:

- Visit trainees at work, and talk to them and their supervisors and the community leaders whom they work with.

- Ask them to show you how they examine a child's eye, and how they counsel a family. Observe how they give a capsule of vitamin A to a child.
- Ask them if they see children with xerophthalmia, how they diagnose it, and what they do.

31.3 RELATING TRAINING TO TRAINEES' NEEDS

When you train people, try to find out *what they already know* and can do and *what they want to learn*. This sounds obvious, but it is not always easy.

Ask trainees before the training

You can visit trainees, or their supervisors, before the training and talk to them about their needs. But they may think that they know about a subject already—for example, breastfeeding or growth monitoring. It is only when they start training that they realize how much there is to learn.

Pre-test and post-test

Sometimes it helps to have a short 'pre-test' at the beginning of a course. You can ask about 20 key questions, to be answered with a simple 'yes' or 'no'. To avoid embarrassment, trainees need not write their names on the papers. They can have a number instead. (At some time you must go through the questions and make sure that everybody knows the right answers.)

Examples

Pale cabbage is a good source of vitamin A.	Yes/No
All babies need glucose water as well as breast milk.	Yes/No
The tongue is a good place to look for paleness due to anaemia.	Yes/No

---

The answers tell you what topics you need to spend time on.

You can repeat the same questions at the end of a course, as part of your evaluation. If most people have the same incorrect ideas at the end of the course as they did at the beginning, then your teaching on that point has not been effective. Try to find out why.

Ask trainees to demonstrate skills

Ask trainees to demonstrate a task. This tells you if they know how to do it correctly or not. For example, ask them to weigh a child; or to role play counselling a mother.

Box 31.2. Example of a programme for a 2-day course on prevention and treatment of vitamin A deficiency

	Content	Method
Day 1		
Lesson 1	Dangers of VAD	Lecture, discussion, pictures
	Signs of xerophthalmia	Photos or slides
Lesson 2	How to examine children's eyes	Demonstration; trainees practise with each other

– – – – – – T E A   B R E A K – – – – – –

| Lesson 3 | Foods which contain vitamin A | Lecture and food demonstration |

– – – – – – M I D D A Y   M E A L – – – – – –

Lesson 4	What Vitamin A foods children eat	Visit health facility
	Examining children's eyes (practical)	1. Ask mothers how often children eat foods with vitamin A.
		2. Practise looking at children's eyes (see VAD in ward if available).
Lesson 5	Availability and cost of Vitamin A foods	Visit market—buy foods to cook on Day 2

– – – – – – T E A   B R E A K – – – – – –

Discussion of visit to hospital and market. Groups display vegetables bought with their prices.

Day 2		
Lesson 1	High-dose vitamin A preparations	Lecture; handout sheet
Lesson 2	How to give a capsule	Demonstration and practice cutting a capsule

– – – – – – T E A   B R E A K – – – – – –

| Lesson 3 | How to feed vitamin A foods to children | Trainees participate in cooking foods. |
| | | Cook the foods bought on Day 1. |

– – – – – – M I D D A Y   M E A L – – – – – –

| Lesson 4 | Counselling families about feeding young children | Role play and discussion |
| Lesson 5 | Course evaluation | Discussion about questionnaire filled in after each lesson. |

It is important not to embarrass them, or tell them if they do something wrong. Praise them for the parts of the task that they do right. But during your training, make sure that they learn to do the task correctly. Give extra time to the parts that they had a problem with.

Feedback during training

Many trainees cannot say what they want to learn before training begins. But they may develop plenty of ideas during the training, both before and after you cover a topic. Some trainers find that just after the midday meal is a good time to get ideas for the next day. It also helps if you keep plenty of time for questions and discussion during the teaching, and if you are available to answer questions during breaks.

Be ready to make time for a topic that you did not plan to do, if trainees want it and if it is relevant.

31.4 TRAINING METHODS AND LEARNING AIDS

Which training methods and learning aids you use depends on whether you are helping trainees to learn facts, attitudes, or skills. Also different methods are suitable for different types of trainees. For example, some trainees enjoy singing and dancing or role play, while others do not.

The 'Things to do' sections of this book give many ideas for training in different topics.

Lectures

Lectures help trainees to learn facts—for example, what is anaemia, and what causes it. But a lecture should not be too long—people may stop learning after about 15–20 minutes.

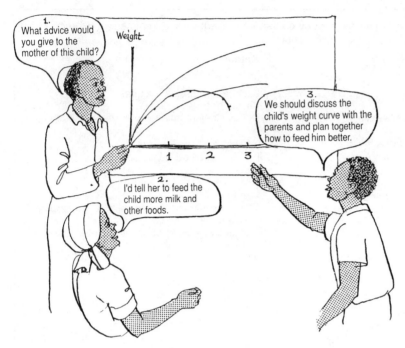

Fig. 31–1 Lectures are more interesting if they are active with questions and discussion.

Always have some sort of learning aid, such as a picture or story or demonstration for a talk or lecture. Lectures are more interesting if they are active—for example, with discussions, and questions. Ask trainees to discuss a question with their neighbour for a minute or two. Ask trainees what they think the learning aid shows.

Pictures, diagrams, and charts

Pictures, diagrams, and charts are useful to:

- give facts and help people remember them;
- summarize information, and emphasize main points;
- explain something complicated (such as the life cycle of a worm);
- explain something you cannot see (such as digestion or the amount of fat in food);
- show a sequence—such as the spread of diarrhoea by poor food handling;
- help people to understand ideas—such as the cycle of undernutrition and infection;
- show differences—such as between the colour of a normal and an anaemic tongue;
- show a problem—for example, a photograph of vegetables in a garden eaten by pests;
- show mistakes—for trainees to point out;

- show a situation for trainees to discuss (including *problem posing*—see Section 26.11).

You can use photographs, drawings, something from a newspaper, a formula advertisement, a poster.

Real objects

Real objects are often the best learning aids. For example, food, a feeding bottle, growth charts showing children's growth lines (make copies at a health centre).

Slides and transparencies

If you have a projector, show slides. These are an important way to show people what things look like when you cannot easily show the real thing, and drawings are not clear enough—for example, soil erosion, cretinism, or a child with kwashiorkor and the same child after treatment. You can sometimes use photographs in the same way.

If you have an overhead projector, show transparencies (acetates). You can draw simple pictures, or trace or copy pictures from books, or you can make charts or diagrams. Keep them clear and simple. If you put words on them, they should be few. Do not write detailed notes which are too small for people to read. Look at them from the back of the room before the lecture to make sure that people can read them.

Videos and films

If you can show videos or films, these can teach facts and demonstrate attitudes; they can show people what things look like and how to do things. But the audience is not active. It is important to follow up a video with discussion and practical work.

Demonstrations

Demonstrations help trainees to learn skills—for example, how to examine a person for anaemia or how to cook enriched porridge. Demonstrate and explain each stage of the task. The trainees then practise the task, while the trainer helps and corrects. Then trainees repeat the task until they do it correctly.

Group discussions

Group discussions can help to change attitudes. They also help trainees to learn decision-making and communication skills. Discussion in small groups of five to eight gives everyone a chance to say something.

Give the group a question or a case history or a nutrition problem to discuss, or a plan to make or ask them to write a story or a song. For example, ask a group:

- to list traditional practices for feeding babies;
- to divide the practices into 'helpful', 'harmless', and 'harmful'.
- to discuss what they would try to do about each type of practice, and how they would do it.

Role play

What role play is. A few trainees each pretend to be someone (such as a mother, father, child, relative, neighbour, nutrition worker) in a particular situation (such as the child becoming sick and undernourished and the mother deciding what to do, or the nutrition worker visiting the family and counselling them). The players act out what those people in that situation would do. There is no prepared script, or planned story, as there is with drama. If trainees have not done role play before, the trainer may need to demonstrate it first.

Uses of role play. Role play helps people to change attitudes. It can help people to learn communication skills, for example, how to counsel families, or how to work with community groups. Role play can be used to present a problem situation—such as a wife not having enough money to buy food for the family. An important part of the learning is the discussion after the role play.

Practical exercises

Practical exercises help trainees to learn skills and facts and to solve problems. For example:

- weighing and examining children;
- practising filling in and interpreting growth charts;
- making weaning foods;
- collecting information about the cost of foods or about the weights of children, and helping to analyse it.

Case studies

Case studies help trainees to learn to solve problems. You can write several case studies on cards—for example, one of the stories in this book or some that you know about.

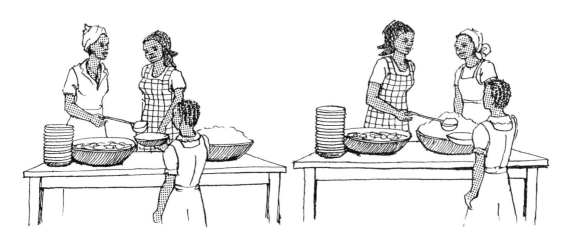

Fig. 31–2 Show a trainee how to do a task, and then let her practise the task.

Trainees take a card and discuss it and suggest solutions which they discuss with the trainer. When they have finished one case, they pass the card on to the next group and take another.

Trainees can also use case studies to practise counselling in pairs or small groups by role play.

Field visits

Field visits help trainees to change attitudes and link what they learn to real life. For example, a 'home visit' to a family or a visit to home gardens, or markets, or to a health centre or hospital to see well and undernourished children.

It is important to discuss before the visit what the purpose is, and what the trainees should do and observe. After the visit, trainees discuss in class what they learned, and how they felt about the people they visited.

Projects and surveys

In some longer courses, trainees may be able to do larger projects, individually, or in pairs or groups. For example:

- Follow up an underweight child and the family for several weeks or months. Even two visits can be very informative.
- Find out how many underweight children there are in a village or block.
- Help to start a vegetable garden at a school or clinic.

Competitions and quizzes

This is a way to reinforce what trainees have learned. For example, divide trainees into two teams. Ask the teams questions in turn. Correct wrong answers and repeat correct ones, explaining them more if necessary.

Score points for right answers. At the end of the quiz, clap the winners.

Preparing learning aids

This is another way to reinforce what trainees have learned. For example, ask students to prepare a chart or a picture showing how much vegetable to add to children's food; or to prepare some foods for a demonstration. However, this is only helpful if the trainer supervises it well.

Handouts

Trainees appreciate handouts which summarize technical points in a lecture or other teaching session, or examples of growth charts, newsletters, photocopies, or other relevant material.

However, handout sheets of lecture notes easily get lost, or muddled, and may not be effectively used or referred to again. It is much better if possible to give trainees an appropriate book which they can refer to during and after the course.

THINGS TO DO

Class exercises

1. Give trainees a list of topics in nutrition that could be the topic for one lesson. Ask them to write the *objective*, *content*, *method*, and *learning aids* that they would use for that lesson. For example:

   a. 'The dangers of bottle feeding.'

   b. 'The symptoms of anaemia in women.'

   c. 'How to enrich a child's porridge.'

Box 31.3.   Hints on how to make training successful

Trainees learn better when:

- Trainers ask for and respect their opinions.
- Training starts from what they know and uses their experience.
- Trainers explain things clearly and in a sensible order.
- Trainees are actively involved in the learning, such as practical tasks, demonstrations, role play, and discussions.
- Trainers use a variety of teaching methods, and there are not too many lectures.
- Trainees see that what they are learning is useful for their work.
- Trainers give immediate feedback—that is, they tell trainees immediately how well they performed on a skill or a test.
- Trainers praise them when they learn a new skill correctly.

d. 'How to visit the family of an undernourished child.'

e. 'Advising families about good and poor value foods.'

2. Ask trainees to choose a topic in nutrition, and to pre-pare pictures, diagrams, or charts which they could use as learning aids to teach the subject. They should be able to say in what way the learning aid would help the trainees—see the list in Section 31.4.

3. Ask trainees to choose a nutrition topic that is import-ant in their area, and a group whom they think it would be useful to train about the topic. Ask them to work through the 'Steps in nutrition training' and to plan how they would train the group.

Make sure that the trainees do not choose too big a topic for the exercise—for example, 'Undernutrition in children' is a very large topic. 'Use of growth charts' might be more appropriate.

USEFUL PUBLICATIONS

Abbatt, F. and MacMahon, R. (1985). *Teaching health care workers.* Macmillan, Basingstoke.

Programme for International Training in Health (1987). *Teaching and learning with visual aids.* Macmillan, Basingstoke.

WHO (1986). *Guidelines for training community health workers in nutrition.* WHO, Geneva.

Appendix 1 Food composition tables

We prepared these food composition tables from the references given below. These are listed in the order of priority in which they were used.

We used values which we considered most accurate but suggest you use local data to supplement or check these values if you can. This is because the nutrient content of food (especially vitamin A and C content) varies according to the variety of the food, and methods of production, handling, processing, and cooking. The composition of foods can also vary because different laboratories estimate nutrient content in different ways.

Codes used in the tables

a. West, C. E., Pepping, F., and Temalilwa, C. R. (1988). *Composition of foods commonly eaten in East Africa.* Department of Human Nutrition, Wageningen Agricultural University, De Driejen 12, 6703 BC Wageningen, Netherlands.

b. FAO (1972). *Food composition tables for use in East Asia.* FAO, Rome.

c. Latham, M. C. (1979). *Human nutrition in tropical Africa.* FAO, Rome.

d. Onwueme, I. C. (1982). *Tropical tuber crops.* Wiley, Chichester.

e. FAO (1989). *Utilization of tropical foods,* Food and Nutrition Paper, no. 47. FAO, Rome.

f. FAO (1984). *Food, nutrition and agriculture tex:book.* FAO, Rome.

g. FAO (in press). *Food and nutrition in management of group feeding programmes,* Food and Nutrition Paper, no. 23. FAO, Rome.

h. WHO (1979). *Health aspects of food and nutrition* (3rd edn). Manila.

i. International Institute for Tropical Agriculture (1989). *Food crops utilization and nutrition—a training manual.* IITA, Ibadan, Nigeria.

j. Manufacturers data.

k. Casey, C. E. and Hambridge, K. M. (1983). In *Lactation: physiology, nutrition and breastfeeding* (ed. M. C. Neville and M. R. Neifert). Plenum Press, New York.

l. Guthrie, H. (1975). *Introductory nutrition.* Mosby & Co., St Louis, Missouri.

m. Holland, B., Welch, A., Unwin I. D., Buss, D. H., Paul, A. A., Southgate, D. A. T. (1991). *McCance and Widdowson's The Composition of Foods* (5th edn). Royal Society of Chemistry and Ministry of Agriculture, Fisheries and Food, Cambridge, UK.

calc Calculated from other values.

The following codes are also used: —, trace; ?, value unknown; ( ), value for sugar plus starch as separate values not found (e.g. 100 g breadfruit contains a total of 23 g of sugar and starch).

1 gram = 1000 mg = 1 000 000 µg;   1000 g = 1 kg.

Table A1.1. Approximate composition of raw foods

Food	% EP	Water (g)	Energy (kcal)	Protein (g)	Fat (g)	Sugar (g)	Starch (g)	Fibre (g)	Iron (mg)	Vit A (RE)	Folate (µg)	Vit C (mg)	References
Dry cereals													
Maize—white													
fresh on cob	70	58	165	5.0	2.1	2.0	32	0.8	3.6	0	?	0	a
flour, wholegrain	100	12	345	10.0	4.5	–	67	1.9	2.5	0	?	0	a
flour, refined, 60–80% extraction	100	12	335	8.0	1.0	3.0	74	0.6	1.1	0	?	0	a
Maize—yellow													
flour, wholegrain	100	12	340	9.3	3.8	5.0	74	1.9	4.2	54	?	3	a, i
Millet—finger, flour	100	13	320	5.6	1.4	0	75	2.6	5.0	4	?	0	a, e
bullrush, flour	100	16	335	11.0	3.5	0	69	2.0	3.0	?	?	0	a, e
Rice polished	100	12	335	7.0	0.5	0	80	0.1	1.0	0	29	0	a, e
parboiled	100	14	335	7.0	0.8	0	80	0.1	1.7	0	29	0	a, e
Sorghum flour, wholegrain	100	11	335	9.5	2.8	1.0	73	2.1	4.5	3	?	0	a, e
Wheat flour, white, 85% extraction	100	12	340	11.0	2.0	2.0	72	0.8	3.6	0	51	0	a
bread, white	100	37	240	7.7	2.0	4.0	47	3.0	1.7	0	28	0	a, j
bread, brown	100	38	235	7.7	2.0	3.0	47	5.0	2.2	0	37	0	a, j
Pasta	100	12	342	12.0	1.8	0	(74)	5.0	2.1	0	34	0	g, m
Chappati (made with fat)	100	29	328	8.1	12.8		(48)	3.7	2.3	0	15	0	m
Starchy roots and fruits													
Breadfruit	66	73	96	1.3	0.3	(23)		1.3	0.7	3	?	12	b
Cassava, fresh	74	60	140	1.2	0.2	5.0	30	1.1	1.0	5	24	31	a, d
dried or flour	100	13	342	1.6	0.5	13.0	69	1.7	2.0	0	?	4	a, d
Cocoyam/taro fresh	84	65	133	1.8	0.3	2.0	21	1.0	2.0	0	?	8	a, d
Plantain/Cooking banana	66	65	130	1.2	0.3	7.0	25	0.5	1.2	0	22	6	a, d, m
Gari	100	13	351	1.0	1.1	(95)		1.9	1.3	130	16	20	a, i
Potato, fresh-round (Irish)	86	78	75	1.7	0.1	1.0	17	0.6	1.1	3	14	21	a, i
sweet	79	69	121	1.6	0.2	3.0	25	1.0	2.0	300*	52	37	a, d
Yam, fresh	84	69	110	1.9	0.2	0.6	27	0.8	0.8	4	?	17	a, d, g
flour	100	14	335	3.4	0.4	0	78	1.6	1.1	0	–	0	a
Dried legumes (seeds)													
Bambara nuts	75	10	345	19.0	6.2	(61)		4.8	12.0	2	?	0	a
Beans, kidney	100	12	320	22.0	1.5	1.0	56	4.4	8.2	3	180	1	a, e
Chickpeas	100	10	325	20.0	3.7	11.0	46	6.7	5.5	11	180	8	a, m
Cowpeas	100	11	320	23.0	1.4	7.0	50	4.8	5.0	3	439	2	a
Groundnuts	70	7	570	25.0	45.0	(23)		2.9	3.8	3	110	1	a, e

In 100 g edible portion of food

Table A1.1. (*contd.*)

	%	Water (g)	Energy (kcal)	Protein (g)	Fat (g)	Sugar (g)	Starch (g)	Fibre (g)	Iron (mg)	Vit A (RE)	Folate (µg)	Vit C (mg)	References
Food	EP												
Dried legumes (seeds) contd.													
Lentils	100	10	325	25.0	1.2	3.0	54	3.9	7.0	10	35	0	a, e
Mungbean	100	10	340	24.0	1.1	2.0	53	4.9	8.9	19	120	5	a, e
Peas	100	11	320	22.0	1.1	3.0	53	5.7	10.0	27	33	0	a, calc
Pigeon peas	100	10	322	20.0	1.3	7.0	51	7.3	5.0	9	100	0	a
Soybeans	100	11	405	38.0	20.0	0	29	4.7	6.1	9	210	0	a, e
Oil seeds													
Coconut, immature fresh	16	68	190	2.0	17.0	?	?	3.7	1.8	0	14	8	a
mature flesh, fresh	48	43	390	3.6	39.0	(35)		6.6	2.5	4	26	2	a
dried	100	2	735	6.0	70.0	(20)		21.0	3.6	0	9	0	e, m
water	100	96	14	0.2	–	(3)		–	–	0	?	–	c, h
milk/cream	100	54	320	5.0	35.0	(6)		?	2.0	0	?	–	h
Melon seeds	75	6	595	26.0	50.0	(15)		4.0	7.4	0	?	–	a
Sesame seeds	100	6	592	20.0	50.0	(22)		4.1	8.1	0	97	2	c, m
Sunflower seeds	50	6	486	13.0	27.7	(51)		2.6	7.6	0	?	0	a, c
Vegetables—fresh unless described differently													
Bean, fresh seeds	100	89	35	2.5	0.2	4.4	2	1.8	1.8	27	36	25	a
Carrots	74	89	35	0.9	0.1	8.2	0	1.4	0.7	1088	8	8	a
Eggplant	78	90	30	1.0	0.2	6.0	0	1.3	1.3	6	29	9	a
Leaves													
pale green	63	91	26	1.7	0.1	4.8	0	1.2	0.7	16	79	54	a
medium green	80	92	25	1.8	0.2	(3)		0.9	1.8	300	50	41	a
dark green	80	80	58	4.5	0.3	(7)		2.0	7.2	550	105	80	a
amaranthus	76	84	45	4.6	0.2	0	7	1.8	8.9	383	85	50	a
baobab	82	77	67	3.8	0.3	(13)		2.8	1.1	?	?	52	a
cabbage	85	79	19	1.4	0.2	(3)		0.7	0.7	64	75	39	b, m
cassava	80	80	50	6.0	1.0	(7)		4.0	7.6	500	?	?310	a, b
cowpea, fresh	95	85	45	4.7	0.3	1.3	5	2.0	5.7	117	135	56	a
dried	100	10	270	28.0	1.8	7.8	30	12.0	35.0	600	690	290	a, calc
pumpkin	77	89	25	4.0	0.2	0.5	2	2.4	0.8	167	?	80	a
sweet potato	80	83	49	4.6	0.2	–	–	2.4	6.2	510	?	70	a
Okra pods	81	89	35	2.1	0.2	(7)		1.7	1.2	32	23	47	a
Onion	94	88	38	1.2	0.1	7.0	2	1.0	0.8	0	14	11	a
Pepper, sweet, green/red	86	86	44	2.0	0.8	7.7	0	2.6	2.6	290/458	24	140	a, c, e
Pumpkin/Squash fruit	77	93	23	1.0	0.1	2.0	3	0.8	1.4	292	8	8	a
Tomato	96	94	22	1.0	0.2	3.0	1	0.6	0.6	74	28	26	a

In 100 g edible portion of food

Table A1.1. *(contd.)*

Food	% EP	Water (g)	Energy (kcal)	Protein (g)	Fat (g)	Sugar (g)	Starch (g)	Fibre (g)	Iron (mg)	Vit A (RE)	Folate (µg)	Vit C (mg)	References
Ripe fruit—fresh unless described differently													
Avocado	50	80	120	1.4	11.0	3.0	1	1.8	1.4	88	22	18	a
Baobab	28	16	280	2.2	0.8	(67)		6.8	7.4	13	?	270	a
Banana	63	77	82	1.5	0.1	17.0	3	0.9	1.4	20	19	9	a
Dates, dried	83	17	295	2.7	0.6	70.0	4	3.9	2.0	5	20	0	a
Guava	81	82	46	1.1	0.4	(5)		5.3	1.3	48	7	325	a
Lemon/lime	59	90	40	0.6	0.8	5.0	3	0.7	0.7	2	10	45	a, g
Mango	72	83	60	0.6	0.2	13.0	2	0.9	1.2	400	7	42	a
Orange/tangerine	75	88	44	0.6	0.4	9.0	1	0.6	0.1	122	37	46	a
Pawpaw	74	91	30	0.4	0.1	6.4	1	0.9	0.6	200	1	52	a, g
Pineapple	55	87	48	0.4	0.1	12.0	0	0.5	0.4	15	11	34	a
Water melon	50	94	22	0.5	0.1	5.1	0	0.4	0.3	42	3	8	a
Sugars													
Honey	100	23	286	0.4	0	76.0	0	0	0.4	0	0	0	f
Jam	100	29	234	0.4	0	69.0	0	–	0.3	–	0	10	f
Sugar, refined white	100	0	400	0	0	100.0	0	0	0	0	0	0	a
cane juice	45	82	54	0.6	0.1	13.0	0	0	2.0	0	0	0	a, c, f
Milk													
Breast milk, mature	100	88	70	0.9	4.2	7.3	0	0	0.04	47	5.2	4	k, m
colostrum	100	87	58	2.3	2.9	5.3	0	0	0.045	89	2	4.4	k, m
Cheese, hard	100	39	384	24.0	32.0	–	0	0	0.5	332	40	–	c, j
Cow's milk, whole fresh	100	87	66	3.5	3.7	4.9	0	0	0.05	52	5	1	k, b
dried	100	4	465	26.0	28.0	38.0	0	0	0.5	288	37	0	a, g, c
skimmed fresh	100	90	38	3.5	0.8	4.4	0	0	0.1	0	6	0	a
dried	100	4	355	36.0	0.8	51.0	0	0	1.0	1500†	50	0	a, g
whole soured	100	87	66	3.5	3.7	4.9	0	0	0.05	52	5	1	calc.
evaporated canned	100	74	140	7.0	8.0	10.0	0	0	0.2	77	8	2	c, g
condensed sweetened canned	100	29	317	7.3	8.0	54.0	0	0	0.2	84	11	2	c, g
Goat's milk, fresh	100	84	84	3.4	4.9	7.0	0	0	0.1	25	?	1	a, c

Table A1.1. *(contd.)*

Food	% EP	Water (g)	Energy (kcal)	Protein (g)	Fat (g)	Sugar (g)	Starch (g)	Fibre (g)	Iron (mg)	Vit A (RE)	Folate (µg)	Vit C (mg)	References
Meat, poultry, and eggs													
Meat without fat—beef, sheep goat, pig, wild animals	100	68	115	22.0	1.9	0	0	0	4.6	–	15	0	g, c
Fat from meat	100	6	846	0	94.0	0	0	0	0	0	0	0	g
Meat with some fat	100	63	235	18.0	18.0	0	0	0	3.6	25	7	0	a
Blood	100	78	80	17.8	0.1	0	0	0	44.0?	21	1	0	g, b
Liver	100	70	135	19.0	4.7	5.0	0	0	10.0	1500*	250	15	a, g
Chicken/Poultry	67	72	140	20.0	6.5	0	0	0	1.1	85	8	0	a, m
Egg—chicken	88	75	140	12.0	10.0	0	0	0	2.0	200	25	0	a
Termites, fresh	100	45	340	20.0	28.0	4.5	0	0	1.0	0	?	?	a
Caterpillars, dried	100	9	390	53.0	15.0	(12)	0	0	2.3	?	?	3	a
Fish and seafood													
Fish flesh, fresh													
fresh water	60	75	115	22.0	3.0	0	0	0	1.7	0	12	0	a, g
sea water	60	81	73	17.0	0.5	0	0	0	1.5	28	12	–	c, m
Fish, dried, large	Varies	14	255	47.0	7.4	0	0	0	4.9	0	?	0	a
small	100	20	320	44.0	16.0	0	0	0	8.5	?	?	0	a
Fish, dried, salted, large (cod)	Varies	32	248	54.5	1.7	0	0	0	2.8	0	?	0	a, b, g
Prawns & shellfish, fresh	Varies	77	94	18.0	1.5	(2)	0	0	1.6	108	65	0	a, c
Sardines canned in oil	100	50	309	20.0	25.0	0	0	0	2.7	58	16	0	c, g
Drinks and liquids													
Beer, commercial (3.9% alcohol)	100	92	30	0.9	0	0	0	0	0.1	0	?	0	h, j
local (3.5% alcohol)	100	90	25	0.2	–	3.0	?	0	0.3	0	–	0	a
Sodas	100	87	45	0	0	12.0	0	0	0	0	0	0	a
Oils and fats													
Animal fat/Lard	100	1	890	0	99.0	0	0	0	0	0	0	0	a, g
Butter	100	21	700	0	77.0	2	0	0	0	731	–	0	a
Cooking fat	100	?	890	0	99.0	0	0	0	0	0	0	0	calc.
Ghee, animal	100	–	898	0	99.8	–	0	0	0.2	760	0	0	m
vegetable	100	–	898	0	99.8	–	0	0	–	680†	0	0	m
Margarine	100	15	745	0	83.0	0	0	0	0	680†	–	0	a
Red palm oil, fresh	100	1	890	0	99.0	0	0	0	0	5000*	0	0	a
old	100	1	890	0	99.0	0	0	0	0	2400*	0	0	a
Vegetable oil	100	0	900	0	100.0	0	0	0	0	0	0	0	a

In 100g edible portion of food

Table A1.1. (*contd.*)

Food	% EP	Water (g)	Energy (kcal)	Protein (g)	Fat (g)	Sugar (g)	Starch (g)	Fibre (g)	Iron (mg)	Vit A (RE)	Folate (µg)	Vit C (mg)	References
Manufactured/commercial foods													
Baby cereals—various	100	–	377	16.0	5.0	30.0	37	?	20.0	750	75	50	j
Baby 'meals' canned/bottled	100	–	380	16.0	7.0	10.0	46	?	20.0	750	75	50	j
Biscuits plain	100	8	407	9.0	7.8	(74)		?	1.5	0	13	0	a, j, m
Doughnut/Mandazi	100	24	390	3.1	18.8	(50)		?	1.2	–	–	0	l
Potato crisps	100	93	36	3.5	1.5	(2)		?	0.6	0	19	0	e, m
Soymilk	100	–	385	0	0	99.5	0	0	0.2	0	0	0	b, h
Sweets/Candy	100	2	546	5.6	37.6	(49)		10.7	1.8	0	40	27	m
Food aid foods													
Bulgur wheat	100	10	354	11.2	1.5	(80)		?	7.8	0	38	0	g
Corn soy blend/Wheat soy blend	100	9	360	20.0	6.0	(60)		?	20.0	500	?	40	g
Corn soy milk/Wheat soy milk	100	9	380	20.0	6.0	(62)		?	18.0	510	200	40	g
High protein biscuits	100	?	450	20.0	20.0	?	?	?	25.0	0	?	63	g
Rolled oats	100	10	363	13.0	7.0	?	?	?	4.0	0	24	0	g
Soy-fortified cornmeal	100	10	392	13.0	1.5	(72)		?	4.8	228	?	0	g
Soy-fortified wheat flour	100	10	355	14.0	1.2	(70)		?	?	0	?	0	g

RE Micrograms retinol equivalents (see Section 4.2)
* Vitamin A content varies.
† If fortified with Vitamin A.
‡ Nutrient content varies with method of preparation.

Table A1.2. Approximate composition of cooked foods (see Table A4.5 for cooking conversion factors)

Cooked food*	In 100 g edible portion of food						Reference
	Water (g)	Energy (kcal)	Protein (g)	Iron (mg)	Vit A‡ (RE)	Vit C‡ (mg)	
Maize, stiff porridge	75	100	2.3	0.3	0	0	calc
thin porridge	87	50	1.4	0.2	0	0	calc
Rice, polished boiled	70	123	2.8	0.3	0	0	g, calc
parboiled boiled	65	134	2.8	0.7	0	0	calc
Pasta, boiled	66	134	4.7	1.2	0	0	calc
Cassava, fresh boiled	60	140	1.2	1.5	–	0	calc
Gari (fermented, dried pounded cassava), boiled	70	121	0.3	?	0	0	i, calc
Plantain, cooked	70	111	0.8	0.9	110	12	f, calc
Potato—round, boiled	78	75	1.7	1.7	–	16	g, calc
fried/chips	47	250–562§	3.8	0.9	0	15	m
—sweet, boiled	69	121	1.6	2.9	440	28	calc
Beans/peas, boiled	65	128	8.8	3.3	–	0	g, calc
Groundnuts, boiled	49	314	13.8	2.1	–	0	calc
roasted	4	585	25.6	?	0	0	g, calc
Soybean, boiled	51	223	20.9	3.4	–	0	calc
Medium green leaves, boiled and drained	48	160	11.5	?	1000	58	calc
Cabbage, boiled	93	23	1.6	?	40	40	b, calc
Chicken, boiled (%EP=67)	61	203	26.0	1.5	110	0	f, calc
Fish, boiled or steamed (%EP=52)	74	118	20.0	1.8	–	0	f, calc

* Percentage edible portion (%EP) = 100 unless stated otherwise.
calc. = Calculated from values for raw foods allowing for different water content. Allowance made for some loss of vitamins during cooking.
‡ The content of vitamin A and vitamin C varies with the cooking method (see Section 6.9).
§ This varies according to how the chips are prepared.

Appendix 2   Energy and nutrient needs

This appendix includes:

- an explanation of energy and nutrient requirements and how we derived the values in Table A2.1 and the table on the back inside cover of this book;
- Table A2.1 showing the daily needs for energy, complete and incomplete protein, fat, iron, iodine and important vitamins for different age and sex groups;
- the references used to calculate or derive the energy and nutrient requirements.

A2.1 USING TABLES OF ENERGY AND NUTRIENT NEEDS

You use tables of energy and nutrient needs to:

- plan diets for groups of people, such as school children;
- advise people about the amounts and types of foods to eat;
- examine diets to find out if they provide enough energy and nutrients. People vary in the amount they eat each day. So it is best to examine nutrient intakes over a period of several days.

A2.2 EXPLANATION OF THE TABLES

Table A2.1 and the table at the back of the book give the *average* individual energy requirements and *'safe levels of intake'* for protein and vitamins for groups of people of different ages and sexes with specified body weights and specified levels of activity. They do not tell us precisely the energy or nutrient needs of an individual.

These weights and activity levels are 'typical' of those in many tropical low-income countries. Even so the values, particularly the energy requirements, are not necessarily appropriate for all these countries because body weights and activity levels differ from place to place.

When possible, you should recalculate the values, particularly those for energy, using local body weights and local activity levels (James and Schofield 1990). For formulae see Chapter 2 and this appendix.

Safe levels of intake

The nutrient needs of people of the same size, sex, and age vary from person to person. 'Safe levels of intake' are the levels which would keep almost all (i.e. 97.5 per cent) normal healthy individuals within a group 'functioning' normally and with adequate body stores of the nutrient. When you plan a diet for a group using 'safe levels', it means that some people in the group will get more of the nutrient than they really need. But it is not harmful to eat these amounts because any excess is excreted (sometimes after being broken into simpler substances, i.e. protein is broken into urea and other waste products) or safely stored in the body (e.g. vitamin A).

When you examine the diet of a group, you may find that the average individual amounts of protein and vitamins eaten are a bit less than those given in Table A2.1. But, because the table gives safe levels, the amounts of nutrients in the diet are probably adequate for most members of the group.

Body weights

We used the 40th centile of WHO reference weights (WHO 1983). These are similar to weights in many low-income countries but give smoother lines when plotted.

Energy requirements

Energy values are *averages* for people of certain types. Because of individual variation they will not necessarily satisfy the requirements for each individual in a group. But we cannot use values which cover the needs of most people in the group (i.e. 'safe levels of intake') because then many people will get too many Calories and be at risk of obesity. When examining diets, the average energy intake for individuals in a group should be about the same as the values in Table A2.1.

Chapter 2 explains how energy needs are calculated.

Protein requirements

Table A2.3 gives the factors used to calculate the safe levels of intake. These values were plotted on a graph

Table A2.1. Daily requirements for energy, protein, fat, iron, iodine, and vitamins for different sex and age groups

Age†	Weight (kg)	Energy (kcal)	Protein (g) Diet** A	B	Fat (g)	Iron (mg) Diet** H	M	L	Iodine (µg)	Vitamin A (RE)	Thiamine (mg)	Riboflavin (mg)	Niacin (mg)	Folate (µg)	Vitamin C (mg)
Children—both sexes															
0–6 months	5.4	585	10	–	–	–	–	–	–	350	–	–	–	19	20
6–12 months	8.8	960	14	–	–	7	11	21	50	350	0.3	0.5	5.4	32	20
0–1 year	7.3	800	12	–	–	7	11	21	50	350	0.3	0.5	5.4	26	20
1–3 years	11.9	1250	14	23	35	5	7	13	70	400	0.5	0.8	9.0	40	20
3–5 years	15.9	1510	18	26	42	5	7	14	90	400	0.7	1.0	10.5	53	20
5–7 years	19.6	1710	20	30	48	7	10	19	90	400	0.8	1.1	12.1	65	20
7–10 years	25.9	1880	26	38	52	8	12	23	120	400	0.9	1.3	14.5	85	20
Boys															
10–12 years	34.0	2170	34	50	60	8	12	23	150	500	1.0	1.6	17.2	110	20
12–14 years	43.2	2360	43	64	66	12	18	36	150	600	1.2	1.7	19.1	140	30
14–16 years	54.5	2620	52	75	73	12	18	36	150	600	1.2	1.8	19.7	180	30
16–18 years	63.6	2820	57	84	78	8	11	23	150	600	1.2	1.8	20.3	200	30
Girls															
10–12 years	35.4	1925	35	52	53	8	11	23	150	500	0.9	1.4	15.5	120	20
12–14 years	44.2	2040	42	62	57	13	20	40	150	600	1.0	1.5	16.4	150	30
14–16 years	51.5	2135	46	69	59	13	20	40	150	550	1.0	1.5	15.8	170	30
16–18 years	54.6	2150	45	66	60	16	24	48	150	500	0.9	1.4	15.2	170	30
If pregnant		+200	+6	+7		26	38*	76*		600	1.0	1.6	17.5	400	50
Men—active															
18–60 years	65.0	2944	49	57	83	8	11	23	150	600	1.2	1.8	19.8	200	30
>60 years	65.0	2060	49	57	56	8	11	23	150	600	1.2	1.8	19.8	200	30
Women—active															
Childbearing age	55.0	2140	41	48	59	16	24	48	150	500	0.9	1.3	14.5	170	30
Pregnant	55.0	2240	47	55	65	26	38*	76*	175	600	1.0	1.5	16.8	400	50
Lactating	55.0	2640	59	68	73	9	13	26	200	850	1.1	1.7	18.2	270	50
>60 years	55.0	1830	41	48	51	6	9	19	150	500	0.9	1.3	14.5	170	30

* Supplements are usually needed to provide enough iron.
† Example to explain how age range is expressed: 1–3 years means 1 year 0 months to 2 years 11 months.
– No value available. Assumption made that breastmilk covers needs.
** See explanation of diets on p. 427.

and then smoothed to give the values in Table A2.1.

Diet A represents a mixed balanced diet with little fibre and plenty of complete protein. The digestibility factor used was 100 per cent and the amino-acid score was 100 for all ages.

Diet B represents diets containing a lot of cereals, starchy roots, and pulses (therefore it is high in fibre) and little complete (animal) protein. The digestibility factor used was 85 per cent and the amino-acid scores were 100 for ages 6 months to 1 year (assuming breast milk would improve protein quality), 70 for ages 1–5 years, 80 for ages 5–17 years, and 100 for adults (WHO 1985).

Fat requirements

These were calculated to provide 25 per cent of average energy requirements. The percentage can safely vary between 20 and 35 per cent.

Iron requirements

The values given are for 'basal requirements' (the amount needed to prevent measurable effects of iron deficiency—not just clinical anaemia) plus an addition for individual variation.

Diet H represents a high iron availability diet (about 15 per cent iron absorbed); diet M a medium iron availability diet (about 10 per cent iron absorbed); diet L a low iron availability diet (about 5 per cent iron absorbed)—see Section 4.10.

The iron requirements during pregnancy are an estimate of the minimum needs over the whole 9 months. Table 4.2 gives iron needs by trimester.

Vitamin and iodine requirements

These were taken from the publications listed at the end of this appendix.

A2.3 FORMULAE AND FACTORS FOR CALCULATING ENERGY AND PROTEIN NEEDS

Formulae used to calculate average individual energy requirements (James and Schofield 1990)

- For ages over 10 years, the average individual energy requirement is Basal metabolic rate (BMR) × Physical activity level (PAL).

- For ages 0–10 years, the average individual energy requirement is Body weight × Energy allowance.

The energy allowance factor allows for the energy needs of frequent infection and desirable levels of activity.

Formulae used to calculate basal metabolic rate (BMR)

	Males	**Females**
10–17+ years	$17.5 \times W + 651$	$12.2 \times W + 746$
18–29+ years	$15.3 \times W + 679$	$14.7 \times W + 496$
30–59 years	$11.6 \times W + 879$	$8.7 \times W + 829$
> 60 years	$13.5 \times W + 487$	$10.5 + W + 596$

where W is the body weight in kilograms.

Table A2.2 gives the BMRs of men and women of different ages and weights. Table A2.3 lists factors for calculating energy and protein needs.

Table A2.2. BMRs of men and women of different weights

Age (years)	Weight (kg)	BMR Men	BMR Women
18–29+	40	1291	1084
	45	1368	1158
	50	1444	1231
	55	1521	1305
	60	1597	1378
	65	1674	1452
	70	1750	1525
30–59+	40	1343	1177
	45	1401	1221
	50	1459	1264
	55	1517	1308
	60	1575	1351
	65	1633	1395
	70	1691	1438
>60	40	1027	1016
	45	1095	1067
	50	1162	1121
	55	1230	1174
	60	1297	1226
	65	1365	1279
	70	1432	1331

Table A2.3. Factors for calculating daily energy and protein needs

Age (years)	Energy allowance (kcal/kg)		Physical activity level (PAL) factor		Protein (g per kg body weight)			
					Male		Female	
	Boys	Girls	Male	Female	Diet*		Diet*	
					A	B	A	B
0+	109	109						
1+	108	108			1.2	2.0	1.2	2.0
2+	104	102			1.15	1.93	1.15	1.93
3+	99	95			1.1	1.85	1.1	1.85
4+	95	92			1.1	1.85	1.1	1.85
5+	92	88			1.0	1.47	1.0	1.47
6+	88	83			1.0	1.47	1.0	1.47
7+	83	76			1.0	1.47	1.0	1.47
8+	77	69			1.0	1.47	1.0	1.47
9+	72	62			1.0	1.47	1.0	1.47
10+			1.76	1.65	1.0	1.47	1.0	1.47
11+			1.72	1.62	1.0	1.47	1.0	1.47
12+			1.69	1.60	1.0	1.47	0.95	1.4
13+			1.67	1.58	1.0	1.47	0.95	1.4
14+			1.65	1.57	0.95	1.4	0.9	1.32
15+			1.62	1.54	0.95	1.4	0.9	1.32
16+			1.60	1.52	0.9	1.32	0.8	1.18
17+			1.60	1.52	0.9	1.32	0.8	1.18
18–59+ light activity			1.55	1.56	0.75	0.88	0.75	0.88
moderate activity			1.78	1.64				
>60 light activity			1.51	1.56				

	Energy (kcal/day)	Protein (g/kg body weight/day)	
		Diet A*	Diet B*
Extra needs for pregnancy			
Light—Moderate activity	100	6	7
Heavy activity	200		
Undernourished women	200–285		
Extra needs for lactation	500	17.5	20.5

* See explanation of diets on p. 427.

A2.4 REFERENCES* AND SOURCES OF MORE INFORMATION

- *Energy* — James, W. P. T. and Schofield, E. C. (1990). *Human energy requirements: a manual for planners and nutritionists.* Published for FAO by Oxford University Press, Oxford.

- *Protein* — WHO (1985). *Energy and protein requirements*, Technical Report Series, no. 724. WHO, Geneva.

- *Iron, vitamin A, and folate* — FAO (1988a). *Requirements of vitamin A, iron, folate and vitamin B_{12}*, Report of a Joint FAO/WHO Expert Consultation. FAO, Rome.

- *Iodine, thiamine, riboflavin, and niacin* — FAO (1988b). *Traditional food plants*, Food and Nutrition Paper, no. 42. FAO, Rome.

- *Vitamin C* — FAO (1970). *Requirements of ascorbic acid, vitamin D, vitamin B_{12}, folate and iron*, Report of Joint FAO/WHO Report Group. FAO, Rome.

- *Body weights* — WHO (1983). *Measuring change in nutritional status.* WHO, Geneva.

* The energy and protein values used in this annex were calculated by FAO (see FAO (in press) *Food and nutrition in management of group feeding programmes.* Food and Nutrition Paper no. 23, FAO, Rome.)

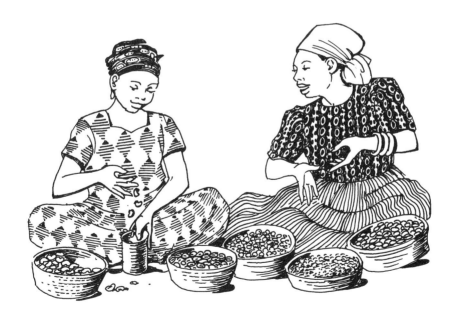

Fig. A2–1 Beans, peas and groundnuts are rich sources of energy, protein, micronutrients, and fibre.

Appendix 3   Useful sources of energy and nutrients

A3.1 FOODS WHICH PROVIDE USEFUL AMOUNTS OF ENERGY AND NUTRIENTS

Energy

*Mainly from **fat***

Oils (e.g. maize, sesame, cottonseed oil)
Fats (e.g. butter, margarine, ghee, lard, cooking fat)
Groundnuts, soybeans
Sesame, sunflower, coconut and other oil seeds and nuts
Fatty meat and fatty fish
Breast milk
Whole milks (animal)
Cheese
Avocado

*Mainly from **starch***

Cereals
Roots
Starchy fruits
Legumes

*Mainly from **sugar***

Sugar
Honey
Sugar-rich foods
Sweet fruits especially when dried

Fibre

Cereals, especially wholemeal cereals
Roots and root vegetables
Legumes
Leafy vegetables and fruits

Protein

Breast milk
Animal milks and milk foods (e.g. yoghurt, cheese)
Eggs
Flesh of animals, birds, and fish
Beans, peas, groundnuts, soybeans

Iron

Haem iron

Liver and other offal
Flesh of animals, birds, and fish

Non-haem iron*

Breast milk
Some dried fruits
Some dark green leaves‡

Also the following where large amounts are eaten:

Cereals (especially fermented and germinated porridges)
Legumes and oil seeds

Iodine

Fish and other foods from the sea
Iodized salt

Calcium

Milk of all kinds and foods made from milk
Fish when the bones are eaten
Beans and peas
Finger millet
Dark green leaves
Water from places where there is lime or chalk in the soil

Zinc

Meat, poultry, fish
Wholegrain cereals
Legumes
Breast milk

---

* Iron absorption is increased if these foods are eaten with foods which provide plenty of vitamin C or with meat or fish.
‡ Much of the iron may be unavailable if the plant contains large amounts of anti-nutrients which interfere with iron absorption.

Vitamin A

Mainly as **retinol**

Liver from animals, birds, and fish
Kidney
Breast milk and colostrum
Animal milk and foods made from the fat of animal
    milk (butter, ghee, cheese)
Eggs
Margarine, dried skimmed milk, and other foods forti-
    fied with vitamin A

As **carotene**

Dark/medium green and orange vegetables (e.g.
    spinach, carrots, pumpkin)
Mangoes, pawpaw, and other orange fruits
Unbleached red palm oil
Yellow maize, yellow sweet potatoes, plantains

Thiamine

Liver
Meat from animals, birds, and fish
Wholegrain cereals
Legumes and oil seeds
Breast milk

Riboflavin

Breast milk
Eggs
Animal milk
Liver, meat, and fish

Niacin

Liver, meat, and fish
Groundnuts
Breast milk
Animal milk
Wholemeal wheat, millet, and rice

Folate

(Folate is easily lost during cooking)

Liver and kidney
Fresh vegetables, especially dark green leaves
Fish
Beans and groundnuts
Breast milk

Vitamin C

(Fresh raw fruits, vegetables, and roots contain more
    vitamin C than cooked ones. When dried these foods
    contain little or no vitamin C except for dried
    baobab.)

Liver
Fruits (especially guava and citrus fruits)
Baobab fruits
Vegetables, e.g. green leaves, peppers, tomatoes
Fresh starchy roots and fruits
Fresh animal milk
Breast milk

Vitamin D

Daylight
Liver
Fat of milks
Egg yolk

Table A3.1.   Nutrients in different types of foods

Food	Rich source of:	Moderate source of:
Cereals	Starch, fibre	Protein, B vitamins, many minerals
Starchy roots and fruits	Starch, fibre	Some minerals, vitamin C if fresh, vitamin A if yellow
Beans and peas	Starch, protein, some minerals, fibre	B vitamins
Oil seeds	Fat, protein, fibre	B vitamins, some minerals
Fats and oils	Fat	Vitamin A if orange
Dark/medium green leaves	Vitamins A, C, and folate	Protein, minerals,
Orange vegetables	Vitamins A and C	Fibre
Orange fruits	Vitamins A and C	Fibre
Citrus fruit	Vitamin C	
Milk	Fat, protein, calcium, vitamins	
Eggs	Protein, vitamins	Fat, minerals (not iron)
Meat	Protein, fat, iron	
Fish	Protein, iron	
Liver	Protein, iron, vitamins	

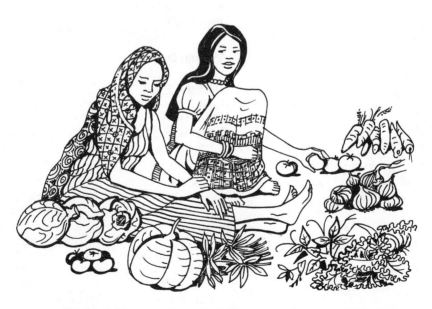

Fig. A3–1 Many vegetables and fruits are rich sources of micronutrients.

Appendix 4 Calculating nutrients in foods

A4.1 WHY WE CALCULATE THE NUTRIENT CONTENT OF FOODS

- To compare the nutrient content of different foods, and to decide which foods are good sources of nutrients and which give best value for money.
- To find out the nutrient value of different weights of raw and cooked foods, and meals.
- To find out the amounts of nutrients a person or group of people eats, and whether this is enough to cover their nutrient needs.
- To plan meals and diets which provide particular amounts of nutrients.

A4.2 CALCULATING THE NUTRIENT CONTENT OF FOODS

To find out the amounts of energy and nutrients in foods we use *food composition tables*. Food composition tables list the amounts of nutrients in 100 g portions of different foods. You can use the tables in Appendix 1. But it is better to use reliable ones prepared for your own country.

Before you use food composition tables you need to understand:

- how food is measured;
- the meaning of 'as purchased' weight, 'edible' weight, and 'per cent edible portion';
- how the proportion of water alters the proportion of other nutrients;
- cooking conversion factors.

Measuring foods

You can measure food:

- by weight—this is most accurate if you have reliable scales;
- by volume using cans, cups, handfuls, etc.;

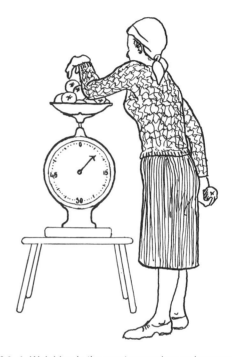

Fig. A4–1 Weighing is the most accurate way to measure a quantity of food.

- by items—for example, numbers of eggs, piles of tomatoes.

To use food composition tables you need to know the weight of food in grams. If you cannot weigh the food, you can estimate the weight by converting volume or item measures into grams using conversion tables like Table A4.4.

'As purchased weight', 'edible weight', and 'per cent edible portion'

These terms are used in food composition tables.

'As purchased' weight of food

This is the weight of a food as we buy or harvest it—for

433

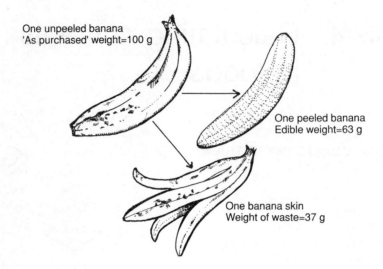

One unpeeled banana
'As purchased' weight=100 g

One peeled banana
Edible weight=63 g

One banana skin
Weight of waste=37 g

Fig. A4–2 'As purchased' food = 'edible' food + waste.

example, the weight of a bunch of unpeeled bananas, a whole fish, or unshelled groundnuts.

The 'as purchased weight' includes the weight of 'waste'. Waste is the part of the food we do not eat such as skin, peel, or bones. 'As purchased' may be shortened to 'AP'. In Fig. A4–2 the 'as purchased weight' of a banana is 100 g.

'Edible' weight of food

This is the weight of food with waste removed—in other words, the weight of food which can all be eaten. For example, the weight of peeled bananas, fish flesh, or shelled groundnuts. In Fig. A4–2 the edible weight of banana is 63 g.

The *'weight of waste'* is the weight of the waste in the 'as purchased' weight. In Fig. A4–2 the weight of waste is 37 g.

The *edible portion* means the part of the food which is edible.

Most food composition tables give the amounts of nutrients in 100 g of the raw edible food—for example, in 100 g of shelled groundnuts or in 100 g peeled bananas. So to use food composition tables you must know the 'edible weights' of the foods.

'Per cent edible portion'

This means the percentage of the 'as purchased' food which is edible. The per cent edible portion is the edible weight of food in 100 g of 'as purchased' food. Look at Fig. A4–2. What is the weight of edible

banana that we get from 100 g 'as purchased' banana? The answer is 63 g. We say the 'per cent edible portion' is 63 per cent.

'Per cent edible portion' can be shortened to '%EP'.

If you know the 'as purchased weight' and the %EP you can work out the edible weight of any food.

For example you buy 200 g of unpeeled bananas. What is the edible weight of these bananas? The answer is

$$200 \text{ g unpeeled} \times \frac{63}{100} = 126 \text{ g peeled.}$$

The formula we use to find out the edible weight from the 'as purchased weight' and the %EP is

$$\text{Edible weight} = \text{'as purchased' weight} \times \frac{\%EP}{100}.$$

(Formula 1)

Here is another example. If you are teaching, you might want to give this to your trainees.

Example

Sofie buys 1 kg of sweet potatoes. After peeling them, what is the edible weight of potatoes? The food composition tables in Appendix 1 tell you that the %EP for sweet potato is 79.

So, using Formula 1,

$$\text{Edible weight of potatoes} = 1000 \text{ g} \times \frac{79}{100} = 790 \text{ g.}$$

Box A4.1.   How to work out the per cent edible portion of local foods

1. Weigh the 'as purchased' food,

e.g. 'As purchased weight' of yams = 600 g.

2. Remove the waste and weigh the food again. This is the 'edible weight',

e.g. Weight of peeled yams = 504 g.

3. Calculate the %EP,

e.g. 600 g unpeeled yams gives 504 g peeled yams.

So 100 g unpeeled yams gives $\dfrac{504\,g}{600\,g} \times 100\,g = 84\,g$ peeled yams.

So %EP for yams = 84%

Or use the formula

$$\%EP = \frac{\text{Weight of edible portion}}{\text{Weight of 'as purchased' food}} \times 100, \textbf{(Formula 2)}$$

e.g.

$$\%EP \text{ for yams} = \frac{504\,g}{600\,g} \times 100 = 84\%$$

For some foods, for example flour and milk, there is no waste. All the food is edible. The 'as purchased weight' equals the 'edible weight'. The 'per cent edible portion' is 100 per cent.

Most food composition tables give values for %EP. Some give per cent waste

$$\%EP = 100\% - \%\text{ waste,}$$

e.g. Fig. A4–2 shows that:

% waste for bananas = 37%

So %EP for bananas =

$$100\% - 37\% = 63\%$$

However, %EPs can vary a lot depending on the quality of the food and how it is prepared. So it is better to work out local values if possible. Box A4.1 shows you how to do this. It is even more accurate to weigh the edible part of the food each time you want to know the nutrient content.

Water content

The water content of a food may vary. For example, dried beans contain much less water than fresh or cooked beans. It is important to understand how the amount of water in food affects the proportion of the other nutrients. The more water in the food, the lower the proportion of other nutrients. This is because the water dilutes the other nutrients.

Figure A4–3 explains this using fish as an example. The figure shows a small fresh fish which weighs 100 g. The fish contains about 12 g protein and 75 g water as well as other nutrients and waste. The per cent protein in this fresh fish is 12 per cent.

Then the fish is dried. This removes 60 g of water so the fish weighs only 40 g. But it still contains 12 g protein. Let us calculate the per cent of protein in the fish now.

40 g fish contains 12 g protein. So:

$$100\,g \text{ fish contains } \frac{12\,g \text{ protein}}{40\,g \text{ fish}} \times 100\,g \text{ fish} = 30\,g \text{ protein.}$$

So the per cent protein in dried fish is 30 per cent.

Cooking conversion factors

Most food composition tables give the nutrient content for only a few cooked foods such as bread. This is because cooking methods, and particularly the amount of water used, vary so much. So to calculate the nutrient content of cooked food you may need to convert a cooked weight of food into its raw weight.

For example, to know the nutrient content of maize porridge you need to know how much maize flour it contains.

Sometimes you want to know how much cooked food

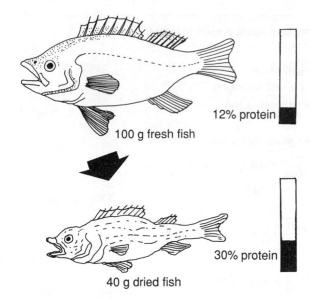

12% protein

100 g fresh fish

30% protein

40 g dried fish

Fig. A4–3 How water content alters the proportion of other nutrients.

you get from a certain weight of raw food. For example, how much porridge you can make from a given weight of maize flour.

To do these calculations you need to know the cooking conversion factors for the particular food.

There are two cooking conversion factors for each food.

1. 'Cooked to raw' factor. This is the weight of raw food in 1 g of cooked food, e.g.

    1 g thick porridge contains 0.29 g maize flour.

The 'cooked to raw' factor is used to convert a given weight (or portion) of cooked food into its equivalent weight of raw food.

2. 'Raw to cooked' factor. This is the weight of cooked food which contains 1 g of raw food, e.g.

    1 g flour gives 3.5 g porridge.

The 'raw to cooked' factor is used to convert a given weight (or portion) of raw food into its equivalent weight of cooked food.

It is best to calculate local conversion factors (see Box A4.2) because they vary with local cooking methods. If this is not possible you can use the ones in Table A4.5 at the end of this appendix.

Box A4.2.   How to calculate local cooking conversion factors

For each food:
1. Weigh the raw food, e.g. 200 g maize flour.
2. Weigh the food after cooking, e.g. 700 g maize porridge.
3. Calculate the 'cooked to raw' cooking factor. This is the grams of raw food in 1 g cooked food, e.g.

    700 g porridge contains 200 g flour.

    So

    $$1\,\text{g porridge contains } \frac{200\,\text{g flour}}{700\,\text{g porridge}} \times 1\,\text{g porridge} = 0.29\,\text{g flour}.$$

So the 'cooked to raw' cooking factor for maize porridge is 0.29
The formula for the 'cooked to raw' factor is:

$$\text{'Cooked to raw' factor} = \frac{\text{weight of raw food}}{\text{weight of cooked food}}. \quad \textbf{(Formula 3)}$$

4. Calculate the 'raw to cooked' cooking factor. This is the grams of cooked food made from 1 g of raw food, e.g.

    200 g flour makes 700 g porridge.

    So

    $$1\,\text{g flour makes } \frac{700\,\text{g}}{200\,\text{g}} \times 1\,\text{g flour} = 3.5\,\text{g porridge}.$$

So the 'raw to cooked' cooking factor for maize porridge is 3.5
The formula for the 'raw to cooked' factor is

$$\text{'Raw to cooked' factor} = \frac{\text{weight of cooked food}}{\text{weight of raw food}}. \quad \textbf{(Formula 4)}$$

A4.3 COMPARING THE NUTRIENT CONTENT OF DIFFERENT FOODS

If you want to compare the nutrient values of different foods and find out which are good sources of particular nutrients:

1. List the foods you want to investigate.
2. Find each food in the food composition tables.
3. Find the column of the particular nutrient you are interested in and write down the amount of the nutrient in 100 g of the food.
4. See which food gives the largest amount of the nutrient.

Example
You want to find out which local foods are good sources of fat. So:

1. List local foods likely to contain fat.
2. Find each food in the food composition tables.
3. Look under the fat column and write down the amount of fat in 100 g of each food.

	g fat in 100 g edible food
Groundnuts, dried	45.0
Milk, fresh	3.7
Margarine	83.0
Maize flour, 95% extraction	4.5

4. Compare the fat contents. The richest source is margarine.

You can find out which foods are good sources of energy, protein, minerals, and vitamins in the same way. You can use this information to find out which foods give best value for money (see Chapter 9).

A4.4 CALCULATING THE NUTRIENT CONTENT OF FOODS AND MEALS

This section explains how to find out the nutrient content of different weights (or portions) of foods and meals.

Nutrients in the edible weight of raw foods

This is how you calculate the amount of energy, protein, or other nutrients in a given weight (or portion) of raw edible food. For example, calculate the amount of protein in 50 g dried beans.

1. Find the food in the food composition tables and then the value for the particular nutrient. This tells you the amount of the nutrient in 100 g of the edible food, e.g.

100 g edible dried beans contains 22 g protein.

2. Calculate the amount of the nutrient in 1 g of the food, e.g.

Amount of protein in 1 g dried beans =

$1\text{ g dried beans} \times \dfrac{22\text{ g protein}}{100\text{ g dried beans}} = 0.22\text{ g protein}.$

3. Calculate the amount of the nutrient in the given weight or portion of the food, e.g.

Amount of protein in 50 g dried beans =

$\dfrac{0.22\text{ g protein}}{1\text{ g dried beans}} \times 50\text{ g dried beans} = 11\text{ g protein}.$

So 50 g dried beans contains 11 g protein.

When you understand this calculation it is quicker to use the following formula:

Amount of nutrient in given weight (portion) of food = $\dfrac{\text{weight of food} \times \text{weight of nutrient in 100 g food}}{100\text{ g}}$

(Formula 5)

So, using Formula 5,

Weight of protein in 50 g dried beans

$\dfrac{50\text{ g}}{100\text{ g}} \times 22\text{ g} = 11\text{ g protein}.$

Nutrients in 'as purchased' raw foods

To calculate the nutrients in 'as purchased' foods:

1. Convert the 'as purchased weight' to the 'edible weight' using Formula 1.
2. Then calculate the amount of the nutrient in the edible weight using Formula 5.

Example
Find the Calories in 250 g of unpeeled bananas

1. Convert the 'as purchased weight' to the 'edible weight'.

'As purchased weight' = 250 g.

%EP for bananas is 63% (from food composition tables)

So, using Formula 1;

Edible weight of banana = $\dfrac{63}{100} \times 250\text{ g} = 158\text{ g}.$

2. Calculate the Calories in 158 g of peeled banana.

100 g edible portion of banana contains 82 kcal (from food composition tables).

So, using Formula 5,

$$\text{kcal in 158 g banana} = \frac{158\,g}{100\,g} \times 82\,kcal = 130\,kcal.$$

So 250 g unpeeled banana contains 130 kcal.

If you are calculating the amounts of energy and nutrients in several foods, you can write the values in a table like Table A4.1. Table A4.1 also shows how you can add together the nutrient values for several ingredients to find out the nutrient content of simple meals and snacks (e.g. bread and margarine).

Nutrients in cooked foods

When calculating the nutrient value of cooked foods, you may need to adjust values for some micronutrients, especially vitamin C and folate, to allow for losses during cooking (see Section 6.2).

Nutrient content of single cooked foods

To find out the nutrient content of a single cooked food (e.g. maize porridge, boiled rice):

1. Weigh the cooked food.

2. Find out the weight of raw food in this weight of cooked food. To do this:

   • Weigh the food before cooking. This is the most reliable method but it is not always possible to do this.

   or

   • Use the 'cooked to raw' cooking conversion factor (explained above).

3. Calculate the nutrient content of this weight of raw food using Formula 5.

Example
To calculate the Calorie content of thick maize porridge

1. Weigh the cooked porridge.

Weight 700 g.

2. Find out the weight of maize flour in the porridge. You can do this by:

   • Weighing the maize flour before cooking.

   200 g flour was used.

   or

   • Multiplying the cooked weight by the 'cooked to raw' cooking conversion factor in Box A4.2.

   'Cooked to raw' factor = 0.29.

   So

   700 g porridge × 0.29 = 203 g flour (or about 200 g).

3. Calculate the Calorie content of 200 g flour using Formula 5.

$$\text{Calorie content of flour} = \frac{200\,g}{100\,g} \times 345\,kcal = 690\,kcal.$$

So the Calorie content of 700 g thick porridge is 690 kcal.

The nutrient content of cooked foods with several ingredients

To calculate the nutrient content of a meal or recipe which contains several ingredients:

1. Weigh all the raw ingredients;

2. Calculate the nutrients in each—see example in Table A4.2.

3. Add up the quantities of Calories and each nutrient. This gives the nutrient content of the whole meal or recipe.

Table A4.1. Nutrient content of different foods

Food	Edible weight (g)	Energy (kcal)	Protein (g)	Iron (mg)	Vitamin A (RE)
Bananas	158	130	2	2	31
Beans	50	160	11	4	0
Snack:					
Bread	210	504	16	4	0
Margarine	15	112	0	0	0
Total snack	225	616	16	4	0

You may want to know the nutrient content of a portion of the meal, for example, a child's portion. To do this:

1. Weigh the total quantity of the cooked meal before serving. In our example, the cooked maize, beans, and onions weighed 3000 g.

2. Weigh the amount given to the child, e.g. 300 g.

3. Calculate the percentage of the total meal which was given to the child, e.g.

$$\frac{300\,\text{g} \times 100}{3000\,\text{g}} = 10 \text{ per cent.}$$

4. Use this percentage to calculate the amounts of nutrients in the child's portion, e.g.

$$2353\,\text{kcal} \times \frac{10}{100} = 235\,\text{kcal.}$$

If you want to know the nutrient content of the food the child actually ate, you must subtract the weight of food not eaten (this is called 'plate waste').

The nutrient content of a person's or a family's daily diet

To do this:

1. Weigh (or estimate the weight) of all the food eaten by a person's or a family's diet over a particular period (usually 24 hours or longer)—see below.

2. Calculate the nutrient content of each food.

3. Add together the values for Calories, for protein, and for other nutrients.

There are several methods for estimating the amounts of foods people eat. These include:

- weighing or estimating the weight of all the foods eaten;
- asking people to record the amounts of all the food they eat;
- recording the amounts of food in a home at the beginning of the weighing period, all the food which is bought, and the food left at the end of the period.

You may need to:

- convert volume measures or numbers of items to weights;
- convert 'as purchased weights' to 'edible weights';
- convert cooked weights to raw weights;
- measure plate waste.

In practice all the methods for finding out the weights of foods eaten are very time-consuming and difficult. People may change their eating habits if someone is watching what they eat, some family members may eat away from home, and it is hard to record everything eaten during 24 hours. Most nutrition workers will not need to do complicated dietary surveys like these. If you do, the references at the end of the chapter will help you.

A4.5 COMPARING THE NUTRIENT CONTENT OF MEALS OR DIETS TO NUTRIENT NEEDS

You may want to know if a group of people are eating enough to cover their needs—for example, if children are eating enough vitamin A. Or you may be asked to say what proportion of daily needs are covered by a particular meal or diet—for example, what proportion of energy needs are covered by a school meal or whether the rations provided to refugees cover their vitamin needs.

Table A4.2. Nutrient content of a simple meal

Food	Weight (g)	Energy (kcal)	Protein (g)	Fat (g)	Vitamin A (RE)
Wholegrain maize, raw	300	1035	28	13	0
Cowpeas, raw	400	1280	92	6	—
Onions, raw	100	38	1	—	0
Total in raw ingredients		2353	121	19	—
Total cooked weight	3000				
Child's portion	300	235	12	2	—

To answer these questions you need to:

1. Calculate the nutrient content of the meal or diet eaten by an average individual in the group.

2. Find out the average individual nutrient needs for the group (see Appendix 2).

3. Compare the nutrients in the food to nutrient needs.

Example

A pre-primary school gives a mug (300 g) of soft sweet porridge as an early morning snack to 150 children aged 3–5 years. The head teacher wants to know what proportion of the children's daily energy needs this provides. To find out:

1. Calculate the energy in one mug of the soft porridge.

   a. Find out the weight of raw maize flour and sugar in each mug of porridge.

   The quantities used to make 150 mugs of porridge are 9 kg maize flour and 1.5 kg sugar

   So the amounts of maize flour and sugar per child are:

$$\frac{9000\,g}{150} = 60\,g\ flour \quad and \quad \frac{1500\,g}{150} = 10\,g\ sugar.$$

   b. Calculate the energy in 60 g flour and 10 g sugar using food composition tables.

$$100\,g\ flour\ gives\ 345\,kcal.$$
$$100\,g\ sugar\ gives\ 400\,kcal.$$
$$60\,g\ flour\ gives\ \frac{345\,kcal}{100\,g} \times 60\,g = 207\,kcal.$$
$$10\,g\ sugar\ gives\ \frac{400\,kcal}{100\,g} \times 10\,g = 40\,kcal$$

The total energy in 1 mug of porridge = 247 kcal.

2. Find out the average individual energy needs of pre-primary school children (ages 3–5 years) from Appendix 2.

$$Energy\ needs\ of\ children = 1510\,kcal/day.$$

3. Calculate the percentage of energy needs supplied by a mug of porridge.

Per cent of energy needs from porridge =
$$\frac{Energy\ in\ porridge}{Energy\ needs} \times 100 = \frac{247}{1510} \times 100 = 16\ per\ cent.$$

So a mug of soft porridge supplies 16 per cent of the children's daily energy needs.

The formula for calculating the proportion of nutrient needs supplied by a meal or diet is:

$$\frac{Nutrient\ content\ of\ meal/diet}{Individual\ daily\ nutrient\ needs} \times 100.\ \textbf{(Formula 6)}$$

You can write the results of these calculations on a table like Table A4.3, especially if you are examining more than one nutrient.

A4.6 PLANNING MEALS AND DIETS

You may need to plan a diet for a particular group of people (e.g. children at boarding school, hospital patients) or a meal containing a certain quantity of Calories, protein, and other nutrients (e.g. a school lunch). To do this prepare a blank table like Table A4.3 and then:

1. Write the amounts of each nutrient which should be supplied to each individual by the diet or meal (see Appendix 2).

Table A4.3. Percentage of daily energy needs supplied by porridge

Food	Weight (g)	Energy (kcal)	Protein (g)	Iron (mg)
For 150 children				
Maize flour	9000			
Sugar	1500			
For 1 child				
Maize flour	60	207	6.0	1.5
Sugar	10	40	0	0
Total		247	6.0	1.5
Average individual needs		1510	26	14
% of needs supplied by porridge		16	23	11

Table A4.4.   Equivalent weights and volumes of foods. The volume of foods can vary according to how tightly it is packed, the shape of the container, etc. So check these values using local foods and measures.

Food	Weight of food (g)		Volume (ml) of 100 g of food
	In 250 ml	In 100 ml	
Cereal flours	150	59	169
Stiff porridge	100	100	100
Soft porridge	100	100	100
Rice, raw	210	85	118
boiled	165	66	152
Cassava flour	130	53	189
Potato, raw diced	160	63	158
cooked diced	180	71	140
Sweet potato, raw diced	140	56	178
cooked mashed	265	107	94
Beans/Peas, raw	200	80	125
cooked	180	72	139
Groundnuts, shelled			
whole raw	160	64	157
flour	120	48	210
paste	265	106	95
Cabbage, raw shredded	75	30	338
Green leaves, raw chopped	75	31	329
cooked	140	55	183
Onions, raw chopped	170	68	148
Tomato, sliced	190	77	131
paste	275	111	91
Banana, mashed	235	95	106
Mango, chopped	170	69	146
Orange sections	190	75	134
Pawpaw, chopped	150	59	169
mashed	250	100	100
Sugar	205	83	121
Meat, ground/minced	240	95	105
Fish, flaked	255	102	99
Milk, fresh	250	100	100
dried skimmed	105	43	236
dried whole	140	55	183
evaporated	265	106	95
condensed sweetened	350	139	72
Margarine	235	95	106
Oil	220	88	114

From FAO (in press). Calculated from values in *Home Economics Research Report*, no. 41, Agricultural Research Service, US Department of Agriculture (1969) and unpublished estimations.

To use Table A4.4 you may need to know the volume of local containers. To find out:

- Fill container to the top with water and carefully measure the volume of water with a measuring container from a laboratory, *or*
- Weigh the container empty and full. The weight of water in grams equals its volume in millilitres, *or*
- Use the following volumes.

Volumes of some local measures (to top of container)
Check these volumes if possible

- 1 teacup or 1 glass holds about 200 ml.
- 1 eating spoon holds about 10 ml.
- 1 teaspoon holds about 5 ml.
- 1 Coke bottle (labelled 193 ml) holds about 200 ml.
- 1 beer bottle (labelled 440 ml) holds about 500 ml.
- 1 can for margarine/cooking fat (labelled 250 g) holds about 250 ml.

2. List the foods you want to use—take into account availability, cost, acceptability, and resources needed for preparation.

3. Adjust the amounts of the main foods until together they supply enough Calories and the meal is not too bulky. These amounts usually supply enough protein.

4. Add other foods as necessary to supply enough micronutrients.

Example
A project manager plans to give a meal of thick maize porridge and beans to young male labourers working on a tree-planting project. He wants the meal to provide 40 per cent of their daily energy needs.

1. Average daily individual energy needs (from Appendix 2) are about 3000 kcal. So 40 per cent of needs is 1200 kcal.

2. The ingredients of the meal are wholemeal maize flour and dry beans.

3. The amounts of maize and beans to supply 1200 kcal are:

260 g maize gives   897 kcal.
100 g beans gives   320 kcal.
So the meal gives   1217 kcal.

Table A4.5. Estimates for cooking conversion factors.
(Check values using local foods and cooking methods)

Raw food/cooked food	Conversion factor	
	'Cooked to raw' (g raw in 1 g cooked)	'Raw to cooked' (g cooked from 1 g raw)
Maize flour/thick porridge	0.29	3.5
Maize flour/thin porridge	0.14	7.0
Dry rice/boiled rice	0.4	2.5
Wheat flour/bread	0.77	1.3
Wheat flour/chapatti	0.63	1.6
Raw potato/boiled potato	1.0	1.0
Dry beans/boiled beans	0.4	2.5
Dry lentils/boiled lentils	0.33	3.0
Dry groundnuts/Boiled groundnuts	0.55	1.8
Raw green leaves/boiled drained leaves	1.67	0.6
Raw cabbage/boiled drained cabbage	1.25	0.8

REFERENCES

Cameron, M. E. and Hofvander, Y. (1983). *Manual on feeding infants and young children*. Oxford University Press, Delhi.

Cameron, M. E. and van Staveren, W. A. (1988). *Manual on methodology for food consumption studies*. Oxford University Press, Oxford.

FAO (in press). *Food and nutrition in management of group feeding programmes*, Food and Nutrition Paper, no. 23. FAO, Rome.

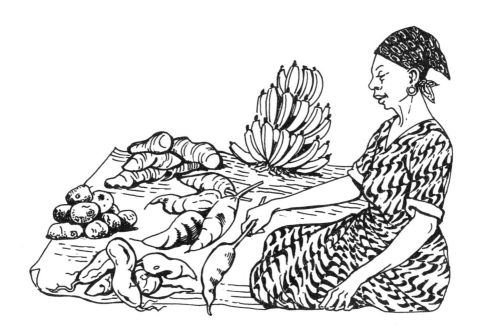

Fig. A4–4 'You can calculate the nutrient values of local foods.'

Appendix 5 Anthropometric reference values

This appendix contains:

Table A5.1. Weights-for-age—girls and boys aged 0–60 months

Table A5.2. Lengths-for-age—girls and boys aged 0–23 months

Table A5.3. Heights-for-age—girls and boys aged 24–60 months

Table A5.4. Weights-for-length—girls and boys of 50–100 cm length aged under 2 years

Table A5.5. Weights-for-height—girls and boys of 80–120 cm height aged 2 years and over

Table A5.6. Weights-for-height—girls and boys of 120–145 cm height (sexes separate)

These tables were derived from values given by WHO (1983).

Table A5.7. Weights-for-heights of adults for different body mass indexes (BMIs) (see Fig. 22–2 and Box 22.1).

Expressing anthropometric indices as per cent of reference value

You may want to express a child's weight (or height or weight-for-height) as a percentage of the reference value. This is useful if the child's measurement is outside the normal range, for example, for children whose weights are below the 3rd centile.

To calculate the percentage of reference weight (or height) use the formula:

$$\% \text{ reference weight-for-age} = \frac{\text{weight of child}}{\text{reference weight-for-age}} \times 100.$$

Example
A child of 27 months weighs 8.9 kg.
Reference weight-for-age at 27 months = 12.7 kg (Table A5.1).

$$\text{So her } \% \text{ of reference weight-for-age} = \frac{8.9}{12.7} \times 100 = 70\%.$$

You can use a similar formula to calculate weights which are different percentages of the reference values to use instead of, or in addition to, centiles.

Example
To find out the 60% of reference weight-for-age values for children aged 12 months.

Reference weight-for-age at 12 months = 9.9 kg (Table A5.1).

So 60% of reference weight-for-age at 12 months =

$$9.9 \text{ kg} \times \frac{60}{100} = 5.9 \text{ kg.}$$

Table A5.1. Weights-for-age—girls and boys aged 0–60 months

Age (months)	Weight (kg)		
	Centile		
	3rd	50th	97th
0	2.4	3.3	4.1
1	3.0	4.2	5.3
2	3.5	5.0	6.4
3	4.1	5.8	7.3
4	4.7	6.4	8.0
5	5.3	7.0	8.7
6	5.8	7.5	9.3
7	6.3	8.0	9.9
8	6.7	8.5	10.4
9	7.1	8.9	10.8
10	7.4	9.2	11.2
11	7.7	9.6	11.6
12	7.9	9.9	11.9
13	8.2	10.1	12.2
14	8.4	10.4	12.4
15	8.5	10.6	12.7
16	8.7	10.8	12.9
17	8.8	11.0	13.2
18	9.0	11.2	13.4
19	9.1	11.4	13.6
20	9.2	11.5	13.8
21	9.4	11.7	14.0
22	9.6	11.9	14.4
23	9.7	12.1	14.5

Table A5.1. (*contd.*)

Age (months)	Weight (kg)		
	Centile		
	3rd	50th	97th
24	9.9	12.2	14.7
25	10.1	12.3	15.3
26	10.2	12.5	15.5
27	10.4	12.7	15.8
28	10.5	12.9	16.1
29	10.6	13.1	16.3
30	10.7	13.3	16.5
31	10.9	13.5	16.8
32	11.0	13.7	17.0
33	11.2	13.9	17.2
34	11.3	14.1	17.5
35	11.4	14.2	17.7
36	11.5	14.4	17.9
37	11.6	14.6	18.1
38	11.8	14.7	18.4
39	11.9	14.9	18.6
40	12.0	15.1	18.8
41	12.1	15.2	19.0
42	12.3	15.4	19.2
43	12.4	15.5	19.5
44	12.5	15.7	19.7
45	12.6	15.9	19.9
46	12.7	16.1	20.1
47	12.9	16.2	20.3
48	13.0	16.4	20.5
49	13.1	16.5	20.7
50	13.2	16.6	20.9
51	13.3	16.8	21.1
52	13.4	17.0	21.3
53	13.6	17.1	21.5
54	13.7	17.3	21.7
55	13.8	17.5	22.0
56	13.9	17.6	22.2
57	14.0	17.7	22.4
58	14.1	17.9	22.6
59	14.3	18.0	22.9
60	14.4	18.2	23.1

Table A5.2. Lengths-for-age—girls and boys aged 0–23 months

Age (months)	Length (cm)		
	Centile		
	3rd	50th	97th
0	46.0	50.2	53.4
1	49.6	54.1	58.6
2	52.7	57.6	62.1
3	55.5	60.3	65.2
4	58.0	62.9	67.8
5	60.0	65.0	70.0
6	61.9	66.9	71.9
7	63.5	68.6	73.3
8	65.0	70.1	75.1
9	65.5	71.4	76.5
10	67.7	72.7	77.8
11	68.9	74.0	79.1
12	70.0	75.2	80.4
13	71.1	76.4	81.7
14	72.2	77.5	82.9
15	73.2	78.6	84.1
16	74.1	79.7	85.2
17	75.1	80.7	86.3
18	75.9	81.7	87.4
19	76.8	82.6	88.5
20	77.7	83.6	89.5
21	78.5	84.5	90.5
22	79.3	85.4	91.5
23	80.1	86.2	92.4
24	80.8	87.1	93.3

Table A5.3. Heights-for-age—girls and boys aged 24–60 months

Age (months)	Height (cm)		
	Centile		
	3rd	50th	97th
24	79.1	85.1	91.0
25	79.7	85.9	92.0
26	80.0	86.7	93.0
27	81.3	87.6	93.9
28	81.9	88.4	94.8
29	82.7	89.1	95.6
30	83.4	89.9	96.5
31	84.1	90.7	97.4
32	84.8	91.5	98.3
33	85.5	92.3	99.1
34	86.1	93.0	99.9
35	86.7	93.8	100.8
36	87.4	94.5	101.7
37	88.0	95.2	102.4
38	88.6	95.9	103.2
39	89.2	96.5	103.8
40	89.9	97.2	104.6
41	90.5	97.9	105.3
42	91.1	98.5	106.0
43	91.7	99.1	106.7
44	92.2	99.8	107.4
45	92.8	100.4	108.1
46	93.4	101.1	108.7
47	94.0	101.7	109.4
48	94.5	102.3	110.1
49	95.1	102.9	110.6
50	95.6	103.5	111.4
51	96.1	104.1	112.0
52	96.6	104.7	112.7
53	97.2	105.3	113.4
54	97.7	105.8	113.9
55	98.2	106.4	114.6
56	98.7	107.0	115.2
57	99.2	107.5	115.8
58	99.7	108.1	116.4
59	100.2	108.6	117.0
60	100.8	109.2	117.7

Table A5.4. Weights-for-length—girls and boys of 50–100 cm length aged under 2 years

Length (cm)	Weight (kg)		
	Centile		
	3rd	50th	97th
50	2.7	3.4	4.2
51	2.8	3.5	4.5
52	2.9	3.7	4.7
53	3.0	3.9	5.0
54	3.2	4.1	5.2
55	3.4	4.3	5.5
56	3.5	4.6	5.8
57	3.7	4.8	6.0
58	4.0	5.1	6.3
59	4.2	5.4	6.6
60	4.4	5.6	6.9
61	4.7	5.9	7.2
62	5.0	6.2	7.5
63	5.2	6.5	7.8
64	5.5	6.8	8.1
65	5.7	7.1	8.5
66	6.0	7.4	8.8
67	6.2	7.6	9.1
68	6.5	7.9	9.4
69	6.8	8.2	9.7
70	7.0	8.5	10.0
71	7.3	8.7	10.3
72	7.5	9.0	10.6
73	7.8	9.2	10.8
74	8.0	9.5	11.1
75	8.2	9.7	11.3
76	8.4	9.9	11.6
77	8.6	10.2	11.8
78	8.8	10.4	12.1
79	9.0	10.6	12.3
80	9.1	10.8	12.4
81	9.3	11.0	12.7
82	9.5	11.2	13.0
83	9.6	11.4	13.2
84	9.8	11.6	13.4
85	10.0	11.8	13.6
86	10.2	12.0	13.8
87	10.4	12.2	14.0
88	10.6	12.4	14.3
89	10.8	12.6	14.5
90	11.0	12.9	14.8
91	11.2	13.0	15.0
92	11.4	13.2	15.3
93	11.6	13.5	15.5
94	11.8	13.7	15.7
95	12.1	14.0	16.0
96	12.3	14.2	16.2
97	12.6	14.5	16.5
98	12.8	14.8	16.8
99	13.0	15.1	17.2
100	13.3	15.4	17.5

Table A5.5. Weights-for-height—girls and boys of 80–120 cm height aged 2 years and over

Height (cm)	Weight (kg)		
		Centile	
	3rd	50th	97th
80	9.0	11.0	13.6
81	9.2	11.1	13.7
82	9.4	11.4	14.0
83	9.6	11.6	14.2
84	9.8	11.8	14.4
85	10.0	12.0	14.7
86	10.2	12.2	14.9
87	10.4	12.5	15.1
88	10.6	12.7	15.3
89	10.8	12.9	15.6
90	11.0	13.1	15.8
91	11.2	13.4	16.1
92	11.4	13.6	16.4
93	11.6	13.8	16.6
94	11.8	14.0	16.9
95	12.0	14.3	17.1
96	12.2	14.5	17.4
97	12.4	14.8	17.7
98	12.6	15.1	18.0
99	12.8	15.3	18.3
100	13.0	15.6	18.6
101	13.2	15.8	18.9
102	13.5	16.1	19.2
103	13.7	16.4	19.5
104	13.9	16.7	19.8
105	14.2	16.9	20.2
106	14.4	17.2	20.5
107	14.6	17.5	20.9
108	14.9	17.8	21.2
109	15.2	18.1	21.6
110	15.4	18.5	22.0
111	15.7	18.8	22.4
112	16.0	19.1	22.8
113	16.3	19.4	23.2
114	16.6	19.8	23.7
115	16.9	20.1	24.1
116	17.2	20.5	24.6
117	17.5	20.9	25.1
118	17.9	21.2	25.6
119	18.2	21.6	26.2
120	18.6	22.0	26.8

Table A5.6. Weights-for-height—girls and boys of 120–145 cm height

Height (cm)	Weight (kg)					
	Girls			Boys		
	Centile					
	3rd	50th	97th	3rd	50th	97th
120	18.3	21.8	26.7	18.8	22.2	26.8
122	19.0	22.7	27.9	19.5	23.0	27.9
124	19.7	23.6	29.3	20.2	23.9	29.2
126	20.5	24.6	30.9	21.0	24.8	30.5
128	21.3	25.7	32.6	21.8	25.7	31.9
130	22.1	26.8	34.6	22.6	26.8	33.5
132	23.0	28.0	36.7	23.4	27.8	35.1
134	23.9	29.4	39.0	24.3	29.0	36.8
136	24.9	30.8	41.6	25.2	30.2	38.7
138	–	–	–	26.0	31.6	40.6
140	–	–	–	27.0	33.0	42.7
142	–	–	–	27.9	34.5	44.9
144	–	–	–	28.8	36.1	47.2

A cut-off point that is often used when measuring weight-for-height is 90% of reference, ie 90% of the 50th centile value. This is higher than the 3rd *centile* value. To calculate 90% of reference weight-for-height, use the following formula:

$$\text{90\% reference weight-for-height}$$
$$= \text{50th centile weight-for-height} \times \frac{90}{100}$$

Example:
90% reference weight for a girl with a height of 132 cm

$$= 28.0\,\text{kg} \times \frac{90}{100} = 25.2\,\text{kg}$$

Table A5.7. Weights-for-heights of adults for different body mass indexes (BMIs) (see Fig. 22–2 and Box 22.1)

Height (cm)	Weight (kg)			
	Body mass index*			
	16	18.5	25	30
146	34	39	53	64
148	35	41	55	65
150	36	42	56	68
152	37	43	58	69
154	38	44	59	71
156	39	45	61	73
158	40	46	62	75
160	41	47	64	77
162	42	49	66	79
164	43	50	67	81
166	44	51	69	83
168	45	52	71	85
170	46	53	72	87
172	47	55	74	89
174	48	56	76	91
176	50	57	77	93
178	51	59	79	95
180	52	60	81	97
182	53	61	83	99
184	54	63	85	102
186	55	64	86	104
188	57	65	88	106
190	58	67	90	108
192	59	68	92	111

Adapted from Truswell (1986).
* Body mass index below 16, malnourished; 16–18.5, possibly malnourished; 18.5–25, probably well nourished; 25–30, possibly obese; over 30, obese.

REFERENCES

Beaton, G., Kelly, A., Kevany, J., Martorell, R., and Mason, J. (1990). *Appropriate uses of anthropometric indices in children*, ACC/SCN Nutrition Policy Discussion Paper, no. 7. ACC/SCN, Geneva.

Truswell, A. S. (1986). *ABC of nutrition. British Medical Journal*, Tavistock Square, London.

WHO (1983). *Measuring change in nutritional status.* WHO, Geneva.

Appendix 6 Sources of reference and teaching materials

This appendix lists the materials and other sources of information which we used to prepare this book and/or which may be useful to nutrition workers, especially trainers and supervisors. It consists of:

A6.1. Bibliography.

A6.2. Learning/teaching materials.

A6.3. Newsletters and annual reports.

A6.4. Journals for nutrition libraries.

A6.5. Organizations associated with nutrition.

A6.6. Addresses for international organizations and sources of materials.

A6.1 BIBLIOGRAPHY

The following are the most important of the publications we consulted. We recommend the items printed in bold because they are easy to obtain and contain information which is reliable and up-to-date at the time at which this book went to the publisher. Many are free or low in cost. In many cases these publications are available from specific organizations. We have indicated this where relevant; full names of organizations and their addresses that do not appear here are given in Section A6.6.

Abbatt, F. and MacMahon, R. (1985). *Teaching health care workers.* Macmillan, Basingstoke. [Available from TALC.]

ACC/SCN (1990a). *Women and nutrition,* Nutrition Policy Discussion Paper, no. 6. ACC/SCN, Geneva. [Available from ACC/SCN.]

ACC/SCN (1990b). Policies to improve nutrition—what was done in the 80s. *SCN News,* no. 6 [Available from ACC/SCN.]

ACC/SCN (1991a). *Controlling iron deficiency,* Nutrition Policy Discussion Paper, no. 9. ACC/SCN, Geneva [Available from ACC/SCN.]

ACC/SCN (1991b). *Managing successful nutrition programmes,* Nutrition Policy Discussion Paper no. 8. ACC/SCN, Geneva [Available from ACC/SCN.

Adamson, P. and Williams, G. (no date). *Facts for life.* Prepared for UNICEF, WHO, and UNESCO by P and LA, Oxford. [Available from TALC and UNICEF Country Offices.]

Aga Khan University (1990). *Cereal based oral rehydration therapy for diarrhoea.* Aga Khan Foundation, Geneva and International Child Health Foundation, Columbia, Missouri. [Available from the Aga Khan Foundation, Box 345, 1211 Geneva 6, Switzerland.]

Akre, J. (Ed.) (1989). *Infant Feeding: The Physiological Basis.* Bull. WHO 67 (supplement).

Alnwick, D., Moses, S., and Schmidt, O.G. (ed.) (1988). *Improving young child feeding in Eastern and Southern Africa.* International Development Research Centre, Ottawa. [Available from International Development Research Centre, Box 8500, Ottawa, Canada.]

Appleton, J. and SCF Ethiopia Team (1987). *Drought relief in Ethiopia—planning and management of feeding programmes.* Save the Children Fund, London. [Available from SCF.]

Beaton, G., Kelly, A., Kevany, J., Martorell, R., and Mason, J. (1990). *Appropriate uses of anthropometric indices in children,* ACC/SCN Nutrition Policy Discussion Paper, No. 7. ACC/SCN, Geneva. [Available from ACC/SCN.]

Berry-Koch, A., Moench, R., Hakewill, P., and Dualeh, M. (1990). Alleviation of nutritional deficiency diseases in refugees. *Food and Nutrition Bulletin,* 12, 26.

Brewster, D. (1989a). Neonatology in the developing world, Part 1. *Tropical Doctor,* 19, 100–4.

Brewster, D. (1989b). Neonatology in the developing world, Part 2. *Tropical Doctor,* 19, 147–51.

Brown, R.C. (1990). Simple system of nutritional surveillance for African communities. *Journal of Tropical Paediatrics,* 36, 162.

Burgess, A. (in press). *Community nutrition in eastern Africa,* AMREF, Nairobi. (Available from AMREF.)

Cameron, M.E. and Hofvander, Y. (1983). *Manual on feeding infants and young children.* Oxford University Press, Delhi. [Available from TALC or AMREF.]

Cameron, M.E. and van Staveren, W.A. (1988). *Manual on methodology for food consumption studies.* Oxford University Press, Oxford.

Casey, C.E. and Hambridge, K.M. (1983). In *Lactation: physiology, nutrition and breastfeeding* (ed. M.C. Neville and M.R. Neifert). Plenum Press, New York.

CFNI (Caribbean Food and Nutrition Institute) (1985). *Nutrition handbook for community workers.* CFNI, Kingston, Jamaica. [Available from Caribbean Food and Nutrition Institute, Box 140, Mona, Kingston, Jamaica.]

***Children in the Tropics* (1989). Nutritional status: inter-**

449

pretation of indicators. *Children in the Tropics*, Vols 181–2. [Available from ICC, Paris.]

Children in the Tropics (1990*a*). Iron and folate deficiency anaemias. *Children in the Tropics*, Vol. 186. [Available from ICC, Paris.]

Children in the Tropics (1990*b*). Childbearing and women's health. *Children in the Tropics*, Vols 187–8. [Available from ICC, Paris.]

Children in the Tropics (1990*c*). Immunity and nutrition. *Children in the Tropics*, Vol. 189. [Available from ICC, Paris.]

Davidson, R. and Eastwood, M.A. (1986). *Human nutrition and dietetics* (8th edn). Churchill Livingstone, Edinburgh.

De Maeyer, E. in collaboration with Dallman, P., Gurney, J.M., Hallberg, L., Sood, S.K., and SriKantia, S.G. (1989). *Preventing and controlling iron deficiency anaemia through primary health care*. WHO, Geneva. [Available from WHO.]

de Ville de Goyet, C. (1991). *Management of nutrition emergencies in large populations*. WHO/UNHCR, Geneva. [Available from WHO and UNHCR.]

Dickson, M. (1983). *Where there is no dentist*. Hesperian Foundation, Palo Alto, California. [Available from TALC.]

Dunn, J. and van der Haar, F. (1990). *A practical guide to the correction of iodine deficiency*. ICCIDD, Adelaide, Australia. [Available from ICCIDD.]

Eastman, S. (1988). *Vitamin A deficiency and xerophthalmia—recent findings and some programme implications*. UNICEF, New York. [Available from UNICEF, New York and HKI.]

FAO (1965). *Requirements of vitamin A, thiamine, riboflavin and niacin*, Report of Joint FAO/WHO Report Group. FAO. Rome.

FAO (1970). *Requirements of ascorbic acid, vitamin D, vitamin B_{12}, folate and iron*, Report of Joint FAO/WHO Report Group. FAO, Rome.

FAO (1972). *Food composition table for use in East Asia*. FAO, Rome.

FAO (1980). *Dietary fats and oils*. Food and Nutrition Series, no. 20. FAO, Rome. [Available from FAO.]

FAO (1982). *Legumes in human nutrition*. FAO, Rome. [Available from FAO.]

FAO (1988*a*). *Requirements of vitamin A, iron, folate and vitamin B_{12}*, Report of a joint FAO/WHO Expert Consultation. FAO, Rome. [Available from FAO.]

FAO (1988*b*). *Traditional food plants*, Food and Nutrition Paper, no. 42. FAO, Rome. [Available from FAO.]

FAO (1989*a*). *Utilization of tropical foods*, Food and Nutrition Papers, no. 47/1 (cereals); 47/2 (roots and tubers); 47/3 (trees); 47/4 (tropical beans); 47/5 (tropical oil seeds); 47/6 (sugars, spices and stimulants). FAO, Rome. [Available from FAO.]

FAO (1989*b*). *Forestry and food security*. Forestry Paper, no. 90. FAO, Rome. [Available from FAO.]

FAO (1990). *Conducting small-scale nutrition surveys: a field manual*, Nutrition in Agriculture, no. 5. FAO, Rome. [Available from FAO.]

FAO (in press). *Food and nutrition in management of group feeding programmes*, Food and Nutrition Paper, no. 23. FAO, Rome. [Available from FAO.]

Fernandes, E.C.M., Oktingati, A., and Maghembe, J. (1985). The Chagga home gardens. *Food and Nutrition Bulletin*, **7**, 29.

Gillespie, S. and Mason, J. (1991). *Nutrition relevant actions*. Nutrition Policy Discussion Paper no. 10 ACC/SCN Geneva. [Available from ACC/SCN.]

Golden, M.H.N. and Ramdath, D. (1985). Free radicals in the pathogenesis of kwashiorkor. In *Proceedings of the 13th International Congress of Nutrition* (ed. T.G. Taylor and N.K. Jenkins), pp. 597–8. International Union of Nutritional Sciences. [Available from John Libbey, 80 Bondway, London SW8 1SF.]

Goode, P. *Edible plants of Uganda,* Food and Nutrition Paper, no. 42/1. FAO, Rome. [Available from FAO.]

Greiner, T. (1988). The complementary foods problem. In *Improving young child feeding in Eastern and Southern Africa* (ed. D. Alnwick, S. Moses, and O.G. Schmidt), pp. 34–8. International Development Research Centre, Ottawa.

Hendrickse, R.G. (1985). *Kwashiorkor: 50 years of myth and mystery. Do aflatoxins provide a clue?* Second P.H. van Thiel Lecture of the Institute of Tropical Medicine, Rotterdam/Leiden. Foris Publications, Dordrecht. [Available from Dr R. Hendrickse, Liverpool School of Tropical Medicine, Pembroke Place, Liverpool.]

Hetzel, B.S. (1988) *The prevention and control of iodine deficiency disorders,* ACC/SCN Nutrition Policy Discussion Paper, no. 3. ACC/SCN, Geneva. [Available from ACC/SCN.]

Hetzel, B.S. (1989). *The story of iodine deficiency*. Oxford University Press, Oxford.

Hofvander, Y. and Underwood, B. (1987). Processed supplementary foods for older infants and young children with special reference to developing countries. *Food and Nutrition Bulletin*, **9**, 1–7.

Hornik, R.C. (1985). *Nutrition education: a state-of-the-art review,* ACC/SCN Nutrition Policy Discussion Paper, no. 1. ACC/SCN, Geneva. [Available from ACC/SCN.]

Horwitz, A., MacFadyen, D.M., Munro, H., Scrimshaw, N.S., Steen, B., and Williams, T.F. (ed.) (1989). *Nutrition in the elderly*. Published for WHO by Oxford University Press, Oxford

IBFAN (1990). *Protecting infant health: a health worker's guide to the international code of marketing of breastmilk substitutes*. IBFAN, Penang, Malaysia. [Available from IBFAN, Box 1045, 10830 Penang, Malaysia.]

ICCIDD (in press). *Laboratory testing for iodine deficiency*. ICCIDD, Adelaide, Australia.

James, W.P.T. and Schofield, E.C. (1990). *Human energy requirements: a manual for planners and nutritionists*. Published for FAO by Oxford University Press, Oxford.

Jansen, A.A.J., Horelli, H.T., and Quinn, V.J. (1987).

Food and nutrition in Kenya—a historical review. Department of Community Health, University of Nairobi, Nairobi. [Available from UNICEF, Kenya.]

Jelliffe, D.B. and Jelliffe, E.F.P. (1978). *Human milk in the modern world.* Oxford Medical Publications, Oxford.

Jelliffe, D.B. and Jelliffe, E.F.P. (1989*a*). *Dietary management of young children with acute diarrhoea.* WHO/UNICEF, Geneva. [Available from WHO.]

Jelliffe, D.B. and Jelliffe, E.F.P. (1989*b*). *Community nutritional assessment with special reference to less technically developed countries.* Oxford Medical Publications, Oxford.

Johns Hopkins University (1990). *Household management of diarrhoea and acute respiratory infections,* Johns Hopkins University Occasional Papers, no. 12. Johns Hopkins University, Baltimore, Maryland.

Kenya Ministry of Agriculture (1981). *Major crops technical handbook.* Ministry of Agriculture, Nairobi.

Kenya Ministry of Health/UNICEF (1986). *Improving young child growth.* Ministry of Health, Nairobi. [Also available from UNICEF, Nairobi.]

Kenya Pediatric Association (1990). *Vitamin A and child health.* **Kenya Pediatric Association. Nairobi. [Available from UNICEF, Nairobi.]**

Kim Wha Young, Lee Yang Cha, Lee Ki Yull, Ju Jin Soon, and Kim Sook He (ed.) (1990). *Proceedings of the 14th International Congress of Nutrition.* International Union of Nutritional Sciences. [Available from the Department of Foods and Nutrition, Ewha Woman's University, 11–1 Daehyun–Dong, Sundaenun–Ku, Seoul 120–750, Korea.]

King, M., King, F., and Martodipoero, S. (1979). *Primary child care.* Oxford University Press, Oxford.

Labbok, M., Koniz–Booher, P., Shelton, J., and Krasovec, K. (1990). *Guidelines for breastfeeding in family planning and child survival programmes.* **Georgetown University Press, Washington, DC. [Available from Institute for Reproductive Health, Georgetown University, Washington, DC 2007, USA.]**

Latham, M. (1981). *Human nutrition in tropical Africa.* FAO. Rome.

Malaŵi Government Food and Nutrition Committee (1990*a*). *Nutrition facts for Malaŵian families.* **Department of Economic Planning and Development, Office of President and Cabinet, Government of Malaŵi, Lilongwe. [Available from Food Security and Nutrition Unit, Box 30122, Lilongwe or UNICEF, Box 30375, Lilongwe.]**

Malaŵi Government (1990*b*). Food security and nutrition policy statement. [Available from Food Security and Nutrition Unit, Box 30122, Lilongwe or UNICEF, Box 30375, Lilongwe.]

McLaren, D.S., Burman, D., Belton, N.R., and Williams, A.F. (ed.) (1991). *Textbook of paediatric nutrition* (3rd edn). Churchill Livingstone, Edinburgh.

McMahon, R., Barton, E., and Piot, M. (1980). *On being in charge.* WHO, Geneva.

Niñez, V. (1985). Household gardens and small-scale food production. *Food and Nutrition Bulletin,* **7,** 1.

Oniang'o, R.K. (1988). *Feeding the child.* **Heineman, Nairobi. [Also available from UNICEF, Nairobi.]**

Open University (1985). *Guide to healthy eating.* Rambletree Pelham, London.

Oxfam (1984). *Oxfam's practical guide to selective feeding programmes,* Practical Guide, No. 1. Oxfam, Oxford.

Oxfam (1991). *Nutrition in emergencies—a practical guide to assessment and response.* Oxfam, Oxford.

Perisse, J., Sizaret, F., and Francois, P. (1969). *FAO Nutrition Newsletter,* **7,** 1.

Pollitt E. (1990). *Malnutrition and infection in the classroom.* **UNESCO, Paris. [Available from UNESCO, Paris.]**

Program for International Training in Health (1987). *Teaching and learning with visual aids.* Macmillan, Basingstoke.

Ritchie, J.A.S. (1983). *Nutrition and familes.* Macmillan, London [Available from TALC.]

Rohde, J.E. (ed.) (1988). Growth monitoring and promotion: international symposium. *Indian Journal of Paediatrics,* **55** (Suppl. 1).

Rosling, J. (1988). *Cassava toxicity and food security.* Published by UNICEF by the International Child Health Unit, Uppsala. [Available from the International Child Health Unit, University Hospital, S–751 85 Uppsala, Sweden.]

Royal College of Midwives (1990). *Successful breastfeeding.* Churchill Livingstone, Edinburgh

Savage King, F. (1992). *Helping mothers to breastfeed* **(revised). AMREF, Nairobi. [Available from TALC or AMREF.]**

Save the Children (1982). *Bridging the gap: a participatory approach to health and nutrition education.* [Available from Save the Children, 54 Wilton Rd, Westport, Connecticut 06880, USA.]

Shaffer, R. (1984). *Beyond the dispensary.* AMREF, Nairobi. [Available from AMREF, Nairobi.]

Sommer, A. (ed.) (1982). *Field guide to detection and control of xerophthalmia.* **WHO, Geneva.**

South Pacific Community Nutrition Training Project Books (1991). [Available from the Community Training Project, Extension Services, University of South Pacific, Box 1168, Suva, Fiji.]

Sserunjogi, L. and Tomkins, A. (1990). Use of fermented and germinated cereals and tubers for improved feeding of infants and children in Uganda. *Transactions of the Royal Society of Tropical Medicine and Hygiene,* **84,** 443–6.

Stephenson, L.S. (1987). *Impact of helminth infections on human nutrition.* Taylor & Francis, London.

Government of the United Republic of Tanzania/UN Economic Commission for Africa/FAO/UNICEF (1975). Workshop on food preservation and storage, Tanzania.

Taylor, T.G. and Jenkins, N.K. (ed.) (1986). *Proceedings of the 13th International Congress of Nutrition.* International Union of Nutritional Sciences. [Available from John Libbey, 80 Bondway, London SW8 1SF.]

Tomkins, A. and Watson, F. (1989). *Malnutrition and infection: a review*, **ACC/SCN Nutrition Policy Discussion Paper, no. 5, ACC/SCN, Geneva. [Available from ACC/SCN.]**

Truswell, A.S. (1986). *ABC of nutrition.* British Medical Journal, Tavistock Square, London.

UNHCR (1990). Policy of UNHCR related to the acceptance, distribution and use of milk products in feeding programmes in refugee situations. [Available from UNHCR, Geneva.]

UNICEF (1986). *Assisting in emergencies: a resource handbook for UNICEF field staff.* UNICEF, New York.

UNICEF (1990). *Strategy for improved nutrition of children and women in developing countries.* **UNICEF, New York. [Available from UNICEF Country Offices.]**

VITAL (1991). *Vital nutrients*, Vitamin A Field Support Project, International Science and Technology Institute, Inc. Arlington. [Available from VITAL, 1601 N. Kent St., Suite 1016, Arlington, Va. 22209, USA.]

Vitamin A Technical Assistance Program/HKI (1990a). Vitamin A reference manual. [Unpublished; available from HKI.]

Vitamin A Technical Assistance Program/HKI (1990b). East, Central and Southern African regional workshop on vitamin A interventions and child survival, 1990. [Unpublished; available from HKI.]

Werner, D. (1979). *Where there is no doctor.* Hesperian Foundation, Palo Alto, California. [Available from TALC and AMREF.]

Werner, D. and Bower, B. (1982). *Helping health workers learn.* **Hesperian Foundation, Palo Alto, California. [Available from TALC and AMREF.]**

West, C.E., Pepping, F., and Temalilwa, C.R. (ed.) (1988). *The composition of foods commonly eaten in East Africa.* Published for the Technical Centre for Agricultural and Rural Development (CTA) and Food and Nutrition Cooperation for East, Central and Southern Africa (ECSA) by Wageningen Agricultural University, Wageningen, the Netherlands.

WFP (1989). *Food aid in emergencies: a handbook for WFP.* WFP, Rome. [Available from Disaster Relief Service, WFP.]

WFPHA (1983a). *Training community health workers.* UNICEF, New York. [Prepared by and available from WFPHA.]

WFPHA (1983b). *Maternal nutrition.* UNICEF, New York. [Prepared by and available from WFPHA.]

WFPHA (1984a). *Improving maternal health in developing countries.* UNICEF, New York. [Prepared by and available from WFPHA.]

WFPHA (1984b). *Program activities for improving weaning practices.* UNICEF, New York. [Prepared by and available from WFPHA.]

WFPHA (1985) *Growth monitoring of preschool children:* *practical considerations for primary health care projects.* UNICEF, New York. [Prepared by and available from WFPHA.]

WFPHA (1986). *Health education.* UNICEF, New York. [Available from WFPHA; prepared for UNICEF and the Aga Khan Foundation by WFPHA.]

WHO (1979). *Health aspects of food and nutrition* (3rd edn). WHO, Manila. [Available from WHO, Box 2932, Manila, Philippines.]

WHO (1981). *Treatment and management of severe protein–energy malnutrition.* WHO, Geneva.

WHO (1983a). *Measuring change in nutritional status.* WHO, Geneva.

WHO (1983b). *Training in recording the child's growth.* WHO, Geneva.

WHO (1984). *Role of food safety in health and development*, Technical Report Series, no. 705. WHO. Geneva.

WHO (1985a). *Energy and protein requirements.* **Technical Report Series, no. 724. WHO, Geneva.**

WHO (1985b). *Prevention of osteoporosis*, WHO, Geneva. ICP/NUT 102/M01.

WHO (1986a). *Guidelines for training community health workers in nutrition.* WHO, Geneva.

WHO (1986b). *The Growth chart—a tool for use in infant and child health care.* WHO, Geneva.

WHO (1988). *Vitamin A deficiency: time for action. Expanded programme on immunization.* WHO, Geneva. [Also available from HKI.]

WHO (1990). *Diarrhoea management training course,* CDD/SER/90.2. WHO, Geneva.

WHO (1991). *Diet, nutrition and the prevention of chronic diseases,* Technical Report Series, no. 797. WHO, Geneva.

WHO/UNICEF (1989). *Promoting, protecting and supporting breastfeeding: the special role of the maternity services. A WHO/UNICEF joint statement.* WHO, Geneva.

WHO/UNICEF/IVACG Task Force (1988). *Vitamin A supplements: a guide to their use in the treatment and prevention of vitamin A deficiency and xerophthalmia.* **WHO, Geneva.**

WHO/UNICEF/United States Agency for International Development/HKI/IVACG (1982). *Control of vitamin A deficiency and xerophthalmia,* WHO Technical Report Series, no. 672. WHO, Geneva.

Wood, C. (ed.) (1986). Dietary salt and hypertension. [Unpublished; available from Royal Society Medical Services, Linacre College, Oxford.]

Young, B, and Durston, S. (1987). *Primary health education.* Longman, Harlow, Essex. [Available from TALC.]

A6.2 LEARNING/TEACHING MATERIALS

Those in bold are especially recommended.

Armstrong, H. (1992). Training Guide in Lactation management. [Available from UNICEF, New York.]

FAO (1984). *Guidelines for training organizers of group feeding programmes: for use in Africa (a training pack).* FAO, Rome. [Available from Food Policy and Nutrition Division, FAO, Rome.]

FAO (1988c). *Field programme management. Food and nutrition: population and nutrition—a training pack.* FAO, Rome. [Available from Food Policy and Nutrition Division, FAO, Rome.]

HKI (1988). *Guidelines for prevention of blindness due to vitamin A deficiency.* HKI, New York. [Available from HKI.]

HKI (1990). *Saving a child from xerophthalmia.* HKI, New York. [Available from HKI.]

HKI (no date). *Know the signs and symptoms of xerophthalmia.* HKI, New York. [Available from HKI.]

HKI/WHO (1988). *Health workers find; treat; prevent vitamin A deficiency.* HKI, New York. [Available from HKI.]

IITA (International Institute for Tropical Agriculture) (1989). Food crops utilization and nutrition—a training manual. [Available from IITA, PMB 5320, Ibadan, Nigeria.]

Kenya Ministry of Health/UNICEF (1987). 'Good growth prevents malnutrition' slides and charts. Slides: 'Using the Kenya child growth chart'; 'Weaning foods and energy in Kenya'; 'Feeding young children in Kenya'; 'Growth monitoring case studies'. Charts: 'Growth monitoring'; 'Child feeding'. [Available from the Division of Family Health, Ministry of Health, Box 43319, Nairobi, Kenya or from UNICEF, Nairobi, Kenya.]

Swaziland Ministry of Health/UNICEF (1988). Training units on growth monitoring and promotion. [Available from Ministry of Health, Box 369, Mbabane, Swaziland or UNICEF, Box 1859, Mbane, Swaziland.]

TALC (various dates). Teaching slides (code letters and date in brackets): 'Protein energy deficiency—signs and causes' (PED; 1990); 'Breastfeeding' (BF; 1989); 'Breastfeeding problems' (BFP; 1985); 'Weaning foods and energy' (WFE; 1985); 'Malnutrition in an urban environment' (MUE; 1979); 'Charting growth in small children' (CHG; 1978); 'Xerophthalmia' (EYX; 1985); 'Common oral diseases' (DNCD; 1985); 'Peridontal disease' (DNPD; 1983). [Available from TALC.]

UNICEF (1990). Nutrition: a UNICEF training package. [Available from UNICEF, New York.]

WHO (1989). Nutrition learning packages. Joint WHO/UNICEF Nutrition Support Programme. [Available from WHO.]

A6.3 NEWSLETTERS AND ANNUAL REPORTS

We recommend the following. Most are free to nutrition workers in low-income countries. The address of the publication follows the title unless the address is that of one of

the organizations in Section A6.6, in which case only the initials of the organization are given.

ARI News. AHRTAG.

Breastfeeding Briefs. Geneva Infant Feeding Association, Box 157, 1211 Geneva 19 Switzerland.

Cobasheca. Community Health Workers' Support Unit, AMREF.

Dialogue on Diarrhoea. AHRTAG.

Footsteps. Tear Fund, 100 Church Rd, Teddington TW11 8QE, UK.

Health Action. AHRTAG

Health Education Network. Box 30125, Nairobi, Kenya.

Health Technology Directions. PATH, 4 Nickerson St., Seattle, WA 98109–1699, USA.

IDD Newsletter. Dr J. T. Dunn, International Council for Control of Iodine Deficiency Disorders, Box 511, University of Virginia Medical Centre, Charlottesville, VA 22908, USA.

IPPF Medical Bulletin. International Planned Parenthood Federation, Box 759. Inner Circle, Regents Park, London NW1 4LQ, UK.

Mothers and Children. Clearing House on Infant Feeding and Maternal Nutrition, American Public Health Association, 1015 15th St. NW, Washington, DC 20005, USA.

NFI Bulletin. Nutrition Foundation of India, 13–37 Gulmohar Park, New Delhi 11004G, India.

Safe Motherhood. Division of Family Health, WHO, Geneva.

SCN News. ACC/SCN.

State of the World's Children. UNICEF annual report available from UNICEF, New York.

TALC Newsletter. Lists of books, slides, and accessories are also available from TALC.

The Helper. Community Health Workers Support Unit, AMREF.

Xerophthalmia Club Bulletin. Dr D.S. McLaren, International Centre for Eye Health, 27 Cayton St., London EC1V 9EJ, UK.

A6.4 JOURNALS FOR NUTRITION LIBRARIES

We recommend the following journals. Many are relatively cheap and some are sent free to selected institutes—but write for prices before ordering. The address of the publication follows the title unless the address is that of one of the organizations in Section A6.6.

Cajanus. Caribbean Food and Nutrition Institute (CFNI), Box 140, Mona, Kingston, Jamaica.

Children in the Tropics. International Children's Centre, Chateau de Longchamp, Bois de Boulogne, 75016 Paris, France.

Contact. Christian Medical Commission, World Council of Churches, 150 route de Ferney, 1211 Geneva 20, Switzerland.

Food, Nutrition and Agriculture. Food Policy and Nutrition Division, FAO, Rome.

Food and Nutrition Bulletin. UNU (United Nations University), toho Seimei Building, 15–1 Shibuya 2-chrome, Shibuya–ku, Tokyo 150, Japan.

Journal of Tropical Paediatrics. Oxford Journals, Oxford University Press, Walton St., Oxford OX2 6DP, UK.

A6.5 ORGANIZATIONS ASSOCIATED WITH NUTRITION

You can find the addresses of national organizations and the local offices of international organizations in the telephone book, in libraries, or by asking colleagues.

Useful foreign and international organizations

- *United Nations.* UNICEF, WHO, FAO, IFAD, WFP, UNDP, UNESCO, World Bank. See section A6.6 for full name.

- *Bilateral aid agencies.* The European Community, many 'Western' countries, and Japan have offices of their official aid agencies in most countries. These agencies can be contacted through their embassies.

- *Non–governmental organizations.* There are many but there is often a national organization to which they all belong. Examples of important ones for nutrition workers are AMREF, Catholic Relief Services, Christian Aid, Helen Keller International, Oxfam, Save the Children Fund (UK) (headquarter addresses below).

A6.6 ADDRESSES FOR INTERNATIONAL ORGANIZATIONS AND SOURCES OF MATERIALS

ACN/SCN (Administrative Committee on Coordination—Subcommittee on Nutrition of the United Nations). The Technical Secretary, ACC/SCN, c/o WHO, Ave Appia, 1211 Geneva 27, Switzerland.

AHRTAG (Appropriate Health Resources and Technology Action Group). 1 London Bridge, London SE1 9SG, UK.

AMREF (African Medical Research Foundation). Box 30125, Nairobi, Kenya.

Christian Aid, Box 100, London, SE17 RT, UK.

CRS (Catholic Relief Services). 1011 First Ave, New York, NY 10022, USA.

FAO (Food and Agriculture Organization). Food Policy and Nutrition Division, FAO, Via delle Terme di Caracalla, 00100 Rome, Italy.

HKI (Helen Keller International). 15 West 16 St, New York, NY 10011, USA.

IBFAN (International Baby Food Action Network for Africa). c/o GIFA, Box 157, 1211 Geneva 19, Switzerland.

ICC (International Children's Centre). Chateau de Longchamp, Bois de Boulogne, 75016 Paris, France.

ICCIDD (International Council for Control of Iodine Deficiency Disorders). The Secretary, ICCIDD, CSIRO Division of Human Nutrition, Kintore Ave, Adelaide 5000, Australia.

IFAD (International Fund for Agricultural Development). 107 Via del Serafico, 00142 Rome, Italy.

IVACG (International Vitamin A Consultative Group). c/o Nutrition Foundation, 888 17th St NW, Washington DC 20006, USA.

Oxfam. 274 Banbury Rd, Oxford OX2 7DZ, UK.

SCF (Save the Children Fund) UK. Mary Datchelor House, 17 Grove Lane, Camberwell, London SE5 8RD, UK.

TALC (Teaching Aids at Low Cost). Box 49, St Albans AL1 4AX, UK.

UNICEF (United Nations Children's Fund). 3 UN Plaza, New York, NY 10017, USA.

UNICEF Regional Office for Eastern and Southern Africa. Box 44145, Nairobi, Kenya.

UNDP (United Nations Development Programme). UN Plaza, New York, NY 10017, USA.

UNESCO (United Nations Education, Scientific and Cultural Organization). Nutrition and Health Education, UNESCO, 7 Place de Fontenoy, 75700, Paris, France.

UNHCR (United Nations High Commissioner for Refugees). Palais de Nations, Box 2500, 1211 Geneva 2, Switzerland.

WFP (World Food Programme). Via Cristoforo Colombo 426, 00145 Rome, Italy.

WFPHA (World Federation of Public Health Associations) HQ: P.O. Box 99, 1211 Geneva 20, Switzerland: American Public Health Association, 1015 15th Street, N.W. Washington D.C. 20005, USA.

WHO (World Health Organization). Nutrition Unit, WHO, Avenue Appia, ch–1211 Geneva 27, Switzerland.

WHO Regional Office for Africa, Box 6, Brazzaville, Congo Brazzaville.

World Bank. 1818 H Street NW, Washington, DC 20433, USA.

Index

Daily requirements of energy, protein, iron, and vitamin A for different sex and age groups (summary of Appendix 2)

Age (years)	Weight (kg)	Energy (kcal)	Protein* (g)	Iron* (mg)	Vitamin A (RE)
Children—both sexes					
0–1	7.3	800	12	21	350
1–3	11.9	1250	23	13	400
3–5	15.9	1510	26	14	400
5–7	19.6	1710	30	19	400
7–10	25.9	1880	38	23	400
Boys					
10–12	34.0	2170	50	23	500
12–14	43.2	2360	64	36	600
14–16	54.5	2620	75	36	600
16–18	63.6	2820	84	23	600
Girls					
10–12	35.4	1925	52	23	500
12–14	44.2	2040	62	40	600
14–16	51.5	2135	69	40	550
16–18	54.6	2150	66	48	500
If pregnant		+200	+7	76**	600
Men—active					
18–60	65.0	2944	57	23	600
> 60	65.0	2060	57	23	600
Women—Active	55.0				
Childbearing age		2140	48	48	500
Pregnant		2240	55	76**	600
Lactating		2640	68	26	850
> 60		1830	48	19	500

* Protein needs assume that all groups (except 0–1-year-old breastfed children) eat very little animal protein, small amounts of vitamin C-rich foods, and large amounts of fibre. Children who are breastfed for 2 years need less protein. Iron needs assume a low iron availability diet is eaten. See explanation in Appendix 2.
** Supplements are usually needed to supply this amount of iron.